COLD SPRING HARBOR SYMPOSIA ON QUANTITATIVE BIOLOGY

VOLUME LIV

COLD SPRING HARBOR SYMPOSIA ON QUANTITATIVE BIOLOGY

VOLUME LIV

Immunological Recognition

COLD SPRING HARBOR LABORATORY PRESS
1989

COLD SPRING HARBOR SYMPOSIA ON QUANTITATIVE BIOLOGY
VOLUME LIV

© 1989 by The Cold Spring Harbor Laboratory Press
International Standard Book Number 0-87969-057-7 (cloth)
International Standard Book Number 0-87969-058-5 (paper)
International Standard Serial Number 0091-7451
Library of Congress Catalog Card Number 34-8174

COLD SPRING HARBOR SYMPOSIA ON QUANTITATIVE BIOLOGY

Founded in 1933 by
REGINALD G. HARRIS
Director of the Biological Laboratory 1924 to 1936

Previous Symposia Volumes

All Cold Spring Harbor Laboratory publications may be ordered directly from Cold Spring Harbor Laboratory Press, Box 100, Cold Spring Harbor, New York 11724. Phone: 1-800-843-4388. In New York (516)367-8423.

Contents

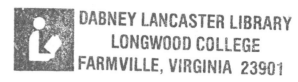

Part 1

B Cells

Recognition by Antibodies

Antigen Recognition by T Cells

Antigen Processing

CONTENTS

Part 2

Signals for Lymphocyte Activation, Proliferation, and Adhesion

Tolerance and Self Recognition

Summary

Appendix

COLD SPRING HARBOR SYMPOSIA ON QUANTITATIVE BIOLOGY

VOLUME LIV

T-cell Clonal Anergy

R.H. Schwartz, D.L. Mueller, M.K. Jenkins, and H. Quill

Laboratory of Cellular and Molecular Immunology, National Institute of Allergy and Infectious Diseases,
National Institutes of Health, Bethesda, Maryland 20892

Two-signal Model for the Induction of a T-cell Proliferative Response

Chemical fixation of splenic antigen-presenting cells (APC) with paraformaldehyde or 1-ethyl-3-(3-dimethylaminopropyl)-carbodiimide (ECDI) destroys their ability to stimulate a proliferative response from interleukin-2 (IL-2)-producing T-cell clones (Jenkins and Schwartz 1987). In addition, exposure of the clones to antigen in the presence of the chemically fixed APC induces in them a hyporesponsive state to subsequent stimulation by normal APC and antigen (Fig. 1A). This induction of proliferative nonresponsiveness requires the correct allelic form of the major histocompatibility complex (MHC) class II molecule and the precise peptide recognized by the antigen receptor of the T-cell clone. These observations suggest that antigen-receptor occupancy is qualitatively normal and that the delivery of some other signal required for T-cell activation has been damaged by the fixation.

This concept is strengthened by experiments in which T-cell clones fail to proliferate in response to peptide presented by planar lipid membranes containing purified MHC class II molecules (Quill and Schwartz 1987). Again, recognition of the correct allelic form of the MHC class II molecule and the appropriate peptide induces the nonresponsive state (Fig. 1B). Thus, antigen-receptor occupancy alone, as achieved in this chemically defined presentation system, appears to be sufficient only for the induction of nonresponsiveness.

More recent studies using a monoclonal antibody against the CD3 ϵ chain of the T-cell antigen receptor have confirmed this interpretation (M.K. Jenkins et al., in prep.). T-cell clones exposed to anti-CD3 adhered to a plastic surface are induced into a nonresponsive state (Fig. 1C). The cells usually give a weak proliferative response during the induction phase, the magnitude of which is dependent on cell density. As shown in Figure 2, the slope of a log-log plot of the number of responding T cells versus response has a value of 2. This suggests that a cell-cell interaction is required to obtain the proliferative response. When this interaction is minimized at low cell density ($< 10^4$ cells per well), receptor occupancy alone leads only to the nonresponsive state.

The need for a cell interaction to obtain a T-cell proliferative response with anti-CD3 suggests that a second signaling event (the costimulatory signal) is required for proliferation. This is demonstrated by the addition of accessory cells (e.g., irradiated T-cell-depleted spleen) to the assay shown in Figure 2 (D.L. Mueller et al., in prep.). These cells, added at a constant number, eliminate the density dependence of the T-cell response (the slope is converted to approximately 1) by providing the costimulatory signal. Equally important, this signal blocks the induction of the nonresponsive state. Figure 3 shows this result for antigen presentation using chemically fixed APC. Addition of allogeneic low-density spleen cells (which cannot present the antigen because they express the wrong allelic product of the MHC class II molecule) prevented ECDI-fixed APC and antigen from inducing nonresponsiveness (Jenkins et al. 1988). Instead, the cells behaved as if they had been preactivated by stimulation with normal APC and antigen. Overall, these results demonstrate that activation of IL-2-producing T-cell clones to divide requires two signals: antigen-receptor occupancy and a costimulatory signal. When the former occurs in the absence of the latter, a different series of events takes place, and the cells not only fail to divide, but enter a state of hyporesponsiveness.

Biochemical Events during the Induction of the Nonresponsive State

Stimulation of IL-2-producing T-cell clones with peptide and chemically fixed APC fails to elicit IL-2, as measured in a bioassay (Jenkins et al. 1987). This is also true at the mRNA level using in situ hybridization (sensitivity of approximately 20 copies of message per cell). In contrast, this form of stimulation is capable of eliciting both γ-interferon and interleukin-3 production, although less than the amounts elicited with normal activation. An examination of early receptor occupancy events revealed that generation of inositol phosphates over the first 90 minutes was significantly lower than normal; however, measurement of intracellular calcium in responding cells revealed normal mean levels of elevation, sustained for at least 20 minutes.

Every mechanism for inducing the nonresponsive state had different quantitative effects on the level of inositol phosphate generation. Most resulted in lower levels than normal, but the response to concanavalin-A stimulation in the absence of accessory cells was identical to that in the presence of accessory cells (Mueller et al. 1989). Since the latter conditions induce a normal proliferative response, and the former induce the non-

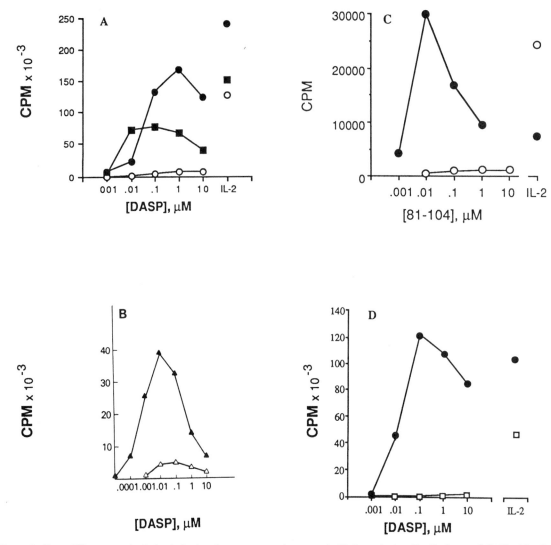

Figure 1. Four different methods for inducing the nonresponsive state in IL-2-producing T-cell clones. (*A*) The T-cell clone A.E7, specific for the antigen pigeon cytochrome *c*, was stimulated with a synthetic peptide analog of the T-cell determinant "DASP" = NH_2-KKANELIAYLKQATK-COOH and B10.A antigen-presenting cells (normal APC = 3000 R irradiated spleen cells) (●) or APC pretreated with 0.5% paraformaldehyde for 15 min at room temperature (○). After 1 day, the T cells were recovered and rested. After 4 more days, they were stimulated with various concentrations of DASP and irradiated B10.A spleen cells (normal APC) or with IL-2 (5% supernatant from the Gibbon cell line, MLA) as a control of viability. The stimulation of T cells not pretreated in any way is shown as the "rested" control (■). The proliferative response (CPM) was measured 3 days later by assessing the incorporation of [³H]thymidine into DNA. Note that pretreatment with chemically fixed APC makes the T cells hyporesponsive to restimulation, compared to rested cells. Pretreatment with normal APC and antigen gives a "preactivated" pattern on restimulation, i.e., an increased maximal response and a shift in the EC_{50} to a larger antigen concentration. See Jenkins et al. (1988) for more details. (*B*) The T-cell F1.A2 was cultured for 24 hr with planar lipid membranes containing the murine MHC class II molecule E^k_β:E^k_α either alone (▲) or in the presence of 10 μM DASP (△). The cells were then recovered and rested. After 8 days, the T cells were restimulated with irradiated B10.A spleen cells (normal APC) and various concentrations of DASP. The proliferative response (CPM) was measured 3 days later. Note that pretreatment with peptide-MHC molecule complexes alone, a pure T-cell antigen-receptor occupancy event, induces a hyporesponsive state lasting at least 8 days. See Quill and Schwartz (1987) for more details. (*C*) The T-cell clone A.E7 (5×10^5 cells/well) was precultured for 24 hr in tissue culture plates precoated with 10 μg/ml anti-CD3 monoclonal antibody 145-2C11 (○) or medium (●). The cells were then recovered and rested in fresh plates without any antibody. After 7 days, surviving cells (20%) were stimulated with either IL-2 or irradiated B10.A spleen cells and various concentrations of the carboxy-terminal cyanogen bromide (CNBr) fragment of pigeon cytochrome *c* (residues 81–104). The proliferative response (CPM) was measured 3 days later. Note that pretreatment with anti-CD3, which binds to the ε chain of the T-cell antigen receptor, induces a hyporesponsive state for antigen restimulation, even though the response to IL-2 is augmented. See M.K. Jenkins et al. (in prep.) for more details. (*D*) The T-cell clone A.E7 was stimulated for 48 hr with 5 μg/ml concanavalin A (□) or medium (●) in the absence of any APC. The cells were treated with α-methylmannoside, recovered on a Ficoll-Hypaque gradient, washed with medium, and rested. After 2 days, the T cells were stimulated with either IL-2 or irradiated B10.A spleen cells and various concentrations of DASP. The proliferative response (CPM) was measured 3 days later. Note that, in the absence of APC, pretreatment with concanavalin A, which binds to many cell-surface glycoproteins including the T-cell antigen receptor, induces the hyporesponsive state. See Mueller et al. (1989) for more details.

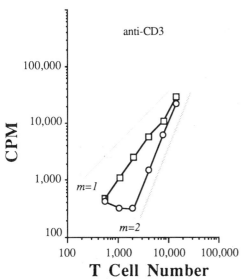

Figure 2. Anti-CD3 stimulation of a T-cell proliferative response requires an interaction with a cell capable of delivering a costimulatory signal. Twofold dilutions of the T-cell clone A.E7 were stimulated in a microtiter plate precoated with 1 μg/ml anti-CD3 monoclonal antibody 145-2C11 either alone (○) or in the presence of 5×10^5 irradiated, T-cell-depleted B10.A spleen cells as a source of costimulatory signal (□). The cells were cultured for 64 hr, and the proliferative response was determined during the final 16 hr by measuring the incorporation of [^{3}H]thymidine into DNA. Note that the log of the response of the T cells alone falls off with a slope of 2.0 (compare to the theoretical stippled line, $m = 2$). In contrast, the addition of a fixed number of APC converts the slope to 1.2 (compare to the theoretical dotted line, $m = 1$). These observations suggest that anti-CD3 stimulation at high cell density depends on the responding T cell interacting with a second cell capable of delivering a costimulatory signal.

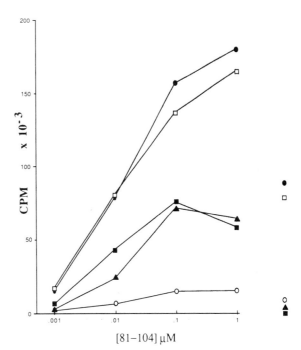

Figure 3. Delivery of the costimulatory signal blocks the induction of nonresponsiveness. The T-cell clone A.E7 was stimulated with either the CNBr fragment 81–104 of pigeon cytochrome c in the presence of irradiated B10.A splenic APC (●: preactivated control); chemically fixed (ECDI) B10.A APC only (■: rested control); chemically fixed B10.A APC and pigeon fragment 81–104 (○: conditions for inducing the nonresponsive state); chemically fixed B10.A APC, pigeon fragment 81–104, and irradiated, allogeneic, low-density (50% Percoll) B10 spleen cells as a source of costimulatory signal (□: experimental group); or chemically fixed B10.A APC and irradiated, low-density B10 spleen cells (▲: allogeneic control). Aliquots of T cells were assayed for their proliferative response 3 days later (plotted as single points for each group in the column at the right of the graph). The remainder of the cells were rested 2 days and then restimulated with various concentrations of pigeon fragment 81–104 and normal irradiated B10.A APC. The proliferative response was assessed 3 days later; dose-response curves for each group are plotted in the left part of the graph. Note that addition of allogeneic APC allowed the T cells to proliferate and blocked induction of the nonresponsive state, i.e., the combination of fixed cells and antigen giving T-cell receptor occupancy, and the allogeneic APC giving delivery of the costimulatory signal, produced an outcome equivalent to activation with normal APC and antigen.

responsive state (Fig. 1D), the results suggest that the costimulatory signal does not influence phosphatidylinositol-4,5-bisphosphate (PtdInsP$_2$) hydrolysis. An examination of later signal transduction events such as activation of protein kinase C by the diacylglycerol generated from PtdInsP$_2$ hydrolysis also failed to reveal any influence of the costimulatory signal. Similar results were observed for stimulation of a tyrosine kinase, an event that might be coupled to receptor occupancy via the CD4 molecule (Veillette et al. 1989).

The critical second messenger for inducing the nonresponsive state appears to be the rise in intracellular calcium (Jenkins et al. 1987). [Ethylenebis(oxyethylenenitrilo]tetraacetic acid (EGTA) blocks the induction of nonresponsiveness stimulated by chemically fixed APC and antigen, except in the presence of excess CaCl$_2$. Furthermore, ionomycin, a calcium ionophore, is capable of inducing the nonresponsive state in a dose-dependent manner (Fig. 4). Maximum effect is achieved when the intracellular calcium is sustained at 400–600 nM for at least 6 hours. The induction of nonresponsiveness by ionomycin is blocked in the presence of cycloheximide (M.K. Jenkins, unpubl.). Cycloheximide also blocks in the planar membrane system (Quill and Schwartz 1987). These results suggest that the induction is an active process involving new protein

synthesis; however, the detailed biochemical events in the process are unknown.

Characterization of the Nonresponsive State

Cells induced into the nonresponsive state remain incapable of responding to T-cell-receptor-mediated stimuli for longer than 1 week. They do respond to IL-2, however, confirming that the cells are viable. This suggests that the primary reason that the cells do not respond to antigen is because they fail to make IL-2. Direct examination of lymphokine production by cells in the nonresponsive state stimulated with normal APC and antigen revealed no measurable IL-2, a small

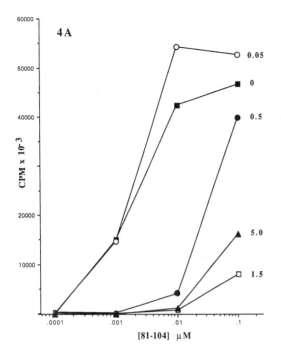

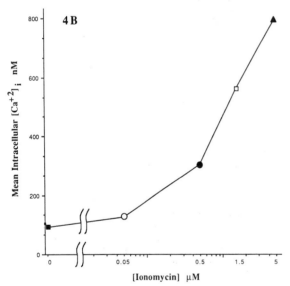

Figure 4. Ionophore-generated increases in intracellular calcium are sufficient to induce the nonresponsive state. (*A*) The T-cell clone A.E7 was preincubated with medium (■) or one of four concentrations of ionomycin: 0.05 μM (○), 0.5 μM (●), 1.5 μM (□), or 5 μM (▲). After 18 hr, the cells were washed, and aliquots were stimulated with various concentrations of the carboxy-terminal CNBr fragment of pigeon cytochrome *c* (residues 81–104) in the presence of irradiated B10.A spleen cells (normal APC). The proliferative response was measured 3 days later (CPM × 10^{-3}). (*B*) In the same experiment, A.E7 cells were preloaded with the calcium-binding dye Indo-1/AM, washed, and stimulated with the same concentrations of ionomycin as in *A*. Steady-state levels of intracellular calcium ion concentrations after ~10–20 min were measured with a FACS II analyzer as described in detail by Jenkins et al. (1987). Note that induction of nonresponsiveness begins at 0.5 μM ionomycin, when the [Ca^{++}]$_i$ is 305 mM, and peaks at 1.5 μM ionomycin, when the [Ca^{++}]$_i$ is 560 nM.

amount of IL-3 (1/8 normal), and substantial amounts of γ-interferon (1/3 normal) after stimulation. The failure to produce IL-2 was confirmed at the mRNA level by in situ hybridization; however, in some experiments, a weak proliferative response was detected, suggesting that very small amounts of IL-2 may still be produced.

The underlying mechanism for the nonresponsive state is not understood. The number of antigen receptors on the cell surface is normal after 2 days. Early activation events such as inositol phosphate generation and increases in intracellular calcium return to normal after 6 days; yet the cells remain unresponsive. Surprisingly, bypassing the antigen receptor, by a combination of direct stimulation of protein kinase C with a phorbol ester (PMA) and increasing intracellular calcium with the ionophore ionomycin, stimulated a comparable response from both normal rested T cells and a cell population induced into the nonresponsive state. This form of stimulation is always suboptimal and, for normal resting cells, involves cryptic delivery of the costimulatory signal by either contaminating APC or the activated T cells (D.L. Mueller et al., in prep.). How this form of stimulation circumvents the nonresponsive state is unknown.

Other T-cell Populations

The detailed study of T-cell clonal anergy has been carried out mainly with IL-2-producing murine T-cell clones (T$_H$1). Experiments with IL-4-producing T$_H$2 clones suggest that their proliferation is not impaired by prior exposure to immobilized anti-CD3 in the absence of accessory cells (M.K. Jenkins et al., in prep.), antigen and chemically fixed APC, nor by exposure to ionomycin (M.K. Jenkins, unpubl.). The same is true for the production of IL-4, one of the growth factors for this type of T-cell clone. Preliminary experiments by Gilbert et al. (1989), however, suggest that T-cell helper function is down-regulated. The biochemical basis for this has not been worked out, but it could involve inhibition of IL-5 or IL-6 production.

In the human, an IL-2-producing clone has also been inactivated from proliferating by exposure to high concentrations of processed antigen (a peptide from influenza hemagglutinin) in the absence of APC (Feldmann et al. 1985). In this case, it has been postulated that the MHC class II molecules expressed on the human T-cell clone present the peptide to other T cells in the culture, thus inactivating them. This presumes that the T-cell clone cannot deliver a costimulatory signal, an assumption that is not supported by other experiments in the literature (Lanzavecchia et al. 1988). The resolution of this paradox may involve differences in lymphokine production by subsets of human T-cell clones or differences in their states of activation.

Are the observations made on T-cell clones applicable to freshly isolated T cells and populations in vivo? T cells from draining lymph nodes of mice immunized with antigen in complete Freund's adjuvant can be

Table 1. Ionomycin Induces a Hyporesponsive State in Freshly Isolated CD4$^+$ T Cells from Antigen-primed Mice

Pretreatment	Proliferative response (Δ CPM) to		
	PPD	Cyt. c	PMA + IL-2
Medium	53,400	28,000	167,000
Ionomycin	1,400	4,100	114,000
% Decrease	97	85	32

B10.A mice were primed with pigeon cytochrome c in complete Freund's adjuvant and T cells prepared from the draining lymph nodes 10 days later by passage over nylon wool columns. CD4$^+$ T cells were isolated by treating the population with complement and monoclonal antibodies against CD8$^+$ cells (83–125), B cells (J11d), and MHC class II-bearing cells (10.2.16 and Y-17). The CD4$^+$ T cells were cultured overnight with either 1 μM ionomycin or medium. The cells were then recovered on a Ficoll-Hypaque gradient and washed, and aliquots were stimulated with normal irradiated B10.A splenic APC and either medium, 20 μg/ml purified protein derivative (PPD) of *Mycobacterium tuberculosis*, 20 μM pigeon cytochrome c fragment 81–104, or 10 ng/ml PMA plus 5% (v/v) supernatant from the Gibbon cell line MLA that constitutively secretes IL-2. After 3 days, the proliferative response was measured as [^{3}H]thymidine incorporation. The data are presented as the difference between antigen-stimulated cultures and the medium control (Δ CPM) or as the percentage decrease in Δ CPM caused by ionomycin. Note that the proliferative responses to antigen are decreased by $\geq$85%, whereas the response to PMA and IL-2 is only reduced by 1/3.

inactivated from proliferating to antigen in vitro by prior exposure to ionomycin for 18 hours (Table 1). The cells still respond to PMA and IL-2. In vivo, ECDI-coupling of antigen to normal spleen cells followed by intravenous injection of the cells into adult mice reduced the subsequent T-cell proliferative response of draining lymph nodes after priming (Miller et al. 1979; Jenkins and Schwartz 1987). The inhibition was both antigen- and MHC class II molecule-specific. Although we cannot be certain that the same mechanism is occurring in vivo that we have detailed in vitro, the observations suggest that even naive T cells can be functionally inactivated (clonal anergy).

Relevance to T-cell Tolerance

The concept of tolerance implies the inability of an organism to eliminate an antigen, whether foreign or self. The mechanisms by which tolerance is thought to occur include (1) deletion of potentially reactive clones of cells, (2) functional inactivation of the clones without deletion, or (3) active suppression of the reactive clones. Evidence exists to support all three mechanisms, although at the T-cell level, the data are strongest for deletion (for review, see Schwartz 1989). It is our opinion that the biochemical underpinnings for each of these mechanisms will turn out to be similar. Clonal anergy, as induced artificially by antigen presentation using chemically fixed cells or planar membranes, results from antigen-receptor occupancy signals in the absence of a costimulatory signal. This is, in essence, the Bretscher and Cohn (1970) two-signal model originally proposed for B-cell activation/inactivation. For T cells, the critical inactivating signal appears to be

initiated by a sustained rise in intracellular calcium, and the inactivation event appears to manifest itself at the level of IL-2 production. Presumably, this inability to secrete IL-2 prevents the expansion of such clones in vivo.

How can clonal anergy be induced in vivo? One way is through MHC class II molecule expression on cells lacking the ability to generate costimulatory activity. For example, keratinocytes are induced to express MHC class II molecules if exposed to γ-interferon (Gaspari et al. 1988). When such cells are used to present antigen to IL-2-producing T-cell clones, they induce the nonresponsive state. Similar observations have been made with β cells from the pancreas of transgenic mice expressing class II molecules under the control of the insulin promoter (Markmann et al. 1988).

Application of these principles to clonal deletion in the thymus would require postulating that the calcium signal in immature T cells leads to cell death rather than anergy. Several groups have shown that calcium levels increased via ionophores or anti-CD3 can lead to apoptosis, a form of cell death involving degradation of DNA by endonucleases (Wyllie et al. 1984; Smith et al. 1989). The normal mechanism would have to involve receptor occupancy in the absence of a costimulatory signal. This could occur if immature thymocytes lack a receptor for the costimulatory activity.

Finally, even the elusive suppressor T cell might inhibit in an analogous manner. Recent experiments with human CD8$^+$ T-cell clones specific for *Mycobacterium leprae* have shown that these cells can suppress a variety of CD4$^+$ T-cell clones specific for the same or other antigens by inducing in them an anergic state (Salgame et al. 1989). The molecular mechanism for this is unknown, but it may involve a soluble lymphokine that either inhibits the delivery of a costimulatory signal or blocks its biochemical pathway inside the cell. Thus, the studies outlined here could provide a general framework for understanding all forms of T-cell tolerance.

ACKNOWLEDGMENTS

We thank Mrs. Chuan Chen and Ms. Lynda Chiodetti for their outstanding technical assistance during the course of these studies.

REFERENCES

Bretscher, P. and M. Cohn. 1970. A theory of self-nonself discrimination. *Science* **169:** 1042.

Feldmann, M., E.D. Zanders, and J.R. Lamb. 1985. Tolerance in T-cell clones. *Immunol. Today* **6:** 58.

Gaspari, A.A., M.K. Jenkins, and S.I. Katz. 1988. Class II major histocompatibility complex-bearing keratinocytes induce antigen-specific unresponsiveness in hapten-specific Th1 clones. *J. Immunol.* **141:** 2216.

Gilbert, K.M., K.D. Hoang, and W.O. Weigle. 1989. Tolerized high density Th clones lose bystander helper activity. *Fed. Proc.* **1691.** (Abstr.).

Jenkins, M.K. and R.H. Schwartz. 1987. Antigen presentation by chemically modified splenocytes induces antigen-specific T cell unresponsiveness *in vitro* and *in vivo*. *J. Exp. Med.* **165**: 302.

Jenkins, M.K., J.D. Ashwell, and R.H. Schwartz. 1988. Allogeneic non-T spleen cells restore the responsiveness of normal T cell clones stimulated with antigen and chemically modified antigen-presenting cells. *J. Immunol.* **140**: 3324.

Jenkins, M.K., D.M. Pardoll, J. Mizuguchi, T.M. Chused, and R.H. Schwartz. 1987. Molecular events in the induction of a nonresponsive state in interleukin 2-producing helper T-lymphocyte clones. *Proc. Natl. Acad. Sci.* **84**: 5409.

Lanzavecchia, A., E. Roosnek, T. Gregory, P. Berman, and S. Abrignani. 1988. T cells can present antigens such as HIV gp120 targeted to their own surface molecules. *Nature* **334**: 530.

Markmann, J., D. Lo, A. Naji, R.D. Palmiter, R.L. Brinster, and E. Heber-Katz. 1988. Antigen presenting function of class II MHC expressing pancreatic β cells. *Nature* **336**: 476.

Miller, S.D., R.P. Wetzig, and H.N. Claman. 1979. The induction of cell-mediated immunity and tolerance with protein antigens coupled to syngeneic lymphoid cells. *J. Exp. Med.* **149**: 758.

Mueller, D.L., M.K. Jenkins, and R.H. Schwartz. 1989. An accessory cell-derived costimulatory signal acts independently of protein kinase *c* activation to allow T cell proliferation and prevent the induction of unresponsiveness. *J. Immunol.* **142**: 2617.

Quill, H. and R.H. Schwartz. 1987. Stimulation of normal inducer T cell clones with antigen presented by purified Ia molecules in planar lipid membranes: Specific induction of a long-lived state of proliferative nonresponsiveness. *J. Immunol.* **138**: 3704.

Salgame, P., R. Modlin, and B.R. Bloom. 1989. On the mechanism of human T cell suppression. *Int. Immunol.* **1**: 121.

Schwartz, R.H. 1989. Acquisition of immunologic self-tolerance. *Cell* **57**: 1073.

Smith, C.A., G.T. Williams, R. Kingston, E.J. Jenkinson, and J.J.T. Owen. 1989. Antibodies to CD3/T-cell receptor complex induce death by apoptosis in immature T cells in thymic cultures. *Nature* **337**: 181.

Veillette, A., M.A. Bookman, E.M. Korak, L.E. Samelson, and J.B. Bolen. 1989. Signal transduction through the CD4 receptor involves the activation of the internal membrane tyrosine-protein kinase p56[lck]. *Nature* **338**: 257.

Wyllie, A.H., R.G. Morris, A.L. Smith, and D. Dunlop. 1984. Chromatin cleavage in apoptosis: Association with condensed chromatin morphology and dependence on macromolecular synthesis. *J. Pathol.* **142**: 67.

The Biology of Human CD2

E.L. Reinherz,*‡ H.-C. Chang,*† L.K. Clayton,*† P. Gardner,§ F.D. Howard,*‡ S. Koyasu,*†
Y.-J. Jin,*† P. Moingeon,*† and P.H. Sayre*

*Laboratory of Immunobiology, Dana-Farber Cancer Institute, and Departments of †Pathology and ‡Medicine,
Harvard Medical School, Boston, Massachusetts 02115; §Department of Medicine,
Stanford University School of Medicine, Stanford, California 94305

Specific antigen recognition by human T lymphocytes involves a set of surface proteins whose various components include a clone-specific heterodimer and the non-covalently associated CD3 γ, δ, ϵ, and ζ subunits (collectively termed T-cell receptor or TCR) as well as a set of "accessory" structures including CD2 and CD4 and/or CD8. The invariant CD2, CD4, and CD8 structures are thought to facilitate T-lymphocyte activation by mediating adhesion between the plasma membrane of a T lymphocyte and its cognate partner (target cells for cytolytic T lymphocytes [CTL] or antigen-presenting cells [APC] for helper T cells). In addition, these structures themselves are involved in providing activation signals.

In this paper, we focus on CD2 and its functional relationship to TCR. The structural basis of signal transduction and adhesion by CD2 will be discussed on the basis of results of functional studies with site-directed mutants and expression of individual protein domains. Furthermore, the contribution of CD2 functions to antigen recognition will be delineated.

The ability of thymus-derived (T) lymphocytes to form spontaneous aggregates or "rosettes" with sheep red blood cells (SRBC) historically served as the earliest marker of human T-lineage cells (Brain et al. 1970; Jondal et al. 1972; Bach 1973; Baxley et al. 1973). Subsequently, an anti-CD2 monoclonal antibody identified the SRBC receptor on human T lymphocytes as a 50–55-kD glycoprotein and provided the initial suggestion that CD2 was involved in mediating intercellular adhesion, since it disrupted the rosetting process (Howard et al. 1981; Kamoun et al. 1981; Bernard et al. 1982). Biochemical, molecular, and functional analyses of CD2 have provided considerable insight into the biology of this molecule.

An in-depth analysis of the CD2 structure and its function is informative from several perspectives. First, CD2, like other cell-surface structures, including lymphocyte function-associated antigen (LFA-1) and probably CD4 and CD8, serves to facilitate cellular adhesion (Fig. 1) between T lymphocytes and their cognate partners (Meuer et al. 1982). Unlike LFA-1 and CD4, however, CD2 is restricted in expression to human T-lineage cells (Reinherz and Schlossman 1980). Second, CD2 subserves a signal transduction role (Meuer et al. 1984). Signal transduction functions are now becoming apparent for other T-cell surface structures,

involving CD4 and CD8, previously thought to have a restricted role as ancillary recognition molecules. For example, the CD4 and CD8 structures were recently shown to be linked to the LCK tyrosine kinase (Rudd et al. 1988; Veillette et al. 1989). Third, the combined adhesion and transduction functions of CD2 facilitate a more efficient T-cell antigen receptor (CD3-Ti) response. This occurs because CD2 optimizes cell–cell contact, thereby increasing the likelihood of TCR triggering, and because its cytoplasmic tail provides signals that synergize with TCR stimulation (Yang et al. 1986). It is likely that a similar role will be played by other adhesion structures as well, even though the precise molecular mechanisms of interaction will differ from CD2. Information obtained about the biology of CD2 should, in principle, provide insight into the function of other adhesion molecules.

Evidence for a central role of the CD2 molecule in T-lymphocyte function was suggested by its expression during early T-cell ontogeny, being represented on > 95% of thymocytes and maintained on virtually all peripheral mature T cells and the vast majority of natural killer (NK) cells. Three epitopes have been identified by monoclonal antibodies on the extracellular segment of CD2: $T11_1$, present on all T cells in close proximity to the SRBC-binding site as defined by a set of monoclonal antibodies that inhibit sheep erythrocyte rosetting; $T11_2$, present on all T cells but distinct from the sheep erythrocyte-binding site; and $T11_3$, preferentially expressed on activated T cells (Meuer et al. 1984). The distribution of $T11_3$ epitope is unusual in that it is expressed only at very low levels on peripheral blood lymphocytes but can be induced within 30 minutes by incubating T lymphocytes with anti-$T11_2$ antibody even at 4°C and in the presence of sodium azide. Therefore, $T11_3$ expression is not dependent on new protein synthesis but rather appears to result from a conformational change in the CD2 molecule following T-lymphocyte activation. Activation of T lymphocytes via the antigen/MHC receptor (CD3-Ti) also results in induction of $T11_3$ expression.

The phenomenon of rosetting between human T lymphocytes and SRBC is dependent on a specific interaction between the CD2 molecule on T cells and a complementary structure on SRBC. The latter, termed the T11 target structure (T11TS), has been biochemically characterized and shown to be a 42-kD glycoprotein

CELL-CELL ADHESION

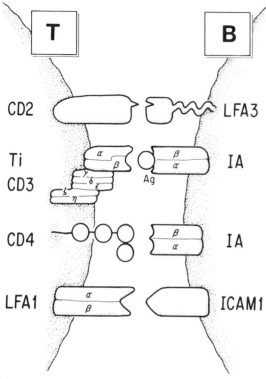

Figure 1. Surface molecules involved in T-cell adhesion and activation. Molecules on the surface of a CD4⁺ T lymphocyte interacting with their specific ligands on a cognate partner. For cytotoxic T cells, CD8 molecules interact in a similar way with MHC class I molecules. The PtdIns-linked and transmembrane forms of LFA-3 are known ligands of CD2.

(Hunig et al. 1986), using antibodies that react with SRBC and block rosettes between SRBC and T lymphocytes. Parallel experiments demonstrated a direct interaction between the human CD2 molecule and the broadly distributed human LFA-3 structure (Dustin et al. 1987a,b; Plunkett et al. 1987; Selvaraj et al. 1987). The LFA-3 molecule has been defined and characterized with monoclonal antibodies selected for their capacity to inhibit cytotoxicity of human CTL lines. LFA-3 is a 55–70-kD molecule expressed on human endothelial, epithelial, and connective tissue cells in most tissues, as well as human T and B lymphocytes, granulocytes, and erythrocytes.

Isolation of LFA-3 cDNAs (Seed 1987; Wallner et al. 1987) revealed two forms of LFA-3, each of which can interact with CD2: a transmembrane form with a short (12 amino acids) carboxy-terminal cytoplasmic tail, and a phosphatidylinositol (PtdIns)-linked form. As expected, a significant degree of primary structural similarity is found between T11TS and LFA-3 (Tiefenthaler et al. 1987), i.e., LFA-3 is the human homolog of sheep T11TS. A broad role for CD2/LFA-3 interaction in mediating adhesion between CD2⁺ T-lineage cells and

LFA-3-expressing cells comes from analysis of T cell-target conjugate formation assays in which adhesion between CD2⁺ human CTL clones and LFA-3-expressing human B-lymphoblastoid cell lines could be inhibited by antibodies against CD2 or LFA-3 (Krensky et al. 1984; Shaw et al. 1986). Furthermore, blocking experiments using monoclonal antibodies directed against the various epitopes of the molecule established that the $T11_1$ epitope is critical for adhesion and therefore identical or close to the LFA-3-binding site. Anti-CD2 antibodies that inhibit sheep-cell rosetting also block a broad range of T-cell functions, including cytotoxicity, helper function, and antigen or mitogen-induced proliferation (Palacios and Martinez-Maza 1982; Krensky et al. 1984; Siliciano et al. 1985; Tadmori et al. 1985; Bolhuis et al. 1986).

CD2 also plays a role in T-lymphocyte activation. Antibodies directed against CD2 extracellular epitopes distinct from the erythrocyte-binding site, especially when used in combination with another CD2 ligand (e.g., a second anti-CD2 antibody or an LFA-3-bearing cell surface), can potently activate T-cell proliferation and CTL and NK cytotoxic effector function (Meuer et al. 1984; Brottier et al. 1985; Siliciano et al. 1985; Bernard et al. 1986; Hunig et al. 1987; Tiefenthaler et al. 1987; Bierer et al. 1988a). Direct evidence that CD2 can transduce activation signals comes from the observation that a combination of anti-$T11_2$ and anti-$T11_3$ monoclonal antibodies induces a series of activation events (polyphosphoinositide turnover, cytosolic calcium increase, i.e., $[Ca^{++}]_i$, IL-2 gene induction, lymphokine production, DNA synthesis, and clonal expansion (Meuer et al. 1984; Alcover et al. 1986; Pantaleo et al. 1987). As will be discussed subsequently, these activation events are virtually indistinguishable from those mediated via the CD3-Ti antigen/MHC receptor complex, implying that common second-messenger pathways are being utilized. In addition, thymocyte activation can be mediated by CD2 (Fox et al. 1985). Furthermore, stimulation of T cells via CD2 and CD3-Ti results in synergistic activation (Yang et al. 1986).

CD2 Protein Analysis and Gene Organization

CD2 was affinity purified from detergent lysates of Jurkat cells, and intact CD2 protein and CNBr fragments were microsequenced. Redundant oligonucleotides based on these sequences were then used to isolate cDNAs. All empirically derived amino acid sequences were found in the translated sequences predicted by the nucleotide analysis of the cDNA. Furthermore, expression of the cDNAs in COS cells resulted in surface CD2 expression, as judged by indirect immunofluorescence with anti-CD2 monoclonal antibodies and rosette formation with SRBCs (Sayre et al. 1987). CD2 has also been cloned by others (Sewall et al. 1986; Seed and Aruffo 1987).

The translated human cDNA sequence (Fig. 2A) predicts an open reading frame of 351 residues, of which the first 24 amino acids comprise a typical hydro-

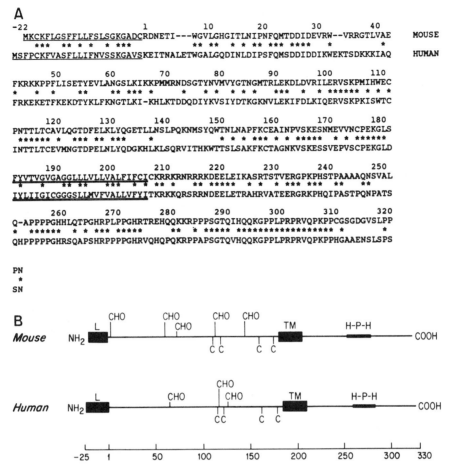

Figure 2. Structural analysis of murine and human CD2. (*A*) Comparison of mouse and human CD2 predicted protein sequence. The alignment is based on the LOCAL algorithm. Asterisks represent identities. The predicted signal peptides and transmembrane segments are underlined. (*B*) Schematic structure of mouse and human CD2. The positions of cysteine residues (C), N-linked carbohydrate addition sites (CHO), the CD2 leader segment (L), the CD2 transmembrane domain (TM), and the proline-rich region containing four histidines (H-P-H) are indicated.

phobic signal peptide that is cleaved from the mature protein. The remaining 327-amino-acid protein has a calculated molecular weight of 36,886 before the addition of sugars. There are three potential N-linked glycosylation sites in the mature protein, consistent with the observed relative molecular weight on SDS-PAGE of approximately 50,000. There is a single 25-amino-acid internal hydrophobic segment that divides the protein into a 185-amino-acid predicted external segment and a 117-amino-acid intracytoplasmic region (Sayre et al. 1987). The large size of the cytoplasmic domain is consistent with a role for the CD2 molecule in signal transduction across the lymphocyte membrane (see below).

Northern analysis with human CD2 cDNA probes reveals 1.3- and 1.7-kb species mRNA in thymocytes, resting T cells, and T-cell tumors (Sayre et al. 1987). The different-sized messages reflect utilization of alternate polyadenylation signals and are identical in their coding region. Phytohemagglutinin-activated peripheral blood T cells have substantially higher (20–50-fold) steady-state CD2 RNA levels than resting T cells, con-

sistent with the enhanced rosetting capacity and increase in CD2 cell-surface protein expression (200,000 copies in activated vs. 20,000 copies in resting T cells) observed for activated T lymphocytes (Meuer et al. 1984).

Human CD2 cDNAs were then used to isolate murine clones encoding a homologous molecule (Clayton et al. 1987). Murine CD2 is 51% identical overall with the human protein. There is a higher degree of similarity with the human cytoplasmic domain (59%) than with its extracellular (47%) or transmembrane (44%) regions (Fig. 2A). A histidine/proline-rich region in the cytoplasmic domain is very highly conserved between human and mouse as well as in the rat CD2 homolog (Williams et al. 1987), which strongly suggests a functional role in CD2 signal transduction for this segment (Fig. 2B).

Genomic DNA clones containing the human and murine CD2 genes were characterized (Diamond et al. 1988; Lang et al. 1988). The human CD2 gene comprises five exons spanning ~12 kb. A leader exon contains the 5'-untranslated region and most of the nucleotides defining the signal peptide (amino acids −24 to −5). Two exons encode the extracellular segment; exon 2 is 321 bp long and codes for four residues of the leader peptide and amino acids 1–103 of the mature protein, and exon 3 is 231 bp long and encodes amino acids 104–180. Exon 4 is 123 bp long and codes for the single transmembrane region of the molecule (amino acids 181–221). Exon 5 is a large 765-bp exon encoding virtually the entire cytoplasmic domain (amino acids 222–327) and the 3′-untranslated region. The murine CD2 gene has a similar organization with exon-intron boundaries essentially identical to the human gene. Substantial conservation of nucleotide sequences between species in both 5′ and 3′ gene-flanking regions equivalent to that among homologous exons suggests that murine and human genes may be regulated in a similar fashion. A recently described T-cell-specific enhancer has been defined several kb 3′ to exon 5 in the human gene (Greaves et al. 1989). Moreover, chromosomal localization of the human (Brown et al. 1987; Clayton et al. 1988) and murine (Sewell et al. 1987; Clayton et al. 1988) CD2 genes shows that they reside in homologous positions in the genome: chromosome 1 at position 1p13 in the human and chromosome 3 in the mouse. Other human genes in this region have their mouse homologs on chromosome 3 (Lalley and McKusick 1985).

The CD2 Extracellular Segment

To begin to define structure–function relationships in the extracellular segment of the transmembrane CD2 molecule, we have used a eukaryotic expression system and a CD2 cDNA to produce milligram amounts of

recombinant soluble CD2 molecules (Sayre et al. 1989). We designed a construct for expression of a soluble fragment of CD2 that would include all the residues encoded by the leader and two extracellular segment exons (exons 1–3). The plasmid pAc373/T11$_{ex2}$ was constructed as described in Figure 3A and encodes 182 amino acids of the predicted CD2 external segment, including all the residues derived from the extracellular exons and part of one codon (for Glu-181) and all of the second codon (for Lys-182) derived from the transmembrane domain exon. This construction thus includes all four extracellular cysteine residues located in domain II of CD2 and thereby avoids problems associated with intermolecular disulfide exchange observed with a previous construction (Richardson et al. 1988).

Plasmid pAc373/T11$_{ex2}$ was used to cotransfect SF9 cells with AcNPV baculoviral DNA. Recombinant baculovirus, termed T11$_{ex2}$-AcNPV, were selected, purified, and used to infect small-scale cultures for metabolic labeling. Immunoprecipitation of radiolabeled supernatants with anti-T11$_1$ (3T4-8B5) verified that T11$_{ex2}$-AcNPV directed the production of a recombinant CD2 molecule in SF9 cells (data not shown). T11$_{ex2}$-AcNPV was therefore used to infect liter cultures for the production of large amounts of protein. T11$_{ex2}$ protein was purified from infected cell supernatants by affinity chromatography on an anti-T11$_1$ column.

T11$_{ex2}$ migrates as a well-demarcated doublet in both reducing and nonreducing conditions in SDS-PAGE (Fig. 3B, lanes a and b). Two well-separated bands at 30–31 kD are seen in the presence of 50 mM of dithiothreitol (DTT) (lane a), which migrate at 27–28 kD in

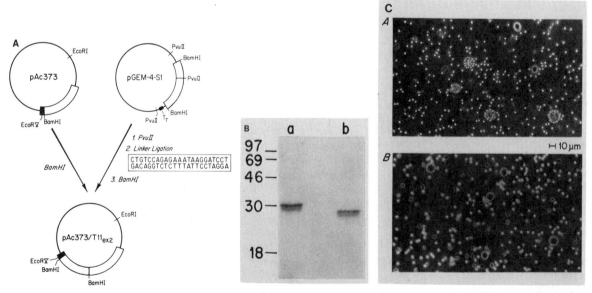

Figure 3. Soluble CD2 protein. (A) Construction protocol for producing and cloning a truncated CD2 cDNA into the pAc373 transfer vector. (B) SDS-PAGE analysis of T11$_{ex2}$ T11$_{ex2}$ (1 μg) purified from large-scale cultures of SF9 cells infected with T11$_{ex2}$ AcNPV was analyzed by Coomassie staining on a 12.5% polyacrylamide gel in the presence of 50 mM DTT (lane a) or in nonreducing conditions (lane b). (C) Rosette inhibition assay. Rosette formation between the Jurkat T-cell line and SRBCs was evaluated in the absence (A) or presence (B) of T11$_{ex2}$ soluble protein.

the absence of reducing agent (lane b). The clear-cut decrease in electrophoretic mobility after reduction with DTT strongly indicates that $T11_{ex2}$ contains intrachain disulfide bridges; it does not form interchain bridges. Although not shown, microsequencing analysis of [^{35}S]cysteine-labeled peptides verifies that there are two sets of intrachain disulfide bonds in $T11_{ex2}$ between the amino-terminal cysteines and carboxy-terminal cysteines.

To investigate the difference between the two bands representing $T11_{ex2}$, 160 pmole of purified protein was separated by SDS-PAGE and blotted onto a polyvinyl difluoride (PVDF) membrane. The upper and lower bands were cut separately from the membrane for amino-terminal sequencing. Each band yielded the CD2 amino-terminal sequence, suggesting that they differ from one another by posttranslational modification. This supposition was verified by deglycosylation experiments (not shown). Although homologies in short stretches of amino acids exist between CD2 and members of the Ig superfamily (Williams et al. 1987), it is unclear whether CD2 is a bona fide member, particularly in view of 2° structural predictions and circular dichroism analyses that raise the possibility of α-helical structures in the CD2 extracellular segment (Clayton et al. 1987; Sayre et al. 1989).

Equilibrium sedimentation analysis demonstrates that $T11_{ex2}$ protein exists as a monomer in solution (Sayre et al. 1989). Other studies show that $T11_{ex2}$ expresses the three epitopes $T11_1$, $T11_2$, and $T11_3$ defined by various anti-CD2 monoclonal antibodies on the native surface CD2 molecule (data not shown). As shown in Figure 3C, $T11_{ex2}$ is able to block rosette formation between Jurkat T cells and SRBC (bottom) (with an IC_{50} concentration of ~1 μM). In addition, $T11_{ex2}$ blocks the binding of an anti-LFA-3 antibody to the corresponding structure expressed on the surface of B-lymphoblastoid cells. The capacity of $T11_{ex2}$ to interact specifically with LFA-3 was further confirmed by directly demonstrating a specific and saturable binding of radiolabeled $T11_{ex2}$ to the LFA-3$^+$ human B cells, JY, which is inhibited by anti-LFA-3 monoclonal antibody. Scatchard analysis of the data indicated a 0.4 μM dissociation constant (K_d) for the CD2/LFA-3 interaction reflecting a relatively low binding affinity between the two molecules when compared to hormone receptor ligand interaction (e.g., for IL-2, $K_d = 10^{-11}$ M). Therefore, it appears that a series of successive low-affinity binding events could be sufficient for two cells to adhere to one another through multimeric interaction that would greatly enhance the avidity of the T cell for its cognate partner. With regard to this point, it should be noted that antigen-stimulated T cells express an order of magnitude more surface CD2 than resting T lymphocytes, thereby presumably enhancing adhesion between presenting (or target) cells and T lymphocytes in areas of ongoing immune responses.

Using enzyme cleavage of a secreted soluble CD2 molecule in conjunction with HPLC separation of the products, it has recently been possible to identify the domain involved in cellular adhesion as being localized to the amino-terminal ~100 amino acids of the molecule (encoded by exon 2) (Richardson et al. 1988). Consistent with this observation, saturation mutation analysis has localized residues comprising and/or affecting the $T11_1$ epitope (known to be identical or very close to the LFA-3-binding site of the molecule) to several discrete stretches of amino acids in this region of the molecule (Peterson and Seed 1987).

Activation Via CD2: Interdependence with the CD3-Ti (α/β) Pathway

In contrast to the TCR (CD3-Ti) complex, which interacts with processed antigen in conjunction with MHC gene products, the CD2 pathway appears to represent an antigen-independent pathway of activation. Interaction of either set of membrane receptors with appropriate mitogenic stimuli, however, results in a virtually identical series of events involving phosphatidylinositol (PtdIns) turnover with subsequent production of 1,4,5 inositol trisphosphate ($InsP_3$) and diacylglycerol. $InsP_3$ is directly implicated in causing a rise in intracellular free calcium ($[Ca^{++}]_i$) (see below), whereas diacylglycerol is an endogenous activator of protein kinase C. Previous studies have suggested that both a rise in intracellular free calcium and phosphorylation events mediated through protein kinase C activation are necessary for IL-2 gene induction (Alcover et al. 1986; Truneh et al. 1985).

Since an increase in cytoplasmic free Ca^{++} appears to be an important early signal in T-lymphocyte activation (Alcover et al. 1986), we questioned whether the recently characterized non-voltage-gated Ca^{++} channels known to be present in the plasma membrane of T cells (Kuno et al. 1986; Pecht et al. 1987) could account for the subsequent rise in Ca^{++} observed following stimulation of T cells through CD2 or CD3-Ti. To characterize the relationship between the Ca^{++} permeable channel and the CD3-Ti and CD2 surface receptors, single-channel recordings were made at Vr from cell-attached patches of human cloned helper T lymphocytes with pipets containing tetrodotoxin (TTX) supplemented isotonic $BaCl_2$ (Gardner et al. 1989). Figure 4A demonstrates representative single-channel inward Ba^{++} currents recorded at Vr following stimulation of the CD3-Ti receptor. Prior to addition of antibody (first trace), infrequent inward current activity was seen (no activity is seen on the demonstrated trace, but rare intermittent activity yielding a very low channel opening probability is often seen in control recordings). Upon addition of anti-CD3 (IgG) antibody to the bathing solution, single-channel inward current activity, seen as downward current deflections, was greatly augmented (second and third traces). Virtually identical results were obtained with anti-CD3 antibody of the IgM isotype and with anti-$T11_{2+3}$ antibodies (Fig. 4B). In contrast, no inward current activity was seen during 6–10-minute recordings from cell-attached

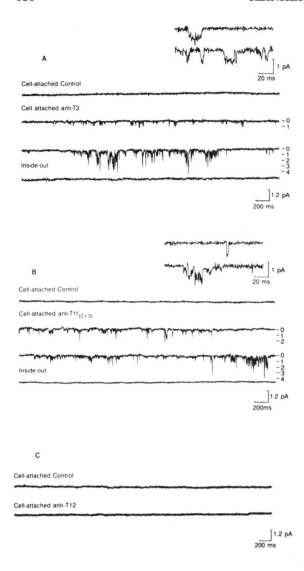

Figure 4. Plasma membrane channels permeable to Ca^{++} ions. Single-channel recording of antibody-induced inward Ba^{++} currents. Currents were recorded from the same membrane patch in cell-attached (first–third traces) and excised inside-out (fourth trace) configurations. The patch pipet contained 110 mM $BaCl_2$, 200 nM TTX, and 10 mM HEPES-KOH (pH 7.3). The bath solution contained 154 mM NaCl, 5.5 mM KCl, 2 mM $CaCl_2$, 1 mM $MgCl_2$, and 10 mM HEPES-NaOH (pH 7.3). Holding potential was 0 mV (equivalent to resting membrane potential Vr, assumed to be approximately -60 mV in the cell-attached configuration) and -60 mV in the inside-out configuration. Current signals were filtered at 1 kHz (-3 db). (A) Anti-CD3. First trace: Current recorded from a membrane patch under control conditions. No unitary inward currents were detected. Second and third traces: Current recorded from the same patch, 20 sec (second trace) and 5 min (third trace) after addition of 300 ng/ml anti-CD3 (IgG) monoclonal antibody to bath solution in which the cell was suspended. Inward currents are seen as downward deflections from base line. Multiple levels are seen in the third trace, indicating presence of at least four active channels in the patch (unitary current levels shown by lines at right of the trace). Inward currents are sometimes attenuated due to brevity of opening event relative to recording bandwidth. Fourth trace: Current recording after excision of membrane patch into inside-out recording configuration. Holding potential was hyperpolarized 60 mV to approximate Vr. Inward currents disappeared immediately after exposure to millimolar Ca^{++} concentration on the cytoplasmic surface. (B) Anti-T11$_2$ + anti-T11$_3$. First trace: Current recorded from membrane patch under control conditions. Second and third traces: Current recorded from the same patch, 20 sec (second trace) and 5 min (third trace) after addition of anti-T11$_2$ + anti-T11$_3$ monoclonal antibodies in a 1:100 dilution to bath solution in which the cell was suspended. Fourth trace: Current recording after formation of an inside-out patch facing millimolar Ca^{++} solutions. Holding potential was hyperpolarized 60 mV to approximate Vr. (C) Anti-T12. First trace: Current recorded from a membrane patch under control conditions. No unitary inward currents were detected. Second trace: Current recorded from the same patch 4 min after addition of 1:100 dilution of anti-T12 monoclonal antibody to bath solution in which the cell was suspended. No inward currents were observed for the entire 8-min recording period.

patches of eight cells exposed to anti-T12 antibody (Fig. 4C).

The unitary Ba^{++} currents had an approximate amplitude of 0.7–0.8 pA (for anti-CD3, unitary amplitude = 0.68 ± 0.15 pA (mean $\pm$ s.d.), $n = 1594$ openings; for anti-T11$_{2+3}$, unitary amplitude = 0.76 ± 0.20 pA, $n = 1797$ openings) at resting potential, and amplitude decreased with increasing membrane depolarization. Although no definitive reversal potential could be ascertained, in part due to limitation of applied voltage to the patch, currents were inward at least 80 mV positive to Vr, suggesting a positive reversal potential. Channel opening induced by anti-CD3 or anti-T11$_{2+3}$ antibodies were characterized by a bursting behavior, i.e., periods of quiescence interspersed with periods of intense bursts of channel activity, often with multiple superimposed levels (Fig. 4A). Single-channel interval analysis, obtained from the infrequent records of patches with few multiple levels, indicated that the antibody-induced channel steady-state kinetics could be described by single-component open-time probability density distributions with very brief open-time constants (for anti-CD3; $\tau_o = 0.41$ ms, $n = 1594$; for anti-

T11$_{2+3}$, $\tau_o = 0.38$ ms, $n = 1797$) and by closed-time distributions that could be fitted by two well-separated constants.

It should be noted that many patches contained no channel activity either before or after antibody addition. This led us to postulate that channels may occur in a clustered but low-density distribution. Elicitation of Ba^{++} currents by anti-CD3 or anti-CD2 antibodies occurred within 20 seconds to approximately 2 minutes after addition of antibody to the bath and persisted for several minutes thereafter. Because our experiments used a static, nonflowing chamber at 20°C, time to onset of current activation cannot be absolutely estimated; however, it appears to be in a reasonable range relative to the time course of sustained cytosolic Ca^{++} increase determined by the previous quin-2 studies (Alcover et al. 1986).

The anti-CD3 and anti-CD2-induced unitary Ba^{++} currents observed across the T-lymphocyte plasma membrane are noteworthy from two points of view. First, since the high-resistance gigaohm seal precludes diffusion of antibody applied in the bathing solution into the membrane directly under the recording pipet, stimulation by anti-CD3 or anti-CD2 antibodies must not interact directly with the channel, but indirectly at sites remote from the channel through an intermediate second messenger. This strongly argues against the possibility that either CD3 or CD2 surface structure includes, or is necessarily directly contiguous with, the ionophore, as previously hypothesized. In fact, addition of InsP$_3$ to excised inside-out patches opens an identical set of channels, consistent with the notion that InsP$_3$ or a related inositide is the second messenger. Second, excision of the patch from the cell attached to the inside-out configuration so that the patch cytoplasmic surface faced solutions containing millimolar Ca^{++} concentrations, followed by imposition of a driving force approximately equal to the normal resting Vr(-60 mV), resulted in immediate abolition of channel opening (Gardner et al. 1989). As shown by Northern blot, the steady-state rise in IL-2 mRNA after CD3-Ti or CD2 stimulation is clearly dependent on the rise of [Ca^{++}]$_i$ resulting from ion movement across this channel: Removal of extracellular Ca^{++} with ethyleneglycol tetraacetic acid abrogates IL-2 gene induction (Gardner et al. 1989).

Because CD3-Ti and CD2 stimulation resulted in an identical set of channel openings, it seems likely that, at least in part, these two receptors work through a common signaling pathway. Therefore, in a parallel series of experiments, we analyzed the interdependence of CD3-Ti and CD2 activation pathways in human T lymphocytes. To address this issue, mutants of the IL-2-producing human T-cell line Jurkat (CD3$^+$, Ti α/β^+, CD2$^+$) have been produced through low-dose gamma irradiation and immunoselection. In this way, it was possible to generate T cells that express only either CD2 or CD3-Ti α/β molecules on their surface. It was shown that CD3-Ti$^-$ mutants fail to be stimulated with monoclonal antibodies directed against either surface molecules to increase phosphoinositide turnover, mobilize calcium, or induce the IL-2 gene (Alcover et al. 1988b). Interestingly, the ability to activate these mutants via CD2 as well as CD3-Ti can be restored following reconstitution of surface CD3-Ti expression upon appropriate DNA transfection (e.g., Ti β subunit cDNA into Ti β^- Jurkat variants). Functional characterization of CD3-Ti$^+$ mutants, lacking detectable surface CD2 as determined by indirect immunofluorescence, immunoprecipitation analysis, and specific radiolabeled antibody-binding assay, established that, as expected, the combination of mitogenic anti-CD2 antibodies failed to stimulate these variants. In contrast, triggering of these CD2$^-$ mutants through CD3-Ti resulted in the normal set of T-lymphocyte-associated activation events including phosphoinositide turnover, elevation in intracellular free calcium, early gene induction events, and IL-2 production (Moingeon et al. 1988). Assuming that the Jurkat cell line is representative of normal cycling mature T cells, these results clearly demonstrate that (1) the CD3-Ti and CD2 pathways of activation are interdependent; (2) the expression of TCR (α/β) components is required for the CD2 transduction function analyzed above (Alcover et al.

1988b); and (3) the presence of the CD2 molecule on the plasma membrane is not a requirement for the expression of a functional CD3-Ti (α/β) receptor (Moingeon et al. 1988). These latter data do not preclude, however, that as yet unidentified signals mediated through the CD2 molecule could influence TCR function. Consistent with the first two points are the independent observations that a recombinant CD2 cDNA-containing baculovirus can induce high-level expression of T11$_1$, T11$_2$, and T11$_3$ epitopes on the surface of gut epithelial cells. However, in this environment, the CD2 protein cannot be triggered to transduce a signal resulting in elevation of [Ca^{++}]$_i$ (Alcover et al. 1988a).

Dissection of the Intracytoplasmic Domain of Human CD2

Comparison of the primary structures of human and murine CD2, deduced from cDNA sequence experiments, established that the highest degree of homology lies in their cytoplasmic domain (Fig. 2A). In particular, two regions are highly conserved between residues 255 and 275 as well as between 286 and 310 (Clayton et al. 1987). The latter region is unique with respect to its multiple proline and basic residues organized in two tandem repeats of the PPPGHR motif within the human sequences. Secondary structure predictions suggest that the intracytoplasmic tail of CD2 has an extended nonglobular conformation. These unusual but conserved features among species including man, mouse, and rat suggest an important role for the CD2 cytoplasmic segment in signal transduction.

To precisely characterize the functional and structural relationship of the cytoplasmic domain of the human CD2 molecule, a series of deletion mutants of the human CD2 cDNA was produced encoding 98, 77, 43, and 18 amino acids of the 117 predicted cytoplasmic CD2 amino acid residues (Chang et al. 1989). Full-length cDNAs as well as the various deletion mutants (obtained by truncation of the wild-type cDNA using the appropriate restriction enzymes) (Fig. 5A) were inserted into the retrovirus expression vector DOL, which contains the neomycin-resistance gene. Defective retrovirus generated upon transfection of a helper-free retrovirus packaging cell line were used to infect the murine T-cell hybridoma 3DO54.8 cell line (specific for ovalbumin in the context of the H-2 [I-A^d] molecule) (Haskins et al. 1983). Neomycin-resistant clones were further selected for surface expression of the human CD2 molecule using an indirect immunofluorescence assay (Fig. 5B). Clones used in subsequent functional studies were designated on the basis of the nature of their CD2 cDNA retroviral insert. CD2FL resulted from retroviral infection with the full-length CD2 cDNA, whereas CD2ΔC98, ΔC77, ΔC43, and ΔC18 resulted from infection with retroviruses containing the entire extracellular and transmembrane segment of CD2 but only 98, 77, 43, or 18 of the 117 cytoplasmic amino acid residues, respectively.

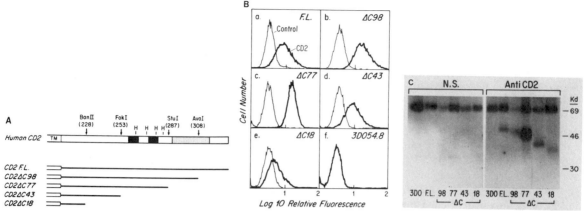

Figure 5. Expression of human CD2 molecules in murine T cells. (*A*) Schematic structure of the transmembrane and cytoplasmic regions of human CD2 and variant molecules. Constructs of full-length and deletion mutants of CD2 are diagramed. The region most conserved between human and mouse CD2 is stippled, and the two repeating PPPGHR segments are marked in black. The H denotes the histidine residues thought to form a putative binding site. The restriction sites that generate the truncated CD2 molecules are marked by arrows with numbers in parentheses corresponding to amino acid residues. (*B*) Flow cytometric analysis of CD2 expression on murine T cells. Indirect immunofluorescence assays were carried out using the anti-T11$_1$ monoclonal antibody (3T4-8B5) (thick line) and compared to an irrelevant antibody (1HT4-4E5) (thin line) as background. Bound antibodies were detected with a 1:40 dilution of fluorescein-coupled goat anti-mouse IgG as a second antibody (Meloy, Springfield, VA). For each sample, 10,000 cells were analyzed on an Epics V cell sorter. Graphs represent the number of cells (ordinate) vs. log 10 fluorescence intensity (abscissa). (*C*) Immunoprecipitation of CD2 from lysates of iodinated cell lines. 10–20 × 10⁶ cells were surface labeled with 1 mCi ^{125}I using the lactoperoxidase method. Immunoprecipitates were obtained from lysates of murine T cells using a nonspecific (NS) antibody (mouse anti-human CD8) or an anti-CD2 antibody (directed against the T11$_1$ epitope) coupled to protein-A-Sepharose beads. Immunoprecipitated material was run under reducing conditions over an SDS 10% polyacrylamide gel. The resulting autoradiogram is shown.

Immunoprecipitation and SDS-PAGE analysis of the corresponding ^{125}I-labeled surface CD2 molecules showed that although no human CD2 was immunoprecipitated from the murine nontransfected 3DO54.8 cell line, a 53-kD band was identified in CD2FL cell lysates (Fig. 5C). Furthermore, parallel analysis of the CD2 proteins expressed by CD2ΔC98, ΔC77, ΔC43, and ΔC18 cells revealed proteins of 51, 47, 43, and 40 kD, respectively (corresponding to the expected truncations). We then examined whether the stimulatory combination of anti-T11$_2$ + anti-T11$_3$ monoclonal antibodies was effective in inducing activation events in CD2FL as well as CD2ΔC cell lines. Figure 6A shows an analysis of alteration in [Ca^{++}]$_i$ after stimulation with anti-T11$_2$ + anti-T11$_3$ in various cell lines as measured with the calcium-sensitive dye indo-1 and flow cytometric analysis in real time. A clear rise in [Ca^{++}]$_i$ (approximately 1 200-nM increment) was observed upon stimulation of CD2FL, CD2ΔC98, and CD2ΔC77 cells. The calcium rise occurs within 2 minutes after adding the stimulating antibodies, most likely corresponding to the time required for expression of the T11$_3$ epitope after anti-T11$_2$ stimulation, a phenomenon observed previously for human T lymphocytes (Alcover et al. 1986). In contrast, CD2ΔC43 and CD2ΔC18 clones were not triggered by anti-T11$_2$ + anti-T11$_3$ antibodies. As expected, the nontransfected line 3DO54.8 was also not stimulated. Given that an immediate [Ca^{++}]$_i$ rise was observed after addition of the Ca^{++} ionophore A23187 (1 μg/ml final concentration), it is clear that cells were loaded with the fluorescent dye. These data establish that a significant rise in [Ca^{++}]$_i$ can be induced through

human CD2 structures expressed on the membrane of murine T cells even in the absence of the carboxy-terminal 40 amino acid residues of the CD2 cytoplasmic segment.

We next examined whether nuclear activation events including IL-2 induction with subsequent IL-2 secretion could be triggered through the human CD2 molecule in murine CD2FL cells. To this end, clones were stimulated, and IL-2 secretion into supernatants was assayed using the IL-2-dependent CTLL-20 cell line. As shown in Figure 6B, supernatants from CD2FL or 3DO54.8 cells stimulated with ovalbumin in the presence of the H-2 (I-A^d)-expressing A20 B lymphoma are able to induce proliferation of the IL-2-dependent CTLL-20 cells in a comparable way. In contrast, the combination of anti-T11$_2$ + anti-T11$_3$ antibodies is effective in inducing IL-2 production by CD2FL cells but not the parental line 3DO54.8. Figure 6C shows that all of the cell lines tested, including CD2FL, 3DO54.8, and the CD2ΔC series, produce a high amount of IL-2 (ranging from 30 to 100 units/ml corresponding to a clonal variation repeatedly observed) when stimulated with ovalbumin in the I-A^d context. This result demonstrates the integrity of the IL-2 synthetic pathway in each clone. Perhaps more importantly, after stimulation with anti-CD2 antibodies, the clones CD2FL, CD2ΔC98, and CD2ΔC77 produce a comparable level of IL-2, whereas transfectants CD2ΔC43 and CD2ΔC18, like the untransfected 3DO54.8, are not triggered through CD2. Taken together, these data show that a full-length human CD2 molecule, as well as a CD2 molecule lacking 19 or 40 carboxy-terminal amino acids from the cytoplasmic domain, is able to

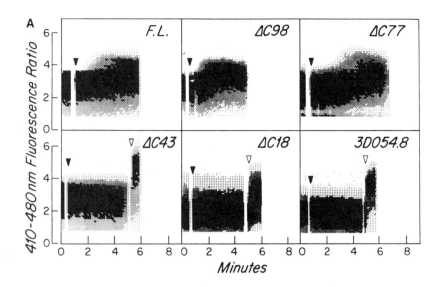

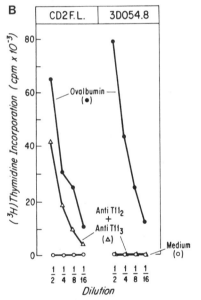

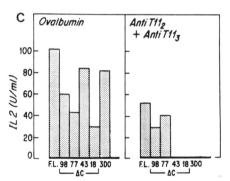

Figure 6. Functional analysis of murine T cells expressing human CD2 molecules. (*A*) Elevation in intracellular free calcium mediated by CD2 stimulation. Cytosolic Ca^{++} concentrations were determined as described previously (Alcover et al. 1988a) by loading 2×10^6 cells for 45 min at 37°C with 2 μg/ml acetylmethyl ester of indo-1 (Molecular Probes, Junction City, OR) in 200 μl of RPMI 1640 + 2% FCS. Cells were diluted tenfold prior to analysis on an Epics V cell sorter. Upon Ca^{++} binding, indo-1 exhibits changes in fluorescein emission wavelengths from 480 to 410 nm. The ratio of 410/480-nm indo-1 fluorescence was recorded vs. real time and expressed in arbitrary units. (One arbitrary unit represents ~ 200 nM [Ca^{++}]$_i$). Black and open arrows correspond to addition of anti-T11$_2$ + anti-T11$_3$ antibodies and calcium ionophore A23187, respectively. (*B*) Effect of culture supernatants from CD2FL or 3DO54.8 on proliferation of CTLL-20 cells. 10^5 cells/well were incubated in 96-well round-bottom plates for 24 hr in the presence of either ovalbumin (1 mg/ml final concentration) plus 10^5 A20-11B lymphoma cells or anti-T11$_2$ + anti-T11$_3$ (ascites 1:100), or culture medium. Since addition of PMA induced a substantial increase in lymphokine production, 5 ng/ml final concentration of PMA was added to all experimental samples including the media control. Subsequently, serial twofold dilutions of supernatants were tested in triplicate for their ability to support the growth of 10,000 cells of the IL-2-dependent murine CTLL-20 cell line. Cultures were pulsed after 24-hr incubation with 1 μCi [^{3}H]thymidine per well and harvested after an additional overnight incubation at 37°C over glass fiber filters on a Mash apparatus. Filters were dried and counted after addition of scintillation fluid on a β counter. Results are expressed as mean of triplicate determinations of cpm of [^{3}H]thymidine incorporated. S.D. were generally < 5–10%; results are representative of five independent experiments. (*C*) IL-2 production upon antigen (ovalbumin) or anti-T11$_2$ + anti-T11$_3$ stimulation. Precise quantification of IL-2 production was obtained by running culture supernatants in parallel to a titration curve of recombinant IL-2 (Biogen Labs, Cambridge, MA). Under these conditions, the limit of detection for IL-2 was < 4 units/ml.

activate T lymphocytes after appropriate perturbation of the CD2 extracellular segment. Interestingly, the CD2ΔC77 clones express human CD2 molecules lacking residues 289–316. The latter corresponds to the segment most conserved among human and murine molecules, with 24 out of 27 residues being identical (Fig. 2A). Presumably, these conserved residues function in another facet of CD2 biology unrelated to IL-2 induction and/or secretion. In contrast, the ΔC43 truncated molecules as well as shorter truncations are nonfunctional with respect to stimulating a rise in $[Ca^{++}]_i$ and IL-2 production.

These data provide unequivocal evidence that the CD2 cytoplasmic domain is involved in signal transduction, as independently suggested by other investigators (Bierer et al. 1988b; He et al. 1988), and that one essential sequence of the cytoplasmic domain necessary for CD2-mediated activation is located between amino acids 253 and 287. This region contains four histidines at amino acid positions 264, 271, 278, and 282 and includes two tandemly repeated segments (PPPGHR, amino acids 260–265 and 274–279) (see Figs. 3A and 8A). These histidine residues could represent a binding site for an ion, cyclic nucleotide, or small regulatory molecule. Site-directed mutagenesis of each of these histidine residues is presently under way.

Segregation of CD2 Adhesion Function: Production of CD2 Adhesion Molecules Lacking Transduction Capability

As noted previously, the CD2 molecule serves to mediate adhesion between T lymphocytes and their cognate cellular partners that express LFA-3 as well as to transduce signals. Although one or both of these functions could be physiologically important for T-cell responses to antigenic stimulation, the contribution of the individual CD2 functions has not been independently examined. To address this issue, we used the above cellular system consisting of murine T hybridomas expressing one or another of the various forms of human CD2 to determine (1) whether the cytoplasmic region of CD2 influences the ability of the extracellular segment to interact with LFA-3 and (2) whether there is a significant contribution of CD2-mediated adhesion per se in the functional recognition of antigen by the T-cell receptor (Moingeon et al. 1989). To examine the interaction of truncated CD2 mutants with LFA-3, a rosetting assay with SRBC was employed. As expected, the parental murine T-cell line, 3DO54.8, which lacks human CD2, does not form rosettes with SRBC. In contrast, 3DO54.8 cells transfected with either the full-length or truncated human CD2 cDNAs (CD2ΔC98 and CD2ΔC43) form rosettes readily detectable as aggregates of SRBC around an individual T lymphocyte. This is the case both for the form of CD2 capable of mediating signal transduction after external segment perturbation such as CD2ΔC98 ($CD2_{trans+}$) and for the truncation CD2ΔC43 ($CD2_{trans-}$), which has lost the capacity to transduce activation signals.

To examine whether truncations of the cytoplasmic region alter the affinity of CD2 for LFA-3, competition analysis was performed by determining the concentration of the water-soluble recombinant CD2 extracellular segment $T11_{ex2}$ (amino acids 1–182) required to half-maximally inhibit SRBC rosetting. Similar competition curves are obtained from CD2FL and CD2ΔC43 with 50% inhibitory concentration of ~0.8 and 0.9 μM, respectively (Moingeon et al. 1989). These data indicate that a truncated CD2 molecule that is unable to transduce activation signals binds to LFA-3 with similar affinity ($K_d \sim 0.9~\mu M$) to the intact, full-length CD2 structure ($K_d \sim 0.8~\mu M$). The latter measurement is in good agreement with K_d determination of the $T11_{ex2}$/LFA-3 interaction as assessed by Scatchard analysis from saturable binding data (Sayre et al. 1989). Thus, the cytoplasmic truncations do not alter the affinity of the CD2 extracellular segment for its ligand, in contrast to results obtained with the adhesion structure, E-cadherin (Nagafuchi and Takeichi 1988).

Having dissociated CD2-mediated adhesion from CD2-mediated activation, it was next possible to independently evaluate the role of adhesion in a physiologic immune response. To this end, we examined the ability of $CD2_{trans-}$ and $CD2_{trans+}$ transfectants to produce IL-2 upon stimulation with the antigen-pulsed I-A^d B-cell line, A20, or the P24A20 variant (schematically depicted in Fig. 7b). The latter is a murine A20 transfectant expressing the human cDNA encoding the PtdIns-linked form of LFA-3. Figure 7a shows an immunofluorescence analysis of LFA-3 expression employing directly fluorescein-isothiocyanate (FITC)-labeled Fab fragment of the anti-LFA-3 monoclonal antibody TS2/A9 on the A20 murine cell line versus the LFA-3 + transfected P24A20 cell derivative. Although not shown, the A20 cell line and P24A20 express identical levels of the I-A^d gene product as judged by indirect immunofluorescence with the anti-I-A^d monoclonal antibody.

As shown in Figure 7c (left panel), the human CD2⁻ parental cell line 3DO54.8 produces equivalent amounts of IL-2 upon ova stimulation, regardless of whether A20 or P24A20 is used as the APC. This result implies that there is no substantial difference in antigen processing by either B-cell line. Individual CD2 transfectants produce differing but reproducible amounts of IL-2 after ova + A20 APC stimulation, reflecting interclonal variability. More importantly, all cell lines expressing the CD2 extracellular segment including CD2ΔC43 produce substantially more IL-2 when stimulated by ova and the P24A20 APCs as opposed to the A20 APCs; 350%, 800%, and 400% for CD2FL, CD2ΔC98, and CD2ΔC43, respectively. The relatively greater increase shown by CD2ΔC98 apparently correlates with the higher level of human CD2 expression on this cell line. LFA-3 expression on the APC, by itself, is not sufficient to augment T-cell responses, since P24A20 has no augmenting effect on IL-2 production by the human CD2⁻ 3DO54.8 cells. Furthermore, the observed augmentation of IL-2 production is linked to

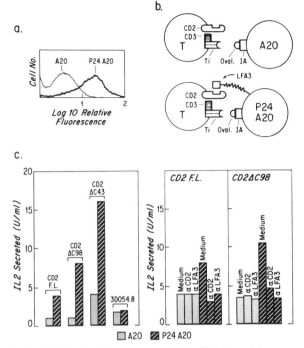

Figure 7. Functional consequence of the CD2/LFA-3 interaction during antigenic stimulation. (*a*) Flow cytometric analysis of human LFA-3 expression on A20 and the transfected P24A20 murine B cells. P24A20 cells were derived from the I-A^d A20 B lymphoma by transfection with 100 μg of *Pvu*I linearized expression plasmid pJOD-S-P24 LFA-3neo, which contains full-length cDNA for the PtdIns-linked form of human LFA-3 as well as the neomycin-resistance gene (B. Wallner, in prep.). Transfectants were obtained by electroporation with Biorad gene pulse (Richmond, CA) at 0.20 μV with capacitance set at 960 microfarads, and selected in culture medium (RPMI 1640 + 10% FCS, 1 mM sodium pyruvate, 2 mM L-glutamine, 1% penicillin-streptomycin, and 50 mM 2-mercaptoethanol) supplemented with 1 mg/ml G418. Neomycin-resistant clones were further selected for LFA-3 surface expression by direct immunofluorescence analysis. Immunofluorescence assays were carried out with the Fab fragment of the anti-LFA-3 TS2/9 monoclonal antibody directly conjugated with FITC. Histograms display fluorescence intensity on a log scale (abscissa) vs. cell number (ordinate). (*b*) Schematic representation of cell–cell interactions. (*c*) Quantitation of IL-2 production by CD2-transfected murine T cells stimulated with antigen-pulsed A20 or P24A20 B cells. CD2-expressing cells (10^5/well) were incubated in 96-well round-bottom plates for 24 hr in the presence of either A20 or P24A20 cells (50,000 cells/well) pulsed with ovalbumin (0.5 mg/ml final concentration). Serial twofold dilutions of supernatant were titrated in triplicate for their ability to support the growth of 10,000 cells of the IL-2-dependent CTLL20 line in parallel to recombinant IL-2 of known specificity. In blocking experiments, anti-CD2 (anti-T11$_1$, 3T48B5 ascites at a 1:400 dilution) or anti-LFA-3 (supernatant at a 1:6 final concentration) monoclonal antibodies were added at the initiation of the assays.

the transfected human CD2 and LFA-3 cDNAs, since reduction of IL-2 secretion to levels stimulated by ova + A20 APCs (see Fig. 7c, right panel) is obtained when CD2FL, CD2ΔC98, or CD2ΔC43 (not shown) is stimulated by ova + P24A20 in the presence of anti-T11$_1$ or LFA-3 monoclonal antibody. Moreover, these antibodies are without effect on the stimulation of

3DO54.8 cells with ova + P24A20 (data not shown). Note that the results presented in Figure 7c (left panel) were obtained using a suboptimal concentration of ovalbumin (0.5 mg/ml). However, 150–300% increases in IL-2 production were also obtained using high (2 mg/ml) or low (0.06 mg/ml) concentrations of antigen. Although we did not test the effects of an APC expressing levels of transmembrane LFA-3 comparable to the PtdIns-linked LFA-3 form used herein, a similar result would be expected, since both bind CD2 (Hollander et al. 1988).

CD2/LFA-3 Adhesion Facilitates Ternary Complex Formation between Antigen/MHC and the TCR

The augmented IL-2 production observed after stimulation of human CD2$^+$ murine T-cell clones by antigen and human LFA-3-expressing APCs probably results from the ability of the CD2/LFA-3 adhesion pair to facilitate more efficient formation of the ternary complex between the TCR and antigen plus the MHC gene product. Although the affinity of monomeric CD2/LFA-3 interactions is low, i.e., micromolar, the increased avidity resulting from multimeric interactions of multiple transmembrane CD2 copies of a given T cell with multiple LFA-3 molecules on the APC is likely great and serves to more optimally oppose surface membranes of the two cell types. Alternatively, if the interaction between LFA-3 and CD2 provides an as yet unrecognized signal that enhances IL-2 responsiveness independently of the known CD2 signaling mechanisms, then an LFA-3/CD2 interaction resulting from an unrelated third-party cell might enhance the functional consequences of TCR triggering, thereby resulting in enhanced IL-2 production. To test this possibility, cDNAs encoding the transmembrane form as well as PtdIns-linked form of LFA-3 were transfected into the I-A^d-negative thymoma cell line R1-1 to yield cell lines termed HT16R1-1 and P24R1-1, respectively (B. Wallner, in prep.). Each of these cell lines was tested for their costimulatory effect on human-CD2-expressing murine T cells in conjunction with ova-pulsed A20. No significant differences were observed in IL-2 production following stimulation by ova + A20 cells, regardless of which third-party cell was added into the assay. Similar results were obtained using the CD2ΔC43 and 3DO54.8 IL-2-producing cell lines (not shown). Thus, the adhesion mediated between CD2 and LFA-3 optimizes the physical interaction between the antigen-responsive T cell and its cognate partners.

We suspect that the present results underestimate the enhancement of antigen response affected by the human CD2/LFA-3 adhesion pair, since it is likely that murine CD2 and LFA-3 are present on 3DO54.8 and A20, respectively. Likewise, that there is not a relatively greater enhancement of IL-2 production when the CD2$_{trans^+}$ clone CD2FL is stimulated by ova + P24A20 versus ova +A20 (350%) as compared to when the CD2$_{trans^-}$ CD2ΔC43 clone is similarly triggered (400%) might be because endogenous murine CD2/murine

LFA-3 interactions have already provided signals that synergize with those resulting from antigen-triggered activation. These data unambiguously define the importance of CD2/LFA-3 adhesion in the interactions of lymphocytes and their cognate partner.

We presume that CD2 and LFA-3 similarly function to increase the interactions between a CTL and its target cell and that adhesion can also be critical for thymocyte/thymic epithelial interactions involved in thymic education and differentiation. In the case of CD4 CTL, this assumption has been shown to be correct. The cognate function of the HIV-1 gp120-specific, Dr4 MHC class-II-restricted human T-cell clone Een217 is illustrative (Siliciano et al. 1988). As shown in Figure 8, panel b, Een217 cells interact poorly with murine fibroblasts transfected with human Dr4 Ia molecules as judged by the small number of T-cell/fibroblast conjugates on the monolayer. In contrast, murine Dr4-transfected fibroblasts also expressing human LFA-3 readily form conjugates with T cells (panel a). The enhanced capacity of LFA-3-transfected fibroblasts to interact with Een217 cells is reflected in their greater ability to present antigen and be susceptible to target lysis by approximately one order of magnitude (S. Koyasu et al., pers. comm.). It is noteworthy, however, that CD2/LFA-3 interaction (even in conjunction with CD4/Ia interaction) is not sufficient to support many

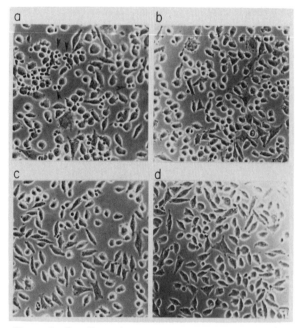

Figure 8. Coordinate interactions of TCR/antigen/MHC, CD4/Ia, and CD2/LFA-3 required to mediate stable intercellular conjugates. The ability of CD2/LFA-3 to facilitate physical T-cell interaction is shown for the HIV-1 gp120 (H3DCG strain)-specific, Dr4-restricted cytolytic T-cell clone Een217 and murine fibroblasts. Conjugates between fibroblast monolayers and T cells were photographed using phase contrast after extensive washing to remove unbound T cells. Panels are as follows: (a and c) Monolayer consists of L cells transfected with Dr4 and LFA-3; (b and d) monolayer consists of L cells transfected with Dr4 alone. In a and b but not c and d, fibroblasts were pulsed with the specific gp120 peptide.

stable conjugates in the absence of specific nominal antigen and the MHC-restricting element (Fig. 8, panels c and d), implying that a coordinated interaction between the TCR/antigen/MHC ternary complex and CD2/LFA-3 and likely including CD4/Ia is required.

Areas Requiring Further Investigation

Role of CD2 in thymocyte development. The presumption that CD2 plays a significant role in thymocyte development is likely correct in view of its (1) expression on the vast majority of thymocytes (Howard et al. 1981); (2) capacity to stimulate an increase in thymocyte IL-2 receptors on both CD3$^+$ and CD3$^-$ (as analyzed by FACS) thymocytes upon triggering by anti-T11$_2$ + anti-T11$_3$ monoclonal antibodies (Fox et al. 1985); and (3) role in mediating adhesion of thymocytes to LFA-3-expressing thymic epithelial cells (Denning et al. 1987a). The latter is likely important in the process of thymic education whereby thymocytes expressing high-affinity self-reactive TCRs are deleted upon TCR cross-linking by self-MHC ($\pm$self-peptides) on epithelial cells. The absence of CD2 on a majority of sheep and chicken CD3 $\gamma\delta$ cells, which might bypass the thymic education process, is consistent with this notion (Mackay et al. 1988). It is also noteworthy that, as with mature thymocytes, CD2/LFA-3 interaction alone does not seem to be sufficient to induce thymocyte proliferation. In vitro studies show that costimulation with anti-CD3 or suboptimal doses of mitogen are required in addition to CD2/LFA-3 interaction for the induction of thymocyte proliferation (Denning et al. 1987a,b; Bierer et al. 1988a). Definitive elucidation of the role of CD2 in thymic development will require analysis of animals whose functional CD2 genes have been deleted. Creation of animals harboring defective CD2 genes may now be possible by the technique of gene targeting using homologous recombination (Thompson et al. 1989).

Significance of synergistic interaction between CD2 and CD3-Ti pathways in facilitating antigen responses in vivo. A costimulatory interaction between CD2 and CD3-Ti resulting in T-cell proliferation has been clearly demonstrated in vitro. Thus, suboptimal concentrations of CD2 or CD3-Ti, which separately fail to trigger T-cell proliferation, are able to activate in concert (Yang et al. 1986). Likewise, suboptimal stimulation of alloreactive T cells by alloantigen incorporated into liposomes fails to induce IL-2 production, whereas the combination of alloantigen and LFA-3 in liposomes can give rise to T-cell activation (Bierer et al. 1988b). The basis for this functional synergy is yet to be explained. Signals emanating from CD2 and CD3-Ti may be complementary in augmenting T-cell response. In this regard, although it is clear that most signals resulting from CD2 and CD3-Ti stimulation are identical, certain differences exist. For example, CD3 ζ phosphorylation on tyrosine residues is not observed after CD2 stimulation (Weissman et al. 1988) but is readily detected after

TCR stimulation. It is also possible that synergy could result from more extensive cross-linking by ligand binding in the event that CD3-Ti and CD2 structures physically coassociated. These two proposed mechanisms need not be mutually exclusive.

CD2 ligands other than LFA-3 and their role in T-lineage activation. In vitro studies suggest that T-cell activation via CD2 is initiated by the combination of an LFA-3-expressing cell and an antibody directed to the T11$_3$ epitope on the molecule, for which no natural ligand has thus far been identified. Likely candidates could be either a soluble factor, membrane-derived molecule, or component of the extracellular matrix. A recent study raised the possibility that CD2 might interact with dextran sulfate as well as with other related sulfated proteoglycans (Parish et al. 1988). Since such sulfated structures are broadly distributed, these interactions might play an important role in adhesion or in positioning of lymphocytes in their lymphoid organs. With regard to a membrane component, one ligand could be CD3-Ti itself, consistent with the functional synergy between CD3-Ti and CD2 noted above and the CD2 dependence on CD3-Ti signaling.

Mechanism of CD2 function in CD3$^-$ cell populations. This requirement of cell-surface CD3-Ti expression for CD2 signaling function is well established for mature T cells. In contrast, it has also been shown that CD2 can transduce activation signals (resulting in cytosolic calcium rise, development of the cytotoxic program, and expression of the β chain of the IL-2 receptor) in cells lacking CD3-Ti on their surface (including CD3$^-$CD2$^+$ NK cells and undifferentiated thymocytes) (Fox et al. 1985; Siliciano et al. 1985). In the case of NK cells, no TCR Ti α, β, γ, or δ transcripts are present in the cell, so low-level CD3-Ti expression is ruled out. Perhaps CD2 can mediate signals directly in these cell populations by interaction with a different transduction pathway or interaction with Fc receptors or a presently unknown molecule functioning in lieu of the TCR components in activating the transduction machinery. Because the entire CD2 cytoplasmic domain is encoded on a single exon, an alternatively spliced CD2 transduction domain seems likely.

ACKNOWLEDGMENT

This work was supported in part by the National Institutes of Health.

REFERENCES

Alcover, A., M.J. Weiss, J.F. Daley, and E.L. Reinherz. 1986. The T11 glycoprotein is functionally linked to a calcium channel in precursor and mature T lineage cells. *Proc. Natl. Acad. Sci.* **83:** 2614.

Alcover, A., H.C. Chang, P.H. Sayre, R.E. Hussey, and E.L. Reinherz. 1988a. The T11 (CD2) cDNA encodes a transmembrane protein which expresses T11$_1$, T11$_2$, and T11$_3$ epitopes but which does not independently mediate calcium influx: Analysis by gene transfer in a baculovirus system. *Eur. J. Immunol.* **18:** 363.

Alcover, A., C. Alberini, O. Acuto, L.K. Clayton, C. Transy, G. Spagnoli, P. Moingeon, P. Lopez, and E.L. Reinherz. 1988b. Interdependence of T3-Ti and T11 activation pathways in human T lymphocytes. *EMBO J.* **7:** 1973.

Bach, J.F. 1973. Evaluation of T cells and thymic serum factors in man using the rosette technique. *Transplant. Rev.* **16:** 196.

Baxley, G., G.B. Bishop, A.G. Cooper, and H.H. Wortis. 1973. Rosetting of human red blood cells to thymocytes and thymus derived cells. *Clin. Exp. Immunol.* **15:** 385.

Bernard, A., C. Gelin, B. Raynal, D. Pham, C. Goose, and L. Boumsell. 1982. Phenomenon of human T cells rosetting with sheep erythrocytes analyzed with monoclonal antibodies: Modulation of a partially hidden epitope determining the conditions of interaction between T cells and erythrocytes. *J. Exp. Med.* **155:** 1317.

Bernard, A., R.W. Knowles, K. Naito, B. Dupont, B. Raynal, H.C. Tran, and L. Boumsell. 1986. A unique epitope on the CD2 molecule defined by the monoclonal antibody 9-1: Epitope-specific modulation of the E-rosette receptor and effects on T cell functions. *Hum. Immunol.* **17:** 388.

Bierer, B.E., A. Peterson, J. Barbosa, B. Seed, and S.J. Burakoff. 1988a. Expression of the T cell surface molecule CD2 and an epitope loss CD2 mutant to define the role of lymphocyte function associated antigen 3 (LFA-3) in T cell activation. *Proc. Natl. Acad. Sci.* **85:** 1194.

Bierer, B.E., A. Peterson, J.C. Gorga, S.H. Herrmann, and S.J. Burakoff. 1988b. Synergistic T cell activation via the physiological ligands for CD2 and the T cell receptor. *J. Exp. Med.* **168:** 1145.

Bolhuis, R.L., R.C. Roozemond, and R.J. van de Griend. 1986. Induction and blocking of cytolysis in CD2 +, CD3 − NK and CD2 +,CD3 + cytotoxic T lymphocytes via CD2 50KD sheep erythrocyte receptor. *J. Immunol.* **136:** 3939.

Brain, P., J. Gordon, and W.A. Willetts. 1970. Rosette formation by peripheral lymphocytes. *Clin. Exp. Immunol.* **6:** 681.

Brottier, P., L. Boumsell, C. Gelin, and A. Bernard. 1985. T cell activation via CD2 (T, gp50) molecules: Accessory cells are required to trigger T cell activation via CD2-D66 plus CD2-9.6/T11$_1$ epitopes. *J. Immunol.* **135:** 1624.

Brown, M.H., P.A. Gorman, W.A. Sewell, N.K. Spurr, D. Sheer, and M.J. Crumpton. 1987. The gene coding for the human T lymphocyte CD2 antigen is located on chromosome 1P. *Human Genet.* **76:** 191.

Chang, H.C., P. Moingeon, P. Lopez, H. Krasnow, C. Stebbins, and E.L. Reinherz. 1989. Dissection of the human CD2 intracellular domain: Identification of a segment required for signal transduction and IL-2 production. *J. Exp. Med.* **169:** 2073.

Clayton, L.K., P.H. Sayre, J. Novotny, and E.L. Reinherz. 1987. Murine and human T11 (CD2) cDNA sequences suggest a common signal transduction mechanism. *Eur. J. Immunol.* **17:** 1367.

Clayton, L.K., H. Ramachandran, D. Pravtcheva, Y.F. Chen, D.J. Diamond, F.H. Ruddle, and E.L. Reinherz. 1988. The gene for T11 (CD2) maps to chromosome 1 in humans and to chromosome 3 in mice. *J. Immunol.* **140:** 3617.

Denning, S.M., D.T. Tuck, K. Singer, and B.F. Haynes. 1987a. Human thymic epithelial cells function as accessory cells for autologous mature thymocyte activation. *J. Immunol.* **138:** 680.

Denning, S.M., D.T. Tuck, L.W. Vollger, T.A. Springer, K.H. Singer, and B.F. Haynes. 1987b. Monoclonal antibodies to CD2 and lymphocyte function associated antigen 3 inhibit human thymic epithelial cell dependent mature thymocyte activation. *J. Immunol.* **139:** 2573.

Diamond, D.J., L.K. Clayton, P.H. Sayre, and E.L. Reinherz. 1988. Exon-intron organization and sequence comparison of human and murine T11 (CD2) genes. *Proc. Natl. Acad. Sci.* **85:** 1615.

Dustin, M.L., M.E. Sanders, S. Shaw, and T.A. Springer. 1987a. Purified lymphocyte function associated antigen 3 binds to CD2 and mediates T lymphocyte adhesion. *J. Exp. Med.* **165:** 677.

Dustin, M.L., P. Selvaraj, R.J. Mattaliano, and T.A. Springer. 1987b. Anchoring mechanisms for LFA-3 cell adhesion glycoprotein at membrane surface. *Nature* **329:** 846.

Fox, D.A., R.E. Hussey, K.A. Fitzgerald, A. Bensussan, J.F. Daley, S.F. Schlossman, and E.L. Reinherz. 1985. Activation of human thymocytes via the 50KD T11 sheep erythrocyte binding protein induces the expression of interleukin 2 receptors on both T3 + and T3 − populations. *J. Immunol.* **134:** 330.

Gardner, P., A. Alcover, M. Kuno, P. Moingeon, C.M. Weyand, J. Goronzy, and E.L. Reinherz. 1989. Triggering of T lymphocytes via either T3-Ti or T11 surface structures opens a voltage insensitive plasma membrane calcium permeable channel: Requirement for interleukin 2 gene function. *J. Biol. Chem.* **264:** 1068.

Greaves, D.R., F.D. Wilson, G. Lang, and D. Kioussis. 1989. Human CD2 3′ flanking sequences confer high level, T cell specific, position independent gene coexpression in transgenic mice. *Cell* **56:** 979.

Haskins, K., R. Kubo, J. White, M. Pigeon, J. Kappler, and P. Marrack. 1983. The major histocompatibility complex restricted antigen receptor on T cells. *J. Exp. Med.* **157:** 1149.

He, Q., A.D. Beyers, A.N. Barclay, and A.F. Williams. 1988. A role in transmembrane signalling for the cytoplasmic domain of the CD2 T lymphocyte surface antigen. *Cell* **54:** 979.

Hollander, N., P. Selvaraj, and T.A. Springer. 1988. Biosynthesis and function of LFA-3 in human mutant cells deficient in phosphatidyl anchored proteins. *J. Immunol.* **141:** 4283.

Howard, F.D., J.A. Ledbetter, J. Wong, C.P. Bieber, E.B. Stinson, and L.A. Herzenberg. 1981. A human T lymphocyte differentiation marker defined by monoclonal antibodies that block E rosette formation. *J. Immunol.* **126:** 2117.

Hunig, T., G. Tiefenthaler, K.H. Meyer zum Buschenfeld, and S.C. Meuer. 1987. Alternative pathway of activation of T cells by binding of CD2 to its cell surface ligand. *Nature* **326:** 298.

Hunig, T., R. Mitnacht, G. Tiefenthaler, C. Kohler, and M. Miyasaka. 1986. T11TS, the cell surface molecule binding to the erythrocyte receptor of T lymphocytes: Cellular distribution, purification to homogeneity and biochemical properties. *Eur. J. Immunol.* **16:** 1615.

Jondal, M., G. Holm, and H. Wigzell. 1972. Surface markers of human T and B lymphocytes. I. A large population of lymphocytes forming non-immune rosettes with sheep red blood cells. *J. Exp. Med.* **136:** 207.

Kamoun, M., P.J. Martin, J.A. Hansen, M.A. Brown, A.W. Siadak, and R.C. Nowinski. 1981. Identification of a human T lymphocyte surface protein associated with the E rosette receptor. *J. Exp. Med.* **153:** 207.

Krensky, A.M., E. Robbins, T.A. Springer, and S.J. Burakoff. 1984. LFA-1, LFA-2, and LFA-3 antigens are involved in CTL target conjugation. *J. Immunol.* **132:** 2180.

Kuno, M., J. Goronzy, C.M. Weyand, and P. Gardner. 1986. Single channel and whole cell recordings of mitogen regulated inward currents in human cloned helper T lymphocytes. *Nature* **323:** 269.

Lalley, P.A. and V.A. McKusick. 1985. Report of the committee gene mapping. *Cytogenet. Cell Genet.* **40:** 536.

Lang, G., D. Wotton, M. Owen, W.A. Sewell, M. Brown, D.Y. Mason, M.J. Crumpton, and D. Kioussis. 1988. The structure of the human CDε gene and its expression in transgenic mice. *EMBO J.* **7:** 1675.

Mackay, C.R., W.R. Hein, M. Brown, and P. Matzinger.

1988. Unusual expression of CD2 in sheep: Implications for T cell interactions. *Eur. J. Immunol.* **18:** 1681.

Meuer, S.C., R.E. Hussey, J.C. Hodgdon, T. Hercend, S.F. Schlossman, and E.L. Reinherz. 1982. Surface structures involved in target recognition by human cytotoxic T lymphocytes. *Science* **218:** 471.

Meuer, S.C., R.E. Hussey, M. Fabbi, D. Fox, O. Acuto, K.A. Fitzgerald, J.C. Hodgdon, J.P. Protentis, S.F. Schlossman, and E.L. Reinherz. 1984. An alternative pathway of T cell activation: A functional role for the 50KD T11 sheep erythrocyte receptor protein. *Cell* **36:** 897.

Moingeon, P., A. Alcover, L.K. Clayton, H.C. Chang, C. Transy, and E.L. Reinherz. 1988. Expression of a functional CD3-Ti antigen/MHC receptor in the absence of surface CD2: Analysis with clonal Jurkat cell mutants. *J. Exp. Med.* **168:** 2077.

Moingeon, P., H.C. Chang, B.P. Wallner, C. Stebbins, A.Z. Frey, and E.L. Reinherz. 1989. CD2 mediated adhesion facilitates T lymphocyte antigen recognition function. *Nature* **339:** 312.

Nagafuchi, A. and M. Takeichi. 1988. Cell binding function of E cadherin is regulated by the cytoplasmic domain. *EMBO J.* **7:** 3679.

Palacios, R. and O. Martinez-Maza. 1982. Is the E receptor on human T lymphocytes a "negative signal receptor?" *J. Immunol.* **129:** 2479.

Pantaleo, G., D. Olive, A. Poggi, W.J. Kozumbo, L. Moretta, and A. Moretta. 1987. Transmembrane signalling via the T11 dependent pathway of human T cell activation. Evidence for the involvement of 1,2 diacylglycerol and inositol phosphates. *Eur. J. Immunol.* **17:** 55.

Parish, C.R., V. McPhun, and H.S. Warren. 1988. Is a natural ligand of the T lymphocyte CD2 molecule a sulfated carbohydrate? *J. Immunol.* **141:** 3498.

Pecht, I., A. Corcia, M. Liuzzi, A. Alcover, and E.L. Reinherz. 1987. Ion channels activated by specific Ti or T3 antibodies in plasma membranes of human T cells. *EMBO J.* **7:** 1935.

Peterson, A. and B. Seed. 1987. Monoclonal antibody and ligand binding sites of the T cell erythrocyte receptor (CD2). *Nature* **329:** 842.

Plunkett, M.L., M.E. Sanders, P. Selvaraj, M.L. Dustin, and T.A. Springer. 1987. Rosetting of activated human T lymphocytes with autologous erythrocytes: Definition of the receptor and ligand molecules as CD2 and lymphocyte function associated antigen 3 (LFA-3). *J. Exp. Med.* **165:** 664.

Reinherz, E.L. and S.F. Schlossman. 1980. The differentiation and function of human T lymphocytes. *Cell* **19:** 821.

Richardson, N.E., H.C. Chang, N.R. Brown, R.E. Hussey, P.H. Sayre, and E.L. Reinherz. 1988. Adhesion domain of human T11 (CD2) is encoded by a single exon. *Proc. Natl. Acad. Sci.* **85:** 5176.

Rudd, C.E., J.M. Trevillyan, J.D. Dasgupta, L.L. Wong, and S.F. Schlossman. 1988. The CD4 receptor is complexed in detergent lysates to a protein tyrosine kinase (PP58) from human lymphocytes. *Proc. Natl. Acad. Sci.* **85:** 5190.

Sayre, P.H., R.E. Hussey, H.C. Chang, T.L. Ciardelli, and E.L. Reinherz. 1989. Structural and binding analysis of a two domain extracellular CD2 molecule. *J. Exp. Med.* **169:** 995.

Sayre, P.H., H.C. Chang, R.E. Hussey, N.R. Brown, N.E. Richardson, G. Spagnoli, L.K. Clayton, and E.L. Reinherz. 1987. Molecular cloning and expression of T11 cDNAs reveal a receptor-like structure on human T lymphocytes. *Proc. Natl. Acad. Sci.* **84:** 2941.

Seed, B. 1987. An LFA-3 cDNA encodes a phospholipid-linked membrane protein homologous to its receptor CD2. *Nature* **329:** 840.

Seed, B. and A. Aruffo. 1987. Molecular cloning of the CD2 antigen, the T cell erythrocyte receptor by a rapid immunoselection procedure. *Proc. Natl. Acad. Sci.* **84:** 3365.

Selvaraj, P., M.L. Plunkett, M. Dustin, M.E. Sanders, S.

Shaw, and T.A. Springer. 1987. The T lymphocyte glycoprotein CD2 binds the cell surface ligand LFA-3. *Nature* **326:** 400.

Sewell, W.A., M.H. Brown, J. Dunne, M.J. Owen, and M.J. Crumpton. 1986. Molecular cloning of the human T lymphocyte surface CD2 (T11) antigen. *Proc. Natl. Acad. Sci.* **83:** 8718.

Sewell, W.A., M.H. Brown, M.J. Owen, P.J. Fink, C.A. Kozak, and M.J. Crumpton. 1987. The murine homologue of the T lymphocyte CD2 antigen: Molecular cloning, chromosome assignment and cell surface expression. *Eur. J. Immunol.* **17:** 1015.

Shaw, S., G.E. Ginther-Luce, R. Quinones, R.E. Gress, T.A. Springer, and M.E. Sanders. 1986. Two antigen independent adhesion pathways used by human cytotoxic T cell clones. *Nature* **323:** 262.

Siliciano, R.F., J.C. Pratt, R.E. Schmidt, J. Ritz, and E.L. Reinherz. 1985. Activation of cytolytic T lymphocyte and natural killer cell function through the T11 sheep erythrocyte binding protein. *Nature* **317:** 428.

Siliciano, R.F., T. Lawton, C. Knall, R.W. Karr, P. Berman, T. Gregory, and E.L. Reinherz. 1988. Analysis of host-virus interactions in AIDS with human T cell clones specific for HIV gp120: Effect of HIV genomic heterogeneity and a mechanism for CD4 + cell depletion. *Cell* **54:** 561.

Tadmori, W., J.C. Reed, P.C. Nowell, and M. Kamoun. 1985. Functional properties of the 50KD protein associated with the E receptor on human T lymphocytes: Suppression of IL-2 production by anti-P50 monoclonal antibodies. *J. Immunol.* **134:** 1709.

Thompson, S., A.R. Clarke, A.M. Pow, M.L. Hooper, and D.W. Melton. 1989. Germline transmission and expression of a corrected HPRT gene produced by gene targeting in embryonic stem cells. *Cell* **56:** 313.

Tiefenthaler, G., M. Dustin, T.A. Springer, and T. Hunig. 1987. Serologic crossreactivity of T11 target structure and lymphocyte function associated antigen 3. *J. Immunol.* **139:** 2696.

Truneh, A., F. Albert, P. Goldstein, and A. Schmitt-Verhulst. 1985. Early step of lymphocyte activation bypassed by synergy between calcium ionophore and phorbol ester. *Nature* **313:** 318.

Veillette, A., M.A. Bookman, E.M. Horak, L.E. Samelson, and J.B. Bolen. 1989. Signal transduction through the CD4 receptor involves the activation of the internal membrane tyrosine protein kinase p56^{LCK}. *Nature* **338:** 257.

Wallner, B.P., A.Z. Frey, R. Tizard, R.J. Mattaliano, C. Hession, M.E. Sanders, M.L. Dustin, and T.A. Springer. 1987. Primary structure of lymphocyte function associated antigen 3 (LFA-3): The ligand of the T lymphocyte CD2 glycoprotein. *J. Exp. Med.* **166:** 923.

Weissman, A.M., P. Ross, E.T. Luong, P. Garcia-Morales, M.L. Jelachich, W.E. Biddison, R.D. Klausner, and L.E. Samelson. 1988. Tyrosine phosphorylation of the human T cell antigen receptor ζ chain: Activation via CD3 but not CD2. *J. Immunol.* **141:** 3532.

Williams, A.F., A.N. Barclay, S.J. Clark, D.J. Paterson, and A.C. Willis. 1987. Similarities in sequence and cellular expression between rat CD2 and CD4 antigens. *J. Exp. Med.* **165:** 368.

Yang, S.Y., S. Chouaib, and B. Dupont. 1986. A common pathway for T lymphocyte activation involving both the CD3-Ti complex and CD2 sheep erythrocyte receptor determinants. *J. Immunol.* **137:** 1097.

Structure-Function Relationships of the Human T Lymphocyte CD2 Antigen

M.H. Brown,* E. Monostori,* M. Gullberg,† R. Zamoyska,‡
G. Lang,§ D. Kioussis,§ and M.J. Crumpton*

*Imperial Cancer Research Fund, Lincoln's Inn Fields, London WC2A 3PX; †Cell and Molecular Biology Institute, University of Umea, Umea, Sweden; ‡ICRF Tumour Immunology Unit, Department of Biology, University College London, London, WC1E 6BT; §National Institute of Medical Research, The Ridgeway, Mill Hill, London NW7 1AA, United Kingdom

T lymphocytes can be activated to express the genes coding for the growth factor interleukin-2 (IL-2) and its receptor by pairs of monoclonal antibodies (MAb) against the CD2 antigen (Meuer et al. 1984; Brottier et al. 1985). There are several lines of evidence indicating that signal transduction via the CD2 molecule contributes to T-cell activation induced by specific antigen (for review, see Bierer et al. 1989). Thus, it has been demonstrated that, in addition to occupation of the T-cell antigen receptor/CD3 antigen (Ti-CD3) complex by specific antigen, the interaction of CD2 with its physiological ligand (namely, the adhesion molecule LFA-3; Hunig 1985; Selvaraj et al. 1987) provides a critical signal for T-cell activation. Murine antigen-specific T-cell hybridomas expressing human CD2 showed enhanced IL-2 production in response to specific antigen and human LFA-3 when present on the same cell (Bierer et al. 1988a; Moingeon et al. 1989). Other experiments in which the CD2 antigen and the Ti-CD3 complex were cross-linked showed that these two receptors synergize to induce T-cell growth (Anderson et al. 1988a; Halvorsen et al. 1988).

An important question is whether the Ti-CD3 complex and the CD2 antigen stimulate separate pathways (i.e., antigen-dependent and -independent pathways, respectively) or whether the CD2 antigen represents an integral part of the antigen-dependent pathway. The close functional coupling between the Ti-CD3 complex and the CD2 antigen that is indicated by several experiments supports the latter view. For instance, activation via CD2 by monoclonal antibodies leads to phosphorylation of the CD3 antigen γ chain (Breitmeyer et al. 1987), which is also induced directly by stimulation through the Ti-CD3 complex (Cantrell et al. 1985, 1987). Also, antigenic modulation of the Ti-CD3 complex from the cell surface results in a refractory response via the CD2 antigen (Meuer et al. 1984). The necessity for Ti-CD3 (Alcover et al. 1988) and, more emphatically, a functional antigen receptor on the surface (Bockenstedt et al. 1988) of the T-leukemic cell line Jurkat for CD2-mediated signal transduction has been demonstrated by transfection experiments. Thus, Jurkat mutants expressing CD2 but not surface Ti-CD3 could not be stimulated via CD2, whereas restoration of Ti-CD3 expression correlated with the ability of CD2

to transduce a positive activation signal. In agreement with these experiments, mouse fibroblasts that do not express the Ti-CD3 complex, when transfected with human CD2, failed to transduce detectable early biochemical responses when stimulated with pairs of mitogenic CD2 monoclonal antibodies (Clipstone and Crumpton 1988). However, there is contradictory evidence against an absolute dependence on Ti-CD3 for CD2-mediated signal transduction (Moretta et al. 1987). Thus, impairment of signal transduction via the Ti-CD3 complex by human immunodeficiency virus (HIV) infection does not lead to defective CD2 signaling (Linette et al. 1988). Moreover, immature CD4⁻ CD8⁻ thymocytes lacking Ti-CD3 respond to stimulation via CD2 (Toribio et al. 1989), and NK cells can be activated via CD2 in the absence of the Ti-CD3 complex (Siliciano et al. 1985), suggesting that, in these instances, the requirement for Ti-CD3 may be satisfied via some other, as yet unidentified, component. The capacity for CD2 to transduce proliferative signals in an antigen-independent fashion has led to speculation on its role in T-cell differentiation (Reinherz 1985). The interaction of CD2 with LFA-3 via their respective extracellular domains in the thymus may well have a part in determining the fate of immature thymocytes.

The functional interaction between CD2 and Ti-CD3 also operates across species barriers. In particular, transfection of human CD2 into murine T-cell hybridomas (Bierer et al. 1988a,b; Chang et al. 1989), or rat CD2 into the human T-leukemia cell line Jurkat (He et al. 1988), resulted in the establishment of a functional CD2 signal transduction pathway. These experiments also formally established a requirement for the cytoplasmic domain of CD2 for signal transduction. The cytoplasmic domain of CD2 is highly conserved among all species in which the CD2 cDNA has been sequenced; namely, human (Sewell et al. 1986; Sayre et al. 1987; Seed and Aruffo 1987), rat (Williams et al. 1987), and mouse (Clayton et al. 1987; Sewell et al. 1987). This conservation of sequence is also apparently shared by more distantly related species, since an antiserum against a conserved peptide from the cytoplasmic domain of human CD2 (Brown et al. 1988) identified CD2 in both sheep (Mackay et al. 1988) and chicken (O. Lassilo and O. Vainio, pers. comm.).

Thus, it is likely that the mechanism of signal transduction via CD2 is similar in different species and that the CD2 cytoplasmic domain interacts with a similarly well conserved intracellular protein(s).

The close functional coupling between the Ti-CD3 complex and CD2 antigen has led to the proposal that the two receptors interact physically. Similar claims have been enumerated previously with respect to other T-cell surface antigens that have a close functional relationship with the Ti-CD3 complex, in particular, CD4 and CD8 (for review, see Emmrich 1988). In fact, positive evidence in support of the latter claims was obtained, based on the ability of these antigens to comodulate and synergize in mitogenesis experiments. Thus, there is a precedent for associations between functionally interacting receptors on the T-cell surface.

In this paper, we present evidence for a physical interaction between the Ti-CD3 complex and the CD2 antigen on the T-cell surface, thereby providing a structural basis for their functional coupling (Brown et al. 1989). We also confirm, by using transgenic mice expressing human CD2 antigen, that signal transduction via CD2 occurs across the human-mouse species barrier. Finally, we present evidence that an inappropriate high level of expression of CD2 can affect T-cell function, and we speculate on the mechanism by which this occurs.

MATERIALS AND METHODS

Materials. Human T lymphoblasts were prepared and expanded with recombinant IL-2 (rIL-2) as described previously (Cantrell et al. 1985).

Mice expressing human CD2 as a transgene were generated by integration of a 28.5-kb fragment of genomic DNA derived from overlapping cosmid clones that encoded the entire CD2 gene (Lang et al. 1988). The transgene was expressed in a T-cell-specific manner, with a distribution comparable to that in humans. Lines of mice were obtained expressing 1–50 copies of the transgene in a copy-dependent fashion. Expression of human CD2 at the cell surface was determined by immunoprecipitation of cell-surface-labeled proteins and by fluorescence-activated cell sorter (FACS) analysis.

Murine T lymphoblasts were generated from spleen cells of a single-copy human CD2 transgenic mouse by stimulation with 5 μg/ml concanavalin A (Con A) and were then expanded by adding 20 ng/ml mouse rIL-2.

The antibodies used were as follows: the human CD3 MAb, UCHT1 from P.C.L. Beverley, ICRF; the human CD2 MAbs OKT11 and MAR206 from A. Moretta (Lausanne, Switzerland); GT2 from A. Bernard (Paris, France); T11$_2$ and T11$_3$ from C. Rudd (Boston, Massachusetts); rabbit anti-CD2 serum (Sewell et al. 1986); the Tac MAb against IL-2 receptor; OKT9 against transferrin receptor; unconjugated and fluorescein isothiocyanate (FITC)-conjugated hamster anti-mouse CD3 MAb 145-2C11 kindly

provided by J. Bluestone (NIH); phycoerythrin (PE)-conjugated anti-mouse CD4 (Becton Dickinson, Cat. No. 1447); FITC-conjugated anti-mouse CD8 (Becton Dickinson, Cat. No. 1353); biotinylated rat anti-mouse Thy-1 MAb YTS154.7; biotinylated rat anti-mouse CD8 MAb YTS169.4 kindly provided by S. Cobbold (Department of Pathology, University of Cambridge, UK); and biotinylated MAb OKT11.

Immunoprecipitation. Human T lymphoblasts prepared using phytohemagglutinin (PHA) (Fig. 1) or MAb OKT3 (Fig. 2) were labeled at the surface by lactoperoxidase-catalyzed iodination (Na^{125}I, IMS30; Amersham International) and lysed at 10^7 cells/ml in 10 mM Tris-HCl buffer (pH 7.2), 0.15 M NaCl containing 1% digitonin (BDH or Sigma) and proteinase inhibitors including 20 mM iodoacetamide (Davies and Brown 1987). Immunoprecipitates were prepared (Davies and Brown 1987) by incubating the lysate for 16 hours at 4°C with the respective monoclonal antibody coupled directly to Sepharose 4B. Precipitates were washed twice in 10 mM Tris-HCl (pH 7.4) 0.15 M NaCl and once in 10 mM Tris-HCl (pH 7.4) prior to analysis on a 15% (Fig. 1) or 10–20% polyacrylamide gel (Fig. 2) by SDS-PAGE. Gels were fixed in 50% methanol and 7% CH$_3$COOH, and labeled bands were revealed by autoradiography. Molecular-weight standards (Bethesda Research Laboratory, Maryland, Figs. 1 and 3; Pharmacia, Sweden, Fig. 2) are stated on the figures.

For phosphorylation studies, mouse T lymphoblasts were washed and cultured for 16–72 hours in RPMI 1640/10% fetal calf serum (FCS) without added IL-2. Cells (2×10^7 to 4×10^7) were labeled for 4 hours at 37°C with 1 mCi of [^{32}P]orthophosphate (Amersham International) in 1 ml phosphate-free E4 medium supplemented with 10% dialyzed FCS. Labeled cells were stimulated for 15 minutes with 1:100 dilution of ascitic fluid containing CD2 MAbs T11$_2$ and T11$_3$. Cells were washed in cold phosphate-buffered saline (PBS) and lysed as described previously (Weissman et al. 1988). Briefly, 3×10^7 cells were lysed in 1 ml of 50 mM Tris-HCl buffer (pH 7.6), containing 0.5% Triton X-100, 300 mM NaCl, 10 mM phenylmethylsulfonyl fluoride and the following phosphatase inhibitors; 0.4 mM sodium vanadate, 10 mM sodium pyrophosphate, 0.4 mM EDTA, and 10 mM sodium fluoride. After 20 minutes on ice, nuclei were removed by centrifuging for 10 minutes in a Beckman microfuge. Postnuclear supernatants were precleared twice with a 10% (w/v) suspension of fixed *Staphylococcus aureus* organisms for 15 minutes and immunoprecipitated for 1 hour at 4°C using a prepared complex of MAb 2C11 against mouse CD3 adsorbed to protein A–Sepharose. Immunoprecipitates were washed three times with the lysis buffer and analyzed either by 12.5% SDS-PAGE under reducing conditions or in two dimensions (nonequilibrium pH gradient electrophoresis vs. SDS-PAGE). Immunoprecipitated polypeptides labeled with ^{32}P were detected by autoradiography.

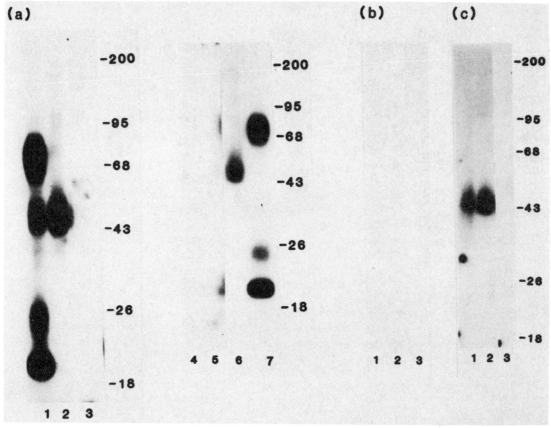

Figure 1. Coprecipitation of the CD2 antigen with the Ti-CD3 complex. (*a*) Immunoprecipitates isolated from T lymphoblasts iodinated at the surface and solubilized in 1% digitonin were prepared with the CD3 MAb UCHT1 (lane *1*), the CD2 MAb OKT11 (lane *2*), and rabbit and mouse normal Ig (lane *3*). Supernatants from the immunoprecipitates analyzed in lanes *1* and *2* were reprecipitated with UCHT1 (lane *4*) or OKT11 (lane *5*), respectively, to show depletion of antigen, and then with the reciprocal antibody OKT11 (lane *6*) and UCHT1 (lane *7*). Precipitates were analyzed under nonreducing conditions. The polypeptides in lanes *1–3* were transferred to Hybond C extra nitrocellulose. (*b*) 16-hr exposure of transfer. (*c*) 16-hr exposure of transfer after blotting with a rabbit antiserum against denatured purified human CD2.

Immunoblotting. Polypeptides separated by SDS-PAGE were transferred electrophoretically in 25 mM Tris–192 mM glycine buffer (pH 8.3) containing 20% (v/v) methanol for 24 hours at 50 V to Hybond C extra (Amersham International). CD2 was detected, using a three-step procedure, by incubating the transfer first with 5% dried skim milk powder and 2% bovine serum albumin (BSA) in PBS (pH 7.2) for 2 hours at 22°C; second, with a rabbit anti-CD2 serum (1:100 dilution in PBS, 0.1% BSA) for 16 hours at 4°C; and third, with ^{125}I-labeled protein A (IM 144; Amersham International) at 0.2 μCi/ml PBS, 0.1% BSA for 16 hours at 4°C. After each step, the transfer was washed in PBS containing 0.05% Tween, and for autoradiography, the moist transfer was wrapped in Saran Wrap.

Proliferation assay. Spleen cells (10^5 cells in 200 μl) from nontransgenic, single- or high-copy human CD2 transgenic mice were stimulated with 20 μg/ml of the CD2 MAb OKT11 with different concentrations of the CD2 MAb GT2, various dilutions of mouse CD3 MAb 2C11, or 5 μg/ml Con A for 4 days. The cultures were pulsed with 1 μCi [^{3}H]thymidine for the last 4 hours, harvested, and counted.

Immunofluorescence analysis. Lymph node or thymus cells (10^6) from nontransgenic or high-copy human CD2 transgenic mice were incubated with 50 μl of biotinylated or directly fluorogen (FITC or PE)-conjugated antibodies for 40 minutes on ice. Samples were washed once in PBS and resuspended in 50 μl of 1/80 dilution of PE-avidin for 10 minutes on ice. Following a further wash in PBS, samples were resuspended in 0.5 ml of PBS/1% BSA/0.05% Na azide for analysis on a Becton Dickinson FACScan flow cytometer using a 488-nm argon ion laser.

RESULTS

Coprecipitation of CD2 Antigen with Ti-CD3 Complex

Analyses of CD2 immunoprecipitates isolated from lysates of surface-labeled human T cells prepared using Nonidet-P40 or Triton X-100 invariably reveal a diffuse band of radioactivity centered at about 50 kD, with no compelling evidence for any associated polypeptides (see, e.g., Fig. 1; Brown et al. 1988). Under the same conditions, immunoprecipitates of the CD3 antigen

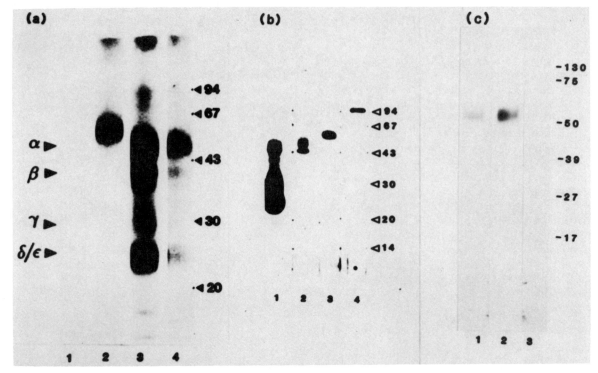

Figure 2. Specificity of coprecipitation of the CD2 antigen with the Ti-CD3 complex. (*a*) Coprecipitation of the Ti-CD3 complex with the CD2 antigen. Immunoprecipitates were prepared from surface ^{125}I-labeled T lymphoblasts, which had been lysed in 1% digitonin, using normal mouse Ig (lane *1*), anti-Tac (lane *2*), the CD3 MAb UCHT1 (lane *3*), and the CD2 MAb MAR206 (lane *4*). (*b*) Specificity of coprecipitation of the CD2 antigen with the Ti-CD3 complex. Immunoprecipitates were prepared as in *a* with MAb UCHT1 (lane *1*), MAb OKT11 (lane *2*), anti-Tac (lane *3*), and the transferrin receptor MAb OKT9 (lane *4*). (*c*) Immunoprecipitates were prepared from digitonin lysates of unlabeled Jurkat cells using MAb UCHT1 (lane *1*), MAb MAR206 (lane *2*), and MAb OKT9 (lane *3*). After SDS-PAGE, the separated polypeptides were electrotransferred to nitrocellulose, and CD2 was detected by immunoblotting, as described in Materials and Methods.

prepared using the MAb UCHT1 contain the CD3 chains and the Ti α and β polypeptides (see, e.g., Fig. 3; Kanellopoulos et al. 1983), although not usually the ζ polypeptide (Klausner et al. 1987). Digitonin has been shown previously (Oettgen et al. 1986) to be more effective than Nonidet-P40 (Triton X-100) at preserving loosely associated molecular complexes and is thus the detergent of choice for exploring possible physical associations of CD2 with the Ti-CD3 complex at the cell surface.

Normal human T lymphoblasts were labeled at the surface by lactoperoxidase-catalyzed iodination before lysis in digitonin and immunoprecipitation with the CD3 MAb UCHT1 or the CD2 MAb OKT11 coupled to Sepharose. The immunoprecipitates were then analyzed by SDS-PAGE under nonreducing conditions. As shown in Figure 1a, lane 1, the CD3 immunoprecipitate contained, in addition to the expected CD3, ϵ (M_r 19,000), δ (M_r 21,000), and γ (M_r 26,000) chains and the disulfide-linked Ti α and β chains (M_r 90,000), a diffuse band of $M_r \sim 50,000$. The mobility of the latter band was identical with that of the CD2 immunoprecipitate in the neighboring lane (Fig. 1a, lane 2), although the band was less intense. Immunoprecipitates of CD3, which had been prepared from lysates previously depleted of the CD2 antigen, no longer

revealed the 50–55-kD band (Fig. 1a, lane 7), thus strengthening the claim that this band represented CD2 that had been coprecipitated with the Ti-CD3 complex. If this was the case, then not all the cell-surface CD2 antigen was associated with the Ti-CD3 complex, because complete deletion of the latter complex did not apparently remove all the CD2 antigen (Fig. 1a, lane 6).

The identity of the 50–55-kD band was unequivocally established as CD2 by an immunoblotting experiment. The iodinated polypeptides shown in Figure 1a were transferred electrophoretically to nitrocellulose. The 50–55-kD bands in both the CD3 (Fig. 1c, lane 1) and CD2 (Fig. 1c, lane 2) immunoprecipitates were visualized after transfer by a rabbit anti-CD2 serum that has been shown previously to be specific for CD2 (Sewell et al. 1986; Brown et al. 1987). Immunoblotting of transfers of CD3 immunoprecipitates prepared from unlabeled Jurkat cells also revealed the presence of the CD2 antigen (Fig. 2c, lane 1). It was concluded from these collective experiments that CD3 immunoprecipitates prepared from digitonin lysates of T lymphoblasts and the T-leukemia cell line Jurkat contain not only Ti, but also the CD2 antigen. Furthermore, densitometric analyses of the separated polypeptides revealed that approximately 40% of the CD2 antigen on the surfaces of T lymphoblasts and Jurkat cells was precipitated with the CD3 antigen.

The interaction of the CD2 antigen with the Ti-CD3 complex appeared to be specific, in that CD2 was not detected in immunoprecipitates of a number of other cell-surface receptors, including the IL-2 receptor (Tac), transferrin receptor (OKT9) (Fig. 2b), LFA-1, and class I antigens (data not shown). The same digitonin lysates as those used for the preparation of the CD3 immunoprecipitates (see Figs. 1 and 2) were employed for the isolation of CD2 immunoprecipitates using a variety of CD2 antibodies against various epitopes, including those located in the extra- and intracellular domains. As illustrated in Figure 2a, lane 4, some evidence for the presence of CD3 polypeptides was provided when the CD2 MAb MAR206 was used for precipitation. However, the coprecipitation of CD3 with CD2 was not reproducible. The reason for our failure to reciprocally coprecipitate the Ti-CD3 complex with the CD2 antigen in a completely satisfying way is not understood.

Phosphorylation of the Murine Ti-CD3 Complex via the Human CD2 Antigen

Transgenic mice expressing the human CD2 antigen in a tissue-specific fashion that mimics the expression of the gene in humans (Lang et al. 1988) provide an opportunity to study the function of the antigen in relation to T-cell development and the functions of the different T-cell subpopulations. However, in order to take advantage of this opportunity, there is an absolute requirement that the expressed transgene reproduces in the mouse background its characteristic biological activities in humans. The latter possibility was investigated initially by determining whether stimulation of the human CD2 antigen on mouse T cells using mitogenic pairs of monoclonal antibodies induced rapid phosphorylation of the mouse CD3 γ and ζ polypeptides; i.e., whether there is a similar coupling of CD2-mediated early biochemical responses in the CD2 transgenic mouse, as has been previously established for human T cells (E. Monostori et al., in prep.).

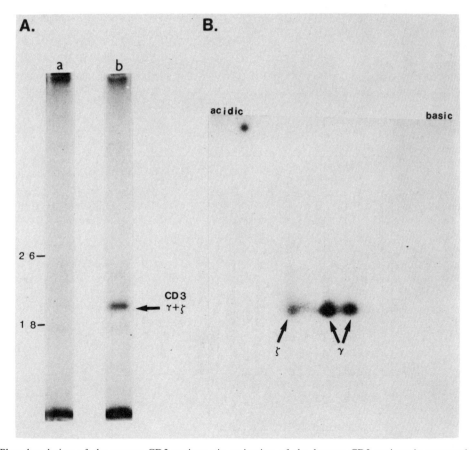

Figure 3. Phosphorylation of the mouse CD3 antigen via activation of the human CD2 antigen in transgenic mice. CD3 immunoprecipitates were isolated using the mouse CD3 MAb 2C11 from ^{32}P-labeled T lymphoblasts generated from spleen cells of single-copy human CD2 transgenic mice that had been either unstimulated (A, lane a) or stimulated (A, lane b, and B) for 15 min with 1:100 dilution of human CD2 MAbs T11$_2$ and T11$_3$. Immunoprecipitates were analyzed (A) in one dimension by SDS-PAGE, or (B) in two dimensions by nonequilibrium pH gradient gel electrophoresis vs. SDS-PAGE under reducing conditions.

Figure 3 shows the results of SDS-PAGE analyses of mouse CD3 immunoprecipitates isolated from ^{32}P-labeled T lymphoblasts derived from a single-copy transgenic mouse that had been stimulated with a mitogenic pair of MAbs ($T11_2$ plus $T11_3$) against human CD2. One-dimensional analysis (Fig. 3A) revealed a 21-kD phosphorylated band in a position coincident with that of the mouse CD3 γ and ζ chains (Klausner et al. 1987). This phosphorylated band was not detected in CD3 immunoprecipitates isolated from cells that had not been incubated with the CD2 MAbs. Because the mouse γ and ζ chains are not resolved by one-dimensional SDS-PAGE, CD3 immunoprecipitates were also analyzed in two dimensions (i.e., nonequilibrium pH gradient electrophoresis followed by SDS-PAGE under reducing conditions; Fig. 3B). Under these conditions, the 21-kD phosphorylated band was resolved into three spots, of which the most acidic corresponded in position to that previously identified for the tyrosine-phosphorylated ζ chain (Klausner et al. 1987), whereas the two other spots were identical in positions with those of the previously described, differentially sialylated forms of the phosphorylated mouse CD3 γ chain (Klausner et al. 1987). Thus, these results indicate that activation of the human CD2 antigen in single-copy transgenic mice induced a pattern of phosphorylation of the CD3 antigen identical to that induced, on the one hand, in human T cells (E. Monostori et al., in prep.) and, on the other hand, in mouse T cells stimulated with specific antigen or mitogenic antibodies against either the mouse CD3 or Thy-1 antigens (Klausner et al. 1987).

Proliferation of Mouse T Lymphocytes via Human CD2

Given the coupling of early biochemical responses, it is of interest to determine whether T cells from CD2 transgenic mice are stimulated to proliferate by human CD2 monoclonal antibodies. As demonstrated in Figure 4, spleen cells from single-copy transgenic mice were stimulated by combinations of OKT11 and GT2 MAbs against human CD2 to grow, as judged by incorporation of [3H]thymidine into DNA. Under the same conditions, spleen cells from nontransgenic mice gave no detectable stimulation of DNA synthesis, whereas cells from single-copy transgenic and normal mice were induced by either Con A or monoclonal antibody against mouse CD3 to give similar proliferative responses.

In contrast to the single-copy transgenic mice, spleen cells from mice carrying multiple (20–30) copies of the human CD2 gene showed a very much reduced stimulation of DNA synthesis when incubated with mixtures of OKT11 and GT2 MAbs (Fig. 4). Furthermore, these cells were not induced to proliferate by Con A or monoclonal antibody against mouse CD3. This reduced capacity to proliferate appeared to be directly related to the number of copies of the human CD2 gene incorporated into the mouse genome, because mice containing an intermediate number of human CD2 genes gave proliferative responses intermediate between those of single-copy and high-copy mice (data not shown). Also, growth responses of T cells from mice with 20–30 copies of human CD2 genes were not restored by addi-

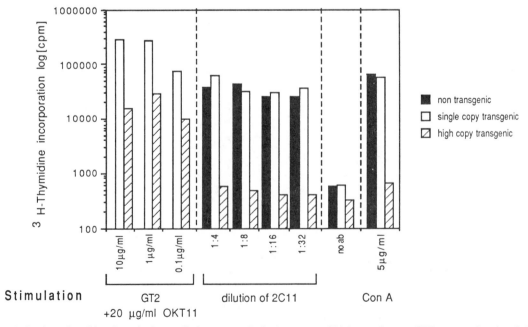

Figure 4. Induction of proliferation of spleen cells from normal, single-copy, and high-copy human CD2 transgenic mice. Spleen cells were stimulated for 4 days with human CD2 MAbs (20 μg/ml MAb OKT11 + different concentrations of MAb GT2), different concentrations of the mouse CD3 MAb 2C11, Con A (5 μg/ml), or medium alone. Cultures were pulsed with 1 μCi [3H]thymidine for the last 4 hr and harvested; radioactivity incorporated into the DNA was measured.

tion of mouse rIL-2 nor by increasing the number of T cells. Thus, it appears that the capacity of cells with multiple human CD2 genes to be activated by polyclonal mitogens is impaired.

T Lymphocyte Subpopulations of Transgenic Mice

This impairment of proliferative responses may, conceivably, be directly related to the increased level of expression of human CD2, or it may indirectly reflect a fundamental change in the nature of the T cells comprising the peripheral compartment. The latter aspect was explored by using immunofluorescence to determine the phenotypes of the T cells of the CD2 transgenic mice. This analysis revealed that the peripheral T cells from high-copy (20–30) transgenic mice possessed a marked reduction (about 50%) in the number of $CD3^+$ and $Thy-1^+$ cells compared with normal mice (Fig. 5A). Furthermore, the proportion of $CD4^+,CD3^+$ cells was preferentially reduced, whereas little change

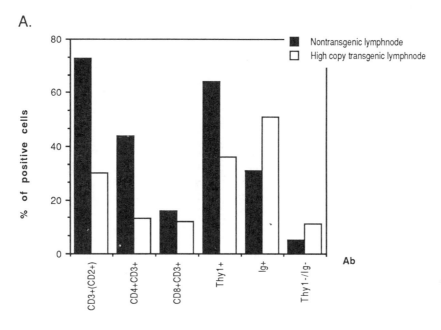

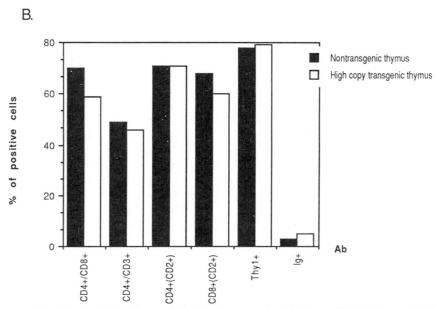

Figure 5. Phenotypes of lymph node (A) and thymus (B) cells from normal and high-copy (20–30) human CD2 transgenic mice. T-cell surface antigens were detected by immunofluorescence using the antibodies and procedures described in Materials and Methods.

in the proportion of CD8$^+$,CD3$^+$ cells was noted. A similar immunofluorescence analysis of thymocytes (Fig. 5B) showed no detectable differences in the numbers of CD4$^+$, CD8$^+$, CD3$^+$, CD4$^+$, CD8$^+$, and Thy-1$^+$ cells, although a more detailed analysis revealed a reduced number of the more mature CD4$^+$ or CD8$^+$ single-positive cells expressing a high level of CD3 (data not shown). These collective results suggest that in the high-copy transgenic mice, there is an impairment in the terminal stage of the thymic differentiation that is particularly apparent in the CD4$^+$ cells, resulting in a reduced number of mature CD4$^+$ cells in the periphery.

DISCUSSION

It is well established that monoclonal antibodies against the human CD2 antigen can stimulate human T lymphocytes to grow in a manner similar to that induced by activation of the Ti-CD3 complex with specific antigen or monoclonal antibodies. This observation has led to speculation that the CD2 antigen functions either as a "receptor" for an antigen-independent pathway of T-cell activation or as an integral part of the antigen-dependent activation pathway. A variety of experimental evidence indicates that there is close functional coupling between the Ti-CD3 complex and the CD2 antigen in the induction of T-cell activation; for instance, CD3 monoclonal antibodies can inhibit CD2-mediated activation (Meuer et al. 1984) and vice versa (Van Wauwe et al. 1981), and CD2 activation stimulates phosphorylation of the CD3 antigen (Breitmeyer et al. 1987; E. Monostori et al., in prep.) in a manner identical to that induced by specific antigen (Cantrell et al. 1987; Klausner et al. 1987). These results lend strong support to the idea that the CD2 antigen functions as part of the antigen-dependent pathway. Furthermore, close functional coupling is a logical consequence of a physical interaction between the Ti-CD3 complex and the CD2 antigen, although interaction is not a prerequisite for functional coupling. Up to now, a variety of studies including cocapping experiments (Reinherz et al. 1982) have not yielded any satisfying evidence in support of an association of CD2 with Ti-CD3 on the T-cell surface. In the present experiments, a mild detergent, digitonin, which has been shown previously to preserve macromolecular associations (Oettgen et al. 1986), was used to lyse surface-iodinated T lymphoblasts. Under these conditions, analyses of immunoprecipitates prepared using the CD3 MAb UCHT1 clearly demonstrated the coprecipitation of not only Ti, but also the CD2 antigen. However, not all of the surface-labeled CD2 antigen was coprecipitated, the results of densitometric analysis suggesting that some 40% of the cell-surface CD2 was associated with the Ti-CD3 complex. In this case, given that there is more CD2 (Meuer et al. 1984) than Ti-CD3 (Cantrell et al. 1985) on the surface of activated cells, it appears that more than one molecule of CD2 is associated with one molecule of Ti-CD3.

On the other hand, the reciprocal experiment failed to provide reproducible evidence for the coprecipitation of the CD3 antigen with CD2 immunoprecipitates. The reason for this lack of reciprocity is not known, but it could reflect the fact that certain CD3 antibodies are more efficient at preserving the CD2/Ti-CD3 association than CD2 antibodies. Similarly, the reason for the disagreement between the results of the present observations and those of previous experiments designed to explore the same question is not known, although the possibility exists that the association of CD2 with Ti-CD3 occurred subsequent to detergent cell lysis. Whether the association occurred before or after lysis, the interaction of CD2 with Ti-CD3 appeared specific, in the context that immunoprecipitates of various other surface antigens did not contain detectable amounts of CD2. The coprecipitation of CD2 with Ti-CD3 may represent an example of interaction on the cell surface between members of the Ig superfamily, as suggested by Anderson et al. (1988b). In this respect, since there is a region of homology between the membrane proximal domains of CD2 and CD4 (Sewell et al. 1986; Williams et al. 1987), the interaction may occur in a manner similar to that suggested for CD4 (Janeway 1989).

The CD2 antigen, through its interaction with its physiological ligand, the cellular adhesion molecule, LFA-3, has been implicated in mediating T-cell responses to antigen (Bierer et al. 1988a; Moingeon et al. 1989) and in T-cell development in the thymus (Reinherz 1985; Vollger et al. 1987). Transgenic mice expressing human CD2 in a tissue-specific fashion provide an attractive approach to describing the molecular bases of regulation of gene expression and of control of tissue expression, but also provide a means of exploring the functional roles of CD2. In the present experiments, T cells derived from transgenic mice expressing a single copy or multiple copies of the human CD2 gene were used to determine whether the human CD2 antigen retains its biological activities in a mouse cellular environment. Retention of activity appeared likely, given the marked conservation in structure of the CD2 cytoplasmic domain across species and the demonstration that human CD2 transfected into murine T-cell hybridomas (Bierer et al. 1988a; Chang et al. 1989) and rat CD2 transfected into human T-leukemia Jurkat cells (He et al. 1988) mediate functional responses. Stimulation of cells from single-copy CD2 transgenic mice with mitogenic pairs of human CD2 monoclonal antibodies reproduced the rapid phosphorylation (within 15 min) of the CD3 γ and ζ chains (Fig. 3) observed previously in similarly stimulated human T cells (E. Monostori et al., in prep.) and in mouse cells stimulated with specific antigen (Klausner et al. 1987). Apart from emphasizing the functional interaction between human CD2 and the murine signal transduction pathway, these results also serve to emphasize the close functional coupling between CD2 and Ti-CD3. If, as has been argued above, the latter coupling derives from the physical association of CD2 with Ti-CD3, then the experiments with transgenic mouse cells suggest that the association is mediated via the CD2 cytoplasmic domain, because this is more highly conserved than the extracellular domain. Besides stimulating rapid phosphorylation, the single-copy CD2 transgenic cells were also induced to proliferate by the human CD2 monoclonal antibodies (Fig. 4). However, T cells from multiple-copy transgenic mice gave a diminished response. Thus, such cells showed much reduced proliferation (about tenfold) when stimulated via the human CD2 antigen and no detectable proliferation when mouse CD3 monoclonal antibody or Con A was used as a polyclonal mitogen (Fig. 4). Because the lack of response was not reversed by addition of IL-2 or by increasing the cell number, it appears that these cells suffer from some intrinsic defect. Given that induction of T-cell activation via CD2 requires expression of Ti-CD3 (Alcover et al. 1988; Bockenstedt et al. 1988) as well as, possibly, a physical association between Ti-CD3 and CD2, it is conceivable that the Ti-CD3/CD2 interaction is perturbed by overexpression of human CD2 such that CD2-induced signal transduction no longer occurs. It is worth noting that a high level of expression of human CD2 in these cells does not in itself lead directly to the promotion of an antigen-independent pathway of activation, assuming that such a pathway exists.

Alternatively, or in addition to the above possibilities, the unresponsiveness of the high-copy T cells was probably related to the reduced number of mature CD4[+] cells in the periphery. The latter effect suggests that high expression of the human CD2 antigen may have interfered with differentiation of T cells in the thymus, possibly through a cross-reaction of the high levels of CD2 with mouse LFA-3. Cross-species interactions between CD2 and LFA-3 have been documented, primarily the description of human CD2 interacting with sheep LFA-3 (Hunig 1985). Also, a role for CD2/LFA-3 interactions in T-cell differentiation in the thymus has been suggested previously (Reinherz 1985).

One particularly interesting aspect of the transgenic mice is that no evidence was obtained by immunohistology (Lang et al. 1988) for the expression of the CD2 transgene in mouse B cells. In contrast, since this work was completed, it has become evident that the mouse CD2 antigen is also expressed on B cells as well as T cells (Yagita et al. 1989). Thus, it appears that the tissue-specific expression of mouse CD2 is controlled differently from that of human CD2.

In summary, the CD2 antigen and the Ti-CD3 complex are closely linked functionally and appear to be associated physically at the cell surface, as judged by analyses of CD3 immunoprecipitates prepared from digitonin-lysates of surface-labeled human T lymphoblasts. The stage at which they become physically associated is not known. A role of the CD2 antigen in the regulation of T-cell differentiation in the thymus is consistent with the apparent deleterious effects on T-cell proliferation of the overexpression of the human CD2 antigen in CD2-multiple-copy transgenic mice.

ACKNOWLEDGMENTS

We thank Neil Clipstone for helpful discussion and Kim Richardson for preparing the manuscript.

REFERENCES

Alcover, A., C. Alberini, O. Acuto, L.K. Clayton, C. Transy, G. Spagnoli, P. Moingeon, P. Lopez, and E.L. Reinherz. 1988. Interdependence of CD3-Ti and CD2 activation pathways in human T lymphocytes. *EMBO J.* **7:** 1973.

Anderson, P., M.L. Blue, C. Morimoto, and S.F. Schlossman. 1988a. Crosslinking CD3 with CD2 using Sepharose-immobilised antibodies enhances T lymphocyte proliferation. *Cell Immunol.* **115:** 246.

Anderson, P., C. Morimoto, J.B. Breitmeyer, and S.F. Schlossman. 1988b. Regulatory interactions between members of the immunoglobulin superfamily. *Immunol. Today* **9:** 199.

Bierer, B.E., B.P. Sleckman, S.E. Ratnofsky, and S.J. Burakoff. 1989. The biologic roles of CD2, CD4, and CD8 in T-cell activation. *Annu. Rev. Immunol.* **7:** 579.

Bierer, B.E., A. Peterson, J. Barbosa, B. Seed, and S.J. Burakoff. 1988a. Expression of CD2 and an epitope loss CD2 mutant to define the role of lymphocyte function-associated antigen-3 (LFA-3) in T cell activation. *Proc. Natl. Acad. Sci.* **85:** 1194.

Bierer, B.E., A. Peterson, J.C. Gorga, S.H. Herrmann, and S.J. Burakoff. 1988b. Synergistic T cell activation via the physiological ligands for CD2 and the T cell receptor. *J. Exp. Med.* **168:** 1145.

Bockenstedt, L.K., M.A. Goldsmith, M. Dusin, D. Olive, T.A. Springer, and A. Weiss. 1988. The CD2 ligand LA-3 activates T cells but depends on the expression and function of the antigen receptor. *J. Immunol.* **141:** 1904.

Breitmeyer, J.B., J.F. Daley, H.B. Levine, and S.F. Schlossman. 1987. The T11 (CD2) molecule is functionally linked to the T3/Ti T cell receptor in the majority of T cells. *J. Immunol.* **139:** 2899.

Brottier, P., L. Boumsell, C. Gelin, and A. Bernard. 1985. T cell activation via CD2 [T,gp50] molecules: Accessory cells are required to trigger T cell activation via CD2-D66 plus CD2-9.6/T11₁ epitopes. *J. Immunol.* **135:** 1624.

Brown, M.H., W.A. Sewell, E. Monostori, and M.J. Crumpton. 1987. Characterisation of CD2 epitopes by western blotting. In *Leucocyte typing III* (ed. A.J. McMichael), p. 110. Oxford University Press.

Brown, M.H., D.A. Cantrell, G. Brattsand, M.J. Crumpton, and M. Gullberg. 1989. The CD2 antigen associates with the T-cell antigen receptor CD3 antigen complex on the surface of human T lymphocytes. *Nature* **339:** 551.

Brown, M.H., W.A. Sewell, D.Y. Mason, J.B. Rothbard, and M.J. Crumpton. 1988. Species conservation of the T cell lymphocyte CD2 cell surface antigen. *Eur. J. Immunol.* **18:** 1223.

Cantrell, D.A., A.A. Davies, and M.J. Crumpton. 1985. Activators of protein kinase C down-regulate and phosphorylate the T3/T-cell antigen receptor complex of human T lymphocytes. *Proc. Natl. Acad. Sci.* **82:** 8158.

Cantrell, D.A., A.A. Davies, M. Londei, M. Feldman, and M.J. Crumpton. 1987. Association of phosphorylation of the T3 antigen with immune activation of T lymphocytes. *Nature* **325:** 540.

Chang, H.-C., P. Moingeon, P. Lopez, H. Krasnow, C. Stebbins, and E.L. Reinherz. 1989. Dissection of the human CD2 intracellular domain. *J. Exp. Med.* **169:** 2073.

Clayton, L.K., P.H. Sayre, J. Novotny, and E.L. Reinherz. 1987. Murine and human T11 (CD2) cDNA sequences suggest a common signal transduction mechanism. *Eur. J. Immunol.* **17:** 1367.

Clipstone, N.A. and M.J. Crumpton. 1988. Stable expression

of the cDNA encoding the human T lymphocyte-specific CD2 antigen in murine L cells. *Eur. J. Immunol.* **18:** 1541.

Davies, A.A. and M.H. Brown. 1987. Biochemical characterization of lymphocyte surface antigens. In *Lymphocytes: Practical approach series* (ed. G. Klaus), p. 229. IRL Press, Oxford.

Emmrich, F. 1988. Crosslinking of CD4 and CD8 with the T cell receptor complex. *Immunol. Today* **9:** 296.

Halvorsen, R., T. Leivestad, G. Gaudernack, and E. Thorsby. 1988. Induction of Interleukin-2 production in CD4$^+$ and CD8$^+$ T-cell subsets after activation via CD3 and CD2. *Scand. J. Immunol.* **28:** 449.

He, Q., A.D. Beyers, N. Barclay, and A.F. Williams. 1988. A role in transmembrane signaling for the cytoplasmic domain of the CD2 T lymphocyte surface antigen. *Cell* **54:** 979.

Hunig, T. 1985. The cell surface molecule recognised by the erythrocyte receptor of T lymphocytes. *J. Exp. Med.* **162:** 890.

Janeway, C.A., Jr. 1989. The role of CD4 in T-cell activation: Accessory molecule or co-receptor. *Immunol. Today* **10:** 234.

Kanellopoulos, J.M., N.M. Wigglesworth, M.J. Owen, and M.J. Crumpton. 1983. Biosynthesis and molecular nature of the T3 antigen of human T lymphocytes. *EMBO J.* **2:** 1807.

Klausner, R.D., J.J. O'Shea, H. Luong, P. Ross, J.A. Bluestone, and L.E. Samelson. 1987. T cell receptor tyrosine phosphorylation. *J. Biol. Chem.* **262:** 12654.

Lang, G., D. Wotton, M.J. Owen, W.A. Sewell, M.H. Brown, D.Y. Mason, M.J. Crumpton, and D. Kioussis. 1988. The structure of the human CD2 gene and its expression in transgenic mice. *EMBO J.* **7:** 1675.

Linette, G.P., R.J. Hartzman, J.A. Ledbetter, and C.H. June. 1988. HIV-1-infected T cells show a selective signaling defect after perturbation of CD3/antigen receptor. *Science* **241:** 573.

Mackay, C.R., W.R. Hein, M.H. Brown, and P. Matzinger. 1988. Unusual expression of CD2 in sheep: Implications for T cell interactions. *Eur. J. Immunol.* **18:** 1681.

Meuer, S.C., R.E. Hussey, M. Fabbi, D. Fox, O. Acuto, K.A. Fitzgerald, J.C. Hodgdon, J.P. Protentis, S.F. Schlossman, and E.L. Reinherz. 1984. An alternative pathway of T-cell activation: A functional role for the 50kd T11 sheep erythrocyte receptor protein. *Cell* **36:** 897.

Moingeon, P., H.-C. Chang, B.P. Wallner, C. Stebbins, A.Z. Frey, and E.L. Reinherz. 1989. CD2-mediated adhesion facilitates T lymphocyte antigen recognition function. *Nature* **339:** 312.

Moretta, A., A. Poggi, D. Olive, C. Bottino, C. Fortis, G. Pantaleo, and L. Moretta. 1987. Selection and characterisation of T-cell variants lacking molecules involved in T-cell activation (T3 T-cell receptor, T44 and T11): Analysis of the functional relationship among different pathways of activation. *Proc. Natl. Acad. Sci.* **84:** 1654.

Oettgen, H.C., C.L. Pettey, W.L. Maloy, and C. Terhorst. 1986. A T3-like protein complex associated with the antigen receptor on murine T cells. *Nature* **320:** 272.

Reinherz, E.L. 1985. A molecular basis for thymic selection:

Regulation of T11 induced thymocyte expansion by the T3-Ti antigen/MHC receptor pathway. *Immunol. Today* **6:** 75.

Reinherz, E.L., S. Meuer, K.A. Fitzgerald, R.E. Hussey, H. Levine, and S.F. Schlossman. 1982. Antigen recognition by human T lymphocytes is linked to surface expression of the T3 molecular complex. *Cell* **30:** 735.

Sayre, P.H., H.-C. Chang, R.E. Hussey, N.R. Brown, N.E. Richardson, G. Spagnoli, L.K. Clayton, and E.L. Reinherz. 1987. Molecular cloning and expression of T11 cDNAs reveal a receptor-like structure on human T lymphocytes. *Proc. Natl. Acad. Sci.* **84:** 2941.

Seed, B. and A. Aruffo. 1987. Molecular cloning of the CD2 antigen, the T-cell erythrocyte receptor, by a rapid immunoselection procedure. *Proc. Natl. Acad. Sci.* **84:** 3365.

Selvaraj, P., M.L. Plunkett, M. Dustin, M.E. Sanders, S. Shaw, and T.A. Springer. 1987. The T lymphocyte glycoprotein CD2 binds the cell surface ligand LFA-3. *Nature* **326:** 400.

Sewell, W.A., M.H. Brown, J. Dunne, M.J. Owen, and M.J. Crumpton. 1986. Molecular cloning of the human T-lymphocyte surface CD2 (T11) antigen. *Proc. Natl. Acad. Sci.* **83:** 8718.

Sewell, W.A., M.H. Brown, M.J. Owen, P.J. Fink, C.A. Kozak, and M.J. Crumpton. 1987. The murine homologue of the T lymphocyte CD2 antigen: Molecular cloning, chromosome assignment and cell surface expression. *Eur. J. Immunol.* **17:** 1015.

Siliciano, R.F., J.C. Pratt, R.E. Schmidt, J. Ritz, and E.L. Reinherz. 1985. Activation of cytolytic T lymphocyte and natural killer cell function through the T11 sheep erythrocyte binding protein. *Nature* **317:** 428.

Toribio, M.-L., A. De La Hera, M.A.R. Marcos, C. Marquez, and C. Martinez-A. 1989. Activation of the interleukin 2 pathway precedes CD3-T cell receptor expression in thymic development. Differential growth requirements of early and mature intrathymic subpopulations. *Eur. J. Immunol.* **19:** 19.

Van Wauwe, J., J. Goossens, W. Decock, P. Kung, and G. Goldstein. 1981. Suppression of human T-cell mitogenesis and E-rosette formation by the monoclonal antibody OKT11A. *Immunology* **44:** 865.

Vollger, L.W., D.T. Tuck, T.A. Springer, B.F. Haynes, and K.H. Singer. 1987. Thymocyte binding to human thymic epithelial cells is inhibited by monoclonal antibodies to CD2 and LFA-3 antigens. *J. Immunol.* **138:** 358.

Weissman, A.M., P. Ross, E.T. Luong, P. Garcia-Morales, M.L. Jelachich, W.E. Biddison, R.D. Klausner, and L.E. Samelson. 1988. Tyrosine phosphorylation of the human T cell antigen receptor ζ-chain: Activation via CD3 but not CD2. *J. Immunol.* **141:** 3532.

Williams, A.F., A.N. Barclay, S.J. Clark, D.J. Paterson, and A.C. Willis. 1987. Similarities in sequences and cellular expression between rat CD2 and CD4 antigens. *J. Exp. Med.* **165:** 368.

Yagita, H., T. Nakamura, H. Karasuyama, and K. Okumura. 1989. Monoclonal antibodies specific for murine CD2 reveal its presence on B as well as T cells. *Proc. Natl. Acad. Sci.* **86:** 645.

Structural Diversity in Domains of the Immunoglobulin Superfamily

A.F. WILLIAMS, S.J. DAVIS, Q. HE, AND A.N. BARCLAY

MRC Cellular Immunology Unit, Sir William Dunn School of Pathology, University of Oxford, OX1 3RE United Kingdom

In recent years, it has become clear that structures related to antibodies function at cell surfaces to control the movement and differentiation of many types of vertebrate cells (for review, see Williams and Barclay 1988; Hunkapiller and Hood 1989). It seems likely that the primitive function of the Ig-related molecules was concerned with cell–cell interactions unrelated to immune mechanisms and that T- and B-cell immunity developed when molecular elements of a self–self recognition system became involved in non-self recognition (Williams 1982, 1987).

The evolutionary and structural basis of the immunoglobulin superfamily (IgSF) rests on gene duplication and divergence of domains of about 100 amino acids that show a characteristic folding pattern to give a structure with two β sheets stabilized by a hydrophobic interior and often by a characteristic disulfide bond between the sheets (for review, see Amzel and Poljak 1979). This structure is called the Ig fold. Molecules are assigned to the IgSF if they contain at least one domain that has sequence patterns suggesting the presence of the core structure of the Ig fold and an evolutionary relationship to the IgSF (Williams and Barclay 1988). In this paper, we will describe any domain of this type as an IgSF domain.

It can be argued that the Ig fold provides a stable platform upon which a diversity of sequences are displayed by varying the amino acids that are exposed on the external faces of the β sheets or on the loops of sequence connecting the β strands. Conserved sequence patterns are seen in the proposed β strands. The functional essence of the IgSF is that a diversity of recognition interactions is seen; however, it is not obvious how the recognition events themselves might lead to conservation of sequence patterns. It may be that a requirement for resistance to proteolysis leads to conservation of the Ig fold and on this stable platform a diversity of recognition determinants can be displayed (Williams 1987).

The Ig fold is a structural type that may allow a greater diversity of sequence than any of the other structural motifs in protein superfamilies involved in cell-surface events. Further diversity comes from the fact that structures consisting of one to eight IgSF domains have been described, and IgSF structures are often found as homo- or heterodimers. It is also common to find that two molecules that are partners in a recognition pair are both members of the IgSF. The essence of the Ig fold can be argued to reside in a core of six β strands that yield the pattern ABE in one β sheet and GFC in the other, as shown in Figure 1 (Lesk and Chothia 1982). These strands come from the beginnings and ends of IgSF domain sequences and, in some cases, it can be argued that the fold consists solely of an ABE:GFC pattern. However, thus far all IgSF domains that have been established by X-ray crystallography have further β strands derived from sequence in the middle of the domain (Amzel and Poljak 1979; Bjorkman et al. 1987). This amounts to one further β strand (strand D) in the case of Ig constant region domains or major histocompatibility complex (MHC) antigen α_3- and β_2-microglobulin domains, or three further strands (C',C'',D) in Ig variable domains. The known and postulated domain types are shown in Figure 1. C-SET sequences are postulated to be of ABE:GFC or ABED:GFC type, but these are further divided into a C1- or C2-SET on the basis of conserved sequence patterns other than those found in the β-strand positions. The C1-SET sequences are found in constant regions of Igs and T-cell receptors and in the MHC antigens, whereas C2-SET sequences are commonly seen in IgSF molecules of nonlymphoid cells. The C2-SET domains have C-type or truncated C-type folds but show sequence patterns in the second half of the domain that are more similar to V-SET than C1-SET sequences. A conserved disulfide bond is usually found between β strands B and F in IgSF domains, but there are now numerous examples of domains suggested to lack the disulfide bond. Thus far, these have been found only in V-SET sequences or in sequences of length such that they might be categorized as short V-SET or long C2-SET domains. The above points have all been reviewed by Williams and Barclay (1988).

Thus far, the Ig-fold has been proven only for Ig V and C domains and the MHC class I IgSF domains. In this paper, we discuss examples of V-SET domains lacking the disulfide bond and truncated C2-SET domains. Furthermore, we propose that there may be some unusual domains that have disulfide bonds within a β sheet. To substantiate these structures, X-ray crystallography is required; toward this goal we describe the use of an expression system that has proved highly effective for the production of extracellular segments of rat CD4. Alternatively, more limited data might be

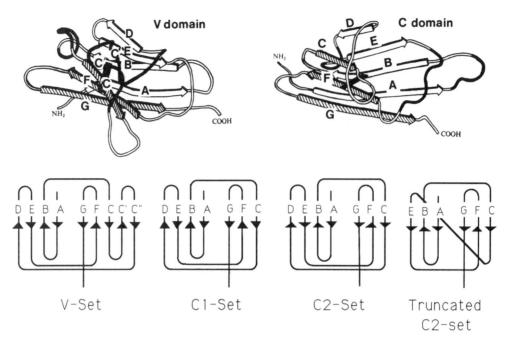

Figure 1. Known and postulated IgSF domain types. In the upper part of the Figure, V and C domain folds as determined by Edmundson et al. (1975) are shown. In the lower part, the various domain types are shown in the schematic form as used by Amzel and Poljak (1979).

obtained by expression of molecules with cysteine residues inserted by site-directed mutagenesis. Preliminary data on the use of this approach are reported.

METHODS

Sequence comparisons. Ig-related domains were identified by eye on the basis of the sequence patterns that have been described previously (Williams and Barclay 1988). To provide an objective assessment, the domains were then compared to a large number of IgSF domains using the ALIGN program of Dayhoff et al. (1983). For these purposes, a domain is defined by identifying cysteine residues likely to form the conserved disulfide bond, or other residues in the equivalent positions, and taking a sequence starting 20 residues before the first cysteine position and ending 20 residues after the second position. No adjustment of sequences in the middle of the domains is made when using the ALIGN analysis. The results are given as standard deviations (s.d.) of the test score away from a mean random score, determined from the same sequences after 100 randomizations. The mutation matrix was used with a bias of 6 and a gap penalty of 6.

Construction and expression of mutated rat CD2 molecules. Rat CD2 was mutated using oligonucleotides; the mutations were confirmed by nucleotide sequencing of a region starting prior to the initiation codon and extending through sequence coding for the first IgSF domain. In the case of the VW mutant (Fig. 5) the full coding sequence has been checked and is the same as for the wild type, apart from the mutations to cysteine at the V and W positions. The constructs were cloned

into the pKG5 neomycin-selectable vector, which was transfected into the human Jurkat cell line by electroporation. All the methods were as in He et al. (1988). Neomycin-resistant cells were selected, and rat CD2 expression was detected with the OX34, OX54, and OX55 monoclonal antibodies (MAbs) which are against noncompetitive determinants of rat CD2 (Clark et al. 1988). Cells were sorted a number of times on the fluorescence-activated cell sorter (FACS) to yield lines that expressed rat CD2 at a level of about 50,000 molecules per cell. The apparent molecular weight of the expressed CD2 was determined by Western blotting or after surface labeling with ^{125}I by the lactoperoxidase method and isolation of CD2 from detergent extracts with OX34 MAb attached to Sepharose 4B beads. The CD2 was run on SDS-PAGE unreduced or after reduction with dithiothreitol in the presence of urea. These methods were essentially as reported by Thomas and Green (1983) and Goding (1986).

Expression of soluble rat CD4 constructs. The expression system of M.I. Cockett, C.R. Bebbington, and G.T. Yarranton of Celltech Ltd., Slough, U.K., was used (in prep.). This is based on the pEE6.HCMV vector that contains the human cytomegalovirus promoter/enhancer (Whittle et al. 1987) plus the glutamine synthetase gene from pSVLGS.1 (Bebbington and Hentschel 1987) cloned into the *Bam*HI site of the construct to allow selection of transfected cells. Plasmid constructs for rat CD4 were prepared by oligonucleotide-directed mutagenesis from a full-length cDNA clone (Clark et al. 1987) and cloned into the *Bcl*I site of pEE6.HCMV. These constructs were transfected by calcium phosphate transformation into CHO-

K1 cells in glutamine-free medium (Gorman 1985; Bebbington and Hentschel 1987). The transfected cells were selected at either 15, 20, or 25×10^{-6} M methionine sulfoximine (MSX). Clones were picked after about 10 days, and supernatants were assayed for the presence of soluble CD4 (sCD4) by inhibition of an indirect radioactive binding assay (Williams et al. 1977). The highest secreting clones were subjected to one round of gene amplification by selecting transfected cells that survived at high levels of MSX. The clone expressing sCD4 (4 domains) was originally selected at 25×10^{-6} M MSX, and the amplified clone selected at 100×10^{-6} M MSX expressed sCD4 at approximately three times the level of the original clone. The sCD4

was purified by affinity chromatography using anti-CD4 monoclonal antibodies and gel filtration (Clark et al. 1987). Further constructs were prepared similarly (see Results and Discussion). A detailed description of the use of this expression system will be published elsewhere (S.J. Davis et al., in prep.).

RESULTS AND DISCUSSION

Unusual IgSF Domains in the MRC OX45 (Blast-1) Antigen

The rat MRC OX45 antigen is a molecule of leukocytes and endothelium that has a structure similar to the CD2 and LFA-3 antigens and also to the first two domains of molecules in the carcino-embryonic antigen family (Killeen et al. 1988). The molecule is anchored to the cell surface by a glycosyl-phosphatidylinositol anchor. A schematic view of this is shown in Figure 2, along with an arrangement of the amino acid sequence into two IgSF domains in the manner used by Amzel and Poljak (1979). The first domain shows a typical V pattern apart from a lack of cysteine residues. The good fit of the pattern is shown by the fact that OX45 domain 1 gives a significant set of ALIGN scores with a variety of V-SET sequences. These are shown in Table 1 along with scores for Thy-1 for comparison.

Domain 2 of OX45 has a truncated C2-SET pattern with two disulfide bonds that have been established and are in accord with the Ig fold (Killeen et al. 1988). The second disulfide bond is in a similar position to the second bond in Thy-1 (Campbell et al. 1981). The human OX45 homolog (Blast-1) has two further cysteine residues in domain 2 (6 Cys in all) in the positions indicated by boxes in Figure 2B (Staunton and Thorley-Lawson 1987). If it is assumed that the other cysteine residues are in disulfide bonds as shown for rat OX45 and that the extra cysteine residues form a disulfide bond, then this bond would be between β strands F and G and thus within the GFC β sheet. A similar extra disulfide bond has been postulated in domain 1 of the MRC OX2 antigen (Clark et al. 1985).

The Possibility of Unusual Patterns in the First Domains of Myelin-associated Glycoprotein and CD33 Antigen

Myelin-associated glycoprotein (MAG) is a five-domain IgSF structure found in myelin and some neurons (Lai et al. 1987a,b), and CD33 is a myeloid antigen whose first two domains are closely related to domains 1 and 2 of MAG (Simmons and Seed 1988). The first domains of these sequences each have two cysteine residues that might be considered to make disulfide bonds in the conserved position of a C2-SET pattern. However, if such domains are postulated, the second half of the sequences lack the typical patterns for β strands E, F, and G, other than the cysteine residues. Such patterns are seen farther upstream in typical format, except that cysteine residues of β strand

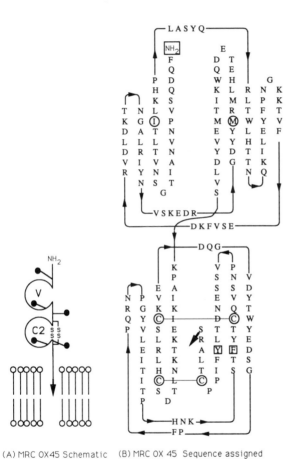

(A) MRC OX45 Schematic View   (B) MRC OX 45 Sequence assigned to beta strands

Figure 2. Model for the MRC OX45 antigen showing the two postulated IgSF domains. (A) Model for the OX45 (Blast-1) antigen showing the two IgSF domains (large circles) plus the carbohydrate sites (?) and the GPI anchor (↓). (B) Sequence of OX45 assigned to β strands as indicated by Killeen et al. (1988) and displayed according to the format used by Amzel and Poljak (1979). The first and second domains are of V-SET and C2-SET type, respectively. The β strands can be compared with the patterns in Fig. 1. In the first domain, the circles mark the positions equivalent to that of the conserved disulfide bond of IgSF domains. In domain 2, established disulfide bonds are indicated. Boxes mark the positions of extra cysteine residues that are found in the human Blast-1 sequence (Staunton and Thorley-Lawson 1987). The arrow on the carboxy-terminal serine residue indicates the position of attachment of the GPI anchor.

Table 1. ALIGN Scores (SD) for Thy-1 and Domains of OX45, MAG, and CD33 Versus V-SET Sequences

| | Thy-1 | OX45 (1) | MAG and CD33 with proposed disulfide bond | | | |
| | | | conventional | | within sheet | |
			MAG	CD33	MAG	CD33
Ig V_κ	5.0	3.8	0.8	1.0	2.6	2.5
Ig V_λ	6.8	3.2	1.3	2.6	3.2	2.6
Ig V_H	3.4	4.4	2.0	0.1	2.8	3.3
TCRα	2.1	3.9	1.3	2.1	2.1	5.0
TCRβ	3.1	2.3	3.1	2.2	4.0	2.8
TCRγ	1.5	3.3	1.0	2.7	2.4	4.0
CD4 (1)	3.0	4.3	0.2	2.5	1.1	2.4
CD8α	5.5	3.9	1.8	0.2	3.5	2.3
CD8β	2.8	3.2	0.3	2.1	2.6	4.2
Poly Ig R (1)	6.2	1.9	4.1	2.1	4.2	4.2
(2)	3.4	1.8	2.5	2.1	3.0	2.1
(3)	6.8	2.4	0.3	2.1	2.4	3.9
OX2 (1)	4.8	3.4	1.1	0.1	2.8	2.5
Thy-1	—	3.2	2.6	0.8	5.5	1.7
P_o	3.7	3.0	2.4	0.7	2.6	3.0
Link	3.4	3.9	3.0	2.6	4.2	3.7

References for sequences are given by Williams and Barclay (1988); conditions for use of the ALIGN program are in the Methods section.

F are missing. The sequences in the β strand F position are CD33:DNGSYFF and MAG:LGGKYYF, to be compared with the pattern DxGxYxC that is common in V and C2-SET sequences (see also β strand F in domain 1 of OX45, Fig. 2B). A V-like domain is shown for MAG in Figure 3A with the above sequence in the β strand F position. The sequence LLL now falls exactly in the conserved β strand E position, and the RLL sequence seems suitable for the base of β strand D.

Good sequence patterns are also available for β strands C', C'', and G, and the assignments are reinforced by equally good patterns in the CD33 sequence (not shown). When the sequence is assigned on the basis of these conserved β strand assignments, the second cysteine falls within β strand E directly above the first cysteine. Thus, it is suggested that these two cysteine residues may form a disulfide bond that is within the sheet, rather than between the β sheets. It should be

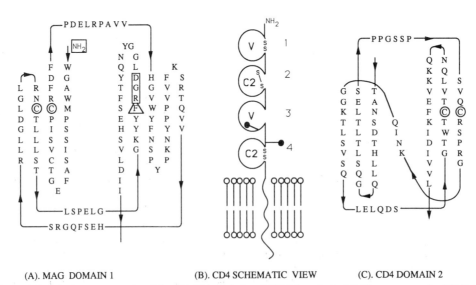

(A). MAG DOMAIN 1   (B). CD4 SCHEMATIC VIEW   (C). CD4 DOMAIN 2

Figure 3. Unusual domain patterns postulated for MAG domain 1 and CD4 domain 2. (*A*) The sequence for MAG domain 1 is shown assigned to a V-SET fold according to the criteria given in the text. (*B*) A schematic model for the CD4 structure with symbols as in Fig. 1. The disulfide bond in domain 2 is indicated to be in an unusual position as shown in C. (*C*) CD4 domain 2 assigned to a C2-SET fold according to the criteria given in the text.

noted that the cysteine positioning follows from the other patterns and was not a primary consideration in assembling the proposed fold.

The MAG domain as in Figure 3A and the similar CD33 domain (not shown) were scored against V-SET sequences using the ALIGN program to yield a significant set of scores as shown in Table 1. In contrast, if the second cysteine residues were assigned to the β strand F positions (the conventional between-sheet assignment), a poor set of scores was obtained (Table 1). If the conventional assignment is made, domain 1 would be much shorter than shown in Figure 3A, and it could be argued that this should be compared with C2-SET sequences rather than V-SET sequences as in Table 1. This was done, and the MAG and CD33 domains were each scored against 42 C2-SET sequences (in total 84 scores) to yield only one score of > 3 s.d. plus 14 that were in the range of 2–3 s.d. (Lai et al. [1987a] previously reported poor scores in similar comparisons.) In contrast, when the domains as shown in Figure 3A were scored against the same C2-SET sequences, 6 of 84 scores of > 3 s.d. were seen, and a further 12 were in the 2–3 s.d. range. These scores are much poorer than those with the V-SET sequences in Table 1, but the results further support an assignment as in Figure 3A rather than a conventional positioning of cysteine residues.

Assignment of MAG domain 1 as in Figure 3A would mean that the domain took up the whole of the exon in this region (Lai et al. 1987b), that there was no extended sequence between domains 1 and 2, and that the RGD sequence indicated within the rectangle in Figure 3A was within the Ig fold rather than being exposed in an extended sequence. It is dubious that an RGD sequence within an Ig fold would be in the same conformation as an RGD sequence in a matrix molecule, and thus the model as in Figure 3A would suggest that the RGD in MAG is not likely to be an integrin-binding site.

The CD4 Domain 2 Fold

The CD4 molecule can be argued to have four IgSF domains, but only the first of these is standard, being a typical V-SET domain (Clark et al. 1987; Maddon et al. 1987). Domain 3 lacks a disulfide bond but is also suggested to be a V-SET sequence. However, the argument for this is much less convincing than for OX45 domain 1 and other V-like sequences that lack the disulfide bond. Domains 2 and 4 are of truncated C2-SET type but again are far from typical. In particular, if the cysteine residues in CD4 domain 2 are placed in the conventional positions, there is not enough sequence to form the ABE:GFC pattern that can be argued to be the minimal core of the Ig fold.

A schematic view of the CD4 structure is given in Figure 3B. This suggests that CD4 may have evolved by gene duplication from a preexisting two-domain structure. All the domains within CD4 are quite diverse in sequence, but there is some indication within the sequence for derivation from a structure like an Ig L chain (or OX2 and OX45 type structures). At the beginning of domains 1 and 3 there are patches of sequences of six residues that are identical within the mouse CD4 sequence (Fig. 4A), and mouse CD4 is the only sequence in the National Biomedical Research Foundation data base with this hexapeptide (the match is supported in the rat and human CD4 sequences with minor variations). At the ends of domains 1 and 3 there are also good matches (Fig. 4A). In domains 2 and 4 a limited, but notable, patch of similarity is the WxC sequence in the β strand F position of each domain. In IgSF domains of all types, the sequence YorFxC is by far the most common in this region. A WxC sequence has not been seen in any IgSF domain other than in CD4 domains 2 and 4. Thus, this patch supports the idea of derivation by duplication of a two-domain structure. However, if the first half of domains 2 and 4 is considered around the cysteine residues, there are no strong matches. If the domains are defined from the first cysteine residues there would be an intervening sequence between domains 1 and 2, whereas domain 4 would follow on very closely from domain 3. An alternative is to argue that the cysteine of domain 2 is not in the β strand B position, but that the match as shown in Figure 4A is the relevant one in this region. If this is done, a strand pattern for domain 2 as shown in Figure 3C can be proposed. The sequence GGSLKLSC is predominant in β strand B sequences of IgV_H domains; this is very similar to the proposed sequence of GQSLTLTL for β strand B in Figure 3C except for the presence of a leucine residue instead of the cysteine. With the proposal in Figure 3C, the disulfide bond is within the sheet between β strands F and C. This is similar to the argument for MAG/CD33 but with the disulfide in the alternative β sheet. With this argument, the first and second halves of CD4 become symmetrical, and each relevant exon encompasses more or less exactly one IgSF fold (Gorman et al. 1987; Maddon et al. 1987). The proposal for CD4 domain 2 as in Figure 3C was compared with other C2-SET sequences, and various favorable alignments were seen. Two of these are shown in Figure 4, B and C.

Human and rat CD4 domain-2 sequences were scored with the ALIGN program against a total of 55 different C2-SET sequences. The domain-2 sequences were either defined as in Figure 3C or with the domain defined in a conventional way with the first cysteine being placed in the β strand B position. The results were that scores of > 3 s.d. were obtained in 15 of 110 tests for the conventional cysteine designation and 29 of 110 for the assignment as in Figure 3C. These scores favor the Figure 3C proposal, but the argument is not as strong as for the MAG/CD33 assignments.

The effects of CD4 mutations on the binding of anti-CD4 monoclonal antibodies or gp120 provide other data to test the proposal in Figure 3C. Mutations in the region of the $P_{121}PG$ sequence of human CD4 domain 2 moderately affect the binding of gp120 to CD4 (Clayton et al. 1988); a similar result is seen with a

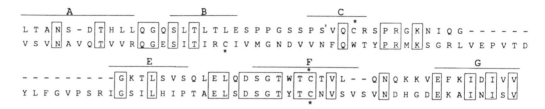

A. Patches of Sequence Similarity within CD4 Sequences Suggesting
   Duplication of a Precursor Two Domain Structure

MOUSE DOMAIN 1	AMINO TERMINUS	Q G K T L V L G K [E G E S A E] L P C
MOUSE DOMAIN 3	START OF EXON	Q S T A I T A Y K S [E G E S A E] F S F
HUMAN DOMAIN 1 ⎫	AT END OF EXONS	K E E V Q L L [V] F G⌐L [T] A N S
HUMAN DOMAIN 3 ⎭	(SHOWN WITH ARROW)	H Q E V N L V [V] M R A⌐T [Q] L Q
HUMAN DOMAIN 2 ⎫	IN PROPOSED BETA	D S [G] T [W] T [C] T V L Q N Q K K V
HUMAN DOMAIN 4 ⎭	STRAND F	E A [G] M [W] Q [C] L L S D S G Q V L
HUMAN DOMAIN 2 ⎫	AROUND PROPOSED BETA	L L [Q] G [Q] S L T [L T] L [E] S P P G S [S P] S V Q C
HUMAN DOMAIN 4 ⎭	STRAND B	A T [Q] L [Q] K N - [L T] C [E] V W G P T [S P] K L M L

B. Alignment of Human CD4 Domain 2 (top) with PDGF Receptor Domain 3

```
           A                    B                    C
                                                     *
L T A [N] S - D [T] H L L Q G [Q] S [L T] L T L E S P P G S S P S'[V] Q C R S [P] R G [K] N I Q G - - - - - -
V S V [N] A V Q [T] V V R [Q] G E [S] I [T] I R C I V M G N D V V N F [Q] W T Y [P R] M [K] S G R L V E P V T D
                                                     *
           E                    F                    G
                                *
- - - - - - - - [G K T] L S V S Q L E [L] Q D S G T [W] T [C] T [V] L - - Q [N] Q K K V E F K [I D] I [V V]
Y L F G V P S R I [G] S I [L] H I P T A E [L] S D S G T [Y] T [C] N [V] S V S V [N] D H G D E K A [I] N [I] S [V]
                                                     *
```

C. Alignment of Rat CD4 Domain 2 (top) with Fc Receptor Epsilon Domain 1

```
           A                    B                    C
V T F N [P] G T R [L L] Q G [Q] S L [T L] I L D S [N] P K V S D P P I E C K [H] K S [S] N I V K
S L D P [P] W I R [I L] T G [D] K V [T L] I C N G [N] N S S Q M N S T K W I [H] N D [S] I S N V

           E                    F                    G
D [S] K A F S T H [S] L R [I Q D S G] I W N [C] T V T L N Q [K] K H S F D M K [L S V] L
K [S] S H W V I V [S] A T [I Q D S G] K Y I [C] Q K Q G F Y [K] S K P V Y - - [L] N [V] M
```

Figure 4. Sequence alignments showing internal homology in the CD4 molecule and suggesting the domain 2 assignment as shown in Fig. 3C. (*A*) Sequence alignments within the CD4 molecule. Human, rat, and mouse sequences from Maddon et al. (1987), Clark et al. (1987), and Gorman et al. (1987). (*B*) Alignment of CD4 domain 2 sequences with other C2-SET sequences. In this case, the domain was taken as the sequence included within the exons encoding domain 2 as determined for human (Maddon et al. 1987) and mouse (Gorman et al. 1987). The PDGF receptor sequence is from Yarden et al. (1986) and the Ig ε Fc receptor is from Kinet et al. (1987). In studies referred to in the text where the CD4 domain 2 sequence was compared with other C2-SET sequences by ALIGN analysis, the domain was defined as starting 20 residues prior to the conserved cysteine position in β strand B and finishing 20 residues after the cysteine in β strand F; i.e., the sequence began and finished two residues before and after the sequences in *B* and *C*.

mutation in Asn-164 in the QNQ region (Mizukami et al. 1988). In the Figure 3C proposal, these sequences are on adjacent loops that would come close to the first domain, which has the main gp120-binding site (Peterson and Seed 1988; Arthos et al. 1989). In contrast, with a conventional cysteine disposition, the PPG sequence would appear to be distant from the first domain and from the QNQ sequence. In the case of MAbs MT151 and OKT4E, there is evidence that binding involves similar regions in the first domain plus Gln-164 in the second domain for MT151 (Mizukami et al. 1988; Peterson and Seed 1988) and Pro-122 for OKT4E (Peterson and Seed 1988). In the Figure 3C proposal, residues 122 and 164 are on adjacent loops at the top end of the molecule, whereas for the conventional model, residue 164 would be on a loop at the top

and residue 122 would be at the back end of the molecule.

Attempts to Study Domain Patterns by Insertion of Cysteine Residues in CD2

If assignments such as those shown in Figures 2 and 3 are correct, then it might be expected that insertion of cysteine residues in appropriate positions would lead to the formation of disulfide bonds. For example, according to Figure 2, it might be expected that replacement of the circled isoleucine and methionine residues with cysteine residues should lead to the formation of a typical conserved disulfide bond. Similarly, in the sequences in Figure 3, A and C, the cysteine residues postulated to be in the novel positions could be mutated out and cysteine residues could be inserted in the conventional positions with the prediction that a disulfide bond should form.

To investigate this approach, mutants have been constructed in domain 1 of rat CD2, and the constructs have been expressed in Jurkat cells. CD2 has a structure similar to OX45 (Fig. 2) and was chosen for these studies in a continuation of experiments in which rat CD2 mutants were expressed to study the role of the cytoplasmic domain of CD2 in signal transduction (He et al. 1988). The scheme for the mutants is given in Figure 5. Mutant V has a cysteine replacing a valine residue in the standard position in β strand F. Mutant VW has the mutant V replacement plus a cysteine replacing isoleucine at the β strand B position. Mutants VX and VY are similar to VW but with the replacements at positions minus two and minus four residues from that expected for the conserved cysteine position. The residues replaced are leucine and isoleucine, respectively, and should point toward the hydrophobic interior of the fold. Mutant VZ has the β strand F replacement plus the substitution of cysteine for tryptophan in the β strand E position.

Assuming that domain 1 of CD2 has an Ig fold, then mutant V should give a stable molecule with one free sulfhydryl buried in the hydrophobic core. This would be a similar case to that of the antibody that has been found to have a cysteine in β strand B and to have tyrosine instead of cysteine at the β strand F position (Rudikoff and Pumphrey 1986). Mutant VW should form a disulfide bond whereas mutants VX and VY should not, but might be expected to give stable domains with two free sulfhydryls buried in the hydrophobic interior. Mutant VZ was constructed to try to mimic the proposed situation for CD4 domain 2 as shown in

Figure 3C. Here the results are unpredictable, since a particular conformation for β strand C might be required for the proposed intrasheet disulfide bond to form.

Analysis of the CD2 mutants is at a preliminary stage, but thus far expression has been achieved in all cases. Labeling of the transfected Jurkat cells with three noncompetitive anti-rat CD2 monoclonal antibodies is shown in Figure 6; for all mutants all three monoclonal antibodies were positive. In each case, the MAB OX34 gave the best labeling, but the MAbs OX54 or OX55 showed relatively weaker labeling on the V, VX, and VZ mutants compared with wild-type, and VW or VY cells. Interpretation of this is at present ambiguous since the antigenic sites for these monoclonal antibodies within the CD2 molecule are unknown. Nevertheless, a key point is that the mutations had no drastic effect on the antigenicity. This is consistent with the possibility that all the residues replaced are inpointing amino acids that are unlikely to be contact residues in an antigenic site.

Molecular analysis was carried out by Western blotting of unreduced extracts, and the apparent molecular weights for all the mutants were the same as in the wild-type, except for the VW mutant, which migrated ahead of the other bands on SDS-PAGE (Fig. 7A). Thus, there was no indication of disulfide-linked multimers for any of the mutants. This is again consistent with the cysteine residues being unexposed at the molecular surface. With reduced samples, positive Western blotting was seen with wild-type CD2, but results were poor with the mutants. It could be that refolding of domain 1 is required for antigenicity and that this does not occur in reduced samples due to the formation of inappropriate disulfide bonds (there are four Cys residues in domain 2 in addition to the inserted residues in domain 1).

The apparent smaller size of the VW mutant might be consistent with the presence of a disulfide bond in domain 1; analysis of ^{125}I surface-labeled material was undertaken in reduced and unreduced conditions in an attempt to further substantiate this possibility. The results are shown in Figure 7B, where it can be seen that the unreduced VW sample migrates ahead of the wild-type, but, unexpectedly, the same result is seen with the reduced sample. A further unusual aspect is that the unreduced form of CD2 runs at a slightly higher apparent molecular weight than the reduced material. This differs from the expectation that an unfolded molecule should appear to be of higher apparent molecular weight than its disulfide-linked form in SDS-PAGE. The full sequence of the VW mutant has been checked, and mutations other than the introduced ones were not found.

To summarize, it is of interest that all the mutants have been expressed, and there is the possibility of a disulfide bond in the VW mutant. However, SDS-PAGE methods have proved inadequate in assessing the mutants for the presence of disulfide bonds or free sulfhydryl groups.

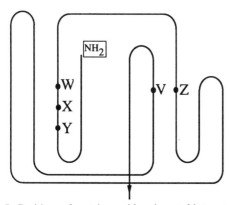

Figure 5. Positions of cysteine residues inserted into rat CD2 domain 1. A schematic V-SET fold is shown to indicate the CD2 domain 1 sequence, which is similar to that of OX45 as shown in Fig. 2. V and W mark the positions that are equivalent to the conserved disulfide bond of IgSF domains, whereas X and Y are, respectively, at positions 2 and 4 residues prior to W. Position Z is located at the site of the conserved tryptophan of β strand C in IgSF domains. In native rat CD2, the residues at these positions are V:Val; W:Ile; X:Leu; Y:Ile; Z:Trp.

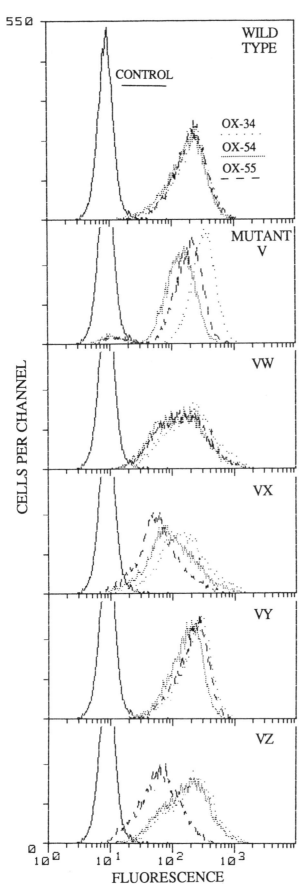

Figure 6. Labeling with anti-CD2 MAbs of human Jurkat cells after transfection with normal or mutated rat CD2. Transfected cells were prepared as in Methods and incubated with tissue culture medium containing MAbs OX34, OX54, or OX55 that react with separate epitopes on rat CD2. The cells were then washed and incubated with fluorescein-labeled rabbit antimouse IgG antibody and then analyzed for fluorescent labeling on a Becton Dickinson FACSCAN instrument. The code for the mutants can be read from Fig. 5.

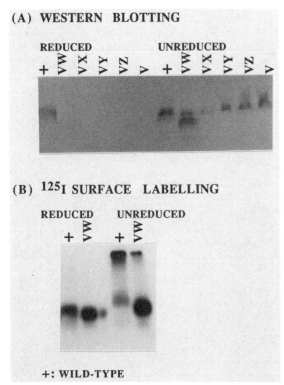

(A) WESTERN BLOTTING

(B) 125I SURFACE LABELLING

+: WILD-TYPE

Figure 7. Analysis of rat CD2 from the transfected Jurkat cells by Western blotting and immunoprecipitation. (*A*) Results of Western blotting with MRC OX34 anti-rat CD2 MAb on nitrocellulose filters with material from SDS-PAGE gels after electrophoresis of extracts in 1% NP-40 detergent plus proteolytic inhibitors (Thomas and Green 1983) from the various cell lines as analyzed in Fig. 6. The samples were prepared either by boiling for 5 min in 3% SDS sample buffer without reduction or by boiling in the presence of buffer plus 50 mM dithiothreitol, 3% SDS, and 8 M urea. The antibody was detected using a peroxidase-conjugated rabbit anti-mouse IgG conjugate. (*B*) Cells with normal rat CD2 or the VW mutant were surface-labeled with ^{125}I according to the method of Goding (1986). Surface proteins were extracted in 1% NP-40 plus proteolytic inhibitors. CD2 was immunoprecipitated with OX34 Sepharose 4B beads (Williams et al. 1987) and bound material was released by boiling for 2 min in nonreducing sample buffer. Some samples were then reduced as above.

Expression of Soluble Rat CD4 in Chinese Hamster Ovary Cells with a New Amplifiable Expression Vector

The ultimate aim in studying the unusual IgSF domains is to determine three-dimensional structure by X-ray crystallography or NMR. One problem in achieving this is the requirement for large amounts of material. In addition, the large number of carbohydrate structures on some molecules may be a problem for crystallization (see, e.g., Fig. 2). In using the cysteine mutagenesis approach outlined above, the availability of large amounts of material would also allow unambiguous determination of disulfide bonds or free sulfhydryl residues by protein chemistry.

In previous studies, expression of soluble cell-surface molecules truncated prior to the transmembrane se-

quence has been reported using the Baculovirus expression system (Hussey et al. 1988; Sayre et al. 1989) or an expression system based on amplification of dihydrofolate reductase (DHFR) (Hakimi et al. 1987; Deen et al. 1988). Levels of expression of the order of 1 mg/l are routinely achieved using the Baculovirus system to express membrane glycoproteins in soluble form. In contrast, very much higher levels of expression of soluble glycoproteins have been achieved using the DHFR-based system. A drawback associated with the latter system is that numerous cycles of gene-amplification via methotrexate selection are required in order to obtain high levels of expression (Hakimi et al. 1987).

We have therefore undertaken the expression of rat CD4 in a glutamine-synthetase-based amplifiable expression system that has been developed at Celltech Ltd. The advantage of this system is that a high level of expression can be obtained after the initial selection, and further gene amplification can be quickly achieved (Bebbington and Hentschel 1987 and in prep.).

The cDNA encoding the CD4 antigen (Clark et al. 1987) was mutated to insert a stop codon adjacent to the transmembrane coding region in a position that disrupted the third potential glycosylation site of the molecule. This yields a form of the molecule containing all four domains of the extracellular sequence (Fig. 3B), referred to henceforth as sCD4. The mutated gene was then ligated into the expression vector. Ten days after transfection of the vector into the CHO-K1 cell line and selection with methionine sulfoximine, 120 clones were obtained, of which about 50% secreted sCD4. Eight of the clones secreted sCD4 at levels of at least 4 mg/l. One clone gave about 16 mg/l sCD4; this clone was subjected to a single round of amplification during culture for 2 weeks in the presence of higher levels of MSX. A subclone secreting about 40 mg/l sCD4 was selected at 100×10^{-6} M MSX.

The same strategy was used to obtain expression of a Gly-179 truncated form of CD4 consisting of the two amino-terminal Ig-related domains at levels of about 4 mg/l; this is called sCD4(half). In contrast, expression of an Asp-103 truncated form consisting of CD4 domain 1 was not detected with a number of anti-CD4 monoclonal antibodies in supernatants from 50 clones. In other studies, the extracellular form of rat CD8 α chain has been expressed at initial levels of about 2 mg/l (B. Classon, unpubl.).

The expressed proteins have been purified to homogeneity by a combination of affinity chromatography with W3/25 or OX35 MAbs and gel filtration (Fig. 8). On SDS-PAGE, the sCD4 had an apparent molecular weight of 46,000 compared with 23,000 for sCD4(half). These values are in accord with the expected sequences plus two- and one-carbohydrate structures, respectively. Both the sCD4 and sCD4(half) molecules migrated as doublets, presumably due to carbohydrate heterogeneity. Amino-terminal sequencing of the sCD4 gave one sequence identical to that expected (Clark et al. 1987). Analysis of peptic peptides from sCD4 has established that the disulfide

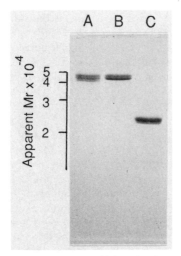

Figure 8. Soluble forms of rat CD4 molecules produced in CHO cells. Three forms of soluble rat CD4 were expressed in CHO cells and run on SDS-PAGE. (*A*) sCD4(mutant), a four-domain form of rat CD4 with a segment of human CD4 spliced into the domain-1 sequence; (*B*) sCD4, the four-domain form of rat CD4; (*C*) sCD4(half), the first two domains of rat CD4. The sCD4 and sCD4(half) forms were purified with a W3/25 monoclonal antibody affinity column, and the sCD4(mutant) was purified using the MAb OX35 (Jefferies et al. 1985). The gels are stained with Coomassie blue.

bonds are formed in the cysteine 1-2, 3-4, and 5-6 positions in accord with data for mouse CD4 (Classon et al. 1986) and that glycosylation occurs at both Asn-159 and -270 in the rat molecule. Attempts are being made to crystallize sCD4 and sCD4(half) in isolation and also in the form of sCD4:Fab complexes.

A mutant construct of sCD4 has also been made with a view to rendering rat CD4 positive for HIV binding and thus confirming by positive results the residues that have been implicated in HIV gp120 binding by mutational analysis of human CD4 leading to loss of function. Specifically, the rat gene codons for YKNK-LLIKGSLE were changed to the human gene codons for NQGSFLTKGPSK, leading to replacement of the proposed C',C'' strands in domain 1 of the rat molecule and a construct called sCD4(mutant). The residues chosen for replacement were selected on the basis of the analysis of the HIV-binding site by Peterson and Seed (1988). The sCD4(mutant) was expressed at about 4 mg/l; the purified form is shown after SDS-PAGE in Figure 8. This form electrophoresed as a triplet rather than a doublet. Thus, the glycosylation of the mutant may differ from the wild-type form, even though no N-linked glycosylation sites were changed in this construct. An analysis of HIV interactions with the sCD4(mutant) is in progress.

ACKNOWLEDGMENTS

We thank Chris Bebbington, Geoff Yarranton, and Paul Stevens of Celltech Ltd. for providing the glutamine synthetase expression system. We are grateful to Keith Gould for oligonucleotide synthesis, to Mike Puklavec for tissue culture, and to Catherine Lee for photography. H.Q. is supported by the Academy of Sciences, China. S.J.D. is supported by the Medical Research Council U.K. AIDS Directed Programme.

REFERENCES

Amzel, L.M. and R.J. Poljak. 1979. Three-dimensional structure of immunoglobulins. *Annu. Rev. Biochem.* **48:** 961.

Arthos, J., K.C. Deen, M.A. Chaikin, J.A. Fornwald, G. Sathe, Q.J. Sattentau, P.R. Clapham, R.A. Weiss, J.S. McDougal, C. Pietropaolo, R. Axel, A. Truneh, P.J. Maddon, and R.W. Sweet. 1989. Identification of the residues in human CD4 critical for the binding of HIV. *Cell* **57:** 469.

Bebbington, C.R. and C.C.G. Hentschel. 1987. The use of vectors based on gene amplification for the expression of cloned genes in mammalian cells. In *DNA cloning* (ed. D.M. Glover), vol. III, p. 163. IRL Press, Oxford.

Bjorkman, P.J., M.A. Saper, B. Samraoui, W.S. Bennet, J.L. Strominger, and D.C. Wiley. 1987. Structure of the human class 1 histocompatibility antigen, HLA-A2. *Nature* **329:** 506.

Campbell, D.G., J. Gagnon, K.B.M. Reid, and A.F. Williams. 1981. Rat brain Thy-1 glycoprotein. *Biochem. J.* **195:** 15.

Clark, M.J., J. Gagnon, A.F. Williams, and A.N. Barclay. 1985. MRC OX-2 antigen: A lymphoid/neuronal membrane glycoprotein with a structure like a single immunoglobulin light chain. *EMBO J.* **4:** 113.

Clark, S.J., W.A. Jefferies, A.N. Barclay, J. Gagnon, and A.F. Williams. 1987. Peptide and nucleotide sequences of rat CD4 (W3/25) antigen: Evidence for derivation from a structure with four immunoglobulin-related domains. *Proc. Natl. Acad. Sci.* **84:** 1649.

Clark, S.J., D.A. Law, D.J. Paterson, M. Puklavec, and A.F. Williams. 1988. Activation of rat T lymphocytes by anti-CD2 monoclonal antibodies. *J. Exp. Med.* **167:** 1861.

Classon, B.J., J. Tsagaratos, I.F.C. McKenzie, and I. Walker. 1986. Partial primary structure of the T4 antigens of mouse and sheep: Assignment of intrachain disulphide bonds. *Proc. Natl. Acad. Sci.* **83:** 4499.

Clayton, L.K., R.E. Hussey, R. Steinbrich, H. Ramachandran, Y. Husain, and E.L. Reinherz. 1988. Substitution of murine for human CD4 residues identifies amino acids critical for HIV-gp120 binding. *Nature* **335:** 363.

Dayhoff, M.O., W.C. Barker, and L.T. Hunt. 1983. Establishing homologies in protein sequences. *Methods Enzymol.* **91:** 524.

Deen, K.C., J.S. McDougal, R. Inacker, G. Folena-Wasserman, J. Arthos, J. Rosenberg, P.J. Maddon, R. Axel, and R.W. Sweet. 1988. A soluble form of CD4 (T4) protein inhibits AIDS virus infection. *Nature* **331:** 82.

Edmundson, A.B., K.R. Ely, E.E. Abola, M. Schiffer, and N. Panagiotopoulos. 1975. Rotational allomerism and divergent evolution of domains in Ig light chains. *Biochemistry* **14:** 961.

Goding, J.W. 1986. Membrane and secretory immunoglobulins: Structure, biosynthesis and assembly. In *Handbook of experimental immunology*. Fourth Edition (ed. D.M. Weir), vol. 1, p. 20.1. Blackwell Scientific Publications, Oxford.

Gorman, C. 1985. High efficiency gene transfer into mammalian cells. In *DNA cloning* (ed. D.M. Glover), vol. 2, p. 142. IRL Press, Oxford.

Gorman, S.D., B. Tourvielle, and J. Parnes. 1987. Structure of the mouse gene encoding CD4 and an unusual transcript in brain. *Proc. Natl. Acad. Sci.* **84:** 7644.

Hakimi, J., C. Seals, L.E. Anderson, F.J. Podlaski, P. Lin, W. Danho, J.C. Jenson, A. Perkins, P.E. Donadio, P.C. Familletti, Y.-C.E. Pan, W.-H. Tsien, R.A. Chizzonite, L. Casabo, D.L. Nelson, and B.R. Cullens. 1987. Biochemical and functional analysis of soluble human interleukin-2 receptor produced in rodent cells. *J. Biol. Chem.* **262:** 17336.

He, Q., A.D. Beyers, A.N. Barclay, and A.F. Williams. 1988. A role in transmembrane signaling for the cytoplasmic domain of the CD2 T lymphocyte surface antigen. *Cell* **54:** 979.

Hunkapiller, T. and L. Hood. 1989. Diversity of the immunoglobulin gene superfamily. *Adv. Immunol.* **44:** 1.

Hussey, R.E., N.E. Richardson, M. Kowalski, N.R. Brown, H.-C. Chang, R.F. Siliciano, T. Dorfman, B. Walker, J. Sodroski, and E.L. Reinherz. 1988. A soluble CD4 protein selectively inhibits HIV replication and syncytium formation. *Nature* **331:** 78.

Jefferies, W.A., J.R. Green, and A.F. Williams. 1985. Authentic T helper CD4(W3/25) on rat peritoneal macrophages. *J. Exp. Med.* **162:** 117.

Killeen, N., R. Moessner, J. Arvieux, A. Willis, and A.F. Williams. 1988. The MRC OX-45 antigen of rat leukocytes and endothelium is in a subset of the immunoglobulin superfamily with CD2, LFA-3 and carcinoembryonic antigens. *EMBO J.* **7:** 3087.

Kinet, J.-P., H. Metzger, J. Hakami, and J. Kochan. 1987. A cDNA presumptively coding for the alpha subunit of the receptor with high affinity for IgE. *Biochemistry* **26:** 4605.

Lai, C., J.B. Watson, F.E. Bloom, J.F. Sutcliffe, and R.J. Milner. 1987a. Neural protein 1B236/MAG defines a subgroup of the Ig superfamily. *Immunol. Rev.* **100:** 129.

Lai, C., M.A. Brow, K.-A. Nave, A.B. Noronha, R.H. Quarles, F.E. Bloom, R.J. Milner, and J.G. Sutcliffe. 1987b. Two forms of 1B236/myelin associated glycoprotein, a cell adhesion molecule for post-natal neural development, are produced by alternative splicing. *Proc. Natl. Acad. Sci.* **84:** 4337.

Lesk, A.M. and C. Chothia. 1982. Evolution of proteins formed by β sheets. II. The core of the Ig domains. *J. Mol. Biol.* **160:** 325.

Maddon, P.J., S.M. Molineaux, D.E. Maddon, K.A. Zimmerman, M. Godfrey, F.W. Alt, L. Chess, and R. Axel. 1987. Structure and expression of the human and mouse T4 genes. *Proc. Natl. Acad. Sci.* **84:** 9155.

Mizukami, T., T.R. Fuerst, E.A. Berger, and B. Moss. 1988. Binding region for human immunodeficiency virus (HIV) and epitopes for HIV-blocking monoclonal antibodies of the CD4 molecule. *Proc. Natl. Acad. Sci.* **85:** 9273.

Peterson, A. and B. Seed. 1988. Genetic analysis of monoclonal antibody and HIV binding sites on the human lymphocyte antigen CD4. *Cell* **54:** 65.

Rudikoff, S. and J.G. Pumphrey. 1986. Functional antibody lacking a variable-region disulphide bridge. *Proc. Natl. Acad. Sci.* **83:** 7875.

Sayre, P.H., R.E. Hussey, H.-C. Chang, T.L. Ciardelli, and E.L. Reinherz. 1989. Structural and binding analysis of a two domain extracellular CD2 molecule. *J. Exp. Med.* **169:** 995.

Simmons, D. and B. Seed. 1988. Isolation of a cDNA encoding CD33, a differentiation antigen of myeloid progenitor cells. *J. Immunol.* **141:** 2797.

Staunton, D.E. and D.A. Thorley-Lawson. 1987. Molecular cloning of the lymphocyte activation marker Blast-1. *EMBO J.* **6:** 3695.

Thomas, M.L. and J.R. Green. 1983. Molecular nature of the W3/25 and MRC OX-8 marker antigens for rat T lymphocytes: Comparisons with mouse and human antigens. *Eur. J. Immunol.* **13:** 855.

Whittle, N., J. Adair, C. Lloyd, L. Jenkins, J. Devine, J. Schlom, A. Raubitschek, D. Colcher, and M. Bodmer. 1987. Expression in COS cells of a mouse–human chimaeric B72.3 antibody. *Protein Eng.* **1:** 499.

Williams, A.F. 1982. Surface molecules and cell interactions. *J. Theor. Biol.* **98:** 221.

———. 1987. A year in the life of the immunoglobulin superfamily. *Immunol. Today* **8:** 298.

Williams, A.F. and A.N. Barclay. 1988. The immunoglobulin superfamily-domains for cell surface recognition. *Annu. Rev. Immunol.* **6:** 381.

Williams, A.F., G. Galfre, and C. Milstein. 1977. Analysis of cell surfaces by xenogeneic myeloma-hybrid antibodies: Differentiation antigens of rat lymphocytes. *Cell* **12:** 663.

Williams, A.F., A.N. Barclay, S.J. Clark, D.J. Paterson, and A.C. Willis. 1987. Similarities in sequences and cellular expression between rat CD2 and CD4 antigens. *J. Exp. Med.* **165:** 368.

Yarden, Y., J. Escobedo, W.-J. Kuang, T. Yang-Feng, T.O. Daniel, S.P.M. Tremble, E.Y. Chen, M.E. Ando, R.N. Harkins, U. Francke, V.A. Fried, A. Ulrich, and L.T. Williams. 1986. Structure of the receptor for platelet-derived growth factor. *Nature* **323:** 226.

Role of CD4 and CD8 in Enhancing T-cell Responses to Antigen

J.R. PARNES,* P. VON HOEGEN,* M.C. MICELI,* AND R. ZAMOYSKA†

*Division of Immunology, Department of Medicine, Stanford University Medical Center,
Stanford, California 94305; †Imperial Cancer Research Fund Tumour Immunology Unit,
Biology Department, University College London, London WC1E 6BT, United Kingdom

T lymphocytes can be divided into two major subsets based on their recognition properties and their expression of either of two cell-surface glycoproteins, CD8 or CD4. In general, T cells that recognize foreign antigen bound to self class I major histocompatibility complex (MHC) proteins express CD8, whereas those that recognize foreign antigen bound to class II MHC proteins express CD4 (Swain 1983). In accord with this functional subdivision, CD8 and CD4 appear to serve as receptors for relatively invariant regions of class I and class II MHC proteins, respectively (Doyle and Strominger 1987; Gay et al. 1988; Norment et al. 1988; Rosenstein et al. 1989). CD8 and CD4 have been called accessory molecules or "co-receptors" based on their ability to increase T-cell responses to antigen. This function may be of major importance in situations where the affinity of the T-cell receptor (TCR) for antigen/MHC is low (Marrack et al. 1983; Biddison et al. 1984; Rojo et al. 1989). To further define the mechanism(s) by which CD8 and CD4 enhance T-cell responses to antigen, we have compared the ability of these proteins to stimulate responses when they can or cannot bind to the same MHC protein as the TCR. We have also examined the functional roles of different domains of these proteins and the function of human CD4 in a mouse system. We find that the ability of CD4 and CD8 to enhance T-cell responsiveness when they cannot bind to the same MHC protein as the TCR is variable and dependent on the specific TCR and its affinity for antigen/MHC. Optimal stimulation of responses occurs when the external domain of these accessory molecules can bind to the same MHC protein as the TCR and when the cytoplasmic tail is capable of interacting with the T-cell-specific tyrosine kinase p56^{lck}. Finally, we demonstrate that hCD4 can stimulate responses of a class-II-restricted, antigen-specific mouse T-cell hybridoma despite the presence of only mouse and not human class II MHC proteins on the antigen-presenting cells.

EXPERIMENTAL PROCEDURES

Expression of CD8 cDNAs in DC27.10. DC27.10 T-hybridoma cells (Gabert et al. 1987) were transfected by protoplast fusion (Oi et al. 1983) with the expression plasmid pHβAPr-neo (Gunning et al. 1987) containing CD8α or CD8α' full-length cDNAs (Zamoyska and

Parnes 1988), or hybrid cDNA molecules encoding assorted CD4 and CD8 extracellular (ext), transmembrane (tm), and cytoplasmic (cyt) domains as described previously (Zamoyska et al. 1989). Transfectants were selected with G418, and expression of CD8 or CD4 external domains was confirmed by specific monoclonal antibody staining.

Functional analysis of DC27.10 cells. Responses to the anti-clonotypic monoclonal antibody Désiré-1 (Hua et al. 1986) were assayed by incubating purified monoclonal antibodies at the concentrations indicated in phosphate-buffered saline on 96-well flat-bottom tissue culture plates for 30 minutes at 4°C. Transfected DC27.10 cells (1×10^5 cells/well) were added in tissue culture media for a final volume of 200 μl and incubated at 37°C. Responses to antigen were measured by incubating 1×10^5 responder cells with either serial dilutions of K^b-transfected L cells or 8×10^5 anti-Thy-1 and complement treated C57BL/6 spleen cells at 37°C in a final volume of 200 μl. Supernatants were harvested at 24 hours and frozen at −20°C until assayed for interleukin-2 (IL-2) content. For both anti-clonotypic and antigen responses, IL-2 was assayed by titrating the supernatants in twofold dilutions with 1×10^4 cytotoxic T-lymphocyte line (CTLL) indicator cells per well in triplicates. CTLL proliferation was assessed in a standard colorimetric assay using cleavage of 3-(4,5-di-methylthiazol-2-yl)-2,5-diphenyl tetrazolium bromide-(MTT) (Mosmann 1983). Total units of IL-2 per well were determined by extrapolation of a plot of supernatant dilution versus optical density (OD), determined as the difference in absorption between 570 nm and 620 nm wavelength.

Expression of CD4 and CD8 genes in BI-141 cells. BI-141 T-hybridoma cells (Reske-Kunz and Rüde 1985) were transfected by electroporation (Smithies et al. 1985) with human or mouse CD4 or mouse CD8α cDNA clones in expression vectors containing the neomycin-resistance gene as described (von Hoegen et al. 1989; C.M. Miceli et al., in prep.). Transfectants were selected with G418 and expression of human CD4, mouse CD4, or mouse CD8α, respectively, confirmed by specific monoclonal antibody staining. Transfectants having comparable levels of TCR, measured by staining with the V$_{β8}$-specific MAb F23.1 (Staerz et al. 1985), were selected for further study.

Functional analysis of BI-141 transfectants.
Transfectants or control BI-141 cells were assayed
for their ability to respond to antigen (beef or pork
insulin) in association with $A_\alpha{}^b A_\beta{}^k$. Responder cells
(1×10^5 per well) were co-cultured in 96-well flat-
bottom tissue culture plates with 1×10^5 MHC class II
$A_\alpha{}^b A_\beta{}^k$-transfected L cells (irradiated with 10,000 rad)
in a final volume of 200 μl tissue culture media, containing threefold serial dilutions of antigen. Triplicate
cultures were incubated at 37°C for 24 hours. Supernatants were then harvested and frozen until assayed for
IL-2 content. IL-2 was analyzed by the ability to support growth of 1×10^4 HT-2 indicator cells (Mosmann
1983), which was assayed by either · [³H]thymidine
incorporation (Reske-Kunz and Rüde 1985) or MTT
cleavage (Mosmann 1983). Proliferation is shown as
incorporated cpm or OD (570–620 nm), respectively.

Inhibition studies. For inhibition experiments with
BI-141 control and transfected cells, purified monoclonal antibodies were added at the onset of cultures at
a final concentration of 100 ng/ml. Recombinant gp120
(Genentech) was added at a final concentration of 6
μg/ml. IL-2 release was analyzed as described above.

RESULTS

Function of the Cytoplasmic Tail of CD8α

To investigate the structural requirements for CD8
function, we have made use of a mouse T-cell hybridoma, DC27.10, that requires CD8 surface expression
for response to the allogeneic class I MHC molecule
K^b. DC27.10 is a cloned line of CD4⁺ helper hybridoma DO-11.10 (specific for I-A^d + ovalbumin) (Kappler et al. 1981) transfected with TCR α- and β-chain
genes encoding a K^b-specific TCR from a CD8⁺ cyto-

toxic T-cell clone (Gabert et al. 1987). In previous
studies, DC27.10 was shown to secrete IL-2 only in
response to an anti-clonotypic monoclonal antibody
specific for the anti-K^b TCR (Désiré-1) and not in
response to K^b until it was transfected with and expressed the mouse CD8α (Ly-2) gene (Gabert et al.
1987). Expression of the CD8β (Ly-3) chain was not
required. We have used this system to examine the role
of the cytoplasmic tail of CD8α. The CD8α gene encodes two forms of protein, α and α', as a result of
alternative patterns of mRNA splicing (Zamoyska et
al. 1985). The two polypeptide chains differ only in
their cytoplasmic tails, with that of α being 28 amino
acids in length as compared to 3 amino acids for α'
(Zamoyska et al. 1985). To determine whether these
polypeptides differ in functional capability, we transfected DC27.10 with cDNA expression vector clones
containing sequence encoding either the α or α' chain
of mouse CD8. Both polypeptides were expressed on
the cell surface in the form of homodimers (data not
shown). Transfectants expressing α or α' were closely
matched for level of surface expression, and the IL-2

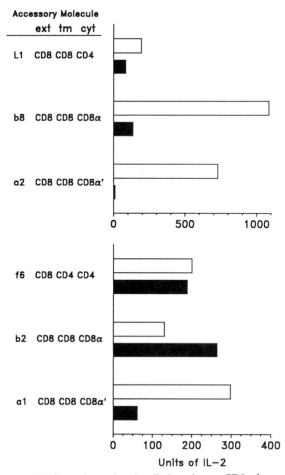

Figure 2. Effect of cytoplasmic tail alteration on CD8α function. Transfected DC27.10 cells expressing the indicated CD8/
CD4 hybrid molecules, CD8α or CD8α', were tested for
response to 10 μg/ml anti-clonotypic MAb Désiré-1 (□) or
1×10^5 K^b-expressing L cells per well (■).

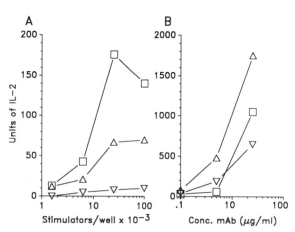

Figure 1. Comparison of CD8α and CD8α' in enhancing the
T-cell response to class I MHC protein. IL-2 production by
DC27.10 T-cell hybridoma cells transfected with cDNA constructs encoding CD8α (□) or CD8α' (△, ▽) was measured
in response to antigen (K^b-expressing L cells) (*A*) or anti-
clonotypic antibody Désiré-1 (*B*). Results are expressed as
units of IL-2 extrapolated from titrating the supernatant on
CTLL indicator cells.

response to the anti-clonotypic monoclonal antibody Désiré-1 was always measured to determine the potential level of responsiveness of the transfectants. As shown in Figures 1 and 2, subclones expressing the α chain secreted much larger amounts of IL-2 at a given antigen (K^b) concentration as compared to those expressing α'.

Function of Hybrid CD8/CD4 Molecules in a Class I MHC-specific T-cell Response

We have further examined the role of the cytoplasmic tail and other portions of the CD8α protein by constructing hybrid cDNA clones encoding the external portion of CD8α and either the transmembrane region and cytoplasmic tail of CD4 or the transmembrane region of CD8α and only the cytoplasmic tail of CD4 (Zamoyska et al. 1989). The reciprocal hybrid constructs, encoding CD4 external to the cell, were also generated. These constructs, as well as clones encoding the full-length CD8α or CD4, were placed into a cDNA expression vector and transfected into a DC27.10 variant that had spontaneously lost expression of the endogenous CD4 gene. In contrast to the decreased functional activity seen when the cytoplasmic tail of CD8α was replaced with that of α', replacement of either the cytoplasmic tail or the transmembrane region and cytoplasmic tail of CD8α with the equivalent regions of CD4 resulted in no loss of response to K^b as compared to the normal CD8α protein (Fig. 2). However, expression on DC27.10 of transfected constructs encoding the external portion of CD4 resulted in complete lack of the ability to stimulate a response to K^b, regardless of whether the transmembrane region and/or cytoplasmic tail was CD4 or CD8 (Table 1). Taken together, these data demonstrate that the lack of function of CD4 in the K^b response was not the result of inability of the CD4 transmembrane region and/or cytoplasmic tail to transmit a necessary signal. Furthermore, the inability of molecules containing CD4 external domains to stimulate transfected DC27.10 responses to antigen was not due to a lack of CD4 ligand on the antigen-presenting cells, since these experiments were done with class-II-expressing, K^b spleen cells as the presenting cells.

The finding that a CD8α molecule with a CD4 cytoplasmic tail was at least as effective as the normal CD8α molecule in stimulating responses to K^b, whereas

CD8α with a foreshortened α' cytoplasmic tail was far less efficient, suggested that there must be some shared function of the cytoplasmic tails of CD4 and CD8α in stimulating antigen responses. Recent studies have demonstrated that both CD4 and CD8 are associated with the T-cell-specific, Src-related tyrosine kinase p56[lck] (Rudd et al. 1988; Veillette et al. 1988). This tyrosine kinase has been shown to phosphorylate the ζ chain of the CD3/TCR complex upon cross-linking of CD4 and is likely to play a role in T-cell activation (Veillette et al. 1989). We therefore examined the possibility that the relative inefficiency of the CD8α' polypeptide in stimulating antigen responsiveness might be a result of failure to associate with p56[lck]. We examined DC27.10 transfectants expressing either the CD8α' chain alone or heterodimers between CD8α' and CD8β and found no association between CD8α' and p56[lck], in contrast to transfectants expressing either the α chain alone or $\alpha\beta$ heterodimers (data not shown; Zamoyska et al. 1989).

Human CD4 Can Enhance Mouse T-cell Responses to Antigen Associated with a Mouse Class II MHC Protein

We have examined the roles of CD4 and CD8 in class-II-restricted antigen responses using a mouse helper-T-cell hybridoma, BI-141, specific for beef insulin in association with the F_1 mouse class II MHC protein $A_\alpha^b A_\beta^k$ (Reske-Kunz and Rüde 1985). This hybridoma had apparently lost expression of CD4 during subcloning. We found previously that cell-surface expression of mouse CD4 (mCD4) after transfection resulted in a much higher response (IL-2 secretion) to beef insulin and a new and much weaker cross-reaction to pork insulin (both in association with $A_\alpha^b A_\beta^k$) (Ballhausen et al. 1988). In the current study, we transfected BI-141 cells with cDNA expression vectors encoding either human CD4 (hCD4) or, as a control, mCD4. hCD4 was expressed on the surface of transfectant clones at levels approximately equal to or slightly lower than seen on human peripheral blood CD4$^+$ cells. These levels were also equivalent to or slightly less than the level of mCD4 on the transfectants expressing mCD4 (data not shown). As illustrated in Figure 3, transfectants expressing hCD4 had a marked enhancement in responsiveness to beef insulin and pork insulin,

Table 1. IL-2 Response of DC27.10 Transfectants to K^b Requires a CD8 External Domain

| Clone | Accessory molecule | | | IL-2 units secreted in response to | |
	ext	tm	cyt	Désiré-1 (1 μg/ml)	K^b spleen cells (8×10^5)
b8.2	CD8	CD8	CD8α	62	69
c27	CD4	CD4	CD4	26	0
k3	CD4	CD4	CD8α	689	0
j1	CD4	CD4	CD8α'	180	0
e9	CD4	CD8	CD8α	167	0

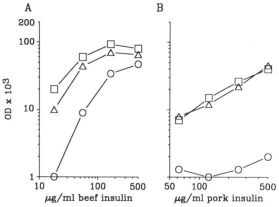

Figure 3. Human CD4 can augment a mouse class-II-restricted antigen response. IL-2 production by BI-141 T-hybridoma cells (○) and by transfectants BI-L3T4D.B3 (mCD4$^+$) (□) and BI-T4.D3 (hCD4$^+$) (△) in response to beef insulin (A) or pork insulin (B) presented on L cells expressing the mouse class II protein $A_\alpha^b A_\beta^k$. IL-2 production was assayed by the ability to support growth of HT-2 cells, measured by MTT cleavage.

and the levels of these responses were indistinguishable from those seen with mCD4. To examine the specificity of this increased response for the hCD4 molecule, we performed monoclonal antibody blocking studies. The data in Figure 4 show that the OKT4B MAb, specific for hCD4, was capable of blocking the response to beef insulin only in a transfectant expressing hCD4 and not in control BI-141 cells or in transfectants expressing mCD4. Similar results have been found with two additional anti-hCD4 MAbs: OKT4D and Leu-3a (von Hoegen et al. 1989). In contrast, MAb GK1.5, specific for mCD4 (Dialynas et al. 1983), could only block the IL-2 response to beef insulin in transfectants expressing

mCD4 and not in hCD4 transfectants or control BI-141 cells. The specificity of the hCD4 effect could be further demonstrated by the ability of soluble gp120, the envelope glycoprotein of HIV-1, to block the response of hCD4 transfectants (Fig. 4), but not control BI-141 cells or mCD4 transfectants. This is in accord with the known ability of gp120 to bind to hCD4 (McDougal et al. 1986) but not mCD4 (Landau et al. 1988). The inhibitory effect of soluble gp120 on the beef insulin response of hCD4 transfectants could be blocked by the simultaneous presence of soluble hCD4, whereas the latter alone had no effect (von Hoegen et al. 1989). We conclude that hCD4 is capable of functionally interacting in a mouse T-cell hybridoma responding to antigen plus mouse class II MHC protein on a mouse antigen-presenting cell.

Function of CD8 in Class-II-restricted Antigen Responses

Since mCD4 was incapable of stimulating antigen responses in the DC27.10 class-I-specific system, we examined the potential of mouse CD8 (mCD8) for stimulating IL-2 secretion in the BI-141 class-II-restricted antigen response. The mCD8α cDNA expression vector clone was transfected into BI-141 cells, and transfectants were selected that expressed surface mCD8α at greater than or equal to physiological levels while maintaining levels of TCR equivalent to the parental line. As shown in Figure 5A, mCD8α expression could stimulate IL-2 secretion in response to beef insulin on $A_\alpha^b A_\beta^k$ antigen-presenting cells, but not as efficiently as mCD4. This was especially evident at the lowest concentrations of beef insulin. The relative inefficiency of mCD8α in stimulating antigen responsive-

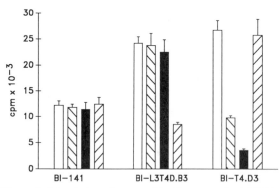

Figure 4. Stimulation of a mouse T-cell response by hCD4 is blocked by specific monoclonal antibody and by gp120. The response of the BI-141 control and transfected T-hybridoma cells to beef insulin presented on L cells expressing $A_\alpha^b A_\beta^k$ was measured with addition at the initiation of culture of 6 μg/ml recombinant gp120 (▨), 100 ng/ml MAb OKT4B (anti-hCD4) (■), or GK1.5 (anti-mCD4) (▩). Concentrations of beef insulin were 500 μg/ml for BI-141 cells (CD4$^-$ control) or 100 μg/ml for BI-L3T4D.B3 (mCD4$^+$) and BI-T4.D3 (hCD4$^+$). Control cultures (□) were without addition. IL-2 production was assayed by the ability to support growth of HT-2 cells, measured by incorporation of [^{3}H]thymidine.

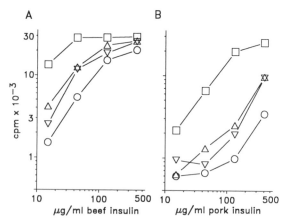

Figure 5. Relative effects of mCD4 and mCD8α in stimulating a class-II-restricted antigen response. The production of IL-2 was measured in response to beef insulin (A) or pork insulin (B) presented by $A_\alpha^b A_\beta^k$-expressing L cells. Responder cells were transfectants BI-L3T4.C5 (mCD4$^+$) (□), BI-Lyt2.D4 (mCD8α^+) (△), and BI-Lyt2.B3 (mCD8α^+) (▽) or untransfected, CD4$^-$/CD8$^-$ control BI-141 cells (○). IL-2 production was assayed as cpm [^{3}H]thymidine incorporated by the IL-2-dependent cell line HT-2.

ness of this T-cell hybridoma was more evident in the response to pork insulin, an antigen for which this hybridoma has a much lower affinity (Fig. 5B). When both mCD4 and mCD8α were transfected into BI-141 cells, the response to antigen was equivalent to that observed for mCD4 single transfectants (M.C. Miceli et al., in prep.). The specificity of the enhanced responses seen in mCD8α transfectants could be shown by the ability of MAb 2.43, specific for the Lyt-2.2 allele of mCD8α, to block the increased response only in transfectants expressing mCD8α and not in mCD4 transfectants. In contrast, GK1.5 (anti-mCD4) blocked responses only in the mCD4 transfectants and not in mCD8α transfectants (M.C. Miceli et al., in prep.). Interestingly, IL-2 secretion by transfectants expressing both mCD4 and mCD8α was blocked effectively only by monoclonal antibody specific for mCD4 and not by that specific for mCD8α (M.C. Miceli et al., in prep.).

DISCUSSION

A role for CD4 and CD8 in T-cell responses was first recognized from a large number of antibody blocking studies (for review, see Parnes 1989). The ability of these proteins to enhance T-cell release of IL-2 has now been shown directly by transfection studies from several laboratories (Dembić et al. 1987; Gabert et al. 1987; Gay et al. 1987; Ratnofsky et al. 1987; Sleckman et al. 1987; Ballhausen et al. 1988). Furthermore, the initial hypothesis that CD4 and CD8 are receptors for relatively invariant portions of class II and class I MHC proteins, respectively, has received strong experimental support from recent binding studies (Doyle and Strominger 1987; Norment et al. 1988; Rosenstein et al. 1989). Data from a number of laboratories have also suggested that CD4 and CD8 can associate with the TCR/CD3 complex, at least under conditions of T-cell activation (Kupfer et al. 1987; O'Neill et al. 1987; Saizawa et al. 1987; Takada and Engleman 1987; Weyand et al. 1987; Anderson et al. 1988; Rojo et al. 1989). These findings have suggested that the stimulation of T-cell antigen responses by CD4 and CD8 might be a result of either or both of two mechanisms: (1) by increasing the avidity of the interaction between T cells and antigen-presenting or target cells by binding to MHC molecules at points of cell-cell contact and (2) by increasing signal transduction, either directly or indirectly (for review, see Parnes 1989). The binding of CD4 or CD8 to class II or class I MHC molecules, respectively, could theoretically be to the same MHC molecule that is presenting antigen to a TCR molecule, and/or to different MHC molecules that are not interacting with a TCR/CD3 complex. Data from several laboratories have provided evidence that CD8 and CD4 can enhance the antigen responsiveness of at least certain T cells in situations where they cannot bind to the same molecule as the TCR (Gay et al. 1987; Ratnofsky et al. 1987; Goldstein and Mescher 1988). We have attempted to further define the role of CD4 and CD8 in antigen responses when these proteins can or cannot

bind to the same MHC molecule as the TCR, and also to determine the importance of the various domains of these proteins in stimulating T-cell function. In the DC27.10 system, we have used hybrid CD8/CD4 molecules to demonstrate that T-cell responses to the class I MHC protein K^b are only detectable when the external portion of the accessory molecule is CD8α, i.e., when it is capable of binding to the same MHC protein as the TCR. Molecules consisting of CD4 external to the cell were nonfunctional, regardless of whether the remainder of the molecule consisted of CD4, CD8α, or CD8α' domains, and regardless of the presence of the CD4 ligand (class II MHC proteins) on the antigen-presenting cells. In contrast, in the BI-141 system, we have demonstrated that an accessory molecule that cannot bind to the same MHC protein as the TCR (i.e., CD8α on a class-II-restricted, antigen-specific T-cell hybridoma) is capable of augmenting the response to antigen. However, the efficiency of CD8α stimulation is far less than that of CD4, which can bind to the same MHC protein as the TCR. Indeed, the effect on the response to pork insulin, for which this TCR has an extremely low affinity, is barely detectable, whereas the stimulation of the response to beef insulin, for which the TCR has a much higher affinity, is more evident. We therefore conclude that CD4 and CD8 function optimally to enhance T-cell responses to antigen when they are capable of binding to the same MHC molecule as the TCR. We further conclude that these proteins can also stimulate T-cell responses when they cannot bind to the same MHC molecule as the TCR; however, this ability is variable and dependent on the specific TCR and its affinity for antigen/MHC.

The results presented here on the differential effectiveness of the CD8α versus CD8α' polypeptide chains indicate that expression of an accessory molecule that can bind to the same MHC molecule as the TCR is not sufficient for optimal enhancement of T-cell antigen responses. Although the α' chain (which has deleted almost all of the CD8α cytoplasmic tail) is clearly able to stimulate transfected DC27.10 cells to respond to K^b, it is far less efficient than the α chain. This may account for the strict developmentally regulated posttranslational control of CD8α' cell-surface expression (Zamoyska and Parnes 1988). Early thymocytes express close to equal amounts of both α and α' chains on the cell surface (as disulfide-linked heterodimers with the β [Ly-3] chain). However, the most mature CD8 single-positive thymocytes and mature peripheral $CD8^+$ T cells retain CD8α'β heterodimers in the Golgi and exclude them from expression on the cell surface (Zamoyska and Parnes 1988). In contrast to the decreased functional activity seen with the physiologically deleted cytoplasmic tail of CD8α', replacement of the CD8α cytoplasmic tail with that of CD4 does not diminish effectiveness in stimulating the response to K^b. Both CD4 and CD8 have been shown to be physically associated with the T-cell-specific tyrosine kinase $p56^{lck}$, which is localized on the inner surface of the cell membrane and is thought to play a role in T-cell activation (Rudd et al. 1988; Veillette et al. 1988). This kinase itself becomes activated and rapidly phosphorylates the ζ chain of the TCR/CD3 complex upon cross-linking of CD4 (Veillette et al. 1989). Notably, we have found that the CD8α' chain does not associate with p56[lck]. Hence, the ability to maximally stimulate T-cell antigen responses when the accessory molecule can bind to the same MHC protein as the TCR correlates with the ability of the accessory molecule to interact with p56[lck]. These findings establish CD8α' as a useful model for an accessory molecule with only a binding or adhesion capability.

Having demonstrated the importance of having an accessory molecule that can bind to the same MHC protein as the TCR, it was somewhat surprising to find that hCD4 was equivalent to mCD4 in stimulating responses to beef and pork insulin by transfected BI-141 cells. The enhanced responses were blocked specifically by monoclonal antibodies specific for human and not mouse CD4 and by gp120 of HIV-1. Although previous studies have demonstrated the ability of hCD4 to increase responses in mouse T-cell hybridomas, in those instances, the ligand for hCD4 was human class II MHC proteins (Gay et al. 1987; Sleckman et al. 1987). This study differs in that the only class II molecules present on the antigen-presenting cells are of mouse origin. It has also been shown previously that human cytotoxic T cells specific for mouse class II MHC proteins can be functionally blocked by monoclonal antibody specific for hCD4 (Swain et al. 1983). However, in that system, hCD4 was expressed on human and not mouse T cells, and other interpretations can be given to the ability of a monoclonal antibody to block function. The current study shows the role of hCD4 more directly, since the function of BI-141 cells expressing or not expressing hCD4 could be directly compared. Assuming that the mechanism by which hCD4 stimulates antigen responses in this system is the same as that by which both hCD4 and mCD4 enhance responses in syngeneic systems, we conclude that hCD4 must be capable of functionally interacting with mouse class II MHC proteins to stimulate mouse T-cell responses.

ACKNOWLEDGMENTS

We are grateful to Richard Flavell for K[b]-transfected L cells; to Ronald Germain for A$_\alpha^b$A$_\beta^k$-transfected L cells; to Jean Gabert and Bernard Malissen for the DC27.10 T-cell hybridoma; to Anne-Marie Schmitt-Verhulst for the MAb Désiré-1; to Wolfgang Ballhausen, Angelika Reske-Kunz, and Tak Mak for the BI-141 T-cell hybridoma; to Genentech, Inc. for soluble gp120 and soluble CD4; to Becton Dickinson for purified Leu-3a monoclonal antibody; and to Patricia Rao for purified OKT4B and OKT4D monoclonal antibodies. This work was supported by National Institutes of Health grants GM-34991, CA-46507, AI-25274, and AI-19512. P.v.H. was supported by a postdoctoral fellowship from the Deutsche Forschungsgemeinschaft. M.C.M. was supported by a postdoctoral training grant (T32 AI-07290) from the N.I.H. and a postdoctoral fellowship from the Arthritis Foundation. J.R.P. is an Established Investigator of the American Heart Association.

REFERENCES

Anderson, P., M.-L. Blue, and S.F. Schlossman. 1988. Comodulation of CD3 and CD4: Evidence for a specific association between CD4 and approximately 5% of the CD3:T cell receptor complexes on helper T lymphocytes. *J. Immunol.* **140:** 1732.

Ballhausen, W.G., A.B. Reske-Kunz, B. Tourvieille, P.S. Ohashi, J.R. Parnes, and T.W. Mak. 1988. Acquisition of an additional antigen specificity after mouse CD4 gene transfer into a T helper hybridoma. *J. Exp. Med.* **167:** 1493.

Biddison, W.E., P.E. Rao, M.A. Talle, G. Goldstein, and S. Shaw. 1984. Possible involvement of the T4 molecule in T cell recognition of class II HLA antigens. *J. Exp. Med.* **159:** 783.

Dembić, Z., W. Haas, S. Weiss, J. McCubrey, H. Kiefer, H. von Boehmer, and M. Steinmetz. 1987. Transfection of the CD8 gene enhances T-cell recognition. *Nature* **326:** 510.

Dialynas, D., Z. Quan, K. Wall, A. Pierres, J. Quintans, M. Loken, M. Pierres, and F. Fitch. 1983. Characterization of the murine T cell surface molecule, designated L3T4, identified by monoclonal antibody GK-1.5: Similarity of L3T4 to the human Leu3/T4 molecule and the possible involvement of L3T4 in class II MHC antigen reactivity. *J. Immunol.* **131:** 2445.

Doyle, C. and J.L. Strominger. 1987. Interaction between CD4 and class II MHC molecules mediates cell adhesion. *Nature* **330:** 256.

Gabert, J., C. Langlet, R. Zamoyska, J.R. Parnes, A.-M. Schmitt-Verhulst, and B. Malissen. 1987. Reconstitution of MHC class I specificity by transfer of the T cell receptor and Lyt-2 genes. *Cell* **50:** 545.

Gay, D., S. Buus, J. Pasternak, J. Kappler, and P. Marrack. 1988. The T-cell accessory molecule CD4 recognizes a monomorphic determinant on isolated Ia. *Proc. Natl. Acad. Sci.* **85:** 5629.

Gay, D., P. Maddon, R. Sekaly, M.A. Talle, M. Godfrey, E. Long, G. Goldstein, L. Chess, R. Axel, J. Kappler, and P. Marrack. 1987. Functional interaction between human T-cell protein CD4 and the major histocompatibility complex HLA-DR antigen. *Nature* **328:** 626.

Goldstein, S.A.N. and M.R. Mescher. 1988. Cytotoxic T cell activation by class I protein on cell-size artificial membranes: Antigen density and Lyt-2/3 function. *J. Immunol.* **140:** 3707.

Gunning, P., J. Leavitt, G. Muscat, S.Y. Ng, and L. Kedes. 1987. A human β-actin expression vector system directs high-level accumulation of antisense transcripts. *Proc. Natl. Acad. Sci.* **83:** 4831.

Hua, C., C. Boyer, A. Guimezanes, F. Albert, and A.-M. Schmitt-Verhulst. 1986. Monoclonal antibodies against an H-2K[b] specific cytotoxic T cell clone detect several clone-specific molecules. *J. Immunol.* **136:** 1927.

Kappler, J., B. Skidmore, J. White, and P. Marrack. 1981. Antigen-inducible, H-2 restricted, interleukin-2 producing T cell hybridomas. *J. Exp. Med.* **153:** 1198.

Kupfer, A., S.J. Singer, C.A. Janeway, Jr., and S.L. Swain. 1987. Coclustering of CD4 (L3T4) molecule with the T-cell receptor is induced by specific direct interaction of helper T cells and antigen-presenting cells. *Proc. Natl. Acad. Sci.* **84:** 5888.

Landau, N.R., M. Warton, and D.R. Littman. 1988. The envelope glycoprotein of the human immunodeficiency virus binds to the immunoglobulin-like domain of CD4. *Nature* **334:** 159.

Marrack, P., R. Endres, R. Shimonkevitz, A. Zlotnik, D. Dialynas, F. Fitch, and J. Kappler. 1983. The major histocompatibility complex restricted antigen receptor on T cells. II. Role of the L3T4 product. *J. Exp. Med.* **158:** 1077.

McDougal, J.S., M.S. Kennedy, J.M. Sligh, S.P. Cort, A. Mawle, and J.K.A. Nicholson. 1986. Binding of HTLV-III/LAV to T4$^+$ T cells by a complex of the 110K viral protein and the T4 molecule. *Science* **231:** 382.

Mossman, T.R. 1983. Rapid colorimetric assay for cellular growth and survival: Application to proliferation and cytotoxicity assays. *J. Immunol. Methods* **65:** 55.

Norment, A., R.D. Salter, P. Parham, V.H. Engelhard, and D.R. Littman. 1988. Cell-cell adhesion mediated by CD8 and MHC class I molecules. *Nature* **336:** 79.

O'Neill, H.C., M.S. McGrath, J.P. Allison, and I.L. Weissman. 1987. A subset of T cell receptors associated with L3T4 molecules mediates C6VL leukemia cell binding of its cognate retrovirus. *Cell* **49:** 143.

Oi, V.T., S.L. Morrison, L.A. Herzenberg, and P. Berg. 1983. Immunoglobulin gene expression in transformed lymphoid cells. *Proc. Natl. Acad. Sci.* **80:** 825.

Parnes, J.R. 1989. Molecular biology and function of CD4 and CD8. *Adv. Immunol.* **44:** 265.

Ratnofsky, S.E., A. Peterson, J.L. Greenstein, and S.J. Burakoff. 1987. Expression and function of CD8 in a murine T cell hybridoma. *J. Exp. Med.* **166:** 1747.

Reske-Kunz, A.B. and E. Rüde. 1985. Insulin-specific T cell hybridomas derived from (H-2^b × H-2^k) F$_1$ mice preferably employ F$_1$-unique restriction elements for antigen recognition. *Eur. J. Immunol.* **15:** 1048.

Rojo, J.M., K. Saizawa, and C.A. Janeway, Jr. 1989. Physical association of CD4 and the T-cell receptor can be induced by anti-T-cell receptor antibodies. *Proc. Natl. Acad. Sci.* **86:** 3311.

Rosenstein, Y., S. Ratnofsky, S.J. Burakoff, and S.H. Hermann. 1989. Direct evidence for binding of CD8 to HLA class I antigens. *J. Exp. Med.* **169:** 149.

Rudd, C.E., J.M. Trevillyan, J.D. Dasgupta, L.L. Wong, and S.F. Schlossman. 1988. The CD4 receptor is complexed in detergent lysates to a protein-tyrosine kinase (pp 58) from human T lymphocytes. *Proc. Natl. Acad. Sci.* **85:** 5190.

Saizawa, K., J. Rojo, and C.A. Janeway, Jr. 1987. Evidence for a physical association of CD4 and the CD3:α:β T-cell receptor. *Nature* **328:** 260.

Sleckman, B.P., A. Peterson, W.K. Jones, J.A. Foran, J.L. Greenstein, B. Seed, and S.J. Burakoff. 1987. Expression and function of CD4 in a murine T-cell hybridoma. *Nature* **328:** 351.

Smithies, O., R.G. Gregg, S.S. Boggs, M.A. Koralewski, and R.S. Kurcherlapati. 1985. Insertion of DNA sequences into the human chromosomal β-globin locus by homologous recombination. *Nature* **317:** 230.

Staerz, U., H.-G. Rammensee, J. Benedetto, and M. Bevan. 1985. Characterization of a murine monoclonal antibody specific for an allotypic determinant on T cell antigen receptor. *J. Immunol.* **134:** 3994.

Swain, S. 1983. T cell subsets and the recognition of MHC class. *Immunol. Rev.* **74:** 129.

Swain, S.L., R.W. Dutton, R. Schwab, and J. Yamamoto. 1983. Xenogeneic human anti-mouse T cell responses are due to the activity of the same functional T cell subsets responsible for allospecific and major histocompatibility-restricted responses. *J. Exp. Med.* **157:** 720.

Takada, S. and. E.G. Engleman. 1987. Evidence for an association between CD8 molecules and the T cell receptor complex on cytotoxic T cells. *J. Immunol.* **139:** 3231.

Veillette, A., M.B. Bookman, E.M. Horak, and J.B. Bolen. 1988. The CD4 and CD8 T cell surface antigens are associated with the internal membrane tyrosine protein kinase p56^{lck}. *Cell* **55:** 301.

Veillette, A., M.A. Bookman, E.M. Horak, L.E. Samelson, and J.B. Bolen. 1989. Signal transduction through the CD4 receptor involves the activation of the internal membrane tyrosine-protein kinase p56$^{lck.}$ *Nature* **338:** 257.

von Hoegen, P., M.C. Miceli, B. Tourvielle, M. Schillham, and J.R. Parnes. 1989. Equivalence of human and mouse CD4 in enhancing antigen responses by a mouse class II-restricted T cell hybridoma. *J. Exp. Med.* (in press).

Weyand, C.M., J. Goronzy, and C.G. Fathman. 1987. Modulation of CD4 by antigenic activation. *J. Immunol.* **138:** 1351.

Zamoyska, R. and J.R. Parnes. 1988. A CD8 polypeptide that is lost after passing the Golgi but before reaching the cell surface: A novel sorting mechanism. *EMBO J.* **7:** 2359.

Zamoyska, R., A.C. Vollmer, K.C. Sizer, C.W. Liaw, and J.R. Parnes. 1985. Two Lyt-2 polypeptides arise from a single gene by alternative splicing patterns of mRNA. *Cell* **43:** 153.

Zamoyska, R., P. Derham, S.D. Gorman, P. von Hoegen, J. Bolen, A. Veillette, and J.R. Parnes. 1989. Inability of CD8α' polypeptides to associate with p56^{lck} correlates with impaired function *in vitro* and lack of expression *in vivo*. *Nature* (in press).

Cross-linking and Conformational Change in T-cell Receptors: Role in Activation and in Repertoire Selection

C.A. Janeway, Jr.,* U. Dianzani,* P. Portoles,* S. Rath,* E.-P. Reich,*
J. Rojo,* J. Yagi,* and D.B. Murphy†

*Section of Immunobiology, Howard Hughes Medical Institute at Yale University School of Medicine,
New Haven, Connecticut 06510; †Laboratory of Immunology, Wadsworth Center,
New York State Department of Health, Albany, New York 12201

Self/non-self discrimination is the most important consequence of immunological recognition. Of cells participating in this central event, the $CD4^+$ T lymphocytes appear to be the most important. In this paper, we use our studies on antigen recognition by cloned T-cell lines to explore two related issues. First, how does the T-cell receptor (TCR) recognize its ligand comprising a peptide fragment of foreign antigen bound to a class II major histocompatibility complex (MHC) molecule? Second, and more difficult, how can the same receptor be selected during its intrathymic ontogeny for the ability to recognize antigen only when presented by self class II MHC molecules?

The receptor for antigen on T cells comprises two highly variable chains termed α and β, bound to an invariant set of chains known as CD3. T cells recognizing antigen presented by class II MHC molecules express the co-receptor molecule CD4 on their cell surface. CD4 is associated in the cell cytoplasm with a tyrosine kinase known as $p56^{lck}$ *(lck)*. Immature thymocytes express both CD4 and CD8, another *lck*-associated cell-surface glycoprotein. CD8 expression is associated with specificity for class I MHC in the TCR. A critical question then is how the association between CD4 expression and class II MHC specificity of the TCR is established. Studies using transgenic mice have clearly established that this association arises during intrathymic ontogeny and is directed by the specificity of the TCR recognizing MHC molecules expressed on thymic cortical epithelial cells. Thus, in explaining positive selection for self-MHC recognition in the thymus, one must also account for the selection for CD4 expression in the case of TCRs with inherent specificity for self class II MHC molecules (for review, see Janeway 1988).

The selective events that occur within the thymus are shown schematically in Figure 1. The TCR plays a critical role in these developmental processes, as outlined in Table 1. Although it is not known whether positive selection precedes, follows, or occurs simultaneously with negative selection during intrathymic ontogeny, this generally accepted picture raises very significant difficulties of interpretation. The central difficulty is the following: If both positive selection and

negative selection involve the interaction of the TCR with class II MHC molecules of self within the thymus, how do these processes differ? The two processes *must* differ in some way, or no T cell that was positively selected for self-MHC recognition would survive negative selection against self-reactivity, and no T-cell repertoire would develop. Two basic hypotheses have been raised to account for these differences. First, it has been suggested that the affinity of the TCR required to generate a positive selective signal differs from that required for negative selection, and that TCRs with a low but not absent affinity for self-MHC molecules would be positively selected but would escape negative selection; we shall term this the affinity hypothesis (Janeway et al. 1976; Blanden and Ada 1978). Alternatively, it has been proposed that the thymic cortical epithelium presents a novel set of peptides associated with class I and class II MHC molecules, such that the actual ligands encountered during positive selection on thymic cortical epithelium differ from those involved in negative selection or expressed elsewhere in the body; we shall term this the altered ligand hypothesis (Janeway 1982; Singer et al. 1986; Marrack and Kappler 1987; Kourilsky and Claverie 1989).

In this paper, we describe a novel monoclonal antibody we have developed that detects a self-peptide bound to a self-class-II MHC molecule to inform us about the distribution of T-cell ligands within the thymus (Murphy et al. 1989). Combining this information with that derived from our analysis of TCR function during T-cell activation in the periphery (Janeway et al. 1989a), we will propose a model to explain how the positive selection signal is delivered to the developing T cell. Our studies of T-cell activation in the periphery suggest that both cross-linking of and conformational change in the TCR are required for optimal signal transduction (Saizawa et al. 1987; Rojo and Janeway 1988). Optimal signal transduction also involves the physical association of CD4 (or CD8) with the TCR (Janeway et al. 1989c). The apparent rarity of self-peptide/self-MHC complexes in thymic cortical epithelium suggests that positive selection could be mediated either by direct, low-affinity recognition of

Table 1. Interaction between TCRαβ and MHC Molecules Is Critical at Four Stages in T-cell Development

1. Positive selection for self-MHC recognition, leading to down-regulation of the co-receptor not recognizing the same MHC class as the TCR

2. Negative selection against direct self-MHC and self-peptide/self-MHC recognition

3. Priming for effector function by specific antigen

4. Recognition of suitable targets and directed secretion of lymphokines during the effector phase

class II MHC by a large number of TCRs, leading to cross-linking but not conformational change, or, alternatively, by high-affinity recognition of very rare peptide/MHC complexes leading to conformational change in single TCRs in the absence of cross-linking, as shown in Figure 2. Either event could transduce a signal sufficient for positive selection, but insufficient

for T-cell activation. A full activating signal, involving both conformational change and cross-linking, is frequently referred to as signal one. Signal one transduction would lead to inactivation or negative selection of developing T cells in this model. Since we are proposing that positive selection is driven by one or the other of these changes, both of which are required to generate signal one, we refer to the signal involved in positive selection as signal one-half.

MATERIALS AND METHODS

The procedures used in these experiments have all been published elsewhere by us. They are referred to in the individual sections in the text.

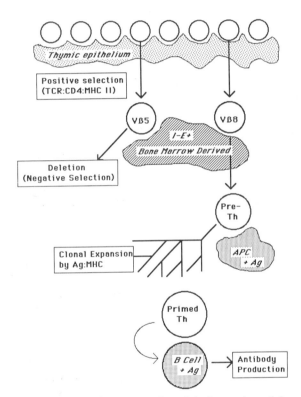

Figure 1. Schematic representation of the interactions of the TCR with ligand during development, activation, and function. The four steps are summarized in Table 1. Positive selection occurs on thymic epithelium and involves the TCR and the co-receptors CD4 and CD8. Positive selection occurs at the CD4, CD8 double-positive stage of T-cell development. Negative selection occurs on any cell, but bone-marrow-derived cells are most effective. Cells expressing $V_\beta 5$ are deleted in mice expressing I-E and the appropriate co-ligand, but cells bearing $V_\beta 8$ are not. Virgin T cells are activated in the periphery by contacting an antigen-presenting cell (APC) expressing peptide/self-MHC molecules. They undergo clonal expansion and differentiation to effector function. Finally, cells that are primed can mediate their effector function (here help to B cells) upon encountering the same ligand on a B-cell surface. For helper T cells, specialized APCs making interleukin-1 are required for clonal expansion; contact with B cells, which express little or no IL-1, leads to production of helper lymphokines and B-cell clonal expansion, but not T-cell clonal expansion.

Rare Ligand, Cross-Linking Only

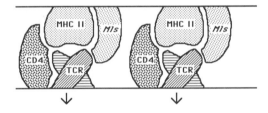

Signal "1/2" = Positive Selection

Rare Ligand: Conformational Change Only

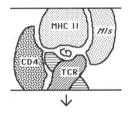

Signal "1/2" = Positive Selection

Figure 2. Signal one-half model of T-cell development. T-cell activation involves both cross-linking of and conformational change in the TCR. On thymic epithelium, we propose that either extensive cross-linking in the absence of conformational change, or conformational change in the absence of cross-linking, generates a signal that positively selects cells bearing self-MHC-restricted TCR. Positive selection involves CD4 co-receptors in the case of class II MHC recognition, and leads to the loss of expression of CD8. Thus, CD4 and CD8 must transduce distinct signals as part of the receptor complex.

RESULTS

Part 1: The Oriented, Clamped Interaction of the TCR with MHC-encoded Ligands

We have extensively analyzed the interaction of the TCR on a single cloned T-cell line, D10.G4.1 (D10), which recognizes a peptide fragment of the protein conalbumin (CA) presented by the syngeneic class II MHC molecule, I-A^k. This TCR also recognizes the allogeneic class II molecules, I-A^{b,d,p,q,v}. We have prepared monoclonal antibodies to many different epitope groupings on the receptor of this cloned T-cell line. Some of the antibodies recognize clonotypic determinants, that is, determinants unique to the D10 cell. Others recognize proteins in the CD3 complex or the V$_\beta$ gene segment encoded region of the TCR (Rojo and Janeway 1988). Using monovalent Fab fragments of these anti-TCR antibodies, we have probed the contribution of these sites to the recognition of different class II MHC ligands by the D10 cloned line (Portoles et al. 1989). These studies have yielded the following results. First, there is strong evidence that the recognition of five different class II MHC molecules is determined by the A$_\beta$ chain of the I-A molecule, as shown by chain recombination studies. Furthermore, the five I-A molecules recognized share a common major sequence in the A$_\beta$ chain different from that of the five I-A molecules not recognized. Finally, antibodies to the TCR V$_\beta$ are extremely efficient at inhibiting antigen plus self-class-II MHC recognition, and are far less effective at inhibiting recognition of non-self-class-II MHC molecules. The interpretation of this result is based on our notion, developed further below, that the TCR always encounters the class II MHC molecule in the same orientation. On this basis, we would argue that the V$_\beta$-encoded portion of the TCR makes contacts with the β chain α helix in the class II model of Brown et al. (1988). This contact is of high affinity for the recognition of specific non-self-class-II MHC by this TCR, and is of lower affinity in the recognition of antigen presented by self-class-II MHC molecules. This conclusion is bolstered by the finding that antibodies directed at hypervariable segments of the TCR are extremely effective at inhibiting recognition of non-self-class-II MHC, and are less effective at inhibiting recognition of antigen presented by self-class-II MHC. This finding implies that the hypervariable portion of the receptor contacts the antigenic peptide and that this contact is of high affinity when the peptide is the specific peptide used to select the cloned T-cell line, and of lower affinity in the recognition of non-self-class-II MHC molecules. Thus, our results suggest that although the TCR always binds to the class II MHC molecule in an identical orientation, different portions of the contacting surface play different roles in the response to distinct ligands.

Role of CD4 in T-cell Activation

The CD4 molecule is expressed on the surface of T cells whose receptors are specific for antigenic peptides presented by class II MHC molecules (Swain 1983). CD4 is known to bind directly to nonpolymorphic regions of the class II MHC molecule (Doyle and Strominger 1987). Two models have been proposed to account for this association. First, it has been proposed that CD4 functions as an accessory molecule, binding directly to class II MHC molecules and increasing the affinity of the TCR (Gay et al. 1986). A second model proposes that CD4 physically associates with the TCR and class II MHC and participates in signal transduction (Janeway et al. 1987; Janeway 1989). This role of CD4 has been termed co-receptor function. Our evidence that CD4 participates in T-cell activation as a co-receptor is summarized below. First, CD4 is observed to localize with the TCR during recognition of antigen class II MHC complexes on APC surfaces (Kupfer et al. 1987). Second, certain anti-TCR antibodies induce a physical association of CD4 with the TCR (Rojo et al. 1989). Significantly, those anti-TCR antibodies that induce a physical association of CD4 with the TCR are approximately 100-fold more potent at inducing T-cell activation than are those antibodies that fail to induce this association. Thus, ligands that could induce the association of CD4 with the TCR, namely by containing class II MHC, would be expected to be at least 100-fold more potent at activating such T cells than ligands that failed to induce such an association, such as those containing class I MHC. It follows that a class I MHC molecule would need to present 100 times as much peptide as a class II MHC molecule in order to activate a CD4$^+$ T cell. Third, antibodies directed at certain epitopes on the TCR or its attendant CD3 complex occupy a site near to where CD4 physically associates, such that antibody to CD4 prevents the physical association of these two molecules and inhibits T-cell activation (Janeway et al. 1987). The antibodies that reveal this phenomenon all bind to a related cluster of epitopes involving V$_\alpha$, C$_\beta$, and the CD3ϵ molecule. The site of these epitopes is noted on the schematic diagram in Figure 3. Fourth, T cells

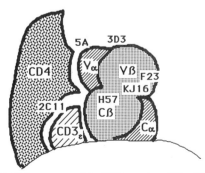

Figure 3. Epitope map of the TCR on cloned T-cell line D10. Each epitope is denoted by an antibody, and the arrangement is based on inhibition of binding of one antibody by the others. Also shown is the docking site of CD4 on the TCR. Certain anti-CD4 antibodies directed at a distinct CD4 epitope inhibit activation of D10 cells by antibodies 5A, H57 anti-C$_\beta$, and 2C11 anti-CD3. These anti-CD4 antibodies inhibit by preventing the physical association of CD4 with the TCR. H57 was a gift from Ralph Kubo, University of Colorado.

expressing both CD4 and CD8 but recognizing a class II MHC ligand are readily inhibited by small amounts of anti-CD4 and can be inhibited only with great difficulty by anti-CD8. The relative ease of inhibition of these two antibodies differs by approximately 100-fold (Jones et al. 1987). Finally, we have shown that direct cross-linking of the TCR to CD4 using hybrid antibodies greatly potentiates activation by anti-TCR antibodies (Janeway et al. 1989c). Taken together, our results suggest first, that the physical association of CD4 with the TCR potentiates signaling by 100-fold and second, that the interaction of CD4 with both the TCR and its class II MHC ligand are stereotopically specific. The consequence of this stereotopic specificity is that the TCR must be oriented to its class II MHC ligand by CD4 itself. Finally, the physical association of CD4 with the TCR is induced only by certain anti-TCR antibodies, suggesting that different antibodies induce different conformational changes in the TCR. This subject will be dealt with in the next part of the paper.

Co-ligands and Their Role in Orienting the TCR

In addition to the role of CD4 and CD8 in orienting and promoting the association of the TCR with their MHC ligands, a second set of molecules may play a role in this alignment process. We term these molecules the co-ligands. To date, most studies of co-ligands such as the Mls loci have involved polymorphisms in internal co-ligands or extrinsic co-ligands such as the staphylococcal enterotoxins (SEs). Properties of the Mls loci and the SEs, both of which can trigger T-cell activation, are contrasted to normal protein antigens in Table 2. The biological properties of the SEs are virtually identical to those of the Mls polymorphic loci: Because SEs are chemically characterized, our studies have focused on these intriguing molecules. SEs appear to activate T cells by binding directly to the outer face of the class II MHC molecule and to the V_β region of the TCR (Janeway et al. 1988, 1989a,b; White et al. 1989; Yagi et al. 1989). These two sites of binding account for the ability of SEs to drive T-cell activation using a variety of class II MHC molecules in an MHC-unrestricted fashion, and to select exclusively for the V_β-encoded portion of the TCR. Direct binding assays reveal binding of intact SEs to both of these structures (Fischer et al. 1989; Fraser 1989; Janeway et al. 1989a; Mollick et al. 1989; Yagi et al. 1989).

The polymorphisms in Mls loci reveal the existence of endogenous co-ligands. Are these aberrancies, or do the products of these polymorphic loci have a function to play in normal T-cell/antigen-presenting cell interaction? To explore this, we have examined the effect of polymorphism in the endogenous co-ligand Mls to alter antigen presentation (Janeway et al. 1983). Our results, confirmed by Hammerling et al. (1988), show that Mls polymorphism can dramatically affect presentation of normal protein antigens to T cells. Furthermore, studies are revealing similar polymorphisms by means of examining the deletion of T cells bearing certain V_β determinants. To date, all such deletional events involve class II MHC molecules and some polymorphic non-MHC product (see White et al. 1989; Kappler et al.; Palmer et al.; both this volume).

Protein antigens are recognized as peptide fragments bound to MHC molecules. Although Mls and the SEs have been termed superantigens (White et al. 1989), we believe the term co-ligand better describes such molecules. We propose that the co-ligands interact with the TCR and the class II MHC molecule as shown in Figure 4. Recent studies by Dellabona et al. (this volume) support the notion that the co-ligands bind to the external face of class II MHC molecules. How widely distributed such co-ligand molecules are, and whether

Table 2. Similarities between the T-cell Responses to Mls and to Staphylococcal Enterotoxins, and Differences with Responses to Protein Antigens

Characteristic of the T-cell response to	Mls-1[a]	SEs	Proteins
High frequency of responding cells	yes (~1:5)	yes (~1:5)	no (~1:10⁴)
Responding T cells CD4⁺	yes	yes	yes[a]
TCR involved in response	yes	yes	yes
T cells of many specificities respond	yes	yes	no
V_β restriction of responding T cells	yes	yes	no[b]
MHC restriction of responding T cells	no	no	yes
Incompetent class II MHC alleles	yes	yes	yes[c]
I-E more involved than I-A	yes	yes	no
Ontogenetic deletion of V_β on CD4⁺8⁺	yes	yes[d]	no
Processing required	?	no	yes
Pulsing APC stimulatory	?	yes	yes
Pulsing T cell stimulatory	?	yes	no
Protein identified	no	yes	yes

Data on T cell responses to Mls and SEs derived from Janeway et al. (1989b).

[a] T cells expressing CD8 respond only to proteins degraded within cells; extrinsic proteins are presented by class II MHC to CD4 T cells.

[b] T-cell responses to protein antigens require all elements of the TCR, whereas those to Mls and SEs appear to require only certain V_β segments (Janeway et al. 1989b; White et al. 1989).

[c] Presentation of proteins is much more restricted in use of allelic forms of class II MHC molecules than is "presentation" of SEs or Mls.

[d] Janeway et al. (1989a).

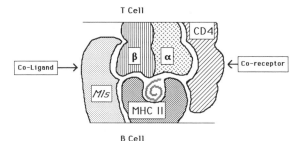

T Cell

B Cell

Figure 4. Complex nature of class II MHC recognition by the TCR. The co-receptor CD4 associates with the α chain of the TCR and some specific site on class II MHC molecules, aligning the TCR and the class II MHC molecule; CD8 is presumed to perform a similar function during class I MHC recognition. Likewise, the co-ligand *Mls* binds to class II MHC away from the peptide-binding cleft and polymorphic sites and to the V_β-encoded portion of the TCR. Normal co-ligands potentiate antigen recognition, presumably by orienting and stabilizing the interaction of the TCR with class II MHC molecules. Note that co-ligands and co-receptors associate with different facets of the TCR and, presumably, of class II MHC as well.

they are required for TCR/MHC interactions is not known. However, the potentiation in T-cell activation achieved through the action of such molecules appears to be at least tenfold, suggesting that co-ligands can play an important role in immunological recognition (Janeway et al. 1983).

The studies summarized here demonstrate that molecules external to the receptor/ligand complex, namely the co-receptor CD4 and co-ligands like *Mls*, can serve to orient the TCR to its class II MHC/peptide ligand. This oriented receptor/ligand pair can derive information from different ligands in different ways, depending on sites of maximal affinity. One disturbing aspect of the picture in Figure 4 is that the complexity of this molecular architecture suggests that these molecular complexes should have significant stability in the absence of specific peptide. Thus, one wonders why T-cell activation is not occurring all the time. One possible explanation for this is given in the next part of this paper.

Part 2: T-cell Activation Involves Cross-linking and Conformational Change in the TCR

We have noted that monoclonal antibodies prepared to different epitopes on the same TCR differ markedly in their ability to activate a cloned T-cell line bearing that receptor. We have measured the amount of antibody needed for half-maximal activation and compared it directly to the amount of antibody binding to the receptor. We find that differences of as great as 500-fold between the amount of antibody bound and the amount required for activation may occur (Rojo and Janeway 1988). How can one explain such differences in potency of antibodies for T-cell activation? Two possibilities have occurred to us. It is possible that the orientation in which TCRs are cross-linked is critical to the activation potential of antibodies. Second, it is

possible that conformational change contributes to activation and that antibodies binding to different epitopes induce distinct conformational changes in the TCR. Our data favor the latter view quite strongly. First, to examine the relative importance of orientation of cross-linking and conformational change, we have used a cross-linking antibody that does not activate the cloned T-cell line of interest to any significant degree. This very low potency antibody, even at high concentrations, gives only minimal activation of the cloned T-cell line D10. However, as shown in Figure 5, the combina-

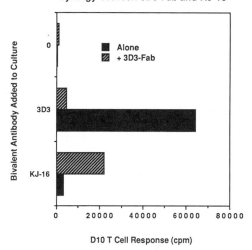

Synergy between 3D3-Fab and KJ-16

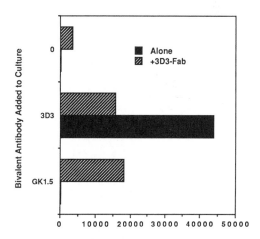

Synergy between 3D3-Fab and GK1.5

Figure 5. Evidence that both conformational change and cross-linking are required for T-cell activation. The non-cross-linking anti-TCR Fab fragment of 3D3 does not activate D10 cells alone, but rather inhibits activation by the cross-linking antibody 3D3. However, when combined with the cross-linking but nonactivating anti-V_β antibody KJ16, good activation is observed, as seen in the upper panel. 3D3-Fab-induced conformational change apparently leads to physical association of CD4 with the TCR, such that bivalent anti-CD4 can now cross-link CD4/TCR complexes to lead to activation, as seen in the lower panel. Data from Rojo and Janeway (1988) and Saizawa et al. (1987).

tion of this cross-linking antibody with the non-cross-linking monovalent Fab fragment of a high-potency antibody, 3D3, gives excellent activation of this cloned T-cell line. Cross-linking is required, since the Fab fragment itself is nonactivating, and, indeed, can inhibit activation by the bivalent form of the same antibody, as shown in Figure 5.

As noted in part 1, high-potency antibodies induce the physical association of CD4 with the TCR. Low-potency antibodies fail to do so. Again, this could be due to conformational change in the TCR, or it could be due to steric effects. If conformational change in the TCR induces a physical association of the TCR with CD4, then the Fab fragment of a high-potency antibody also ought to induce physical association of CD4 with the TCR. To test this, the Fab fragment of the high-potency antibody 3D3 was added to D10 cells, and we then attempted to cross-link the TCR with the bivalent anti-CD4 antibody GK1.5. Again, as seen in Figure 5, the combination of nonactivating stimuli led to potent T-cell activation (Saizawa et al. 1987). Thus, our results are consistent with the hypothesis that activation of T cells occurs optimally when both conformational change and cross-linking occur. We would propose that the presence of a foreign peptide bound to self-class-II MHC molecules augments signaling through the TCR in two distinct ways. First, it stabilizes the complex of TCR/class II MHC molecule, allowing stable colocalization of CD4 to the TCR. Second, it transmits conformational information through the TCR, increasing the fit between CD4 and the TCR and possibly transducing information down the TCR molecule itself. Thus, we would conclude that T-cell activation by peptide/self-class-II MHC complexes involves both cross-linking and conformational change in the TCR. These two changes, taken together, transduce the complete signal for T-cell activation known as signal one. Our studies have not addressed the issue of signal two, the second signal derived from antigen-presenting cells required to get T-cell clonal expansion (see Janeway, this volume). In our system using cloned D10 cells, signal two consists of interleukin-1 (Kaye et al. 1984).

Part 3: The Distribution of a TCR Ligand

One of the great difficulties in understanding positive and negative selection of the TCR repertoire is that ligands potentially influencing that repertoire cannot be directly detected. We are able to detect the distribution of MHC molecules, and this has shown that class II MHC molecules are richly represented on thymic cortical epithelial cells, on thymic medullary cells, and with certain cells in the periphery. However, it is now clear that cell-surface MHC molecules are normally associated with self-peptides, and it is the distribution of specific self- and non-self-peptide/class II MHC complexes that is critical to understand.

We have recently produced a monoclonal antibody specific for a peptide derived from the class II molecule I-E bound to the class II molecule I-A^b. To date, the specific peptide bound has not been identified. Never-

theless, there is a good deal of evidence to support the contention that this monoclonal antibody does detect a self-peptide presented by a self-class-II MHC molecule (Murphy et al. 1989). These data are as follows: First, L cells transfected with either the I-A^b or the I-E^b molecules are not recognized by this antibody. Second, mice that fail to express the I-E molecule also fail to express this determinant, whereas mice with an identical genetic background expressing the I-E molecule are highly positive for the determinant. Third, biochemistry demonstrates the precipitation of the A$_\alpha$ and A$_\beta$ chains, together with a distinctive set of lower molecular weight materials. Fourth, epitope mapping of the binding site of the antibody demonstrates that it binds across the peptide-binding groove in the Brown et al. (1988) model of the class II MHC molecule. It binds to approximately 12% of the I-A^b molecules on B cells expressing I-E molecules.

If one accepts that the monoclonal antibody recognizes a typical self-peptide/self-class-II MHC ligand such as those recognized by autoreactive T cells, then one can use the antibody to examine the tissue distribution of such complexes. Interestingly, this complex is widely distributed on class-II-positive cells of hematopoietic origin. However, it is essentially absent from thymic cortical epithelial cells. Indirect evidence also suggests the absence from thymic medullary cells of epithelial origin. These thymic epithelial cells express both of the class II molecules, I-A^b, which presents the peptide, and the peptide donor, I-E^b. Thus, these results suggest that the processing and presentation of self-peptides differs between cells of hematopoietic origin and other cell types that express class II MHC molecules. Consistent with this result is our recent observation that L cells transfected with both I-A^b and I-E^b react weakly or not at all with our antibody (S. Rath et al., unpubl.).

If the class II molecules present on thymic epithelium are not presenting the self-peptides presented in the periphery, what are they presenting? Furthermore, how does this distinction in presentation arise? Whatever the answer, the net effect of this difference is that the class II molecules in the thymic cortex express either a totally different set of ligands or express very low levels of those ligands found in the periphery. This area needs extensive work, and our data only reveal that the peptides presented in these two sites are different, not the means by which they differ. Nevertheless, such findings have important implications for selective events in the thymus, especially since positive selection is believed to occur only by contact with thymic cortical epithelial cells (Lo and Sprent 1986). These issues will be dealt with in the next part.

Part 4: Negative and Positive Selection of the TCR Repertoire during Thymic Development—The Half-signal Model

The selective events that occur in the thymus during T-cell development play a critical role in the behavior of the immune system. Generally, it is considered that two selective events occur: positive selection for those T cells able to recognize antigen only when it is presented by the MHC molecules expressed on thymic cortical epithelium, and negative selection against T cells able to respond in the periphery to self-MHC or self-peptides presented by self-MHC molecules. The process of negative selection is essential for the maintenance of self-tolerance. Recently, a third class of ligand has been found to play a critical role in negative selection in the mouse. The unknown product of the *Mls* loci, and the SEs, as well as other molecules, appear to bind directly to class II MHC and to the V_β gene segment encoded portion of the TCR. By cross-linking these two molecules, T-cell activation is achieved. We refer to these structures as co-ligands. Polymorphism in co-ligands and/or MHC molecules can lead to T-cell activation in the periphery and to its counterpart, deletion during T-cell development in the thymus.

Negative selection. For negative selection to be effective in maintaining self-tolerance, it seems likely that T cells must be negatively selected at a lower threshold for activation than that existing in the periphery. Furthermore, the signal for negative selection should be identical to that required for T-cell activation; the difference in outcome reflects the differentiation state of the responding cells. However, natural in vivo co-ligands cannot be measured quantitatively, either in the periphery or in the thymus. To approach the question of thresholds required for negative selection as opposed to thresholds required for activation, we have used the artificial co-ligand SEB to compare these two parameters. In brief, our findings show that approximately 100-fold less SEB is required for clonal deletion in thymic organ cultures as compared to the concentration required for T-cell activation in vivo. The two dose response curves are roughly parallel, thus demonstrating a very significant window between tolerance induction and activation. Indeed, the window appears to be embarrassingly wide. However, it must be noted that this measurement only covers the co-ligand portion of the deleting element and ignores the contribution of the class II MHC molecule. It is quite possible that class II MHC molecules in contact with developing T cells are expressed at a higher level in thymic epithelium than they are in the periphery, and thus that the net concentration of that SEB bound to the appropriate class II MHC molecule may be higher in thymic organ culture than it is in peripheral T-cell cultures. Also, it should be noted that the thymus deletion experiments are carried out in organ culture at high cell density, whereas T-cell activation studies are carried out in dissociated lymphoid cells at lower cell density. Nevertheless, there is obviously a striking difference between tolerance induction and T-cell activation in terms of ligand densities (Yagi and Janeway 1989).

Recently, we have also examined a system in which co-ligand-directed deletion of V_βs may have a practical consequence. The non-obese diabetic (NOD) mouse is an interesting model for human insulin-dependent diabetes mellitus. This animal develops diabetes sponta-

neously around 4 months of age. NOD mice do not express a functional I-E gene, whereas NOD mice made transgenic to express such a gene do not get diabetes. Thus, the I-E gene somehow protects the mouse from diabetes (Nishimoto et al. 1987). Using cloned T-cell lines specific for pancreatic β cells and able to transfer disease, we asked whether this effect of I-E is on the target tissue or whether it affects the developing T-cell repertoire. Our cloned T-cell lines will damage I-E$^+$ β cells and will respond to I-E$^+$ β-cell stimulation in vitro. Thus, I-E does not appear to protect the target or alter its specificity. However, our diabetogenic T-cell clones all express TCRs encoded in $V_\beta 5$, a set of V_β genes all of which are deleted during intrathymic ontogeny in I-E$^+$ but not in I-E$^-$ mice. We have examined (NOD × BALB/c) F$_1$ mice and have found that $V_\beta 5$ expression is significantly decreased in these mice as compared to NOD mice. Thus, negative selection by co-ligands appears to play a role protecting NOD mice from this particular autoimmune disease (Reich et al. 1989).

Negative selection is a highly sensitive and effective mechanism for preserving self-tolerance. It appears to be significantly more sensitive than T-cell activation, as would be predicted for a major mechanism protecting the host from autoimmune attack.

Positive selection. The original finding that T cells develop within the thymus only if their receptors can recognize the MHC molecules expressed on thymic cortical epithelium has been amply confirmed by studies carried out using TCR transgenic mice (see von Boehmer et al. 1989). One of the hallmarks of this positive selective event is the selective expression of CD4 in the case of class II MHC recognizing TCR, and CD8 in the case of class I receptors. However, although these cells recognize foreign antigens presented by self-MHC in the periphery, they show no detectable response to self-MHC alone. Nevertheless, it appears to be self-MHC alone that selects for their expansion in the thymus. How do we explain this? One way to explain this result is to state simply that the activation properties of the TCR are different in these two sites, leading to positive selection but not proliferation in the thymic cortex, but leading to proliferation in the periphery. A difficulty with all such models is that if the same ligand is encountered in the thymus and the periphery, one would expect either autoimmunity or the total absence of a T-cell repertoire as the result of negative selection. Thus, one is forced to postulate either that the set of ligands presented by the thymic cortical epithelial cell is unique or that thresholds of affinity required for positive selection are set well below those required for negative selection or T-cell activation in the periphery. Given that the threshold for negative selection is also set significantly below that for activation in the periphery, it is difficult to imagine that a threshold set far lower than this would be effective in selecting cells for recognition of self-MHC.

We propose an alternative hypothesis to explain positive selection in the thymic cortex (Table 3). This ex-

Table 3. Proposed Basis for T-cell Repertoire Selection in the Thymus: The Half-signal Model

1. The density of peptide/MHC ligands on thymic cortical epithelial cells is very low relative to peripheral cells or cells in thymic medulla.

2. Negative selection involves precisely the same receptor/ligand interactions as activation in the perhipery, but is set at a lower threshold to avoid autoreactivity.

3. Positive selection occurs on thymic cortical epithelial cells, which have a very low ligand density, except for MHC molecules themselves.

4. Low ligand density could lead to low-affinity binding of the TCR/co-receptor complex to MHC alone, generating cross-links but not conformational change. Alternatively, rare peptide/MHC complexes could bind to single TCR/co-receptor complexes, generating conformational change in the absence of cross-links. Either process could give rise to the signal for positive selection.

planation is based on the distribution of self-peptide/self-MHC complexes in the thymus, as described in part 3 of this report; on the clamped and oriented nature of the TCR ligand interaction exemplified in Figure 4; and on the evidence that both cross-linking of and conformational change in the TCR are required for signal one. Studies on the distribution of the T-cell self-MHC ligand suggest that the density of individual peptide/MHC complexes in the thymus will be extremely low. At the same time, the structures shown in Figure 4 suggest that the TCR can interact effectively with class II MHC ligands in the absence of peptide, but that such interactions do not normally lead to T-cell activation and therefore go undetected. However, such extensive cross-linking in the absence of peptide might indeed transduce a partial signal for activation, which we will refer to as signal one-half. We use this terminology since it appears to be half of the required signal one. If the structure shown in Figure 4 and in the top panel of Figure 2 requires a certain low threshold of affinity of the TCR for the class II MHC molecule independent of the peptide bound by that molecule, cross-linking could occur and lead to perceptible signaling and positive selection, and yet fall short of delivering the full signal one, which would be tolerogenic at this stage in T-cell development. An alternative mechanism for positive selection is shown in the bottom panel of Figure 2, in which rare peptide/MHC complexes binding to the TCR with high affinity cause conformational change in the receptor but cannot cross-link due to their low frequency and, therefore, do not cause full signal-one transduction and tolerance induction. This model also predicts that full cross-linking and conformational change of the receptor in developing thymocytes leads to deletion. We suggest that either extensive cross-linking in the absence of conformational change, or, alternatively, conformational change in the absence of cross-linking, delivers an incomplete signal for T-cell activation, which is translated into positive selection by the T cell. We have previously suggested that the TCR hypervariable regions themselves would provide a rich source of peptides for this positive selection process within the thymus (Janeway 1982). One virtue of using hypervariable peptides from the TCR as a source of positive-selecting peptides is the unlikelihood of reencountering such peptides in the periphery. However, nothing is really known about

either an involvement of selecting peptides in positive selection or the source of such peptides.

DISCUSSION

Our data obtained studying the cloned T-cell line D10.G4.1 have indicated that activation of this cloned T-cell line involves both cross-linking of its receptor and conformational change in the receptor molecule. In addition, activation involves the association of CD4 with the TCR complex. These events lead to the accumulation of further proteins making up the TCR/ligand complex, as depicted in Figure 4. The great extent of contacts postulated in this model suggests the TCR might be able to stabilize itself in interacting with class II MHC molecules alone under appropriate conditions. Using antibodies like KJ16, we can ask what are the consequences of cross-linking the TCR in the absence of full T-cell activation. Should distinctive biochemical changes accompany the binding of KJ16 or of the 3D3 Fab fragment, those biochemical changes could also be sought in the developing thymus, in order to attempt to understand the process of positive selection. The model shown in Figure 2 suggests two ways in which an incomplete activating signal could be delivered to the TCR. When these two signals are combined, leading to full T-cell delivery of signal one, immature T cells are deleted. This deletion within the thymic cortex has recently been demonstrated for two TCR transgenic mice, recognizing L^d (Sha et al. 1988) or H-Y:D^b (Kisielow et al. 1988). It appears that negative selection could happen either before or after positive selection, depending largely on the site in which the deleting ligand is expressed. Although it might appear more efficient to delete autoreactive T cells prior to positive selection, what is essential is that only a fraction of positively selected T cells is deleted, and not whether deletion occurs either before or after positive selection. One argument in favor of later deletional events is that the more mature thymocytes have activation properties comparable to those encountered in the periphery, and it is activation by peripheral self molecules that one wants to avoid.

We propose that the thymic cortical epithelium has a unique distribution of peptide/MHC complexes, bearing a random assortment of self-peptides. Such self-peptides might be directly involved in positive selection by inducing conformational change in the TCR without cross-linking, or they could be irrelevant, allowing cross-linking to occur in the absence of conformational change. Either of these incomplete changes in the state of the TCR could lead to the unique signal that must be involved in positive selection. Finally, both models incorporate CD4 recognition of class II MHC, since one of the major consequences of positive selection is the selective expression of CD4 or CD8, depending on the restriction specificity of the TCR. This model is open to direct biochemical test, and it is hoped that it will lead to new insights into the central question of positive selection of T cells in the thymus.

SUMMARY

TCRs undergo a series of interactions with ligands during development. We have characterized the interaction of a TCR with its ligand and the attendant co-receptor and co-ligand structures. This characterization has led to the model in which the TCR not only binds to class II MHC, but also binds to CD4 co-receptors and co-ligands such as *Mls*. We have shown that both cross-linking and conformational change in the TCR are required for optimal T-cell activation. Finally, we have used the observation that a particular self-peptide found abundantly associated with class II MHC in the periphery is essentially lacking from thymic cortical epithelium to argue that positive selection for self-MHC recognition may occur by a novel process in the thymic cortex. A TCR recognizing class II MHC with low affinity could either be multiply cross-linked in the absence of conformational change, which here would be driven by a unique peptide, or could be conformationally changed without cross-linking due to the rarity of the individual high-affinity peptide on thymic cortical epithelial cells. Either proposal leads to a partial signal one delivered via the TCR, which we refer to as signal one-half. This signal one-half would induce the cell to repress its other co-receptor molecule and to undergo maturation events such as up-regulation in TCR expression. Such cells are then rigorously screened for activating interactions with autologous structures, such as *Mls*. The threshold for clonal deletion is set very low to avoid autoreactivity. By this combination of signaling events, a mature TCR repertoire is generated that has the functional characteristics observed in immune systems.

ACKNOWLEDGMENTS

The authors thank Elizabeth Cluggish for the preparation of this manuscript; Pat Conrad, Cara Wunderlich, and Denise Scaringe for technical assistance; and their many colleagues who have shared ideas and reagents with them over the years.

REFERENCES

Blanden, R.V. and G.L. Ada. 1978. A dual recognition model for cytotoxic T cells based on thymic selection of precursors with low affinity for self H-2 antigens. *Scand. J. Immunol.* **7:** 181.

Brown, J.H., T. Jardetzky, M.A. Saper, B. Samraoui, P.J. Bjorkman, and D.C. Wiley. 1988. A hypothetical model of the foreign antigen binding site of class II histocompatibility molecules. *Nature* **332:** 845.

Doyle, C. and J.L. Strominger. 1987. Interaction between CD4 and class II MHC molecules mediates cell adhesion. *Nature* **330:** 256.

Fischer, H., M. Dohlsten, M. Lindvall, H.-O. Sjogren, and R. Carlsson. 1989. Binding of staphylococcal enterotoxin A to HLA-DR on B cell lines. *J. Immunol.* **142:** 3151.

Fraser, J.D. 1989. High-affinity binding of staphylococcal enterotoxins A and B to HLA-DR. *Nature* **339:** 221.

Gay, D., C. Coeshott, W. Golde, J. Kappler, and P. Marrack. 1986. The MHC-restricted antigen receptor on T cells. IX. Role of accessory molecules in recognition of antigen plus isolated I-A. *J. Immunol.* **136:** 2026.

Hammerling, U., M. Toulon, M. Chun, S. Palfree, and M. Hoffman. 1988. Bidirectionality of mixed lymphocyte stimulation (Mls) response. Effects of *Mls^b* stimulator cells on *Mls^a* helper cells. *J. Immunol.* **140:** 2543.

Janeway, C.A., Jr. 1982. Selection of self-MHC recognizing T lymphocytes: A role of idiotypes? *Immunol. Today* **3:** 261.

———. 1988. T cell development: Accessories or coreceptors? *Nature* **335:** 208.

———. 1989. The role of CD4 in T cell activation: Accessory molecule or co-receptor? *Immunol. Today* **10:** 234.

Janeway, C.A., Jr., H. Wigzell, and H. Binz. 1976. Hypothesis: Two different V_H gene products make up the T cell receptors. *Scand. J. Immunol.* **5:** 993.

Janeway, C.A., Jr., J. Chalupny, P.J. Conrad, and S. Buxser. 1988. An external stimulus that mimics *Mls* locus responses. *J. Immunogenetics* **15:** 161.

Janeway, C.A., Jr., S. Haque, L.A. Smith, and K. Saizawa. 1987. The role of the murine L3T4 molecule in T cell activation: Differential effects of anti-L3T4 on activation by monoclonal anti-receptor antibodies. *J. Mol. Cell. Immunol.* **3:** 121.

Janeway, C.A., Jr., P.J. Conrad, J. Tite, B. Jones, and D.B. Murphy. 1983. Efficiency of antigen presentation differs in mice differing at the Mls locus. *Nature* **306:** 80.

Janeway, C.A., Jr., P. Portoles, J.M. Rojo, U. Dianzani, J. Yagi, S. Rath, and S. Buxser. 1989a. The interaction between the T cell receptor: CD4 complex and its class II MHC ligand. *UCLA Symp. Ser. Mol. Cell. Biol.* (in press).

Janeway, C.A., Jr., J. Yagi, P.J. Conrad, M.E. Katz, B. Jones, S. Vroegop, and S. Buxser. 1989b. T cell responses to *Mls* and to bacterial proteins that mimic its behavior. *Immunol. Rev.* **107:** 61.

Janeway, C.A., Jr., J. Rojo, K. Saizawa, U. Dianzani, P. Portoles, J. Tite, S. Haque, and B. Jones. 1989c. The co-receptor function of murine CD4. *Immunol. Rev.* **109:** 77.

Jones, B., P.A. Khavari, P.J. Conrad, and C.A. Janeway, Jr. 1987. Differential effects of antibodies to Lyt-2 and L3T4 on cytolysis by cloned, Ia-restricted T cells expressing both proteins. *J. Immunol.* **139:** 380.

Kaye, J., S. Gillis, S.B. Mizel, E.M. Shevach, T.R. Malek, C.A. Dinarello, L.B. Lachmann, and C.A. Janeway. 1984. Growth of a cloned helper T cell line induced by a monoclonal antibody specific for the antigen receptor. Interleukin 1 is required for the expression of receptors for Interleukin 2. *J. Immunol.* **133:** 1339.

Kisielow, P., H. Bluthmann, U.D. Staerz, M. Steinmetz, and H. von Boehmer. 1988. Tolerance in T cell receptor transgenic mice involves deletion of nonmature CD4^+8^+ thymocytes. *Nature* **333:** 742.

Kourilsky, P. and J.-M. Claverie. 1989. MHC restriction, alloreactivity, and thymic education: A common link? *Cell* **56:** 327.

Kupfer, A., S.J. Singer, C.A. Janeway, Jr., and S.L. Swain. 1987. Co-clustering of CD4 (L3T4) molecules with the

T-cell receptor is induced by specific direct interaction of helper T cells and antigen-presenting cells. *Proc. Natl. Acad. Sci.* **84:** 5888.

Lo, D. and J. Sprent. 1986. Identity of cells that imprint H-2-restricted T-cell specificity in the thymus. *Nature* **318:** 672.

Marrack, P. and J. Kappler. 1987. The T cell receptor. *Science* **238:** 1073.

Mollick, J.A., R.G. Cook, and R.R. Rich. 1989. Class II MHC molecules are specific receptors for Staphylococcus enterotoxin A. *Science* **244:** 817.

Murphy, D.B., D. Lo, S. Rath, R.L. Brinster, R. Flavell, A. Slanetz, and C.A. Janeway, Jr. 1989. A novel MHC class II epitope expressed in thymic medulla but not cortex. *Nature* **338:** 765.

Nishimoto, H., H. Kikutani, K.-I. Yamamura, and T. Kishimoto. 1987. Prevention of autoimmune insulitis by expression of I-E molecules in NOD mice. *Nature* **328:** 432.

Portoles, P., J.M. Rojo, and C.A. Janeway, Jr. 1989. Asymmetry in the recognition of antigen:self class II MHC and non-self class II MHC molecules by the same T cell receptor. *J. Mol. Cell. Immunol.* **4:** 129.

Reich, E.-P., R.S. Sherwin, O. Kanagawa, and C.A. Janeway, Jr. 1989. An explanation for the protective effect of I-E in murine diabetes. *Nature* (in press).

Rojo, J. and C.A. Janeway, Jr. 1988. The biological activity of anti-T cell receptor variable region monoclonal antibodies is determined by the epitope recognized. *J. Immunol.* **140:** 1081.

Rojo, J.M., K. Saizawa, and C.A. Janeway, Jr. 1989. Physical association of CD4 and T cell receptor can be induced by anti-T cell receptor antibodies. *Proc. Natl. Acad. Sci.* **86:** 3311.

Saizawa, K., J. Rojo, and C.A. Janeway, Jr. 1987. Evidence for a physical association of CD4 and the CD3:α:β T cell receptor. *Nature* **328:** 260.

Sha, W., C. Nelson, R. Newberry, D. Kranz, J. Russel, and D. Loh. 1988. Positive and negative selection on an antigen receptor on T cells in transgenic mice. *Nature* **336:** 73.

Singer, A., T. Mizuochi, T.I. Munitz, and R.E. Gress. 1986. Role of self antigens in the selection of the developing T cell repertoire. *Prog. Immunol.* **6:** 60.

Swain, S.L. 1983. T cell subsets and the recognition of MHC class. *Immunol. Rev.* **74:** 129.

von Boehmer, H., H.S. Teh, and P. Kisielow. 1989. The thymus selects the useful, neglects the useless, and destroys the harmful. *Immunol. Today* **10:** 57.

White, J., A. Herman, A.M. Pullen, R. Kubo, J. Kappler, and P. Marrack. 1989. The Vβ specific superantigen Staphylococcal enterotoxin B: Stimulation of mature T cells and clonal deletion in neonatal mice. *Cell* **56:** 27.

Yagi, J. and C.A. Janeway, Jr. 1989. Ligand thresholds at different stages of T cell development. *Int. Immunol.* (in press).

Yagi, J., J. Baron, S. Buxser, and C.A. Janeway, Jr. 1989. Bacterial proteins that mediate the association of a defined subset of T cell receptor:CD4 complexes with class II MHC. *J. Immunol.* **143:** (in press).

Problems in the Physiology of Class I and Class II MHC Molecules, and of CD45

A.G. Fisher, L.K. Goff, L. Lightstone, J. Marvel, N.A. Mitchison,
G. Poirier, H. Stauss, and R. Zamoyska
*Imperial Cancer Research Fund, Tumour Immunology Unit,
University College London, London WC1E 6BT, United Kingdom*

The decade that separates this Symposium from the previous one devoted to immunology in this series has been marked by intense activity in research on T cells. Much of that research has concentrated on the glycoproteins that guide and mark these cells. Although progress in delineating the structure of these molecules has been rapid, our understanding of how they function under physiological conditions has lagged, and we still have much to learn. This paper deals with four topics in that area, where in each an important problem can be posed, but where in no case is the answer yet known.

Do MHC Class I Molecules Loaded with Viral Epitopes Pass from Tissue Cells to Dendritic Cells?

The evolution of specialized MHC class I molecules and the parallel evolution of specialized antigen-presenting cells pose a dilemma for the immune system. That dilemma is between maintaining the rule of local-loading of class I molecules and taking full advantage of specialized presentation. On the one hand, class I molecules have as their only known function the guidance or "docking" of cytotoxic T cells in defense against viruses, and they therefore need to take up antigenic epitopes in a strictly local fashion. Were they to acquire epitopes indiscriminately from other cells, uninfected bystander cells would suffer cytotoxic attack. Apparently in order to avoid that possibility, an extraordinary mechanism has evolved whereby class I molecules take up epitopes only from viral proteins that are synthesized within that cell, the so-called "cytosolic" or "endogenous" route of loading (Townsend et al. 1985; Braciale et al. 1987; Chain et al. 1989). What makes this mechanism so unusual is that viral proteins do not need a leader sequence to let their degradation products reach the outer surface of the cell. The route is not confined to virus-encoded proteins, since peptide epitopes encoded by the cell itself also load onto class I molecules, where they haven been detected as minor alloantigens, such as H-Y.

On the other hand, specialized antigen-presenting cells have developed adaptations that enable them effectively to activate cytotoxic T cells. These adaptations include adhesion molecules such as the now famous trio of LFA-1, LFA-3, and ICAM-1, plus others that may yet be discovered. They include also cytoskeletal adap-

tations, of which the most important seems to be formation of dendrites, as the following observations argue: Macrophages and interdigitating dendritic cells both express the trio of adhesion molecules, but only dendritic cells form clusters with T cells, and they are the cells that activate T cells most effectively. Secretion of soluble mediators may represent a third adaptation. IL-1 is secreted by macrophages and probably helps activate T cells, although whether it does so directly or via an effect on dendritic cells is debatable (Koide and Steinman 1987).

This argument can be taken too far: The activation process cannot be very much more efficient than the final targeting process, as otherwise activated cytotoxic cells would accumulate that could not interact with their targets. Perhaps activation is more difficult to achieve than targeting, but that argument is circular: A high threshold of activation could be a consequence rather than a cause of using superefficient antigen-presenting cells.

There is another reason to expect interdigitating dendritic cells to activate cytotoxic T cells, concerned with their special ability to implement epitope linkage. This argument is based on the scheme of cell interaction set out in Figure 1, which has been developed in several of our recent publications (Dexter et al. 1987; Mitchison 1989). On the left is the well-established pathway of T-B interaction that depends on juxtaposition of the two cells in a "conjugate" or "two-cell-type cluster"; for an excellent recent review of this topic, see Vitetta et al. (1989). It is now generally agreed that this interaction fulfills two major functions: (1) to coordinate the immune response by implementing epitope linkage, so that the response can be spread from one epitope to another of an invading organisms; and (2) to allow one of the partners, the T cell, to take care of self-tolerance and thus leave the other free to hypermutate. On the right is a pathway more recently established for the T-helper/T-cytotoxic interaction, which fulfills the same function of implementing epitope linkage, but does so by a somewhat different mechanism. As long as the number of antigenic particles in the input does not exceed the number of antigen-presenting cells, each such cell will tend to take up a single particle, and a three-cell-type cluster will form that involves helper and cytotoxic epitopes derived from the same particle.

T-B and T-T regulatory interactions: how the immune system implements linkage of epitopes

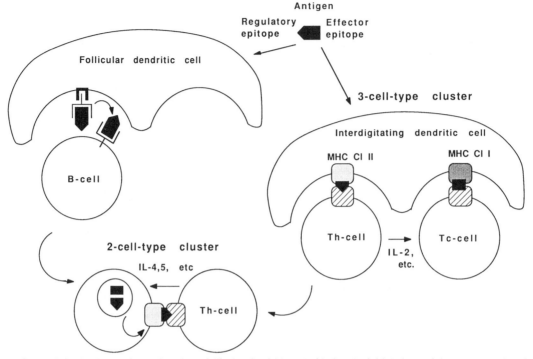

Figure 1. On the left, B cells acquire antigen from follicular dendritic cells (during the initial phase of the response, B cells may acquire antigen directly). Follicular dendritic cells retain configurationally intact antigen by means of Fc-receptors (and other receptors not shown) for long periods, thus meeting the needs of B cells, and spread a dense network of dendrites across areas traversed by B cells. Epitope linkage is implemented by a B cell using its sIg receptor to acquire antigen and the loading antigenic fragments onto its own MHC class II molecules. On the right, interdigitating dendritic cells present MHC-bound peptides, but probably do not retain antigen for long periods and are spaced apart from one another in areas traversed by T cells. Epitope linkage is thought to be implemented by processing of single antigenic particles so that their epitopes are retained within a single three-cell-type cluster (Mitchison and O'Malley 1987).

For a presenting cell to perform this task efficiently, it must fulfill four conditions: (1) It must express both MHC class I and class II molecules; (2) it must be able to activate T cells efficiently; (3) it must be located in the T-cell area of lymphoid tissue, so as to encounter T cells; and (4) the presenting cells must be spaced far enough apart from one another to ensure that the clusters do not overlap, and thus lose the benefits of epitope linkage. Only interdigitating dendritic cells meet the bill. The extent to which these cells are spaced apart from one another is well illustrated by a histological study with two newly developed monoclonal antibodies (Breel et al. 1987); and in a normal human lymph node cortex they are the only cells that stain strongly for HLA-DR (the point is worth emphasizing, since activated human T cells also express class II, but do so to a lesser extent than dendritic cells).

The above are reasons for expecting interdigitating dendritic cells to excel at activating virus-specific cytotoxic T cells, and we now need to inquire how isolated populations of these cells actually perform. This kind of experiment is becoming easier to conduct as methods of isolating these cells improve (Macatonia et al. 1989) and as these new markers become available. In three recent studies, with a herpesvirus (Hengel et al. 1987), with a retrovirus (Kast et al. 1988), and with influenza

virus (Macatonia et al. 1989), isolated dendritic cells performed significantly better than macrophages, particularly in activating the unprimed precursors of cytotoxic T cells. For the purposes of this discussion, it is important to know whether this superiority applies to the class I interaction with the cytotoxic precursors themselves, rather than to a class II interaction with helper T cells that may also be involved. The latter possibility was examined in one of these studies by sorting for CD8 T cells at the beginning of the experiment (Hengel et al. 1987), but interpretation of the results is unclear because killed virus was used. In summary, the available evidence suggests that dendritic cells are indeed superior as inducers of a primary cytotoxic T-cell response, but critical evidence on the point is still lacking.

The evolutionary dilemma still stands then, albeit with these various provisos attached. Figure 2 illustrates four possible solutions. In the first, activation of cytotoxic T cells occurs only at infected tissue cells, and dendritic cells are simply not involved, whereas in the second, the reverse applies. These solutions avoid the dilemma and assume that conventional mechanisms operate with different viruses striking various kinds of balance between these two possibilities. Human immunodeficiency virus grows extensively in dendritic

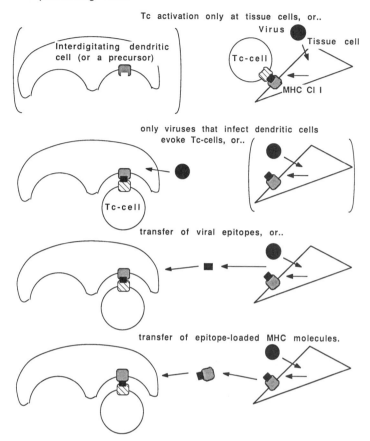

How the immune system may reconcile local loading of MHC Class I molecules with using professional antigen-presenting cells

Tc activation only at tissue cells, or..

only viruses that infect dendritic cells evoke Tc-cells, or..

transfer of viral epitopes, or..

transfer of epitope-loaded MHC molecules.

Figure 2. Four ways in which the benefits of antigen presentation by interdigitating dendritic cells might be reconciled with the local loading of MHC class I molecules. The bottom line illustrates the transfer of loaded class I molecules proposed here as a likely mechanism.

cells, whereas a more experienced virus such as influenza may have learned not to do so (Knight and Macatonia 1988). In the third possibility, viral proteins are processed in tissue cells to yield peptides able to load onto class I molecules, and these peptides then pass to dendritic cells. This has the virtue that class I molecules are known to be able to pick up exogenous peptides (Townsend et al. 1986), but it has the drawbacks that small peptides (1) might get lost on the way and (2) would be dangerous to have drifting about while activated cytotoxic T cells are on the prowl. In the fourth possibility, class I molecules load up with virus-derived epitopes in the infected cell and then pass as an entire assembly to dendritic cells.

We find this last possibility attractive. Obviously, the process of transfer might take place in various ways; for instance, transfer could take place during juxtaposition of an infected tissue cell with a dendritic cell precursor, such as the Langerhans cell of skin; or class I molecules might be shed into body fluids as a component of membrane vesicles from the infected tissue cell. Cultured spleen cells can shed in this way, because H-2 class I molecules (and class II molecules also) have been detected in supernatants in the form of particles associated with membrane lipid (Emerson and Cone 1981). Whether such particles reach the circulation is

doubtful, since rat plasma contains readily detectable class I molecules, but these are exclusively in the form of <70-kD molecules (Singh et al. 1988). Afferent lymph would be worth a look, perhaps in the sheep.

We particularly like this hypothesis because it fits so well with information that we have been accumulating about the coprocessing of alloantigens in the immune system. This is illustrated in Figure 3 and dates back to our contribution to the previous Cold Spring Harbor Symposium (Lake and Mitchison 1977). All the experiments illustrated in the figure were performed with two alloantigens (or sets of alloantigens in the case of the undefined minor histocompatibility antigens [Mhas]) that were presented to the immune system either together or on separate cells during a cell transfer. Regulatory T cells (helper T cells) recognized one alloantigen(s), and effector cells (B cells or cytotoxic T-cell precursors) recognized the other, and we found in all four experiments that the two need to be administered on the same cell in order to obtain a maximum response. Evidently, then, host-presenting cells can pick up assemblies of molecules from transferred cells, and this, we consider, lends support to the loaded-class-I-transfer hypothesis. The objection might be raised that the transferred cells themselves were doing the presenting, rather than serving as a source of antigen for other

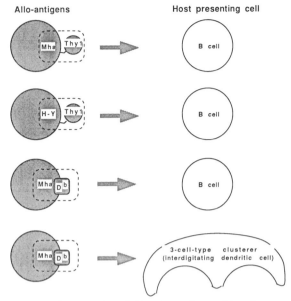

Figure 3. Coprocessing of alloantigens detected in cell transfer experiments. In each case, the antigen recognized by helper T cells is shown on the left, and the antigen recognized by effector cells (B or cytotoxic T-cell precursor) on the right. They are handled by antigen-presenting cells as a single physically linked structure, as indicated by the dashed enclosures. References: first experiment (Lake and Mitchison 1977; Lake et al. 1989); second experiment (Mitchison and Pettersson 1983); third experiment (unpubl.); fourth experiment (Mitchison 1983; Mitchison and O'Malley 1987).

presenting cells. This seems unlikely, particularly when the antigenic cells are Thy-1$^+$ thymocytes and therefore presumably MHC class II$^-$ as in the first two experiments shown in the figure. We emphasize, however, that these experiments do not directly demonstrate that donor MHC molecules are transferred to host antigen-presenting cells with donor Mhas already loaded into them. Our own restriction experiments (Mitchison and O'Malley 1987) have shown that these donor Mhas are in fact presented to host T-helper cells in the context of host class II molecules. So the model that these experiments provide for loaded-class-I-transfer is only indirect; what they do establish is that chunks that include membrane glycoproteins can pass from cell to cell.

The present position, then, is that a transfer mechanism has considerable attraction as a means of resolving the conflicting needs of local class I loading and of specialized presentation. It is not entirely clear that such a mechanism is required; nor is it clear how it might work. Our hypothesis has the merit of making clear-cut predictions that could fairly easily be tested by means, for instance, of class-I-restricted H-Y-specific T-cell clones.

Do Antigen-presenting Cells in the Thymus Load Their MHC Class II Molecules in the Normal Way?

We have attempted to classify self-proteins into three groups: *high concentration*, those that induce self-toler-

ance in both B and helper T cells; *intermediate concentration*, those that induce self-tolerance in helper T cells but not in B cells; and *low concentration*, those that induce self-tolerance in neither cell (Mitchison 1985; Griffiths et al. 1987). In this classification, "concentration" refers loosely to the effective concentration in the vicinity of the lymphocyte, and not to any absolute value in body fluids. Hemoglobin (Reichlin 1972; Howard and Mitchison 1975) is one of the oldest-established members of the first group, although its concentration in normal plasma is very low (presumably B cells are exposed to higher concentrations of hemoglobin in local regions of erythrocyte damage).

More recently, a similar question about effective concentration has begun to be asked, but from a different point of view: Do MHC class II molecules become charged with epitopes of self-proteins under normal conditions? Thus, in the case of F liver protein, for instance, the question has been asked whether freshly isolated antigen-presenting cells hold enough F-derived epitopes in their class II molecules to enable them to stimulate proliferation of T cells primed against F. For this purpose, it is necessary to prime T cells by some stratagem, such as using a mouse that is defective or variant for the protein in question.

Information can now be lined up for the first three proteins that have been scrutinized from both points of view, namely, F liver protein, C5, and hemoglobin. The first two both tolerize helper T cells but not B cells, and therefore belong to the intermediate-concentration group (Harris et al. 1982; Griffiths et al. 1987). Hemoglobin, as mentioned above, tolerizes both types of cells. Neither of the first two normally charges class II molecules to a detectable extent (Winchester et al. 1984; Lin and Stockinger 1989), whereas hemoglobin does so (Lorenz and Allen 1988). Thus, the agreement is good, on the basis of this tiny sample.

The failure of these intermediate-concentration self-proteins to charge class II molecules in this way raises an interesting problem: How is self-tolerance achieved during the normal maturation of T cells in the thymus? If not enough protein gets into class II molecules to stimulate primed T cells, surely it must be even more difficult for antigen-presenting cells of the thymus to fulfill their task of negatively selecting unprimed T cells so as to achieve self-tolerance.

This difficulty does not so far arise for "high-concentration" proteins. As for class I molecules, the position is unclear. In a sense, all known self-molecules that can stimulate cytotoxic T cells, such as H-Y or the Mhas, belong to the "high-concentration" category, even though they cannot be detected in body fluids, because they induce self-tolerance in B cells in the few instances where this has been tested and are detectable on normal antigen-presenting cells. However, a strong ascertainment bias is at work here, and if we knew how to detect self-proteins that do not normally charge class I molecules, we might well be able to find them. A reasonable approach would be to look for novel class-I-restricted responses against cells manipulated so as to overexpress a self-nucleoprotein.

The "peptidic self" hypothesis, as we understand it, solves this problem by postulating unusual properties in the antigen-presenting cells of the thymus: They are unusually good at expressing self-peptides (for class I presentation) and at collecting self-proteins (for class II presentation) (Kourilsky et al. 1987). Right or wrong, these ideas have the virtue of being testable, for instance, by exposing organ cultures of thymus to F protein and looking for induction of tolerance.

Can Membrane Glycoproteins Transduce Signals by Perturbing Locally a Phosphorylation Equilibrium?

This question is prompted by recent studies on the CD45 (T200 or LCA) glycoprotein of man, rats, and mice (and presumably other mammals). This molecule has attracted interest because of its unique cytoplasmic domain and also because its isoforms mark subpopulations of T cells. In this section, we deal with the first topic, and in the next, with the second. Previous studies in man (Merkenschlager et al. 1988) and rat (Arthur and Mason 1986; Powrie and Mason 1989) prompted us to study CD45 on mouse T cells (Dexter et al. 1987; Marvel and Mayer 1988), and this field is now expanding (Bottomly 1988). For this purpose, we used three monoclonal antibodies from the American Type Culture Collection, RA3-3A1, RA3-2C2, and 14.8 directed against CD45R, and one monoclonal antibody, M1-93, that recognizes all the isoforms and is therefore directed against CD45. The three CD45R monoclonals immunoprecipitate the two largest isoforms (220, 205 kD), therefore recognize the membrane-distal A segment, and are consequently designated as specific for "CD45RA" in conformity with the new human nomenclature (Johnson et al. 1989). Each of the three can block one another's binding and therefore recognize adjacent epitopes. RA3-3A1 is particularly useful for immunoprecipitation, whereas the other two stain and stimulate T cells well, with RA3-2C2 slightly the better in this respect. The ensuing discussion refers to data obtained only with RA3-2C2.

Our first study of freshly isolated mouse T cells used a fluorescence analyzer equipped with a mercury arc, which revealed $<10\%$ of mouse mature T cells as $CD45R^+$ (Dexter et al. 1987; Marvel and Mayer 1988). This low figure was suspect, since the same antibody stimulated T cells to proliferate rather effectively when used in synergy with suboptimal doses of phytohemagglutinin. In more recent studies, we have used an analyzer equipped with a laser (Becton Dickinson Facscan), and this yields an overall figure for mouse spleen T cells of $\sim 20\%$ CD45RA$^+$, with a slightly higher frequency in the CD8 than the CD4 populations, but with both having unequivocally positive cells. T cells stain less brightly than B cells, and it is likely that a fraction greater than 20% express some CD45RA molecules.

This antibody, when applied on its own to B-depleted mouse spleen cells, induces only a low proliferative response but synergizes well with a suboptimal dose of phytohemagglutinin. Cell depletion studies and supplementation with lymphokines indicate that this

synergistic C45RA-mediated response utilizes (1) the adherent cell stimulation pathway and (2) the IL-2/IL-2R pathway (Marvel et al. 1989). There is nothing unusual in this; what is of greater interest is the antagonism between the CD45 signal and the CD3 signal.

Attention was drawn to this interaction by studies on human CD45 that showed (1) that within its large cytoplasmic domain this molecule has two consensus tyrosine phosphatase sequences (Tonks et al. 1988), (2) that this domain is in fact active as a tyrosine phosphatase (Charbonneau et al. 1988), and (3) that cross-linking via antibodies plus avidin of this phosphatase with the known tyrosine-phosphatase inducer CD3 silences the signal otherwise transduced by the latter molecule (Ledbetter et al. 1988).

We now report that we have verified this finding for the mouse T cell, using essentially the same methods as those used previously for human T cells. A biotinylated monoclonal antibody to CD3 could induce a Ca^{++} flux when tested in the presence of avidin and a non-biotinylated antibody to CD45. When the CD45 antibody was itself biotinylated, so that under the same conditions the CD3 and CD45 molecules became cross-linked, the flux was inhibited.

This finding leads us to postulate the signaling mechanism illustrated in Figure 4. This mechanism could operate when either a phosphatase or the corresponding kinase becomes aggregated at the cell–cell contact region as a result of binding to a ligand on the opposite cell. This would locally perturb the equilibrium level of phosphorylation, and that could initiate a signal. Note that no conformational change is involved nor any "switching on " of individual molecules; what matters is the behavior of populations of glycoproteins in relation to one another.

It is too early to gauge how important a mechanism of signal transduction this may be. Possibly it operates only as a secondary mechanism to modulate signals

Signal transduction without conformational change: aggregation of a transmembrane protein might locally perturb the equilibrium between a phosphokinase and a phosphatase

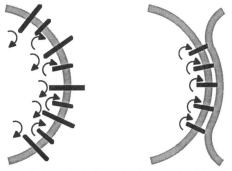

Figure 4. A hypothetical mechanism of signal-transduction operative with CD45 and CD3. In an unperturbed lymphocyte on the left, the larger CD45 molecules intermingle with smaller CD3 molecules and thus establish an equilibrium level of phosphorylation. On the right, ligand-induced aggregation of CD3 takes place at a cell–cell interface, and the level of phosphorylation rises locally. This is read by the lymphocyte as a signal for activation.

transduced by the more conventional mechanism of conformational change. We simply do not know, and we shall be unlikely to find out until events at the cell–cell interface in physiological interactions have been worked out in detail: a tough task, but worthwhile.

Do Most Cells in the Thymus (the Majority of the CD4CD8 Double-positive Population) Have the Phenotype of a Doomed Cell?

Most of the interest in CD45 as a marker has centered on the transition from C45RA to CD45RO (i.e., from expression of the larger isoforms to the smallest) that accompanies the activation of human and rat T cells (Merkenschlager et al. 1988; Powrie and Mason 1989). We have not yet studied this transition in the mouse, having been delayed while trying to separate CD45RA cells. Functional differences between CD45RA and CD45RO subpopulations have also attracted some interest, but the subject has become confused because of the difficulty of sorting out activation (or "memory") versus function: For a recent discussion of this vexed topic see our recent review (Mitchison 1988).

So far, the most interesting findings with the marker have been made in the thymus. In both man and mouse, the majority of thymic lymphocytes are CD45RO, an apparent paradox insofar as virgin T cells emerging from the thymus in man are believed to express CD45RA and to become CD45RO only upon activation as described above. Do developing T cells undergo a series of changes in phenotype, or can a minor linkage of CD45RA cells be traced all the way through the processes of maturation and selection in the thymus? This question is posed in Figure 5 and is further discussed below in the light of our present information about the mouse thymus. Much the same question can be posed for the human thymus, where a recent study opts for the second hypothesis (minor lineage) on the basis of information of a somewhat different nature from ours (Pilarski et al. 1989). The great advantage of the mouse lies in the opportunity it provides for recolonization experiments, such as can be performed with the Owen-Jenkinson culture system (Dexter et al. 1987).

We have three kinds of data, one of which is derived from three-color fluorimetric analysis using CD4, CD8, and CD45RA as markers. This establishes that the CD4CD8 double negatives, which make up the earliest population in the thymus, express the CD45RA phenotype, as also does the single-positive (CD4 or CD8) mature thymic emigrant population. The intermediate population of CD4CD8 double-positive cells, which includes most cells in the thymus, is CD45RA$^-$ (CD45RO). This summary is subject to two major provisos. Neither the double negatives nor the single positives are uniformly CD45RA$^+$; in each case, only 10–20% score as positive under our conditions of examination, and these grade into the negatives without

bimodality. Among the single positives only the CD8$^+$ display this phenotype, whereas the CD4$^+$ are $<1\%$ CD45RA$^+$.

Our second source of data is recolonization experiments with thymus subpopulations. Like other investigators, we find that only CD4CD8 double-negative cells can repopulate a thymic lobe in culture, and we find that separation experiments with CD45RA monoclonal antibodies when performed on the total thymic cell population do not yield meaningful information. However, by starting with a population that has been depleted of CD4 and CD8 cells (CD4CD8 double negatives), meaningful separations can be performed with CD45RA monoclonal antibody. Panning on this antibody yields populations enriched or depleted for expression of the molecule, and the former repopulates $\sim$ tenfold better and the latter $\sim$ tenfold worse than the unfractionated CD4CD8-depleted population. This finding is a relief to us, because it removes some of our concern that the CD45RA$^+$ fraction within the CD4CD8 double-negative population may be too small to be meaningful.

Our third source of data is phenotyping performed by our colleague David Andrew with his new 95K marker "STB1" (Andrew 1989). This marker has a somewhat different distribution to S7 (Gulley et al. 1988), but the two monoclonals may nevertheless recognize different epitopes on the same glycoprotein. The glycoprotein has a size near to that of Ly-24 (Trowbridge 1986) but has a distribution so different that we think they must be different molecules. Within the thymus, the distribution of STB1 has features in common with that of CD45RA. The CD4CD8 double negatives and single positives both express high levels of STB1, with $\sim$95% of cells staining brightly. The CD4CD8 double positives express low levels, with a tailing, non-bimodal distribution.

Our interpretation of these data starts from the discovery made by our colleague Laurie Smith that CD4 single-positive, mature T cells are derived from CD4CD8 double-positive precursors (Smith 1987). This conclusion has been confirmed by other workers, albeit grudgingly (Fowlkes et al. 1988). The double positives are themselves derived from the double-negative stem-cell population that alone has the capacity to regenerate a normal thymic population, possibly with an intermediate stage at which they turn on expression of CD8 before that of CD4 (Crispe and Bevan 1987). With this background understanding of lineage, we can now formulate in detail the two hypotheses illustrated in Figure 5. On the left, the lineage runs through cells with a phenotype characteristic of most of the CD4CD8 double positives, i.e., the majority phenotype. Two shifts in phenotype occur; one from that of the double-negative stem cells, and then another back to that of the single-positive mature cells. On the right, the lineage runs through a minor fraction of the CD4CD8 double-positive population that has the same phenotype, with respect to CD45RA and STB1, as the stem and mature cells, and no shift occurs in this line-

PHENOTYPE-SHARING BETWEEN THYMIC STEM-CELLS (DOUBLE NEGATIVE) AND MATURE THYMIC EMIGRANT T CELLS (SINGLE POSITIVE)

Phenotype is shared in this way for (i) CD45RA (with provisos), and (ii) p95 (STB1, ?=S7, ??=Ly-24).

Hypothesis 1
Two phenotype shifts, on pathway to mature T cells

Hypothesis 2
One phenotype shift, on pathway to death

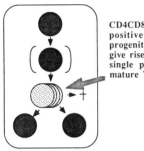
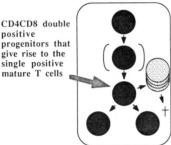

CD4CD8 double positive progenitors that give rise to the single positive mature T cells

Figure 5. Lineages in the thymus. Differentiation from a CD4CD8 double-negative stem cell, possibly via a CD8 single-positive cell, to a CD4CD8 double-positive cell (this population is split into a minor and a major fraction according to hypothesis 2) and thence to mature single-positive emigrant T cells. Cell death is indicated by a cross.

age. The latter hypothesis is attractively simple, but we have no direct evidence of the existence of such a minor population. A straightforward extension of this hypothesis is that the majority phenotype (CD45RA⁻, STB1-low) is acquired when the double positives fail selection (either positive or negative selection) and become doomed to die. These cells continue to cycle, so this extension leads us to postulate a curiously slow process of apoptosis: a jolly death, with plenty of opportunity to reproduce beforehand.

SUMMARY

1. Co-processing of alloantigens suggests that epitope-loaded MHC class I molecules may pass from tissue cells to dendritic cells.
2. Antigen-presenting cells in the thymus need some special trick in order to load their MHC class II molecules with epitopes from "intermediate concentration" self-proteins in order to induce self-tolerance in developing cells.
3. Cell–cell interactions may transmit signals simply by rearranging surface glycoproteins and thus locally perturbing a phosphorylation equilibrium.
4. The CD45 and STB1 phenotype of most cells in the thymus may be characteristic of a doomed cell.

REFERENCES

Andrew, D. 1989. STB1, a mouse lymphocyte marker as found on T cell and B cell sub-populations. *Cell. Immunol.* (in press).

Arthur, R.P. and D. Mason. 1986. T cells that help B cell responses to soluble antigen are distinguishable from those producing interleukin 2 on mitogenic or allogeneic stimulation. *J. Exp. Med.* **163:** 774.

Breel, M., R.E. Mebius, and G. Kraal. 1987. Dendritic cells of the mouse recognised by two monoclonal antibodies. *Eur. J. Immunol.* **17:** 1555.

Bottomly, K. 1988. A functional dichotomy in CD4⁺ T lymphocytes. *Immunol. Today* **9:** 268.

Braciale, T.J., L.A. Morrison, M.T. Sweetser, J. Sambrook, M.J. Gething, and V.L. Braciale. 1987. Antigen presentation pathways to class I and class II MHC-restricted T lymphocytes. *Immunol. Rev.* **98:** 95.

Chain, B.J., N.A. Mitchison, T.J. Mitchison, D.H. Davies, and J. Marcinkiewicz. 1989. Antigen processing: Current issues, exceptional cases (Thy 1 alloantigen, MHC class II-restricted cytolytic T cells) and implications for vaccine development. *J. Autoimmun.* (suppl.) **2:** 45.

Charbonneau, H., N.K. Tonks, K.A. Walsh, and E.H. Fischer. 1988. The leukocyte common antigen (CD45: A putative receptor-linked protein tyrosine phosphatase. *Proc. Natl. Acad. Sci.* **85:** 7182.

Crispe, I.N. and M.J. Bevan. 1987. Expression and functional significance of the Jlld marker on mouse thymocytes. *J. Immunol.* **138:** 2013.

Dexter, M., J. Marvel, M. Merkenschlager, N.A. Mitchison, D. Oliveira, C. O'Malley, L. Smith, L. Terry, and E. Timms. 1987. Progress in T cell biology. *Immunol. Lett.* **16:** 171.

Emerson, S.G. and R.E. Cone. 1981. I-Kᵏ and H-2Kᵏ antigens are shed as supramolecular particles in association with membrane lipids. *J. Immunol.* **127:** 482.

Fowlkes, B.J., R.H. Schwartz, and D.M. Pardoll. 1988. Deletion of self-reactive thymocytes occurs at a CD4⁺8⁺ precursor stage. *Nature* **334:** 620.

Griffiths, J.A., N.A. Mitchison, N. Nardi, and D.B.G. Oliveira. 1987. F protein. In *Immunogenicity of protein antigens: Repertoire and regulation* (ed. E. Sercarz and J. Berzofsky), vol. 2, p. 35. CRC Press, Boca Raton.

Gulley, M.L., L.C. Ogata, J.A. Thorson, M.O. Dailey, and J.D. Kemp. 1988. Identification of a murine pan-T cell antigen which is also expressed during the terminal phases of B cell differentiation. *J. Immunol.* **140:** 3751.

Harris, D.E., L. Cairns, F.S. Rosen, and Y. Borel. 1982. A natural model of immunologic tolerance. Tolerance to murine C5 is mediated by T cells, and antigen is required to maintain unresponsiveness. *J. Exp. Med.* **156:** 567.

Hengel, H., M. Lindner, H. Wagner, and K. Heeg. 1987. Frequency of herpes simplex virus-specific murine cytotoxic T lymphocyte precursors in mitogen and antigen-driven primary in vitro T-cell responses. *J. Immunol.* **139:** 4196.

Howard, J.G. and N.A. Mitchison. 1975. Immunological tolerance. *Prog. Allergy* **18:** 43.

Johnson, P., L. Greenbaum, K. Bottomly, and I.S. Trowbridge. 1989. Identification of the alternatively spliced exons of murine CD45 (T200) required for reactivity with B220 and other T200-restricted antibodies. *J. Exp. Med.* **169:** 1179.

Kast, W.M., C.J.P. Boog, B.O. Roep, A.C. Voordouw, and C.J.M. Melief. 1988. Failure or success in the restoration of virus-specific cytotoxic T lymphocyte response defects by dendritic cells. *J. Immunol.* **146:** 3186.

Knight, S.C. and S.E. Macatonia. 1988. Dendritic cells and viruses. *Immunol. Lett.* **19:** 177.

Koide, S. and R.M. Steinman. 1987. Induction of murine interleukin 1: Stimuli and responsive primary cells. *Proc. Natl. Acad. Sci.* **84:** 3802.

Kourilsky, P., G. Chaouat, C. Rabourdin-Combe, and J.M. Claverie. 1987. Working principles in the immune system implied by the "peptidic self" model. *Proc. Natl. Acad. Sci.* **84:** 3400.

Lake, P. and N.A. Mitchison. 1977. Regulatory mechanisms in the immune response to cell surface antigens. *Cold Spring Harbor Symp. Quant. Biol.* **41:** 589.

Lake, P., N.A. Mitchison, E.A. Clark, M. Khorshidi, I.

Nakashima, J.S. Bromberg, M.R. Brunswick, T. Szensky, K.B. Sainis, G.H. Sunshine, L. Favilla-Castillo, J.N. Woody, and D. Lebwohl. 1989. The regulation of antibody responses to antigens of the cell surface: Studies with Thy-1 H-2 antigens. In *Cell surface antigen Thy-1: Immunology, neurology and therapeutic applications* (ed. A.E. Reif and M. Schlesinger), p. 367. Marcel Dekker, New York.

Lin, R.H. and B. Stockinger. 1989. T cell immunity or tolerance as a consequence of self antigen presentation. *Eur. J. Immunol.* **19:** 105.

Ledbetter, J.A., N.K. Tonks, E.H. Fischer, and E.A. Clark. 1988. CD45 regulates signal transduction and lymphocyte activation by specific association with receptor molecules on T or B cells. *Proc. Natl. Acad. Sci.* **85:** 8628.

Lorenz, R.G. and P.M. Allen. 1988. Direct evidence for functional self-protein/Ia molecule complexes in vivo. *Proc. Natl. Acad. Sci.* **85:** 5220.

Macatonia, S.E., P.M. Taylor, S.C. Knight, and B.A. Askonas. 1989. Primary stimulation by dendritic cells induces antiviral proliferative and cytotoxic T cell responses in vitro. *J. Exp. Med.* **169:** 1255.

Marvel, J. and A. Mayer. 1988. CD45R gives immunofluorescence and transduced signals on mouse T cells. *Eur. J. Immunol.* **18:** 825.

Marvel, J., G. Poirier, and E. Lightstone. 1989. Anti-CD45RA antibodies increase the proliferation of mouse T cells to PHA through the IL-2/IL-2R pathway. *Eur. J. Immunol.* (in press).

Merkenschlager, M., L. Terry, R. Edwards, and P.C.L. Beverley. 1988. Limiting dilution analysis of proliferative responses in human lymphocyte populations defined by the monoclonal antibody UCHL1: Implications for differential CD45 expression in T cell memory formation. *Eur. J. Immunol.* **18:** 1653.

Mitchison, N.A. 1983. Linked help in the cytotoxic T cell response revealed by adoptive transfer. *Transplant. Proc.* **15:** 2121.

———. 1985. Four intermediate concentration proteins and their message for self-tolerance, autoimmunity, and suppressor epitopes. *Clin. Immunol. Newslett.* **6:** 12.

———. 1988. Suppressor activity as a composite property. *Scand. J. Immunol.* **28:** 271.

———. 1989. T cells in transplantation immunity. *Immunol. Lett.* **21:** 15.

Mitchison, N.A. and C. O'Malley. 1987. Three cell type clusters of T-cells with antigen presenting cells best explain the epitope linkage and non-cognate requirements of the in vivo cytolytic response. *Eur. J. Immunol.* **17:** 579.

Mitchison, N.A. and S. Pettersson. 1983. Does clonal selection occur among T cells? *Ann. Immunol. Inst. Pasteur.* **134D:** 37.

Pilarski, L.M., R. Gillitzer, H. Zohr, K. Shortman, and R. Scollay. 1989. Definition of the thymic generative lineage by selective expression of high molecular weight isoforms of CD45 (T200). *Eur. J. Immunol.* **19:** 589.

Powrie, F. and D. Mason. 1989. The MRC Ox-22⁻CD4⁺ T cells that help B cells in secondary immune responses derive from naive precursors with the MRCDx-22⁺CD4⁺ phenotype. *J. Exp. Med.* **169:** 653.

Reichlin, M. 1972. Localising antigenic determinants in human haemoglobin with mutants. Molecular correlations of immunological tolerance. *J. Mol. Biol.* **64:** 485.

Singh, P.B., R.E. Brown, and B. Roser. 1988. Class I transplantation antigens in solution in body fluids and in the urine. Individuality signals to the environment. *J. Exp. Med.* **168:** 195.

Smith, L. 1987. CD4⁺ murine T cells develop from CD8⁺ precursors *in vivo. Nature* **326:** 798.

Tonks, N.K., H. Charbonneau, C.D. Diltz, E.D. Fischer, and K.A. Walsh. 1988. Demonstration that the leucocyte common antigen CD45 is a protein tyrosine phosphatase. *Biochemistry* **27:** 8695.

Townsend, A.R.M., F.M. Gotch, and J. Davey. 1985. Cytotoxic T cells recognise fragments of influenza nucleoprotein. *Cell* **42:** 457.

Townsend, A.R.M., J.B. Rothbard, F.M. Gotch, G. Bahadur, D.C. Wraith, and A.J. McMichael. 1986. The epitopes of influenza nucleoprotein recognized by cytotoxic T lymphocytes can be defined with short synthetic peptides. *Cell* **44:** 959.

Trowbridge, I.S. 1986. Cell surface receptors and differentiation. In *Receptors in recognition and developmental processes* (ed. R.M. Gorczynski), p. 267. Academic Press, New York.

Vitetta, E.S., R. Fernandez-Botran, C.D. Myers, and V.M. Sanders. 1987. Cellular interactions in the humoral immune response. *Adv. Immunol.* **45:** 1.

Winchester, G., G.H. Sunshine, N. Nardi, and N.A. Mitchison. 1984. Antigen presenting cells do not discriminate between self and non-self. *Immunogenetics* **19:** 487.

Studies on the Leukocyte-common Antigen: Structure, Function, and Evolutionary Conservation

R.J. Matthews, J.T. Pingel, C.M. Meyer, and M.L. Thomas

Department of Pathology, Washington University School of Medicine, St. Louis, Missouri 63110

The leukocyte-common antigen (L-CA, CD45) is a family of large-molecular-weight glycoproteins expressed on the surface of all cells of hematopoietic origin except erythrocytes and platelets. The function of this family of molecules has not been well understood; however, studies using antibodies against L-CA have implicated the family in lymphocyte activation and proliferation (for review, see Thomas 1989). We recently developed a mouse T-cell clone that is deficient in the surface expression of L-CA (Pingel and Thomas 1989). This clone is impaired in certain aspects of proliferation, implicating L-CA in the regulation of lymphocyte cell division. Here, we correlate our functional studies with our previous results on the structure of the L-CA family and present a model to account for these results.

Leukocyte-common Antigen Structure

The L-CA glycoprotein consists of a heavily glycosylated, amino-terminal external domain, a single-membrane-spanning region, and a large cytoplasmic domain. L-CA is encoded by a single structural gene located in a region that is syntenic between humans and mice and is on chromosome 1 for both species (Ralph et al. 1987; Hall et al. 1988; Saga et al. 1988; Johnson et al. 1989). The family is generated by differential splicing of three consecutive exons, which results in a potential for eight different mRNAs; six of these have been isolated as cDNAs (Barclay et al. 1987; Ralph et al. 1987; Saga et al. 1987; Streuli et al. 1987; Thomas et al. 1987; Jackson and Barclay 1989). The differential splicing events are precisely controlled through cell lineage differentiation and cellular activation, and these steps are conserved through mammalian evolution. The immediate amino-terminal region of the mature glycoprotein is encoded by six exons, 3–8, and encodes potential O-linked carbohydrate sites. Exons 4–6 are the differentially spliced exons; each encodes approximately 50 amino acids. Therefore, different leukocytes are controlling the O-linked carbohydrate region of L-CA by using exons 4–6 as developmental cassettes to add or delete potential O-linked carbohydrate sites. Since L-CA is an abundant cell-surface molecule, the differential splicing may greatly alter the types and amounts of carbohydrate presented by different leukocytes.

The remaining portion of the external domain is encoded by exons 9–15 and encodes approximately 300 amino acids. This area can be divided into three separate regions: two distinct cysteine clusters and a short spacer region. The cysteine clusters presumably represent separate domains, and it is possible that the second cluster may be divided into two further subdomains. A schematic representation of the external domain of humans, mice, and rats is shown in Figure 1. The locations of the cysteine residues are conserved, as are many of the sites of potential N-linked carbohydrates.

The cytoplasmic domain of L-CA is approximately 700 amino acids in length and is encoded by exons 17–33. It contains two tandem homologous domains, each of approximately 300 amino acids, as evidenced by both protein sequence homologies and genomic structure. The two subdomains are approximately 35% homologous. Recently, Charbonneau et al. (1988) reported a sequence of a protein tyrosine phosphatase, PTPase 1b, isolated from human placenta and presumably cytoplasmic, and noted the homology of PTPase 1b to each of the cytoplasmic subdomains of L-CA. This group confirmed this observation by showing that L-CA has tyrosine phosphatase activity (Tonks et al. 1988). Streuli et al. (1988) described another membrane protein, LAR, whose distribution, unlike L-CA, is not restricted to cells of hematopoietic origin. The cytoplasmic domain of LAR is similar to L-CA and also consists of two subdomains. The two cytoplasmic subdomains of L-CA and LAR as well as PTP 1b all share approximately 35% homology (Fig. 2), and each presumably is a tyrosine phosphatase with distinct regulation and substrate specificity. This finding suggests that L-CA is part of a larger family of tyrosine phosphatases important in the regulation of cell growth.

Conservation through Vertebrate Evolution of the L-CA Tyrosine Phosphatase Domain

Comparison of human, mouse, and rat L-CA protein sequence shows that the overall homology for the external domain is very low with only approximately 35% of the residues identical. In contrast, sequence comparison for cytoplasmic domain shows a remarkable degree of conservation; 85% identical residues and over 90% when accounting for conservative replacements. This observation was extended into other vertebrates. Southern blot analysis identifies fragments from other vertebrate species that hybridize to a probe containing sequence for the cytoplasmic domain of

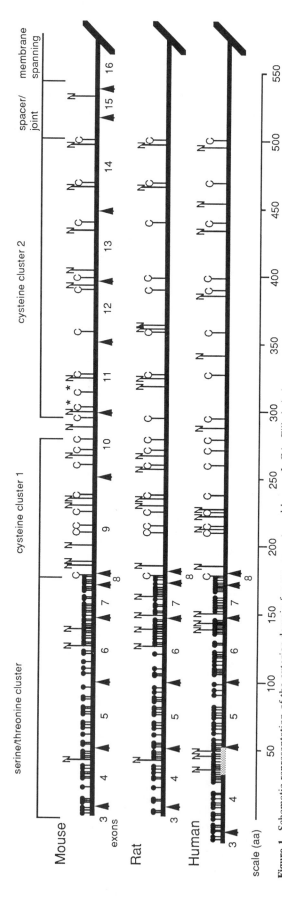

Figure 1. Schematic representation of the exterior domain for mouse, rat, and human L-CA. Filled circles represent positions of serine/threonines in the O-linked glycosylation region, N represents sites of N-linked glycosylation, C represents cysteine residues, and asterisks denote the cysteine residues only found in the mouse sequence. Arrows designate exon/exon junctions. The scale is in amino acids.

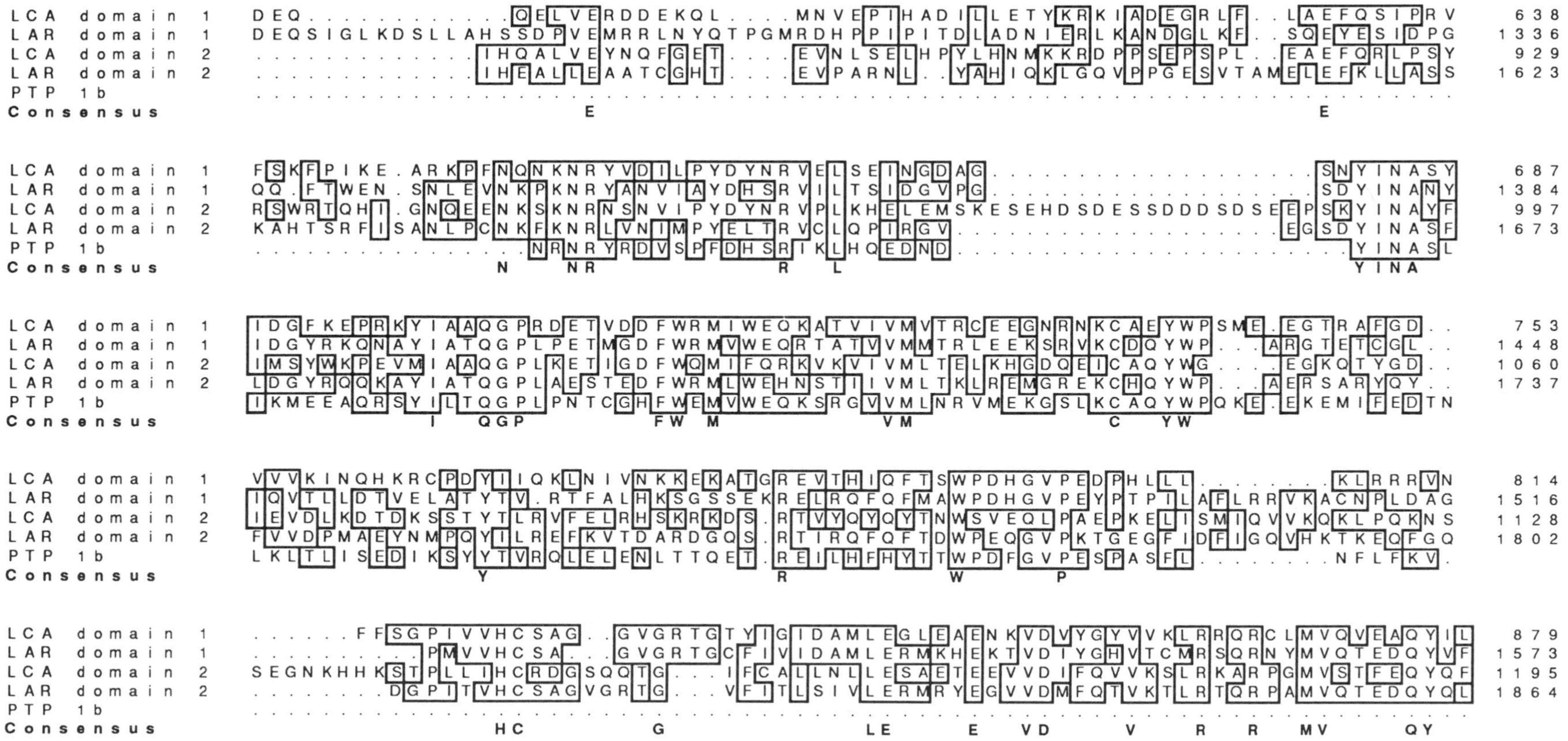

Figure 2. Sequence comparison of the two putative tyrosine phosphatase domains for human L-CA and LAR and the single domain of PTPase 1b. Identical residues are boxed, and the single-letter amino acid code is used. Numbers designate the position in the mature protein of the amino acid. Sequences are from L-CA (Ralph et al. 1987); LAR (Streuli et al. 1988), and PTPase 1b (Charbonneau et al. 1988).

human L-CA. Figure 3A shows a Southern blot for mouse and green iguana (*Iguana iguana*) genomic DNA hybridized to pHLC-1 (Ralph et al. 1987). The filter was washed under stringent conditions (52°C in $0.1 \times SSC$, 0.1% SDS), thus indicating that the fragments that hybridized do encode L-CA sequence rather than other tyrosine phosphatases. This result was confirmed by sequence analysis. Oligos were derived for the boundaries of human exon 25 and used to prime green iguana genomic DNA in a polymerase chain reaction. The sequence was determined for the amplified fragment and is shown in Figure 3B. There were three changes between human and green iguana. Two of these are conservative replacements; the sequence is much more closely related to human L-CA than any other known tyrosine phosphatase, thus indicating that the sequence is derived from green iguana L-CA. It appears likely, therefore, that the sequence of the L-CA tyrosine phosphatase domain is highly conserved throughout vertebrate evolution. This implies that the interactions of the domain are under tight evolutionary constraint and emphasizes the importance of the tyrosine phosphatase activity.

Analysis of an L-CA-defective T-lymphocyte Clone

To investigate L-CA function, we derived from the A.E7 mouse T-helper-cell clone subclones that were deficient in the expression of surface L-CA. We recently reported these observations, and just a synopsis is presented here (Pingel and Thomas 1989). The A.E7 clone is CD4[+], I-E[k]-restricted, and specific for pigeon cytochrome *c* (Matis et al. 1983). The L-CA-deficient subclones (L-CA[−]) were derived by mutagenizing A.E7 cells with N-methyl-N'-nitro-nitrosoguanidine and selecting for cells lacking surface L-CA by treating with I3/2.3, an antibody directed against a common determinant on L-CA, and rabbit complement. Cells that failed to express surface L-CA were isolated by limiting dilution. These cells were completely negative for L-CA, as determined by flow cytometry analysis (Fig. 4A) and surface-labeled immunoprecipitation.

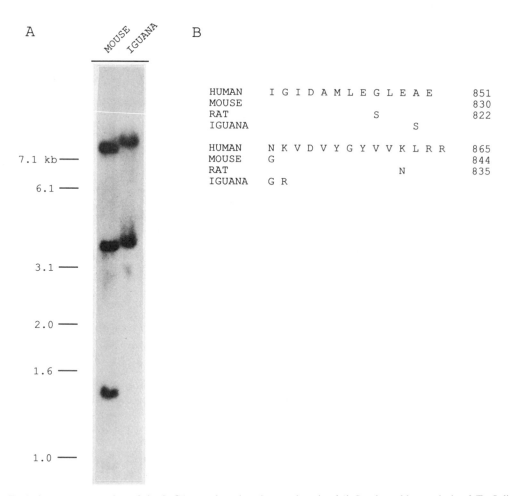

Figure 3. Evolutionary conservation of the L-CA tyrosine phosphatase domain. (*A*) Southern blot analysis of *Taq*I-digested mouse and green iguana genomic DNA hybridized with human pHLC-1 cDNA. (*B*) Protein sequence of exon 25 for human, mouse, rat, and green iguana. The single amino acid code is used. Only amino acid substitutions are shown, otherwise, sequences are identical to the human sequence.

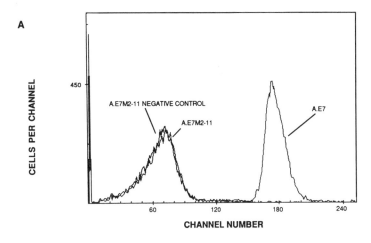

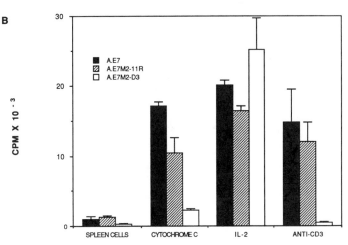

Figure 4. Analysis of L-CA-deficient T-cell clone. (*A*) Flow cytometry of the parent, A.E7 clone, and the L-CA-deficient A.E7M2-11 clone, stained with I3/2.3 antibody (Trowbridge 1978) and fluoresceinated secondary antibody. The negative control was A.E7M2-11 stained with secondary antibody alone. (*B*) [^{3}H]Thymidine incorporation of A.E7, A.E7M2-D3 (L-CA-deficient), and the revertant A.E7M2-11R, stimulated with either spleen cells, cytochrome *c*, 5% supernatants from phorbol-ester-stimulated EL4 cells or anti-CD3. Incorporation was measured 72 hr poststimulation from a 24-hr pulse.

However, the subclones did express normal size mRNA, and when labeled biosynthetically, a protein could be detected by immunoprecipitation. Examination of other cell-surface molecules by flow cytometry revealed no apparent defect. The T-cell antigen receptor (TCR), CD3, CD4, IL-2 receptor, LFA-1, Thy-1, and Pgp-1 (CD44) were all expressed. Therefore, the defect appears to be specific for L-CA and affects the proper processing of the molecule that allows surface expression.

The L-CA$^-$ cells were unusual in several aspects. They tended to be larger and more spherical, and there appeared to be more cell death in these cultures, as evidenced by more cellular debris and a much slower growth rate than the parent. The number of cells obtained at the end of biweekly passages was at least fourfold less for the L-CA$^-$ cultures than for the parent clone. The abnormally slow growth rate was examined in more detail and is shown for the L-CA$^-$ clone, A.E7M2-D3, in Figure 4B. Proliferation induced by 100 μg/ml antigen in the presence of irradiated syngeneic spleen cells leads to a burst of proliferation in the L-CA$^+$ A.E7 parent line, as measured by [^{3}H]thymidine incorporation at day 3 poststimulation; little, if any, proliferation is seen with the A.E7 L-CA$^-$

subclone. In five separate experiments, the proliferation of the mutant clones was less than 10% of the response of the parent. Similarly, unlike the parent clone, L-CA$^-$ cells failed to proliferate in response to anti-CD3, even though both the parent and the mutant express CD3 in approximately equivalent amounts. In the experiment shown in Figure 4B, 2 μg/ml anti-CD3 was used to precoat wells, and proliferation was measured at 72 hours. In contrast, the L-CA$^-$ clones would proliferate in response to IL-2, either recombinant IL-2 or in the form of 5% supernatants from phorbol-myristate-acetate-stimulated EL4 cells, as shown in Figure 4B. The response, however, of the L-CA$^-$ cells to IL-2 was usually somewhat diminished; in five separate experiments, the average response of the mutant cells was 75% of the response of the parent.

A spontaneous revertant, A.E7-M2-11R, was obtained that expressed L-CA in equivalent amounts to the parent. The revertant regained the ability to respond to antigen and anti-CD3 and proliferated as well as the parent in response to IL-2 (Fig. 4B). Since a double revertant for two separate mutations is an unlikely event, the ability of the revertant cells to proliferate in response to antigen or anti-CD3 is most likely due to reexpression of L-CA.

Potential Modes of Action of the L-CA Family

The L-CA family is generated by differential splicing of three exons leading to forms that differ in their amino-terminal region and resulting in variation of potential O-linked carbohydrate sites. The different family members are presented in cartoon form in Figure 5A. The data from the analysis of L-CA⁻ T-cell clones indicate that the expression of surface L-CA is required for antigen-induced proliferation and suggest that the requirement is the dephosphorylation of a critical tyrosine residue.

Presumably, interactions of the external domain lead to the activation of the tyrosine phosphatase domain,

and the tyrosine phosphatase domain is brought into close proximity to potential substrates. A possible model to account for the structural and functional activity of L-CA is presented in Figure 5B. The main points of the model are that interactions of the external domain with specific ligands, such as cell-bound lectins, leads to activation of the tyrosine phosphatase domain and relocalization such that the phosphatase may interact with potential substrates. The expression of different variable exons may dictate which cells activate various leukocyte populations. Although the variable exons encode potential O-linked carbohydrate sites, they are not necessarily glycosylated differently. Expression of different exons may cause different sets of

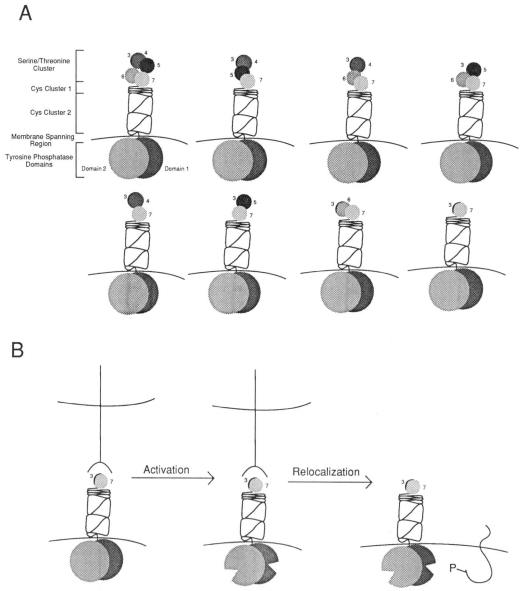

Figure 5. Model of L-CA and potential interactions with other molecules. (*A*) Cartoon of L-CA family members. The numbers represent the exons encoding the O-linked carbohydrate region. Exons 4, 5, and 6 are differentially spliced. (*B*) Binding of L-CA with other cell-surface molecules. Binding leads to activation of the tyrosine phosphatase domains and relocalization with potential tyrosine phosphatase substrates.

surface lectins to be recognized by the spatial arrangement of the carbohydrates, or the interactions may be a combination of both N- and O-linked carbohydrate and protein. Another level of control may be the sets of glycosyltransferases that various leukocytes express, thereby changing the interactions even though different cells may express the same protein form. An example of differential L-CA carbohydrate expression and tissue localization may be demonstrated with peanut agglutinin binding. Peanut agglutinin binds a subset of mouse lymph node B cells that localize to germinal centers (Rose et al. 1980; Butcher et al. 1982). The major binding molecule on peanut-agglutinin-positive B cells appears to be the high-molecular-weight form of L-CA (De Petris and Takacs 1983), thus correlating differential lectin binding of L-CA and tissue localization. Additionally, it has been amply demonstrated that both common and restricted antibodies to L-CA can modulate phytohemagglutinin-induced proliferation in both human and mouse T cells, therefore indicating that at least part of the phytohemagglutinin-induced proliferation signal is mediated through L-CA (Ledbetter et al. 1985; Bernabeu et al. 1987; Marvel and Mayer 1988).

L-CA does not appear to associate with other surface molecules on the same cell in an uninduced state; however, when L-CA is capped using secondary antibodies, other surface molecules are cocapped (Bourguignon et al. 1978). The mechanism by which other molecules cocap is unknown; however, it appears that L-CA interacts with the cytoskeletal component fodrin (Suchard and Bourguignon 1987), and this may be important in bringing other cell-surface molecules that are potential substrates in close contact with the tyrosine phosphatase domain.

The substrates of the tyrosine phosphatase domains are not known; however, in this regard, the observations of Ostergaard et al. (1989) may be of critical importance. Their data indicate that the phosphotyrosine at position 505 in the tyrosine kinase *lck* is a potential substrate for L-CA. This observation has implications in the role that L-CA plays in the regulation of cell growth. *lck* is a member of the *src* gene family that is expressed in the T-lymphocyte lineage, and position 505 of *lck* is part of a sequence that is highly conserved in all members of the *src* gene family. This position is thought to play a regulatory role in the activity of these proteins (Hunter 1987). It is possible, therefore, that one function of L-CA is to activate members of the *src* gene family, and the deficient step in the L-CA⁻ T-cell clones is the ability to activate *lck*. It should be noted that L-CA has two potential tyrosine phosphatase domains that are only 35% homologous, and, therefore, each domain will most likely interact with different sets of substrates. Not in all leukocytes, such as macrophages and neutrophils, will activation of L-CA necessarily lead to signals for proliferation, but activation of L-CA may be important in other signaling events, such as transcriptional activity.

ACKNOWLEDGMENTS

We thank Matt Haffner for preparation of figures and Dr. Randy Junge and Mrs. Barbara Dressel of the St. Louis Zoo for providing us with a range of vertebrate tissues. This work was supported by grant AI-26363 from the U.S. Public Health Service and grants from the Council for Tobacco Research. M.L.T. is the recipient of an Established Investigator Award from the American Heart Association.

REFERENCES

Barclay, A.N., D.I. Jackson, A.C. Willis, and A.F. Williams. 1987. Lymphocyte specific heterogeneity in the rat leukocyte common antigen (T200) is due to differences in polypeptide sequences near the NH₂-terminus. *EMBO J.* **6:** 1259.

Bernabeu, C., A.C. Carrera, M.O. De Landázuri, and F. Sánchez-Madrid. 1987. Interaction between the CD45 antigen and phytohemagglutinin. Inhibitory effect on the lectin-induced T cell proliferation by anti-CD45 monoclonal antibody. *Eur. J. Immunol.* **17:** 1461.

Bourguignon, L.Y.W., R. Hyman, I. Trowbridge, and S.J. Singer. 1978. Participation of histocompatibility antigens in capping of molecularly independent cell surface components by their specific antibodies. *Proc. Natl. Acad. Sci.* **75:** 2406.

Butcher, E.C., R.V. Rouse, R.L. Coffman, C.N. Nottenburg, R.R. Hardy, and I.L. Weissman. 1982. Surface phenotype of Peyer's patch germinal center cells: Implications for the role of germinal centers in B cell differentiation. *J. Immunol.* **129:** 2698.

Charbonneau, H., N.K. Tonks, K.A. Walsh, and E.H. Fischer. 1988. The leukocyte common antigen (CD45): A putative receptor-linked protein tyrosine phosphatase. *Proc. Natl. Acad. Sci.* **85:** 7182.

De Petris, S. and B. Takacs. 1983. Relationship between mouse lymphocyte receptors for peanut agglutinin (PNA) and *Helix pomatia* agglutinin (HPA). *Eur. J. Immunol.* **13:** 831.

Hall, L.R., M. Streuli, S.F. Schlossman, and H. Saito. 1988. Complete exon-intron organization of the human leukocyte common antigen. *J. Immunol.* **141:** 2781.

Hunter, T. 1987. A tail of two *src*'s: Mutatis mutandis. *Cell* **49:** 1.

Jackson, D.I. and A.N. Barclay. 1989. The extra segments of sequence in rat leukocyte common antigen (L-CA) are derived by alternative splicing of only three exons and show extensive O-linked glycosylation. *Immunogenetics* **29:** 281.

Johnson, N.A., C.M. Meyer, J.T. Pingel, and M.L. Thomas. 1989. Sequence conservation in potential regulatory regions of the mouse and human leukocyte-common antigen gene. *J. Biol. Chem.* **264:** 6220.

Ledbetter, J.A., L.M. Rose, C.E. Spooner, P.G. Beatty, P.J. Martin, and E.A. Clark. 1985. Antibodies to common leukocyte antigen p220 influence human T cell proliferation by modifying IL 2 receptor expression. *J. Immunol.* **135:** 1819.

Marvel, J. and A. Mayer. 1988. CD45R gives immunofluorescence and transduces signals on mouse T cells. *Eur. J. Immunol.* **18:** 825.

Matis, L.A., D.L. Longo, S.M. Hedrick, C. Hannum, E. Margoliash, and R.H. Schwarz. 1983. Clonal analysis of the major histocompatibility complex restriction and the fine specificity of antigen recognition in the T cell proliferative response to cytochrome c. *J. Immunol.* **130:** 1527.

Ostergaard, H.L., D.A. Shackelford, T.R. Hurley, P. Johnson, R. Hyman, B.M. Sefton, and I.S. Trowbridge. 1989. Expression of CD45 alters phosphorylation of the *lck* tyrosine protein kinase in murine lymphoma T cell lines. *Proc. Natl. Acad. Sci.* (in press).

Pingel, J.T. and M.L. Thomas. 1989. Evidence that the leukocyte-common antigen is required for antigen induced T lymphocyte proliferation. *Cell* (in press).

Ralph, S.J., M.L. Thomas, C.C. Morton, and I.S. Trowbridge. 1987. Structural variants of human T200 glycoprotein (leukocyte-common antigen). *EMBO J.* **6:** 1251.

Rose, M.L., M.S.C. Birbeck, V.J. Wallis, J.A. Forrester, and A.J.S. Davies. 1980. Peanut lectin binding properties of germinal centers of mouse lymphoid tissue. *Nature* **284:** 364.

Saga, Y., J.-S. Tung, F.-W. Shen, and E.A. Boyse. 1987. Alternative use of 5′ exons in the specification of Ly-5 isoforms distinguishing hematopoietic cell lineages. *Proc. Natl. Acad. Sci.* **84:** 5364.

Saga, Y, J.-S. Tung, F.-W. Shen, T.C. Pancoast, and E.A. Boyse. 1988. Organization of the Ly-5 gene. *Mol. Cell. Biol.* **8:** 4889.

Streuli, M., L.R. Hall, Y. Saga, S.F. Schlossman, and H. Saito. 1987. Differential usage of three exons generates at least five different mRNAs encoding human leukocyte common antigens. *J. Exp. Med.* **166:** 1548.

Streuli, M., N.X. Krueger, L.R. Hall, S.F. Schlossman, and H. Saito. 1988. A new member of the immunoglobulin superfamily that has a cytoplasmic region homologous to the leukocyte common antigen. *J. Exp. Med.* **168:** 1523.

Suchard, S.J. and L.Y.W. Bourguignon. 1987. Further characterization of fodrin-containing transmembrane complex from mouse T-lymphoma cells. *Biochim. Biophys. Acta.* **896:** 35.

Thomas, M.L. 1989. The leukocyte common antigen family. *Annu. Rev. Immunol.* **7:** 339.

Thomas, M.L., P.J. Reynolds, A. Chain, Y. Ben-Neriah, and I.S. Trowbridge. 1987. B-cell variant of mouse T200 (Ly-5): Evidence for alternative mRNA splicing. *Proc. Natl. Acad. Sci.* **84:** 5360.

Tonks, N.K., H. Charbonneau, C.D. Diltz, E.H. Fischer, and K.A. Walsh. 1988. Demonstration that the leukocyte common antigen CD45 is a protein tyrosine phosphatase. *Biochemistry* **27:** 8696.

Trowbridge, I.S. 1978. Interspecies spleen-myeloma hybrid producing monoclonal antibodies against mouse lymphocyte surface glycoprotein, T200. *J. Exp. Med.* **148:** 313.

Cell Membrane Molecule I-J Transduces a Negative Signal for Early T-cell Activation Induced via the TCR

Y. Asano,* T. Nakayama,* H. Kishimoto,* T. Komuro,* K. Sano,*
N. Utsunomiya,† M. Nakanishi,† and T. Tada*

*Department of Immunology, Faculty of Medicine, and †Department of Physical Chemistry, Faculty of
Pharmaceutical Sciences, University of Tokyo, 7-3-1 Hongo, Bunkyo-ku, Tokyo 113, Japan

I-J was first described as a marker of T-suppressor cells (T_S) and suppressor factors (T_SF) controlled by a gene of the mouse major histocompatibility complex (MHC) (Murphy et al. 1976; Tada et al. 1976; for review, see Murphy 1987). Several T-cell hybridomas expressing I-J or producing the I-J-bearing T_SF were produced, and a number of monoclonal anti-I-J antibodies were established in several laboratories (Kanno et al. 1981; Waltenbaugh 1981; Kurata et al. 1984). Subsequent studies have, however, revealed that the I-J gene could not be encoded within the MHC by molecular cloning analyses (Steimetz et al. 1982; Kobori et al. 1984, 1986) and that the I-J transcript was not detected in T-cell hybridomas expressing I-J on their surface by cosmid probes covering the whole stretch of I region of MHC (Kronenberg et al. 1982). The compelling evidence thus indicated that I-J is not a direct product of an MHC gene but is indirectly controlled by the MHC.

Subsequent studies using radiation bone marrow chimeras and transgenic mice revealed that the I-J phenotype of T cells undergoes systematic adaptive alterations under chimeric and transgenic conditions according to the environmental MHC where T cells are developed from bone marrow stem cells of different MHC genotype (Sumida et al. 1985; Uracz et al. 1985; Flood et al. 1986; Asano et al. 1987). In T cells of $H-2^{kxb}F_1$, the T-helper (T_H) cell population having A^k-restricted specificity carried I-J^k, whereas T_H cells having A^b-restricted specificity did not express I-J^k (Asano et al. 1987). Experiments utilizing fully allogeneic chimeras demonstrated that I-J^k epitopes are expressed on T_H cells differentiated in $H-2^k$ but not in $H-2^b$, regardless of the origin of bone marrow stem cells. These observations indicate that I-J is an acquired trait adaptively expressed on T cells according to the environmental MHC.

The question arises as to whether the I-J epitope is merely an idiotypic determinant of the class-II-restricted T-cell receptor (TCR) heterodimer, which reflects the acquired MHC-restriction specificity. If not, what is the molecular entity of I-J, and what is the role in the immune response? In this paper, we describe the recent biochemical characterization of the molecule and its role in early T-cell activation.

METHODS

The procedures involved in establishing and maintaining T-cell clones are the same as those described in a previous publication (Asano and Hodes 1983). The methods of immunoprecipitation and gel analysis have been described previously (Nakayama et al. 1989). The measurement of intracellular Ca^{++} by stopped-flow fluorocytometry has been described previously (Utsunomiya and Nakanishi 1986; Utsunomiya et al. 1986, 1989).

RESULTS AND DISCUSSION

Expression of I-J on T-cell Clones

I-J expression on cloned T cells has been described in detail previously (Nakayama et al. 1988). We established IL-2-dependent T-cell clones of $L3T4^+$, $Ly-2^-$ with T_H and T_S functions. The T_S subtype was defined by the criteria where cells do not produce both IL-2 and IL-4, lack the helper activity for H-2-compatible B cells, and inhibit the antibody response of histocompatible T and B cells (Asano and Hodes 1983; Y. Asano, unpubl.). Two other $L3T4^-$, $Ly-2^+$ T_S clones, one of which produced a T_SF upon stimulation by antigen and appropriate antigen-presenting cells (APC), were also included. These clones originated from splenic T cells from $H-2^k$, $H-2^b$, $H-2^{kxb}F_1$, and radiation bone marrow chimeras produced by semi-allogeneic combinations. Antigen and MHC-restriction specificities were established by in vitro stimulation with antigen (keyhole limpet hemocyanin [KLH] or fowl gamma globulin [FGG]) presented by APC of $H-2^k$ or $H-2^b$. Some clones were found to react with the self class II antigen alone without requiring the presence of external antigens. Properties of these T-cell clones are summarized in Table 1.

The I-J^k expression of these T-cell clones was determined by (1) inhibition of antigen-induced proliferation by an anti-I-J^k monoclonal antibody (MAb) (JK10-23), (2) inhibition of the helper activity in the in vitro secondary antibody response by the anti-I-J^k, and (3) direct immunofluorescence staining. As listed in Table 1, all the $H-2^k$ class-II-restricted T-cell clones were found to be positive in the I-J^k expression in one

Table 1. Expression of I-J^k Epitope on T-cell Clones

Code	Origin	Specificity	Function	I-J^k expression
MS-S2	C3H	A^k	Th	+
9-5	F$_1$[2]	A^k + KLH	Ts	+
9-16	F$_1$	E^k + KLH	Th	+
28-4	F$_1$	A^k + KLH	Th	+
23-1-8	F$_1 \rightarrow$ C3H	A^k + KLH	Th	+
23-2	F$_1 \rightarrow$ C3H	E^k + KLH	Th	+
25-11-20	B6$\rightarrow$F$_1$	A^k + KLH	Ts	+
25-18-5	B6$\rightarrow$F$_1$	E^k + KLH	Ts	+
2-19-2	B10	A^b + FGG, A^{bm12}	Th	−
8-4	F$_1$	A^b + KLH	Ts	−
8-5	F$_1$	A^b + KLH	Th	−
24-2	F$_1 \rightarrow$ B6	A^b + KLH	Th	−
24-15-1	F$_1 \rightarrow$ B6	A^b	Th	−
40-5	B10.A(5R)	E^k + KLH	Ts	+
40-12	B10.A(5R)	A^b + KLH	Ts	+
44-11	B10.A(3R)	A^b + KLH	Ts	−
3D10[1]	C3H	A^k + KLH	Ts	+
13G2[1]	B6	A^b + casein	Ts	−

[1]L3T4$^-$ Ly-2$^+$.

[2]B6C3F$_1$.

or more of the above criteria. The proliferative response of both T_H and T_S clones with H-2^k-restriction specificity was strongly inhibited by the addition of anti-I-J^k, whereas the response of H-2^b-restricted clones from H-2^b, F$_1$, and chimeras were inhibited by anti-I-J^k. Both A^k- and E^k-restricted T-cell clones were inhibitable by the identical anti-I-J^k.

However, the expression of I-J^k is not primarily determined by the genotype of the T-cell clones. Those T-cell clones derived from F$_1$, H-2$^b \rightarrow$ F$_1$, and F$_1 \rightarrow$ H-2^k chimeras were found to express the same I-J^k epitope, regardless of their genotypic origin. On the other hand, T-cell clones with H-2^b-restriction specificity derived from F$_1 \rightarrow$ H-2^b chimera were found to be negative for I-J^k, even though the genotype may predict the expression of I-J^k. A T_SF-producing Ly-2$^+$ T_S clone 3D10 was also positive for I-J^k. Two T-cell clones from B10.A(5R) having either A^b- or E^k-restriction specificity were found to be I-J^k-positive, whereas a clone from B10.A(3R) having A^b-restriction specificity was I-J^k-negative. These results extended the previous observation (Asano et al. 1987) indicating that the I-J epitope is expressed on T cells adaptive to the environmental MHC in radiation bone marrow chimeras.

A crucial question is whether the I-J epitope is the idiotypic marker of TCR, reflecting the acquirable MHC restriction specificity of T cells. Since some of the T-cell clones can be stained with the anti-I-J^k, we studied by microfluorometry whether the I-J epitope is associated with the TCR/CD3 complex. The TCR/CD3 complex was modulated by incubating T cells with anti-CD3 antibody (145-2C11; Leo et al. 1987) at 37°C overnight, and then the cells were stained with anti-I-J^k. The staining with anti-CD3 became completely negative after incubation, whereas the anti-I-J^k staining was unchanged (Nakayama et al. 1988). The result indicates that the I-J epitope is not associated with the

TCR heterodimer and that I-J is not an idiotypic determinant on TCR.

Biochemical Identification of the I-J Molecule in Gel Electrophoresis

Nonidet P-40 lysates of ^{125}I-surface-labeled cloned T cells were immunoprecipitated with anti-I-J^k (JK10-23) or control antibodies including F23.1 (irrelevant anti-TCR monoclonal antibody of the same immunoglobulin [Ig] subclass to JK10-23; Staerz et al. 1985) and 6623 (pan-reactive rabbit anti-mouse TCR antiserum; Kubo and Roehm 1986). Immunoprecipitates were analyzed by two-dimensional (nonreducing/reducing) SDS-polyacrylamide gel electrophoresis (SDS-PAGE).

Figure 1 illustrates the electrophoretic mobilities of the I-J molecule precipitated from a T-cell clone MS-S2 in the two-dimensional gel. The anti-I-J precipitated a molecule that migrated as an off-diagonal spot in the gel. Such a spot was not seen with irrelevant MAb F23.1 of the same IgG$_{2a}$ subclass. The off-diagonal spot in the two-dimensional gel was M_r 44K, resulting from the reduction of an M_r 86K species (Fig. 1a). An on-diagonal spot of 44K was also precipitated from some but not all T-cell clones with anti-I-J^k. The I-J molecule was distinct from either α or β chain of the TCR from the same T-cell clone: This particular T-cell clone MS-S2 gave α and β chain spots separately (42K, 36K, and 32K), none of which corresponded to the I-J molecule observed in Figure 1a. Furthermore, by sequential immunoprecipitation, anti-I-J^k could precipitate the 44K molecule after extensive clearance of TCR heterodimer with the rabbit anti-TCR 6623 (Fig. 1d).

Further biochemical characterization of the I-J molecule was performed by nonequilibrium pH gradient electrophoresis (NEPHGE). The I-J molecule from

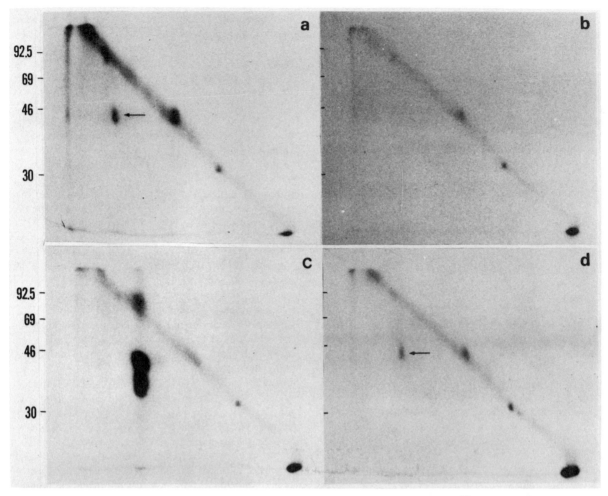

Figure 1. Two-dimensional SDS-PAGE of I-J molecule and TCR from a T-cell clone MS-S2. ^{125}I-surface-labeled cells were solubilized with Nonidet P-40. Immunoprecipitations were prepared with (a) JK10-23 (anti-I-J^k MAb, IgG$_{2a}$), (b) F23.1 (an irrelevant anti-TCR V$_\beta$ MAb, IgG$_{2a}$), (c) 6623 (pan-reactive rabbit anti-TCR serum), and (d) JK10-23 after preclearance with 6623. Precipitates were analyzed by two-dimensional (non-reducing/reducing) SDS-PAGE.

MS-S2 showed a single homogeneous species migrating in the position of pH 5.3 to 6.4 with M_r 44K, which again suggested the homodimeric nature of the molecule. The TCR α and β chains from the same T-cell clone migrated with the expected basic and acidic mobilities, respectively, and did not overlap with the I-J chain (Nakayama et al. 1989). Deglycosylation experiment of the I-J molecule showed that the I-J subunit is only lightly glycosylated with two glycosylation sites and that the protein backbone is M_r 41K, which is larger than TCR α and β chains from the same clone. The I-J is also distinguished from other previously described homodimeric T-cell antigens such as A1 (Nagasawa et al. 1987), YE1/48 (Chan and Takei 1988), and CD28 (Yokoyama et al. 1988).

Role of I-J in Negative Signal Transduction

The anti-I-J^k (JK10-23) was capable of inhibiting various functions of MHC-restricted normal and cloned T$_H$ and T$_S$ including helper activity and antigen-

induced T-cell proliferation (Asano et al. 1987; Nakayama et al. 1988). We have recently studied the effect of anti-I-J on early intracellular signal transduction in T cells induced by antigenic stimulation.

MHC-restricted cloned T$_H$ cells were loaded with Ca^{++}-sensitive fluorophore Fura 2AM (Grynkiewitz et al. 1985) and were stimulated with specific antigens and APC. The increase of intracellular Ca^{++} ([Ca^{++}]$_i$) was measured by stopped-flow fluorography. The cells were treated by incubation with monoclonal antibodies against I-J^k (JK10-23), I-J^b (WF8.D2.4; Waltanbaugh 1981), or L3T4 (GK1.5; Dialynas et al. 1983) prior to stimulation with antigen and APC. Figure 2 shows that treatment of the A^k-restricted T$_H$ clone 23-1-8 with anti-I-J^k monoclonal antibody inhibited the Ca^{++} response induced by the subsequent stimulation with antigen-pulsed APC. Anti-I-J^b (WF8.D2.4), a monoclonal antibody raised against the similar molecule of H-2^b haplotype, was unable to inhibit the Ca^{++} response of this clone. The inhibitory effect of the anti-I-J was MHC-specific: The [Ca^{++}]$_i$ response of T$_H$ clone 23-1-8

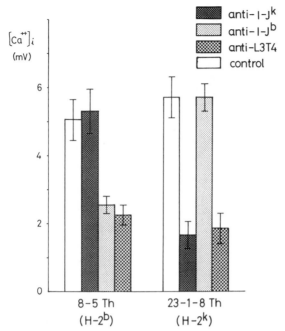

Figure 2. Treatment of cloned T_H cells with anti-I-J MAb inhibits the antigen-induced increase of $[Ca^{++}]_i$. Cloned T_H cells (8–5, KLH-specific and A^b-restricted; 23-1-8, KLH-specific and A^k-restricted) were labeled with a Ca^{++}-sensitive fluorophore Fura 2AM. These T cells were pretreated with an appropriate concentration of anti-I-J^k (JK10-23), anti-I-J^b (WF8.D2.4), or anti-L3T4 (GK1.5) MAb for 30 min on ice. After washing, these cells were stimulated with T-cell-depleted KLH-pulsed APC. $[Ca^{++}]_i$ was measured as stopped-flow fluorescence.

was not inhibitable by anti-I-J^b. The $[Ca^{++}]_i$ responses of an A^b-restricted T_H cell clone 8-5 derived from (C57BL/6 × C3H)F$_1$ was inhibited by anti-I-J^b but not by anti-I-J^k. The degree of inhibition by anti-I-J was, in general, comparable to that caused by anti-L3T4 (Fig. 2). The major portion of $[Ca^{++}]_i$ response was abrogated by the addition of ethylenglycol-bis (β-aminoethyl ether)-$N,N,N'N'$-tetraacetic acid (EGTA) into the medium, indicating that the method utilized in this study primarily detects the influx of Ca^{++}.

The inhibition of Ca^{++} influx by anti-I-J requires the cross-linking of membrane I-J molecules. Monovalent

Fab fragments of anti-I-J monoclonal antibody were inactive in the inhibition of Ca^{++} response (Fig. 3). The addition of rabbit anti-mouse Ig to this reaction mixture could induce the inhibition of Ca^{++} influx. The results indicate that the ligation of the surface I-J molecules transduces a negative signal for early signal transduction in T cells.

The anti-I-J monoclonal antibody was unable to inhibit the Ca^{++} response of T-cell clones induced by anti-CD3 (Fig. 4). A^k-restricted T_H clone 23-1-8 was stimulated with anti-CD3, anti-TCR$\alpha\beta$ (H57-597; Kubo et al. 1989), or antigen-pulsed APC. The pretreatment of the clones with anti-I-J did not inhibit the Ca^{++} influx induced by anti-CD3, but was able to inhibit the responses induced by antigen-pulsed APC and anti-TCR monoclonal antibody. The response to concanavalin A (Con A) was not inhibited by anti-I-J (data not shown). Thus, anti-I-J was found to inhibit an early process subsequent to the recognition of antigen via the TCR heterodimer but not the consequence of signal transduction induced via the CD3 complex. This suggests the presence of a second messenger that transduces a T-cell activation signal from TCR to the CD3 complex, and the I-J-derived signal seems to inhibit this particular process. Alternatively, the signal transduced through the TCR by specific ligand or anti-TCR monoclonal antibody involves a different pathway from that generated by stimulation with anti-CD3, and such a pathway without participation of CD3 is the target of the negative signal via the I-J receptor.

CONCLUSION

I-J has been an enigmatic molecule for several years primarily because of its adaptive nature to MHC (Sumida et al. 1985; Uracz et al. 1985; Flood et al. 1986; Asano et al. 1987; Asano and Tada 1989). Its epigeneic expression on MHC-restricted T cells in the radiation bone marrow chimeras according to the host MHC suggests that I-J is generated through an interaction with a self-ligand present in the maturation environment of the T cells. It has been known that the restriction specificity of TCR of most T_H cells is determined by thymic selection (Bevan and Fink 1978;

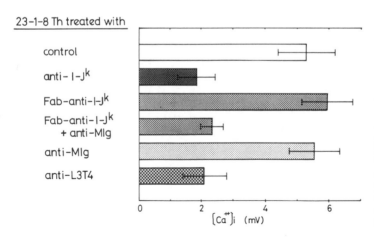

Figure 3. Cross-linking of I-J molecules on T_H cells is required for the inhibition of the antigen-induced increase of $[Ca^{++}]_i$. Fura-2-loaded T_H cells (23-1-8) were pretreated with anti-I-J^k (JK10-23) or Fab fragment of the anti-I-J^k. For cross-linking of the surface-bound Fab fragments, the T_H cells were first pretreated with the Fab fragments and then preincubated with rabbit anti-mouse immunoglobulin. The treated T cells were subsequently stimulated with KLH-pulsed B10.A APC. Monovalent Fab fragments of anti-I-J MAb did not inhibit the Ca^{++} response, but the cross-linking of Fab resulted in inhibition.

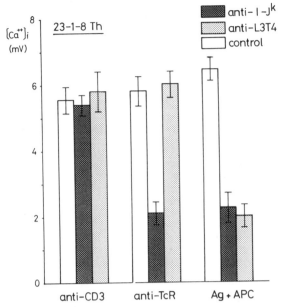

Figure 4. Ca^{++} influx caused by specific activation through TCR but not by anti-CD3 MAb is blocked by anti-I-J. Fura-2-loaded cloned T_H (23-1-8) cells were pretreated with anti-I-J^k (JK10-23) or anti-L3T4 (GK1.5). These T cells were stimulated with anti-CD3 MAb (145-2C11), anti-TCR$\alpha\beta$ (H57-597), or antigen-pulsed B10.A APC. Anti-I-J failed to inhibit the increase of $[Ca^{++}]_i$ induced by anti-CD3. The same treatment resulted in the suppression of Ca^{++} influx stimulated by anti-TCR or specific antigen.

Singer et al. 1982; Marrack et al. 1988). I-J is another example showing a similar adaptive process to the self-MHC. In view of the present finding, we think that I-J plays a role in both selection and maintenance of the T-cell repertoire: It has been reported that strong proliferative signals generated via the TCR result in an apoptosis of developing thymocytes (Smith et al. 1989). The signal from the I-J receptor may limit such intrathymic overproliferation of positively selected T cells and rescue the MHC-restricted T cells. It may serve as a device to limit the expansion of auto-MHC-reactive T cells in the peripheral lymphoid pool that have escaped from the thymic negative selection.

ACKNOWLEDGMENTS

This work was supported by grants from the Ministry of Education, Science and Culture, and the life science research projects of the Institute of Physical and Chemical Research, Japan. The authors thank Drs. R.T. Kubo, J.A. Bluestone, E.M. Shevach, R. Nagasawa, F. Takei, and C. Waltenbaugh for their willingness to provide us with their antibodies used in this study.

REFERENCES

Asano, Y. and R.J. Hodes. 1983. T cell regulation of B cell activation. Cloned Lyt-1$^+$2$^-$ Ts cells inhibit the major histocompatibility complex-restricted Th cell interaction with B cells and/or accessory cells. *J. Exp. Med.* **158:** 1178.

Asano, Y. and T. Tada. 1989. Generation of T cell repertoire. Two distinct mechanisms for generation of T suppressor cells, T helper cells, and T augmenting cells. *J. Immunol.* **142:** 365.

Asano, Y., T. Nakayama, M. Kubo, J. Yagi, and T. Tada. 1987. Epitopes associated with MHC restriction site of T cells. III. I-J epitope on MHC-restricted T helper cells. *J. Exp. Med.* **166:** 1613.

Bevan, M.A. and P. Fink. 1978. The influence of thymus H-2 antigens on the specificity of maturing killer and helper cells. *Immunol. Rev.* **42:** 3.

Chan, P.-Y. and F. Takei. 1988. Characterization of a murine T cell surface disulfide-linked dimer of 45-kDa glycopeptides (YE1/48 antigen). Comparison with T cell receptor, purification, and partial amino acid sequences. *J. Immunol.* **140:** 161.

Dialynas, D.P., D.B. Wilde, P. Marrack, A. Pierres, K.A. Wall, W. Harvan, G. Otten, M.R. Loken, M. Pierres, J.W. Kappler, and F.W. Fitch. 1983. Characterization of the murine antigenic determinant, designated L3T4a, recognized by monoclonal antibody GK1.5: Expression of L3T4a by functional T cell clones appears to correlate primarily with class II MHC antigen-reactivity. *Immunol. Rev.* **74:** 29.

Flood, P.M., C. Benoist, D. Mathis, and D.B. Murphy. 1986. Altered I-J phenotype in E$_\alpha$ transgenic mice. *Proc. Natl. Acad. Sci.* **83:** 8308.

Grynkiewicz, G., M. Poenie, and R.Y. Tsien. 1985. A new generation of Ca^{2+} indicators with greatly improved fluorescence properties. *J. Biol. Chem.* **260:** 3440.

Kanno, M., S. Kobayashi, T. Tokuhisa, I. Tekei, N. Shinohara, and M. Taniguchi. 1981. Monoclonal antibodies that recognize the product controlled by a gene in the I-J subregion of the mouse H-2 complex. *J. Exp. Med.* **154:** 1290.

Kobori, J.A., E. Strauss, K. Minard, and L. Hood. 1986. Molecular analysis of the hotspot of recombination in the murine major histocompatibility complex. *Science* **234:** 173.

Kobori, J.A., A. Winoto, J. McNicholas, and L. Hood. 1984. Molecular characterization of the recombination of six major histocompatibility complex (MHC) I-region recombinants. *J. Mol. Cell. Immunol.* **1:** 125.

Kronenberg, H., M. Steinmetz, J.A. Kobori, E. Kraig, J.A. Kapp, C.W. Pierce, C.M. Sorensen, G. Suzuki, T. Tada, and L. Hood. 1982. RNA transcripts for I-J polypeptides are apparently not encoded between the I-A and I-E subregions of the murine major histocompatibility complex. *Proc. Natl. Acad. Sci.* **79:** 5704.

Kubo, R.T. and N. Roehm. 1986. Preparation and characterization of a "pan-reactive" rabbit anti-mouse T-cell receptor antiserum. *Mol. Immunol.* **23:** 869.

Kubo, R.T., W. Born, J.W. Kappler, P. Marrack, and M. Pigeon. 1989. Characterization of a monoclonal antibody which detects all murine $\alpha\beta$ T cell receptor. *J. Immunol.* **142:** 2736.

Kurata, A., K. Yamauchi, T. Watanabe, M. Nonaka, R. Abe, K. Okumura, and T. Tada. 1984. Is there multiplicity in I-J subregion products? *J. Mol. Cell. Immunol.* **1:** 267.

Leo, O., M. Foo, D.H. Sachs, L.E. Samelson, and J.A. Bluestone. 1987. Identification of a monoclonal antibody specific for a murine T3 polypeptide. *Proc. Natl. Acad. Sci.* **84:** 1374.

Marrack, P., D. Lo, R. Brinster, R. Palmiter, L. Burkly, R.H. Flavell, and J.W. Kappler. 1988. The effect of thymus environment on T cell development and tolerance. *Cell* **53:** 627.

Murphy, D.B. 1987. The I-J puzzle. *Annu. Rev. Immunol.* **5:** 405.

Murphy, D.B., L.A. Herzenberg, K. Okumura, L.A. Herzenberg, and H.O. McDevitt. 1976. A new I subregion (I-J) marked by a locus (Ia-4) controlling surface determinants on suppressor T lymphocyte. *J. Exp. Med.* **144:** 699.

Nagasawa, R., J. Cross, O. Kanagawa, K. Townsend, L.L. Laner, J. Chiller, and J.A. Allison. 1987. Identification of a novel T cell surface disulfide-bonded dimer distinct from the $\alpha\beta$ antigen receptor. *J. Immunol.* **138:** 815.

Nakayama, T., R.T. Kubo, H. Kishimoto, Y. Asano, and T. Tada. 1989. Biochemical identification of I-J as a novel dimeric surface molecule on mouse helper and suppressor T cell clones. *Int. Immunol.* **1:** 50.

Nakayama, T., R.T. Kubo, M. Kubo, I. Fujisawa, H. Kishimoto, Y. Asano, and T. Tada. 1988. Epitopes associated with MHC restriction site of T cells. IV. I-J epitopes on MHC-restricted cloned T cells. *Eur. J. Immunol.* **18:** 761.

Singer, A., K.S. Hathcock, and R.J. Hodes. 1982. Self-recognition in allogeneic chimeras. Self-recognition by T helper cells from thymus-engrafted nude mice is restricted to thymic H-2 haplotype. *J. Exp. Med.* **155:** 339.

Smith, C.A., G.T. Williamson, R. Kingston, E.J. Jenkinson, and J.J.T. Owen. 1989. Antibodies to CD3/T-cell receptor complex induce death by apoptosis in murine T cells in thymic cultures. *Nature* **337:** 181.

Staerz, J.D., H. Rammansee, J. Benedetto, and M. Bevan. 1985. Characterization of a murine monoclonal antibody specific for an allotypic determinant on T cell antigen receptor. *J. Immunol.* **134:** 3944.

Steinmetz, M., K. Minard, S. Horvath, J. McNicholas, J. Frelinger, C. Wake, E. Long, B. Mach, and L. Hood. 1982. A molecular map of the immune response region from the major histocompatibility complex of the mouse. *Nature* **300:** 35.

Sumida, T., T. Sado, M. Kojima, H. Ono, K. Kamisaku, and M. Taniguchi. 1985. I-J as an idiotype of the recognition component of antigen-specific suppressor T cell factor. *Nature* **316:** 738.

Tada, T., M. Taniguchi, and C.S. David. 1976. Properties of the antigen-specific suppressive T-cell factor in the regulation of antibody responses in the mouse. IV. Special subregion assignment of the gene(s) that codes for the suppressive T cell factor in the H-2 histocompatibility complex. *J. Exp. Med.* **144:** 713.

Uracz, W., Y. Asano, R. Abe, and T. Tada. 1985. I-J epitopes are adaptively acquired by T cells differentiated in the chimeric condition. *Nature* **316:** 741.

Utsunomiya, N. and M. Nakanishi. 1986. A serine protease triggers the initial step of transmembrane signaling in cytotoxic T cells. *J. Biol. Chem.* **261:** 16514.

Utsunomiya, N., N. Tsuboi, and M. Nakanishi. 1986. Early transmembrane events in alloimmune cytotoxic T-lymphocyte activation as revealed by stopped-flow fluorometry. *Proc. Natl. Acad. Sci.* **83:** 1877.

Utsunomiya, N., M. Nakanishi, Y. Arata, M. Kubo, Y. Asano, and T. Tada. 1989. Unidirectional inhibition of early signal transduction of helper T cells by cloned suppressor T cells. *Int. Immunol.* **1:** 460.

Waltenbaugh, C. 1981. Regulation of immune responses by I-J gene products. I. Production and characterization of anti-I-J monoclonal antibodies. *J. Exp. Med.* **154:** 1570.

Yokoyama, W.M., F. Koning, P.J. Kehn, G.M.B. Pereira, G. Stingl, J.E. Coligan, and E.M. Shevach. 1988. Characterization of a cell surface-expressed disulfide-linked dimer involved in murine T cell activation. *J. Immunol.* **141:** 369.

Interleukin-2 Receptor β Chain: Molecular Cloning and Functional Expression of the Human cDNA

T. Taniguchi,* M. Hatakeyama,* S. Minamoto,* T. Kono,* T. Doi,*
M. Tsudo,† M. Miyasaka,† and T. Miyata‡

*Institute for Molecular and Cellular Biology, Osaka University, Yamadaoka 1-3, Suita-shi, Osaka 565, Japan;
†Tokyo Metropolitan Institute of Medical Science, Bunkyo-ku, Tokyo 113, Japan;
‡Department of Biology, Kyushyu University Faculty of Science, Higashi-ku, Fukuoka 812, Japan

Ample evidence has been accumulated that lymphokines (or cytokines), a class of soluble mediators driving intercellular communications, play a key role in the regulation of the immune system. They induce proliferation, differentiation, and activation of target cells through interaction with specific receptor(s). Interleukin-2 (IL-2), the first of a series of lymphokines to be discovered and completely characterized, is known to play a pivotal role in the antigen-specific clonal proliferation of T lymphocytes (T cells) (Fig. 1). IL-2 also acts on other cell types such as B lymphocytes (B cells), macrophages, natural killer cells (NK cells), and immature thymocytes (for review, see Smith 1980, 1988; Taniguchi et al. 1986). Furthermore, recent studies provided evidence that IL-2 functions on neural cells such as oligodendrocytes (Benveniste and Merrill 1986). These biological properties have opened new possibilities for clinical application of IL-2 (Rosenberg et al. 1985). On the other hand, dysregulation of the IL-2 system in certain neoplastic T-cell transformation has been documented by a number of studies, in particular, for adult T-cell leukemia by a lymphotropic retrovirus, HTLV-1 (for review, see Wong-Staal and Gallo 1985; Yoshida and Seiki 1987; Taniguchi 1988).

Despite extensive studies of the IL-2 system in the context of basic and clinical immunology, little is known about the molecular mechanism(s) underlying the IL-2-mediated signal transduction. The receptor for IL-2 is quite unique in that three forms of IL-2 receptor (IL-2R) can be detected: high-, intermediate-, and low-affinity forms with the respective dissociation constants (K_d values) of about 10^{-11}M, 10^{-9}M, and 10^{-8}M (Robb et al. 1984; Smith 1988). Following the initial expression studies for the cloned human IL-2Rα cDNA, it became evident that IL-2Rα constitutes the low-affinity form, which is nonfunctional per se in the IL-2 internalization and signal transduction both in lymphoid and nonlymphoid cells (Greene et al. 1985; Hatakeyama et al. 1985). Furthermore, the IL-2Rα participates in the formation of the functional, high-affinity IL-2R in association with a specific membrane component(s) of lymphoid cells (Hatakeyama et al. 1985; Kondo et al. 1986; Robb 1986). Subsequently, such a component was identified to be a novel IL-2 receptor chain, termed IL-2Rβ chain (IL-2Rβ or p70-75) (Sharon et al. 1986; Tsudo et al. 1986; Dukovich et al. 1987; Teshigawara et

al. 1987). In fact, IL-2R of the cells expressing the IL-2Rβ but not IL-2Rα manifests the intermediate-affinity form; the same IL-2R form can also be detected in cells expressing high-affinity IL-2R when they are treated by monoclonal antibody against IL-2Rα (Tsudo et al. 1986; Teshigawara et al. 1987). These observations strongly suggest that the functional high-affinity IL-2R is formed by the association of the two receptor components, IL-2Rα and IL-2Rβ chains. Despite extensive studies on the IL-2 system, only limited information has been available about the molecular nature of the IL-2Rβ chain thought to be responsible for the IL-2-mediated signal transduction.

As an essential step to gain further insight on the molecular basis of the functional (i.e., high-affinity) IL-2R and on the mechanism of IL-2-mediated signal transduction, we have isolated the cDNAs encoding the human IL-2Rβ chain.

EXPERIMENTAL PROCEDURES

Preparation of cDNA libraries and screening of the IL-2Rβ-specific clones. Essentially, we applied the expression cloning strategy established by Seed and colleagues (Seed 1987; Seed and Aruffo 1987) for the cDNA library preparation and screening, by using the monoclonal antibodies Mik-β1 and Mik-β2, both of which were raised against IL-2Rβ chain (Tsudo et al. 1989). A few sets of cDNA libraries were prepared by using the poly(A)$^+$ RNA from YT, a human leukemic cell line that expresses high levels of IL-2Rβ (Yodoi et al. 1985). In the cDNA synthesis, however, random primer (Amersham) was used rather than oligo(dT) primer. Screening of the COS cells expressing the antigenic epitope(s) for Mik-β1 and/or Mik-β2 (Tsudo et al. 1989) has been carried out essentially according to the procedure described previously (Seed and Aruffo 1987; see Results section for details).

Plasmid constructions and expression of the IL-2Rβ chain cDNA. Expression vectors were constructed by the following procedures. pIL-2Rβ30 (see Results section) was digested with HindIII (cleavage site is located within the polylinker regions of CDM8; Seed 1987) and, after filling in both ends, a BamHI linker was attached and religated. The resulting plasmid was then

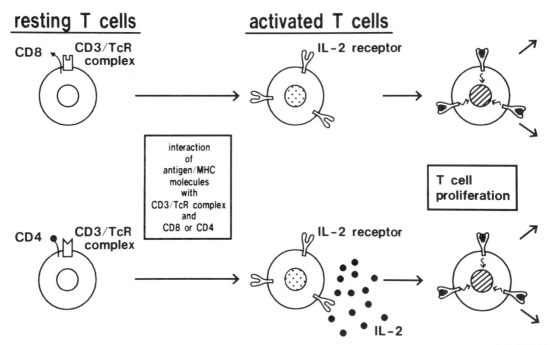

Figure 1. Simplified view of the IL-2 system. Upon activation by the interactions of antigen/MHC complex with CD3/T-cell antigen receptor complex, and with CD4 or CD8 molecules, the resting T cells acquire growth competence. Cellular activation signals lead to the induction of IL-2 and the functional IL-2 receptor complex.

digested with *Bam*HI, and the 1.8-kb DNA fragment that contains the entire coding sequence for the β chain was introduced into the *Bam*HI-cleaved p1013 vector containing the mouse *lck* promoter (generously provided by R. Perlmutter, University of Washington) to construct pLCKRβ. The human IL-2α expressing vector, pSVIL2Rneo, was obtained from pSVIL2R-3 (Hatakeyama et al. 1985) by replacing the Eco-gpt with the neo-resistance gene. Transfection of the expression plasmids into Jurkat cells was carried out by electroporation, as described previously (Potter et al. 1984). Transfected cells were selected in the RPMI 1640 medium containing 10% fetal calf serum and G418 (1.5 mg/ml). To obtain cells expressing cDNAs for human IL-2Rα and IL-2Rβ chains simultaneously, a Jurkat-derived clone, Jα-5, transfected with pSVIL2Rneo, was cotransfected with pLCKRβ and a plasmid containing the hygromycin-resistance gene, pHyg (kindly provided by F. Grosveld, MRC, London, England). The transfected cells were selected with 200 μg/ml hygromycin. For flow cytometric analysis, 5×10^5 cells were treated with antibody (1:500 dilution of ascites) at 4°C for 30 minutes. After washing, cells were stained with fluorescein-conjugated goat anti-mouse IgG. The stained cells were analyzed on a FACS 440 flow cytometer (Becton Dickinson). The ^{125}I-labeled IL-2 binding assay and Scatchard plot analysis were carried out as described previously (Hatakeyama et al. 1985). The recombinant human IL-2 was kindly provided by Takeda Chemicals Co., Ltd. (Osaka, Japan).

RESULTS

Isolation of the cDNA Encoding the IL-2Rβ Chain

We describe below the detailed process of the cDNA isolation. The plasmid DNA representing 5.6×10^6 independent colonies was prepared by the standard procedure, and one milligram of DNA was used for the first DNA transfection. Actually, the DNA was divided into 100 tubes (therefore, each tube contained 10 μg of DNA), and they were each transfected into 3.5×10^5 monkey COS cells in a tissue culture dish (60-mm polystyrene dish, Corning). The transfection was done using the standard DEAE-dextran procedures (Seed and Aruffo 1987). The transfected COS cells were then treated with a cocktail of Mik-β1 and -β2 antibodies (400-fold diluted ascites for each antibody) and subjected to the standard panning procedure. The dish used for panning was the FALCON 60-mm dish, coated with anti-mouse IgG as described previously (Seed and Aruffo 1987). In this first round of panning, 100 IgG-coated dishes were used. After panning, Hirt extract was prepared by the standard procedure (Seed and Aruffo 1987), and the recovered plasmids were introduced into *Escherichia coli*. By this procedure, 3.7×10^6 colonies were obtained. Those bacterial colonies were fused with COS cells by the standard protoplast fusion procedures (Seed and Aruffo 1987). In these fusion experiments, 26 Corning dishes, each containing 5×10^5 COS cells, were used. After the fusion, the COS cells were subjected to panning as described above, and Hirt extract was prepared. About 32,000 bacterial colonies were obtained from the Hirt extract. The fusion and panning procedures were repeated, and about 32,000 bacterial colonies were obtained from the subsequent Hirt extract. The same procedures were repeated once again, obtaining about 28,000 bacterial colonies (in the meantime, there may be a dramatic enrichment of the objective clones). The same procedures were repeated once again, and about 6,000 colonies were obtained. From these colonies, 30 colonies were picked randomly, and the cDNA inserts were analyzed. Of these, only 7 colonies contained plasmids from which cDNA inserts can be excised by the restriction enzyme XhoI. The vector-derived XhoI sites are located at both sides of the cDNA (Seed 1987). All other plasmids had lost such cleavage sites due to DNA rearrangements; in fact, all were much smaller in size than the original vector. Thus, they were considered to be nonspecific products. On the other hand, all of the 7 colonies were derived from the same mRNA, as confirmed by the conventional restriction enzyme cleavage analysis and DNA blot analysis. Of these, one plasmid, termed pIL-2Rβ30, contained longer cDNA than the other 6 plasmids, which turned out to be identical to each other (designated pIL-2Rβ9). In this procedure, therefore, we isolated two independent cDNA clones, IL-2Rβ9 and pIL-2Rβ30; each of the expression products specifically reacted with the antibodies. A typical expression profile of the product by pIL-2β30 in COS cells is shown in Figure 2. The two clones, pIL-2Rβ9 and pIL-2Rβ30, contained cDNA inserts of 1.3 kb and 2.3 kb, respectively, and the cDNAs cross-hybridized with each other. Subsequent sequence analysis of the cDNAs revealed that they represent the same mRNA. In fact, RNA blotting analysis revealed that the mRNA is approximately 4 kb in size (Hatakeyama et al. 1989). Subsequently, we screened other YT cDNA libraries by using the cloned cDNAs as probes, and several independent cDNA clones that together cover the entire mRNA for the IL-2Rβ chain were isolated. Thus pIL-2Rβ6 and pIL-2Rβ19 were obtained by screening the cDNA libraries with the pIL-2Rβ9 cDNA insert as the probe (Hatakeyama et al. 1989).

Primary Structure of the Human IL-2Rβ Chain

The complete nucleotide sequences of the cloned cDNAs were determined (Hatakeyama et al. 1989). The cDNA contains a large open reading frame that encodes a protein consisting of 551 amino acids. No significant homology with other known proteins was found in the Protein Sequence Database (National Biomedical Research Foundation, Washington, D.C.) or in our own data base for the recently published sequences. Thus, neither IL-2Rα chain nor IL-2Rβ chain belongs to the immunoglobulin superfamily (Cosman et al. 1984; Leonard et al. 1984; Nikaido et al. 1984; Hatakeyama et al. 1989). The mature form of the IL-2Rβ chain appears to consist of 525 amino acids, of which 214, 25, and 286, respectively, constitute the extracellular, membrane-spanning, and cytoplasmic regions (Fig. 3).

The extracellular region contains 8 cysteine residues, 5 of which are found in the amino-terminal half and are interspaced rather periodically by 9–12 amino acids. It is likely that disulfide linkages between the cysteine residues impart a stable configuration for ligand binding. Interestingly, the predicted number of amino acids within the extracellular region of the IL-2Rβ chain (214) is almost comparable in number to that of the IL-2Rα chain (219) (Fig. 3). Such size similarity may be significant in considering the conformation of the heterodimeric receptor complex that is quite unique for this receptor, since both α and β chains individually interact with distinct sites of the same IL-2 molecule (Collins et al. 1988).

The cytoplasmic region of the β chain is far larger than that of the α chain, which is only 13 amino acids long. The consensus sequences of tyrosine kinase (Gly-x-Gly-x-x-Gly) (Hanks et al. 1988) are absent in the β chain. However, we note the presence of a triplet, Ala-Pro-Glu(293–295), that has been implicated as the consensus motif for a catalytic domain of some protein kinases (Hanks et al. 1988). The possibility for the cytoplasmic region of the β chain to have a protein kinase activity is yet to be tested. The primary structure of this region revealed yet another interesting feature: a rather strong bias for certain characteristic amino acids. This region is rich in proline (24/286) and serine (30/286) residues. The proline-rich structure may impart a nonglobular conformation to this region that may be

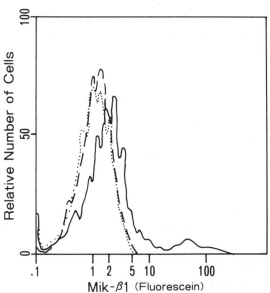

Figure 2. Expression of the human IL-2Rβ chain cDNA in COS cells. COS cells were transfected with clone pIL-2β30, stained indirectly with antibodies, and analyzed by FACS as described previously (Minamoto et al. 1989). (Solid line) Transfected cells were treated by Mik-β1; (broken line) transfected cells were treated by anti-Tac (a monoclonal antibody against the human IL-2Rα chain; (dotted line) transfected cells were stained with fluorescein-conjugated goat-anti-mouse IgG alone.

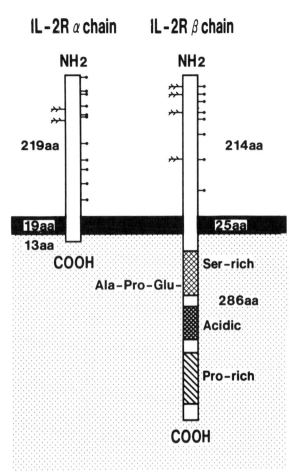

IL-2R α chain   IL-2R β chain

Figure 3. Schematic representation of the human IL-2Rα and IL-2Rβ chains. Symbols on the right and left sides of each column represent the cysteine residues and N-glycosylation sites, respectively. For details of the IL-2Rβ chain structure, see Hatakeyama et al. (1989).

important in coupling of the receptor molecule with other signal transducer(s). The predominant serine residues may be the major target for phosphorylation, which could also modulate the receptor function (Fig. 3). In addition, the cytoplasmic region is notably biased for negatively charged amino acids. In fact, this region contains 40 such amino acids (i.e., glutamic and aspartic acids), whereas only 18 amino acids account for the positively charged residues (i.e., lysine and arginine). Such a bias is particularly notable in the middle portion (amino acids 345–390) of the cytoplasmic region (Fig. 3). Thus, the cytoplasmic region of the β chain may be quite acidic. Taken together, some, if not all, of these unique characteristics may be responsible for driving further the downstream signal transduction pathway(s).

Functional Expression of the IL-2Rβ Chain cDNA

A series of cDNA expression studies were carried out in order to examine if the cDNA product binds IL-2 and indeed manifests the properties of the native IL-2Rβ chain that have been demonstrated and/or suggest-ed in previous studies. A cDNA expression plasmid was constructed in which expression of the cDNA spanning the entire coding region was directed by the mouse *lck* gene promoter (pLCKRβ) (Hatakeyama et al. 1989). The plasmid pLCKRβ was introduced into the human T-cell leukemia Jurkat, which is known to be devoid of surface molecules that bind human IL-2. Stable transformant clones expressing the cDNA product were obtained, as judged by FACS analysis. One of these was termed Jβ-8. In addition, we introduced the same gene into the Jurkat transformant clone, Jα-5, which expresses the transfected, human IL-2Rα chain cDNA. The resulting transformant, Jαβ-10, was found to express both α and β chains (Hatakeyama et al. 1989). When the IL-2 binding studies were carried out with ^{125}I-labeled recombinant human IL-2, the following binding profiles were obtained by Scatchard plot analyses (Fig. 4). Actually, the Jβ-8 cells, expressing the β chain cDNA, displayed intermediate affinity to IL-2 with an estimated K_d value of about 2 nM. Furthermore, the Jαβ-10 clone expressing both α and β chains displayed both high- and low-affinity receptors with respective K_d values of 16 pM and 20 nM. The high-affinity IL-2R complex was completely abolished following treatment of the cells by Mik-β1 antibody (Fig. 4). Essentially, the results obtained with these clones were reproducible (Hatakeyama et al. 1989).

In contrast to the IL-2Rβ expressed on the Jurkat T-cell line and a mouse T-lymphoma line, EL4 (Hatakeyama et al. 1989), the IL-2Rβ expressed on nonlymphoid cells such as NIH-3T3, L929, and COS cells failed to display significant IL-2 binding ability (Hatakeyama et al. 1989; S. Minamoto, unpubl.). It is possible that another lymphoid-specific component(s) is involved in maintaining a functional conformation for IL-2Rβ. Further work will be required to clarify this point.

DISCUSSION

In this paper, we report the isolation and expression of a cDNA encoding the human IL-2Rβ chain. The availability of the cDNAs for IL-2 (Taniguchi et al. 1983), IL-2Rα chain (Cosman et al. 1984; Leonard et al. 1984; Nikaido et al. 1984), and IL-2Rβ chain (Hatakeyama et al. 1989) will make it possible to elucidate the intricacies of the IL-2 system. The functional IL-2 receptor complex is unique in that two structurally distinct membrane components, the IL-2Rα and IL-2Rβ chains, both bind IL-2 independently. Our preliminary data support the notion that IL-2 binding to both α and β chains is important for the IL-2-mediated signal transduction (i.e., cell growth) (T. Doi et al., in prep.). At present, little is known about the cascade of biochemical events triggered by cytokines interacting with their homologous receptors. Our findings on the structure of the IL-2Rβ chain demonstrate the presence of a large cytoplasmic region that most likely is involved in driving the IL-2 signal pathway(s). The particular acidic nucleus as well as the serine-rich re-

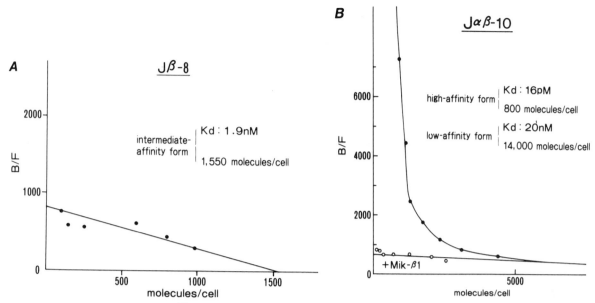

Figure 4. Scatchard plot analysis of ^{125}I-labeled IL-2 binding to the transfectants expressing the human IL-2Rα and/or IL-2Rβ chain cDNAs. (*A*) The Jurkat-derived clone Jβ-8, expressing the IL-2Rβ chain cDNA. (*B*) The Jurkat-derived clone Jαβ-10, expressing both IL-2Rα and IL-2Rβ chain cDNAs. The binding data in the absence (●) or presence (○) of 1:100-diluted ascites of Mik-β1. The number of IL-2 binding sites per cell and the receptor affinity were determined by computer-assisted analysis of the IL-2 binding data.

gion, both found in the cytoplasmic region, may suggest coupling to other cytoplasmic signal transducers. The availability of the expression system in which the cDNA-encoded β chain can deliver growth signal (T. Doi et al., in prep.) will allow us to dissect further the functional domains of the receptor. The mouse homolog of the IL-2Rβ chain has also been cloned recently. The murine IL-2Rβ chain consists of 539 amino acids, and the structure appears to be highly homologous to that of the human β chain (T. Kono et al., in prep.). Thus, by using the mouse system, it will be possible to make various experimental approaches to elucidate the role of the IL-2 system in the development and regulation of the immune system.

ACKNOWLEDGMENTS

We are indebted to Drs. E. Barsoumian and B. Seed for invaluable advice and to Ms. Y. Maeda for excellent assistance. We also thank Drs. J. Yodoi, T. Uchiyama, R. Perlmutter, and F. Grosveld for YT cell, anti-Tac antibody, p1013, and pHyg, respectively. This work is supported in part by a grant-in-aid for special Project Research, Cancer Bioscience from the Ministry of Education, Science and Culture of Japan and the Nissan Science Foundation.

REFERENCES

Benveniste, E.N. and J.E. Merrill. 1986. Stimulation of oligodendroglial proliferation and maturation by interleukin-2. *Nature* **321:** 610.
Collins, L., W.-H. Tsien, C. Seals, J. Hakimi, D. Weber, P.

Bailon, J. Hoskings, W.C. Greene, V. Toome, and G. Ju. 1988. Identification of specific residues of human interleukin-2 that affect binding to the 70-kDa subunit (p70) of the interleukin-2 receptor. *Proc. Natl. Acad. Sci.* **85;** 7709.
Cosman, D., D.P. Cerretti, A. Larsen, L. Park, C. March, S. Dower, S. Gillis, and D. Urdall. 1984. Cloning, sequence and expression of human interleukin-2 receptor. *Nature* **312:** 768.
Dukovich, M., Y. Wano, J.B. Thuy, P. Katz, B.R. Cullen, J.H. Kehr, and W.C. Greene. 1987. A second human interleukin-2 binding protein that may be a component of high-affinity interleukin-2 receptors. *Nature* **327:** 518.
Greene, W., R.J. Robb, P.B. Svetlik, G.M. Rusk, J.M. Depper, and W.J. Leonard. 1985. Stable expression of cDNA encoding the human interleukin-2 receptor in eukaryotic cells. *J. Exp. Med.* **162:** 363.
Hanks, S.K., A.M. Quinn, and T. Hunter. 1988. The protein kinase family: Conserved features and deduced phylogeny of the catalytic domains. *Science* **241:** 42.
Hatakeyama, M., S. Minamoto, T. Uchiyama, R.R. Hardy, G. Yamada, and T. Taniguchi. 1985. Reconstitution of functional receptor for human interleukin-2 in mouse cells. *Nature* **318:** 467.
Hatakeyama, M., M. Tsudo, S. Minamoto, T. Kono, T. Doi, T. Miyata, M. Miyasaka, and T. Taniguchi. 1989. Interleukin-2 receptor β chain gene: Generation of three receptor forms by cloned human α and β chain cDNA's. *Science* **244:** 551.
Kondo, S., A. Shimizu, M. Maeda, Y. Tagaya, J. Yodoi, and T. Honjo. 1986. Expression of functional human interleukin-2 receptor in mouse T cells by cDNA transfection. *Nature* **320:** 75.
Leonard, W.J., J.M. Depper, G.R. Crabtree, S. Rudikoff, J. Pumphrey, R.J. Robb, M. Kronke, P.B. Svetlik, N.J. Peffer, T.A. Waldmann, and W.C. Greene. 1984. Molecular cloning and expression of cDNAs for the human interleukin-2 receptor. *Nature* **311:** 626.
Minamoto, S., S. Itoh, T. Kono, T. Doi, and M. Hatakeyama. 1989. Ligand-dependent selection of the receptor gene: Segregation of IL-2 binding activity and anti-Tac reactivity

by a single amino acid alteration in the Tac antigen. *Immunol. Lett.* **20:** 139.

Nikaido, T., A. Shimizu, N. Ishida, H. Sabe, K. Teshigawara, M. Maeda, T. Uchiyama, J. Yodoi, and T. Honjo. 1984. Molecular cloning of cDNA encoding human interleukin-2 receptor. *Nature* **311:** 631.

Potter, H., L. Weir, and P. Leder. 1984. Enhancer-dependent expression of human κ immunoglobulin genes introduced into mouse pre-B lymphocytes by electroporation. *Proc. Natl. Acad. Sci.* **81:** 7164.

Robb, R.J. 1986. Conversion of low-affinity interleukin 2 receptors to a high-affinity state following fusion of cell membranes. *Proc. Natl. Acad. Sci.* **83:** 3392.

Robb, R.J., W.C. Greene, and C.M. Rusk. 1984. Low and high affinity cellular receptors for interleukin-2. Implications for the level of Tac antigen. *J. Exp. Med.* **160:** 1126.

Rosenberg, S.A., M.T. Lotze, L.M. Muul, S. Leitman, A.E. Chang, S.E. Ettinghause, Y.L. Matory, J.M. Skibber, E. Shiloni, J.T. Vetto, C.A. Seipp, C. Simpson, and C.M. Reichert. 1985. Observations on the systematic administration of autologous lymphokine-activated killer cells and recombinant interleukin-2 to patients with metastatic cancer. *N. Engl. J. Med.* **313:** 1485.

Seed, B. 1987. An LFA-3 cDNA encodes a phospholipid-linked membrane protein homologous to its receptor CD2. *Nature* **329:** 840.

Seed, B. and A. Aruffo. 1987. Molecular cloning of the CD2 antigen, the T-cell erythrocyte receptor, by a rapid immunoselection procedure. *Proc. Natl. Acad. Sci.* **84:** 3365.

Sharon, M., R.D. Klausner, B.R. Cullen, R. Chizzonite, and W.J. Leonardo. 1986. Novel interleukin-2 receptor subunit detected by cross-linking under high-affinity conditions. *Science* **234:** 859.

Smith, K.A. 1980. T-cell growth factor. *Immunol. Rev.* **51:** 1171.

———. 1988. Interleukin-2: Inception, impact and implications. *Science* **240:** 1169.

Taniguchi, T. 1988. Regulation of cytokine gene expression. *Annu. Rev. Immunol.* **6:** 439.

Taniguchi, T., H. Matsui, T. Fujita, C. Takaoka, N. Kashima, R. Yoshimoto, and J. Hamuro. 1983. Structure and expression of a cloned cDNA for human interleukin-2. *Nature* **302:** 305.

Taniguchi, T., H. Matsui, T. Fujita, M. Hatakeyama, N. Kashima, A. Fuse, J. Hamuro, C. Nishi-Takaoka, and G. Yamada. 1985. Molecular analysis of the interleukin-2 system. *Immunol. Rev.* **92:** 121.

Teshigawara, K., H.-M. Wang, K. Kato, and K.A. Smith. 1987. Interleukin-2 high-affinity receptor expression requires two distinct binding proteins. *J. Exp. Med.* **165:** 223.

Tsudo, M., F. Kitamura, and M. Miyasaka. 1989. Characterization of the interleukin-2 receptor β chain using three distinct monoclonal antibodies. *Proc. Natl. Acad. Sci.* **86:** 1982.

Tsudo, M., R.W. Kozak, C.K. Goldman, and T.A. Waldmann. 1986. Demonstration of a non-Tac peptide that binds interleukin-2: A potential participant in a multi-chain interleukin-2 receptor complex. *Proc. Natl. Acad. Sci.* **83:** 9694.

Wong-Staal, F. and R.C. Gallo. 1985. Human T-lymphotropic retroviruses. *Nature* **317:** 395.

Yodoi, J., K. Teshigawara, T. Nikaido, K. Fukui, T. Noma, T. Honjo, M. Takigawa, M. Sasaki, N. Minato, M. Tsudo, T. Uchiyama, and M. Maeda. 1986. TCGF (IL-2)-receptor inducing factor(s). I. Regulation of IL-2 receptor on a natural killer-like cell line (YT cells). *J. Immunol.* **134:** 1623.

Yoshida, M. and M. Seiki. 1987. Recent advances in the molecular biology of HTLV-1: *Trans*-activation of viral and cellular genes. *Annu. Rev. Immunol.* **5:** 541.

Immune Dysfunctions and Activation of Natural Killer Cells in Human IL-2 and IL-2/IL-2 Receptor L-chain Transgenic Mice

Y. Ishida,* M. Nishi,*# O. Taguchi,† K. Inaba,‡
N. Minato,§ M. Kawaichi,* and T. Honjo*

*Department of Medical Chemistry, Kyoto University Faculty of Medicine, ‡Department of Zoology,
Kyoto University Faculty of Science, Kyoto 606; †Laboratory of Experimental Pathology, Aichi Cancer Center
Research Institute, Nagoya 464; §Department of Medicine, Jichi Medical School, Tochigi 329-04, Japan

Interleukin-2 (IL-2), a glycoprotein formerly called T-cell growth factor, is secreted by peripheral helper T cells when they recognize antigenic peptides in association with protein products of the major histocompatibility complex (MHC). Secreted IL-2 then binds to its receptor expressed on antigen-stimulated peripheral T cells and induces their proliferation (Smith 1988).

The interleukin-2 receptor (IL-2R) consists of at least two polypeptide chains, namely the light (L) chain (p55) and the heavy (H) chain (p75) (Tsudo et al. 1986; Robb et al. 1987; Teshigawara et al. 1987). The L and H chains bind IL-2 with low (K_d, 10 nM) and intermediate (K_d, 100 pM) affinities, respectively. IL-2 first binds to the L chain, and the IL-2/L-chain complex then quickly associates with the H chain on the cell surface to form the ternary complex of IL-2, the L chain, and the H chain, which gives rise to the high-affinity binding site (K_d, 10 pM) and transduces the growth signal (Kondo et al. 1987; Ogura et al. 1988; Saito et al. 1988).

The L chain, which alone cannot transduce the growth signal (Sabe et al. 1984; Greene et al. 1985), is expressed transiently on peripheral T cells only when they are stimulated by antigens or mitogens (Waldmann 1986). On the other hand, the H chain is believed to transduce the growth signal by itself at a higher concentration of IL-2 (Siegel et al. 1987; Tsudo et al. 1987; Wang and Smith 1987), and is constitutively expressed on T cells in a limited number (Nishi et al. 1988; Tsudo et al. 1989).

There is no doubt that IL-2 and its receptor are indispensable for the growth of mature T cells in vitro. However, it is still controversial whether they play other important roles in vivo. If IL-2 is involved in regulation of T-cell growth and differentiation in vivo, the constitutive expression of IL-2 and its receptor in animals would bring about T-cell abnormalities. In addition, the constitutive expression of the IL-2R L chain on T cells may cause some T-cell malignancies, as proposed for a mechanism of leukemogenesis of adult

T-cell leukemia (Yodoi et al. 1983; Depper et al. 1984; Maeda et al. 1987).

To test these possibilities, we produced transgenic mice expressing human IL-2 constitutively (Ishida et al. 1989a) and then mated them with transgenic mice expressing human IL-2R L chain constitutively (Nishi et al. 1988) to obtain mice that express both the ligand and the receptor constitutively (Ishida et al. 1989b).

EXPERIMENTAL PROCEDURES

RNase protection assay. RNA (20 μg) isolated from the individual organs was hybridized overnight with a ^{32}P-labeled antisense in vitro transcript of human IL-2, followed by digestion with RNase A and T1. The protected fragments were separated on a polyacrylamide/urea gel and exposed to an X-ray film.

Histological and cytological examinations. Sections were stained routinely with hematoxylin and eosin. For Thy-1$^+$ dendritic epidermal cell (DEC) staining, the fixed epidermis was incubated with fluorescein isothiocyanate (FITC)-labeled anti-Thy-1 monoclonal antibody (MAb). Morphology of spleen cells was assessed after depositing cells on microscope slides with a cytocentrifuge and staining with Wright and Giemsa stain. For the immunological staining, the following reagents were used: FITC-anti-Thy-1.2 MAb, phycoerythrin (PE)-anti-CD4 MAb, FITC-anti-CD8 MAb, biotinylated anti-mouse CD3 MAb, and PE-streptavidin. Dead cells were excluded from analysis using a combination of low-angle and sideway light scatter.

Immunological assays. Spleen cells of human IL-2 transgenic mice were stimulated with mitomycin-C-treated dendritic cells prepared from spleens of CD2 F_1 mice (H-2^d) (mixed leukocyte reaction). [^{3}H]Thymidine was added in the last 12 hours of the culture period of the kinetic study, and incorporated radioactivities were measured by liquid scintillation counting. For the assay of cytotoxic T lymphocyte (CTL) activity, spleen cells were primed by culturing with allogenic dendritic cells (H-2^d) for 5 days and used as effector cells. The

---

Present address: Department of Molecular Biology, Research Institute of Scripps Clinic, La Jolla, California 92037.

[51]Cr-labeled P815 (H-2^d) cells were used as target cells. Mitogen responses were assayed by culturing spleen cells with anti-CD3 MAb (Leo et al. 1987), concanavalin A (Con A), or lipopolysaccharide (LPS), and the kinetics of their proliferative responses were analyzed as described previously (Ishida et al. 1989a). Natural killer (NK) cell activity was measured with ^{51}Cr-labeled YAC-1 cell line (H-2^a) as the NK target. Target cells were added to effector spleen cells and incubated for 4 hours. In some experiments, the P815 cell line was also used as a target.

RESULTS

Skin and Lung Lesions in Human IL-2 Transgenic Mice

The complete human IL-2 cDNA with its own translational start and stop codons and polyadenylation signal was fused to the constitutive murine MHC class I (H-2K^d) promoter (Fig. 1A). The construct DNA, which is similar to the one containing human IL-2R L-chain cDNA (Nishi et al. 1988), was microinjected into fertilized eggs of C57BL/6 mice to obtain transgenic mice. Expression of the transgene as human IL-2

mRNA was detected in the thymus, spleen, bone marrow, lung, skin, and muscle of the transgenic mice by using a specific RNase protection assay (Fig. 1,B and C). Enzyme-linked immunosorbent assay for human IL-2 detected 30–570 pM human IL-2 protein in the sera of most transgenic mice, but not in the sera of normal control mice (data not shown).

All the transgenic mice began to suffer from alopecia around 8 weeks of age (Fig. 2,A and B). Then the body weight of the mice decreased gradually, and all of them died within a year after birth. Histological examinations of 11-week-old transgenic mice showed several alterations in their skin tissues (Fig. 2,C and D). The hair roots of the mice disappeared at the alopecic sites, and the epidermis and hair follicles were markedly thickened. The skin of the younger (5 weeks old) transgenic mice showed only slight histological changes (data not shown), but contained a markedly increased number of Thy-1$^+$ DECs as compared with the age-matched normal mice (Fig. 2,G and H). In addition to the dermatological changes, we found severe pneumonia in the transgenic mice at the age of 11 weeks (Fig. 2,E and F). A wide range of diffuse infiltration of neutrophils and focal infiltration of lymphocytes in the lung were found. The lymphoid tissues, including the

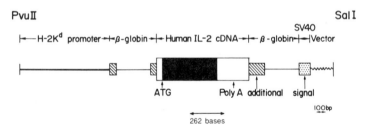
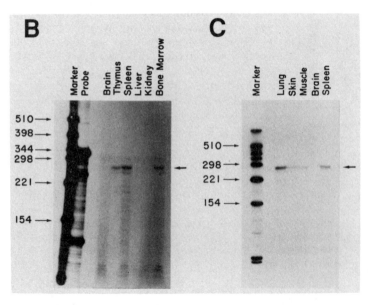

Figure 1. Construction and expression of the transgene in human IL-2 transgenic mice. (A) The transgene H-2K^d·h·IL-2 was constructed as described previously (Ishida et al. 1989a). The antisense probe (262 bases) used for the RNase protection assay is shown as a horizontal arrow below the construct. Translated and untranslated regions of human IL-2 cDNA are indicated by black and open rectangles, respectively. (B, C) RNA from various tissues of human IL-2 transgenic mice was analyzed by the RNase protection assay using the probe shown in A. Arrows indicate the expected size (262 bases) of the protected probe.

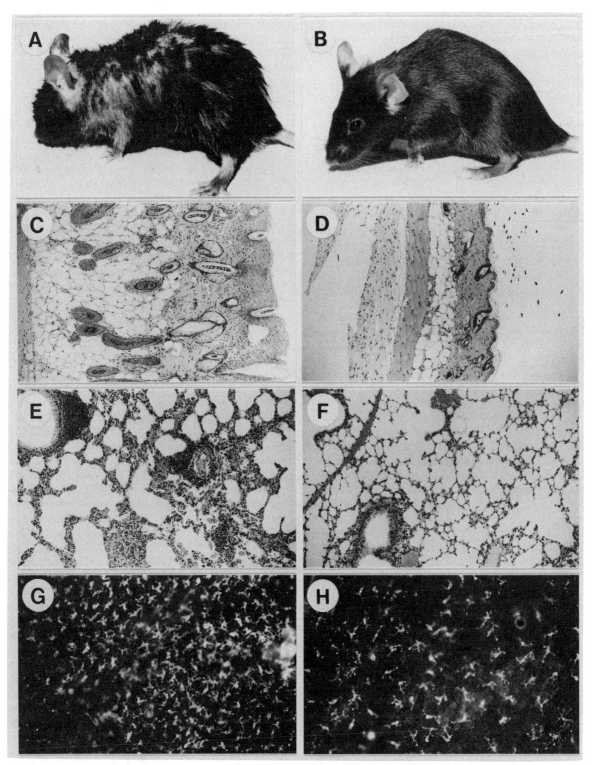

Figure 2. Phenotype of human IL-2 transgenic mice. (*A*) Alopecia of a human IL-2 transgenic mouse. (*B*) A normal C57BL/6 mouse. (*C*) Histology of the skin lesion in human IL-2 transgenic mice. (*D*) Normal skin histology. (*E*) Histology of pneumonia in human IL-2 transgenic mice. (*F*) Normal lung histology. (*G*) Thy-1$^+$ DEC in the epidermal sheet of human IL-2 transgenic mice immunohistologically stained with an anti-Thy-1.2 antibody. (*H*) Thy-1$^+$ DEC in normal mice. Thy-1$^+$ cells in *G* and *H* were negative for both CD4 and CD8 antigens (data not shown). Ages of mice used were 11 weeks (*A–F*) and 5 weeks (*G* and *H*). Magnifications, 67× (*C–F*) and 152× (*G* and *H*).

697

thymus, spleen, and lymph nodes of the mice, did not show any sign of histological abnormality at the age of 11 weeks.

To elucidate the primary cause of the skin lesion in human IL-2 transgenic mice, we performed reciprocal skin transplantations between human IL-2 transgenic and normal mice. When transplanted, the transgenic skin looked healthy, because the transgenic mice examined were too young (5–6 weeks old) to show any skin lesions. However, transgenic skin grafts transplanted to normal mice became alopecic, whereas normal skin grafts transplanted to transgenic mice remained hairy when the surrounding skin of the transgenic mice became alopecic (data not shown). The result indicates that the tissue of the transgenic skin itself, but not mobile components like lymphocytes, contains agents responsible for the skin lesion of the mice.

Unaltered Distribution of Lymphocyte Subsets and Absence of Autoimmune Symptoms in Human IL-2 Transgenic Mice

We investigated whether human IL-2 transgenic mice had distorted proportions of lymphocyte subsets in the thymus and spleen, but we found no significant difference between the human IL-2 transgenic and normal control mice (data not shown).

We next examined whether autoimmune reactions were involved in the lesions in the skin and lungs of human IL-2 transgenic mice. First, we could not detect autoreactive antibodies in the sera of the transgenic mice by immunohistochemical techniques (data not shown). Second, we injected the transgenic spleen cells intravenously into sublethally irradiated (750 rad) normal C57BL/6 mice (1.5×10^7 cells/mouse), but we could not transfer any pathological lesions found in the donor transgenic mice to the recipient mice, indicating the absence or very low frequency of autoreactive T cells in the spleen of the transgenic mice (data not shown). All these results suggest that the lesions in the skin and lungs of the mice may not be due to typical autoimmune reactions.

Immune Dysfunctions in Human IL-2 Transgenic Mice

We then examined the possibility that human IL-2 transgenic mice might suffer from immunodeficiency. The results of in vitro functional analyses of the transgenic spleen cells are shown in Figure 3. Although human IL-2 transgenic mice had almost normal proportions of lymphocyte subsets in the spleen, the proliferative response of their spleen cells in the allogenic mixed leukocyte culture was markedly lower than that of the control mice (Fig. 3A). The CTL activity after priming in the allogenic mixed leukocyte culture was also reduced in the transgenic mice (Fig. 3B). In addition, the IgG response by spleen cells of the transgenic mice that had been immunized with sheep red blood

cells was markedly reduced (data not shown). In contrast, the mitogenic responses of the transgenic spleen cells to polyclonal lymphocyte activators like anti-CD3 MAb, Con A, or LPS were almost indistinguishable from those of normal controls (Fig. 3,C–E). Despite these lymphocyte dysfunctions, we found that the NK activity of human IL-2 transgenic spleen cells was not impaired as compared with the control spleen cells (Fig. 3F).

Phenotypes of Human IL-2/IL-2R L-chain Transgenic Mice

We have already reported some properties of human IL-2R L-chain transgenic mice (Nishi et al. 1988). Unstimulated spleen cells of the mice had about 120 high-affinity binding sites for IL-2 per cell and proliferated in vitro in the presence of exogenous recombinant human IL-2, indicating the constitutive expression of the H chain of IL-2R in unstimulated normal spleen cells (Nishi et al. 1988). We have not observed any abnormality in this transgenic mouse, probably because endogenous murine IL-2 has orders of magnitude weaker binding affinity to the human IL-2R than to the murine counterpart.

To further study the effects of the constitutive expression of IL-2 and its receptor, we produced "hybrid" mice, which carried both human IL-2 and IL-2R L-chain transgenes, by crossing the two parental strains (Ishida et al. 1989b). The hybrid mice always showed severe growth retardation, which became apparent about a week after birth. In addition, their gait was disturbed or ataxic (i.e., wide-based and staggering) and they easily fell down while walking. These hybrid mice died by 4 weeks of age without exception.

Histological studies on 3-week-old hybrid mice revealed interstitial pneumonia with focal infiltration of lymphocytes (Fig. 4,A and B). The thymus and spleen of the hybrid mice of that age were far smaller than those of the control mice, and profound lymphocyte depletions were found histologically in the cortex of the thymus (Fig. 4,C and D) and in the red pulp of the spleen (Fig. 4,E and F) of the hybrid mice. In addition to these histological changes, the hybrid mice selectively lost Purkinje cells in the cerebellum without any sign of inflammation (Fig. 4,G and H), which might be associated with the ataxic gait of the mice. Histological studies on 2-week-old hybrid mice did not show any severe damage to the thymus, spleen, and cerebellum, although interstitial pneumonia was already seen at this age. The results indicate that the damage in the thymus, spleen, and cerebellum took place mainly after birth.

Expansion of NK Cells in the Spleen of Human IL-2/IL-2R L-chain Transgenic Mice

The most striking cellular immunological abnormality found in the hybrid mice was the increase in the proportion and number of Thy-1$^+$/CD3$^-$ cells in the

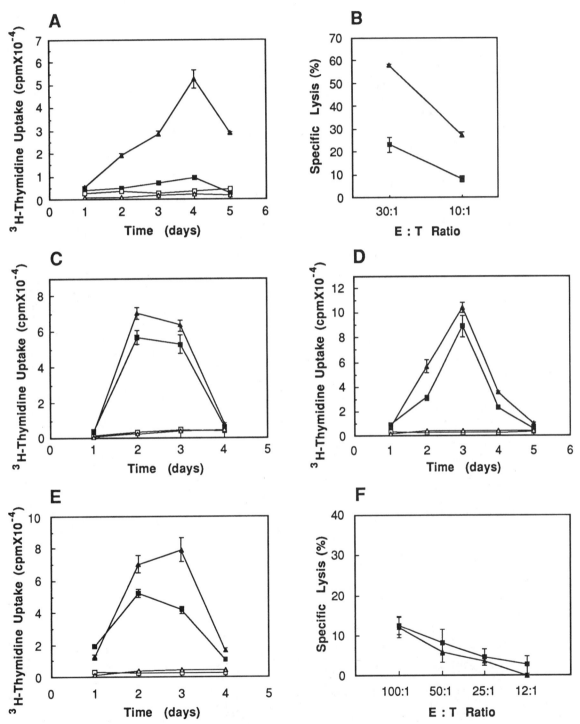

Figure 3. Immunological functions of spleen cells of human IL-2 transgenic mice. The kinetics of the proliferative responses against allogenic stimulator cells (*A*), anti-CD3 MAb (*C*), Con A (*D*), and LPS (*E*) are shown. CTL activity against allogenic P815 cells (*B*) and NK activity against NK-sensitive YAC-1 cells (*F*) are also shown. Unfractionated spleen cells were used as responders or effectors as described in Experimental Procedures. (■) IL-2 transgenic spleen cells; (▲) normal spleen cells; (□) IL-2 transgenic spleen cells without stimulators; (△) normal spleen cells without stimulators. Means of data from three mice are plotted with standard deviations (vertical bars) except for the responses without stimulators, which had deviations too small to show.

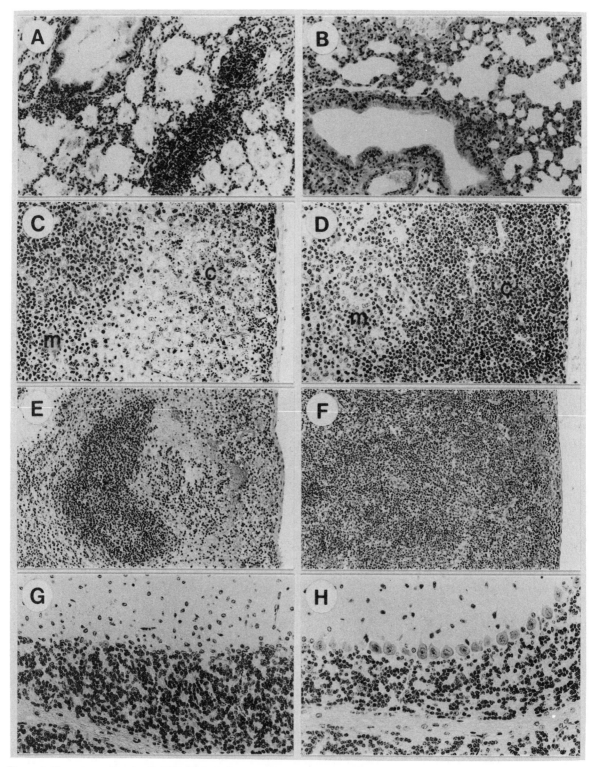

Figure 4. Phenotype of human IL-2/IL-2R L-chain transgenic mice. (*A*) Histology of pneumonia in the hybrid mice. (*B*) Normal lung histology. (*C*) Histology of lymphocyte depletion in the cortex of the hybrid thymus. (*D*) Normal thymus histology. (*E*) Histology of lymphocyte depletion in the hybrid spleen. (*F*) Normal spleen histology. (*G*) Histology of the selective loss of Purkinje cells in the cerebellum of hybrid mice. (*H*) Normal cerebellum histology. In *C* and *D*, *c* and *m* indicate cortex and medulla, respectively. Mice analyzed were 3 weeks old. Magnifications, 133 × (*A* and *B*), 214 × (*C, D, G,* and *H*), and 105 × (*E* and *F*).

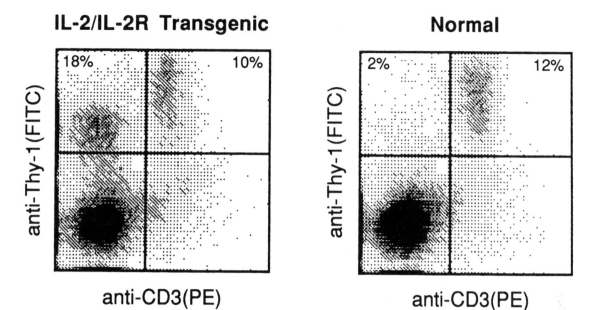

Figure 5. Expansion of Thy-1$^+$/CD3$^-$ cells in the spleen of human IL-2/IL-2R L-chain transgenic mice. Whole spleen cells of the mice (2 weeks old) were stained with optimal concentrations of FITC-anti-Thy-1.2 MAb and biotinylated anti-mouse CD3 MAb followed by PE-streptavidin. Fluorescence intensities of cells are indicated as dot matrices with logarithmic scales.

spleen, as shown in Figure 5. About 18% of the spleen cells of 2-week-old hybrid mice were phenotypically Thy-1$^+$/CD3$^-$, whereas the age-matched normal spleen did not contain a significant proportion of cells with this phenotype. The Thy-1$^+$/CD3$^-$ cells were also rare in the spleen of the parental (IL-2 or IL-2R) transgenic mice. Another staining experiment showed that the spleen of 2.5-week-old hybrid mice contained a larger proportion of Thy-1$^+$ cells ($\sim$28%) than that of normal mice (Table 1). However, the sum ($\sim$11%) of CD4$^+$ and CD8$^+$ cells was far less than the total Thy-1$^+$ cells, indicating that there were a larger number of Thy-1$^+$/CD4$^-$8$^-$ cells ($\sim$17%) in the spleen of the hybrid mice (Table 1). Since mature CD4$^+$ and CD8$^+$ T cells always express the CD3 complex on their surface (Clevers et al. 1988), the two populations (Thy-1$^+$/CD3$^-$ and Thy-1$^+$/CD4$^-$8$^-$ cells) detected independently in the spleen of the hybrid mice are most likely identical. Hybrid mice had almost normal proportions of thymocyte subsets as compared with age-matched normal C57BL/6 mice, although the number of thymocytes in the hybrid mice was significantly smaller (Table 1).

We also performed morphological analysis on the hybrid spleen cells. The spleen of 2.5-week-old hybrid mice contained a larger proportion of large granular lymphocytes (LGL) ($\sim$28%) as compared with the normal control ($\sim$7%). It was then examined whether the expanded Thy-1$^+$/CD3$^-$ cells were morphologically LGL. We collected the Thy-1$^+$/CD3$^-$ cells and Thy-1$^+$/CD3$^+$ cells separately from the spleen of the hybrid mice by using a fluorescence-activated cell sorter, and assessed the morphology of each population. More than 95% of the Thy-1$^+$/CD3$^-$ cells were morphologically LGL (Fig. 6A). In contrast, the Thy-1$^+$/CD3$^+$

cells in the hybrid spleen were not LGL, but ordinary lymphocytes without granules (Fig. 6B).

When analyzed functionally, spleen cells of the hybrid mice showed markedly elevated NK activity (Fig. 7) as well as defects such as found in the IL-2 transgenic mice (data not shown). Not only a common NK target, YAC-1 cells (Fig. 7A), but also P815 cells (Fig. 7B) were killed by the hybrid spleen cells. Such NK activity of the hybrid spleen cells is extraordinarily elevated as compared with normal spleen cells. Spleen cells of normal mice (including nude mice) at the age of 2–3 weeks usually have only marginal NK activity, and they cannot kill P815 cells at all. We next examined which of the two Thy-1$^+$ populations (Thy-1$^+$/CD3$^-$ or Thy-1$^+$/CD3$^+$ cells) in the spleen of the hybrid mice bore the strong NK activity. The sorted Thy-1$^+$/CD3$^-$ LGL showed very strong NK activity, whereas the Thy-1$^+$/

Table 1. Distribution of Lymphocyte Subsets in Human IL-2/IL-2R L-chain Transgenic Mice

		Percentage of cells	
		transgenic	normal
Thymus	CD4$^-$8$^-$	4.0 ± 0.1	2.7 ± 0.5
	CD4$^+$8$^+$	87.1 ± 0.8	85.1 ± 2.2
	CD4$^+$8$^-$	7.1 ± 0.7	7.7 ± 0.8
	CD4$^-$8$^+$	1.8 ± 0.3	4.4 ± 1.8
Spleen	Thy-1$^+$	28.2 ± 3.9	11.5 ± 0.1
	CD4$^+$8$^-$	4.6 ± 0.4	5.2 ± 0.4
	CD4$^-$8$^+$	6.3 ± 0.5	3.2 ± 0.2

Mean percentages from three mice (2.5 weeks old) are shown with ± standard deviations. Mean numbers of nucleated cells per organ of these mice were 4.5 ± 0.2 × 10^7/transgenic thymus, 11.3 ± 0.9 × 10^7/normal thymus, 3.6 ± 0.4 × 10^7/transgenic spleen, and 4.3 ± 0.9 × 10^7/normal spleen. Washed cells were stained with the fluorescein-labeled antibodies and analyzed by flow cytometry.

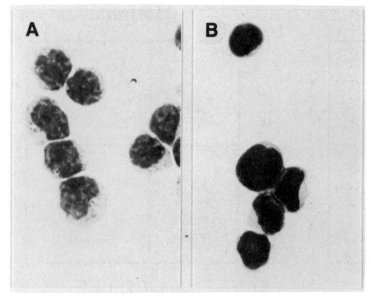

Figure 6. Morphology of Thy-1$^+$/CD3$^-$ cells (A) and Thy-1$^+$/CD3$^+$ cells (B) collected separately from the spleen of human IL-2/IL-2R L-chain transgenic mice.

CD3$^+$ cells, which represent ordinary T cells, had negligible NK activity (data not shown).

The absence of the CD3 complex on the cell surface of the expanded LGL in the hybrid mice suggests that they have neither the $\alpha\beta$- nor $\gamma\delta$-type of T-cell receptor (TCR). To confirm this observation, we analyzed the rearrangement of TCR genes in the LGL of hybrid mice that were selectively expanded in vitro from the spleen of the mice by culture with IL-2. With the use of the C_β and C_γ probes, only discrete germ-line bands of the expected intensity were detected in the Thy-1$^+$/CD3$^-$ LGL-enriched hybrid spleen cells, whereas germ-line bands with decreased intensity and rearranged bands (for the C_γ probe) were seen in the CD3$^+$ cell-enriched spleen cells of the normal mice (data not shown). These results indicate that the expanded LGL in the hybrid mice have not rearranged the TCR genes and, as a consequence, do not express TCR molecules on their surface.

DISCUSSION

Possible Defects Responsible for Immune Dysfunctions in Human IL-2 Transgenic Mice

Since IL-2 is well established to stimulate T cells in vitro, we first expected that the constitutive expression of IL-2 in mice would cause some kind of "hyperimmune" state like autoimmunity. However, we could not find any typical signs of autoimmunity in the mice, but, unexpectedly, we observed several immune dysfunctions. One possibility to explain the mechanism of these immune dysfunctions in the IL-2 transgenic mice is that the mice may have a skewed T-cell repertoire. If the frequency of T cells recognizing a particular antigen is extremely low among the IL-2 transgenic T-cell population, the T cells as a whole would be much less efficient in responding to the antigen, although they could respond to polyclonal T-cell activators as strongly as the normal T-cell population. A defect in the an-

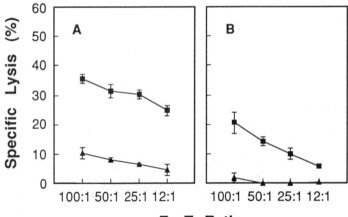

Figure 7. Elevated NK activity of spleen cells of human IL-2/IL-2R L-chain transgenic mice. The NK activity of unfractionated spleen cells of the transgenic mice (■) and normal controls (▲) was examined using either NK-sensitive YAC-1 cells (A) or relatively NK-resistant P815 cells (B) in various effector:target (E:T) ratios. Means of data from three mice (2 weeks old) are plotted with standard deviations (vertical bars).

tigen-nonspecific cell-to-cell interaction is another possible explanation of immune dysfunctions in human IL-2 transgenic mice. Cell-to-cell interaction is required for proliferative response and cytotoxicity against allogenic antigens and antibody production against the in vivo immunized antigen, but not for the response to soluble polyclonal activators. However, this is not so likely because the NK activity of the transgenic spleen cells was not impaired at all as compared with normal controls: Cell-to-cell contacts are believed to be essential in the cytolytic process by NK cells. We will discuss later another possibility of negative feedback by the constitutive expression of IL-2.

Skin and Lung Lesions in Transgenic Mice

Thy-1$^+$ DEC were reported to bear the cytolytic activity (Kuziel et al. 1987) and to have the capacity to respond to IL-2 under certain conditions (Nixon-Fulton et al. 1986). Since we detected human IL-2 mRNA in the skin of the IL-2 transgenic mice, it is reasonable to assume that the IL-2 transgenic skin cells themselves would secrete IL-2 which, in turn, activates Thy-1$^+$ DEC in situ to affect the neighboring skin cells. In addition to the skin lesion, all the human IL-2 and IL-2/IL-2R L-chain transgenic mice suffered from pneumonia with infiltration of lymphocytes. Although the exact mechanism for the pneumonia development is unknown, several immune dysfunctions found in the mice may cause a kind of immunodeficient state in the transgenic mice, which could result in the infection in their lungs. Alternatively, in situ activation of cytolytic cells (such as NK cells) in the lungs of the mice may be the primary cause of the pneumonia development, since we detected human IL-2 mRNA in the lungs of IL-2 transgenic mice. In fact, the majority of the lymphocytes infiltrating the lungs of the IL-2/IL-2R L-chain transgenic mice were morphologically LGL (data not shown).

Expansion of NK Cells but Not T Cells in Human IL-2/IL-2R L-chain Transgenic Mice

Since LGL expanded in the spleen of the hybrid mice had the Thy-1$^+$/CD3$^-$4$^-$8$^-$ phenotype, the germ-line configuration of TCR genes, and strong NK activity, they can be regarded as classic NK cells of non-T-cell lineage (Hersey and Bolhuis 1987; Hercend and Schmidt 1988). Recent studies (Nishi et al. 1988; Tsudo et al. 1989) showed that both LGL (or NK cells) and ordinary T cells (especially CD8$^+$ T cells) expressed the H chain of IL-2R constitutively even at the resting state. According to these findings, T cells as well as NK cells of the hybrid mice are expected to express high-affinity binding sites for IL-2 and to proliferate efficiently in response to IL-2. Therefore, we first expected the expansion of ordinary Thy-1$^+$/CD3$^+$ T cells in the hybrid mice carrying the IL-2 as well as IL-2R L-chain transgenes. Unexpectedly, however, we could not detect the expansion of ordinary T cells in the hybrid

mice, but instead we observed a remarkably increased number of Thy-1$^+$/CD3$^-$ NK cells in the spleen. These results suggest that NK cells in the hybrid mice have apparent advantages for selective proliferation as compared with ordinary T cells in these mice. There are three major possibilities that we should consider seriously: (1) The continuous activation of the IL-2/IL-2R pathway in vivo in the hybrid mice might have triggered negative feedback reactions in T cells but not in NK cells. (2) It is also possible that T cells but not NK cells might require an additional signal for their long-term proliferation in vivo that could be transduced by the TCR complex. (3) T cells may require a growth factor other than IL-2 for the proliferation in vivo.

We have never observed any incidence of leukemia or lymphoma in the hybrid mice. This may be partly due to the shortened life span of the hybrid mice.

Other Abnormalities in Human IL-2/IL-2R L-chain Transgenic Mice

We found that the spleens of hybrid mice at the age of 3 weeks were smaller than normal, which was probably due to lymphocyte depletion from the organ. Because NK cells were reported to have the capacity to kill syngeneic lymphocytes (Hansson et al. 1979), ordinary lymphocytes in the spleen of the hybrid mice might have been killed by the expanded Thy-1$^+$/CD3$^-$ LGL with elevated NK activity. Although profound lymphocyte depletion was also observed in the cortex of the thymus of 3-week-old hybrid mice, we could never detect the expansion of Thy-1$^+$/CD3$^-$ LGL in the thymus of the mice (data not shown). This suggests that the mechanisms of lymphocyte depletion in the spleen and thymus of the mice might be different.

The ataxic movement of the hybrid mice is most likely due to the decreased number of Purkinje cells. Although the histology of the cerebellum of hybrid mice at the age of 2 weeks was almost normal, we found that hybrid mice at the age of 3 weeks selectively lost more than half of the Purkinje cells in their cerebella. Patients treated with high-dose recombinant IL-2 occasionally showed psychological reactions such as confusion (Lotze et al. 1986), suggesting that IL-2 may have some effects on the central nervous system. In fact, astrocytes or oligodendrocytes in the brain were shown to proliferate and to mature in response to IL-2 (Merrill et al. 1984; Benveniste and Merrill 1986). Although we could not detect mRNA of human IL-2 or IL-2R L-chain in the brain of the transgenic mice (Nishi et al. 1988), a localized expression of the transgenes could allow activation of the IL-2-responsive cells in the brain of the hybrid mice, which may somehow result in the loss of Purkinje cells. Another possibility is that Purkinje cells may be extremely susceptible to NK-specific factors (Herbermann et al. 1986) produced by increased Thy-1$^+$/CD3$^-$ LGL in the hybrid mice. At this stage, however, it is fair to say that we have no reasonable explanation for the specific loss of Purkinje cells in the hybrid mice.

ACKNOWLEDGMENTS

We are grateful to Dr. K. Onoue for his generous supply of human IL-2 cDNA clone and to Dr. M. Honda for his measurement of serum IL-2. We acknowledge Dr. K. Kuribayashi for his help in the NK assay and Dr. Y. Nishizuka for the pathological diagnosis. We also thank S. Okazaki and J. Kuno for excellent technical assistance, and M. Sugiura for typing the manuscript. This investigation was supported by grants from the Ministry of Education, Science and Culture of Japan.

REFERENCES

Benveniste, E.N. and J.E. Merrill. 1986. Stimulation of oligodendroglial proliferation and maturation by interleukin-2. *Nature* **321:** 610.

Clevers, H., B. Alarcon, T. Wileman, and C. Terhorst. 1988. The T cell receptor/CD3 complex: A dynamic protein ensemble. *Annu. Rev. Immunol.* **6:** 629.

Depper, J.M., W.J. Leonard, M. Krönke, T.A. Waldmann, and W.C. Greene. 1984. Augmented T-cell growth factor receptor expression in HTLV-I infected human leukemic T cells. *J. Immunol.* **133:** 1691.

Greene, W.C., R.J. Robb, P.B. Svetlik, C.M. Rusk, J.M. Depper, and W.J. Leonard. 1985. Stable expression of cDNA encoding the human interleukin 2 receptor in eukaryotic cells. *J. Exp. Med.* **162:** 363.

Hansson, M., R. Kiessling, B. Andersson, K. Kärre, and J. Roder. 1979. NK cell-sensitive T-cell subpopulation in thymus: Inverse correlation to host NK activity. *Nature* **278:** 174.

Herbermann, R.B., C.W. Reynolds, and J.R. Ortaldo. 1986. Mechanism of cytotoxicity by natural killer (NK) cells. *Annu. Rev. Immunol.* **4:** 651.

Hercend, T. and R.E. Schmidt. 1988. Characteristics and uses of natural killer cells. *Immunol. Today* **9:** 291.

Hersey, P. and R. Bolhuis. 1987. "Nonspecific" MHC-unrestricted killer cells and their receptors. *Immunol. Today* **8:** 233.

Ishida, Y., M. Nishi, O. Taguchi, K. Inaba, N. Minato, M. Kawaichi, and T. Honjo. 1989a. Effects of the deregulated expression of human interleukin-2 in transgenic mice. *Int. Immunol.* **1:** 113.

Ishida, Y., M. Nishi, O. Taguchi, K. Inaba, M. Hattori, N. Minato, M. Kawaichi, and T. Honjo. 1989b. Expansion of natural killer cells but not T cells in human interleukin-2/interleukin-2 receptor (Tac) transgenic mice. *J. Exp. Med.* (in press).

Kondo, S., M. Kinoshita, A. Shimizu, Y. Saito, M. Konishi, H. Sabe, and T. Honjo. 1987. Expression and functional characterization of artificial mutants of interleukin-2 receptor. *Nature* **327:** 64.

Kuziel, W.A., A. Takashima, M. Bonyhadi, P.R. Bergstresser, J.P. Allison, R.E. Tigelaar, and P.W. Tucker. 1987. Regulation of T-cell receptor γ-chain RNA expression in murine Thy-1⁺ dendritic epidermal cells. *Nature* **328:** 263.

Leo, O., M. Foo, D.H. Sachs, L.E. Samelson, and J.A. Bluestone. 1987. Identification of a monoclonal antibody specific for a murine T3 polypeptide. *Proc. Natl. Acad. Sci.* **84:** 1374.

Lotze, M.T., A.E. Chang, C.A. Seipp, C. Simpson, J.T. Vetto, and S.A. Rosenberg. 1986. High-dose recombinant interleukin 2 in the treatment of patients with disseminated cancer. *J. Am. Med. Assoc.* **256:** 3117.

Maeda, M., N. Arima, Y. Daitoku, M. Kashihara, H. Okamoto, T. Uchiyama, K. Shirono, M. Matsuoka, T. Hattori, K. Takatsuki, K. Ikuta, A. Shimizu, T. Honjo, and J. Yodoi. 1987. Evidence for the interleukin-2 dependent expansion of leukemic cells in adult T cell leukemia. *Blood* **70:** 1407.

Merrill, J.E., S. Kutsunai, C. Mohlstrom, F. Hofman, J. Groopman, and D.W. Golde. 1984. Proliferation of astroglia and oligodendroglia in response to human T cell-derived factors. *Science* **224:** 1428.

Nishi, M., Y. Ishida, and T. Honjo. 1988. Expression of functional interleukin-2 receptors in human light chain/Tac transgenic mice. *Nature* **331:** 267.

Nixon-Fulton, J.L., P.R. Bergstresser, and R.E. Tigelaar. 1986. Thy-1⁺ epidermal cells proliferate in response to concanavalin A and interleukin 2. *J. Immunol.* **136:** 2776.

Ogura, T., M. Konishi, N. Suzuki, S. Kondo, H. Sabe, and T. Honjo. 1988. Molecular mechanism for the formation of the high-affinity complex of interleukin 2 and its receptor. *Mol. Biol. Med.* **5:** 123.

Robb, R.J., C.M. Rusk, J. Yodoi, and W.C. Greene. 1987. Interleukin 2 binding molecule distinct from the Tac protein: Analysis of its role in formation of high-affinity receptors. *Proc. Natl. Acad. Sci.* **84:** 2002.

Sabe, H., S. Kondo, A. Shimizu, Y. Tagaya, J. Yodoi, N. Kobayashi, M. Hatanaka, N. Matsunami, M. Maeda, T. Noma, and T. Honjo. 1984. Properties of human interleukin-2 receptors expressed on non-lymphoid cells by cDNA transfection. *Mol. Biol. Med.* **2:** 379.

Saito, Y., H. Sabe, N. Suzuki, S. Kondo, T. Ogura, A. Shimizu, and T. Honjo. 1988. A larger number of L chains (Tac) enhance the association rate of interleukin 2 to the high affinity site of the interleukin 2 receptor. *J. Exp. Med.* **168:** 1563.

Siegel, J.P., M. Sharon, P.L. Smith, and W.J. Leonard. 1987. The IL-2 receptor β chain (p70): Role in mediating signals for LAK, NK, and proliferative activities. *Science* **238:** 75.

Smith, K.A. 1988. Interleukin-2: Inception, impact, and implications. *Science* **240:** 1169.

Teshigawara, K., H. Wang, K. Kato, and K.A. Smith. 1987. Interleukin 2 high-affinity receptor expression requires two distinct binding proteins. *J. Exp. Med.* **165:** 223.

Tsudo, M., F. Kitamura, and M. Miyasaka. 1989. Characterization of the interleukin 2 receptor β chain using three distinct monoclonal antibodies. *Proc. Natl. Acad. Sci.* **86:** 1982.

Tsudo, M., R.W. Kozak, C.K. Goldman, and T.A. Waldmann. 1986. Demonstration of a non-Tac peptide that binds interleukin 2: A potential participant in a multichain interleukin 2 receptor complex. *Proc. Natl. Acad. Sci.* **83:** 9694.

Tsudo, M., C.K. Goldman, K.F. Bongiovanni, W.C. Chan, E.F. Winton, M. Yagita, E.A. Grimm, and T.A. Waldmann. 1987. The p75 peptide is the receptor for interleukin 2 expressed on large granular lymphocytes and is responsible for the interleukin 2 activation of these cells. *Proc. Natl. Acad. Sci.* **84:** 5394.

Waldmann, T.A. 1986. The structure, function, and expression of interleukin-2 receptors on normal and malignant lymphocytes. *Science* **232:** 727.

Wang, H. and K.A. Smith. 1987. The interleukin 2 receptor: Functional consequences of its bimolecular structure. *J. Exp. Med.* **166:** 1055.

Yodoi, J., T. Uchiyama, and M. Maeda. 1983. T-cell growth factor receptor in adult T-cell leukemia. *Blood* **62:** 509.

Regulation of the Biological Effects of IL-4 on Murine T and B Cells

R. FERNANDEZ-BOTRAN, V.M. SANDERS, AND E.S. VITETTA

Department of Microbiology, University of Texas Southwestern Medical Center at Dallas, Texas 75235

Considerable evidence has accumulated to suggest that cytokines are pleiotropic, i.e., they act on a variety of target cells and exert a number of different effects (for review, see O'Garra et al. 1988; Vitetta et al. 1989). Commonly, a single cytokine has more than one effect on the same cell type. Moreover, it is not unusual for cytokines to have similar effects on one cell type and different or even opposite effects on another cell type. In combination, cytokines can have both synergistic and antagonistic effects (Sporn and Roberts 1988; Vitetta et al. 1989). Little is known about the molecular mechanisms underlying the pleiotropism, multiple activities, or interactions of cytokines. It also remains unclear how the activities of cytokines are regulated in vivo.

Interleukin-4 (IL-4) is a T-cell-derived lymphokine with multiple activities on a variety of cells (for review, see Paul 1987; Vitetta et al. 1989). IL-4 plays a central role in the humoral immune response by regulating B-cell activation, proliferation, and isotype switching (for review, see Paul 1987; O'Garra et al. 1988; Vitetta et al. 1989). In addition, IL-4 is a growth factor for activated T-helper (T_H) cells and mast cells and can act on thymocytes, cytotoxic T cells, macrophages, and progenitor cells from a variety of hematopoietic cell lineages (for review, see Paul 1987; O'Garra et al. 1988; Vitetta et al. 1989). In B cells, different IL-4-mediated activities are highly dose-dependent (Severinson et al. 1987; Lebman and Coffman 1988; Snapper et al. 1988). Paradoxically, however, only a single class of IL-4 receptors (IL-4Rs) has been identified on both hematopoietic and nonhematopoietic cells (Nakajima et al. 1987; Ohara and Paul 1987; Park et al. 1987; Lowenthal et al. 1988). In our studies, we have attempted to obtain insight into the mechanisms regulating the action of IL-4 on T and B cells by analyzing the structure of IL-4Rs. This has been done by cross-linking ^{125}I-labeled IL-4 at different concentrations to both types of cells. We have also studied the effects of IL-4 on the modulation of high-affinity IL-2 receptors expressed on T cells. In addition, we have obtained evidence for the presence of a soluble IL-4-binding protein (IL-4-BP) in mouse serum and ascites that could play an important role in the regulation of IL-4 activity in vivo.

EXPERIMENTAL PROCEDURES

Animals. (DBA/2 × C57BL/6)F$_1$ (BDF$_1$) and BALB/c mice, 8–10 weeks of age, were bred in our animal facility at the Department of Microbiology, University of Texas Southwestern Medical Center at Dallas.

Cells. The IL-2/IL-4-responsive T-cell line, HT-2 (Watson 1979), was maintained in the presence of recombinant IL-2 (rIL-2) (Fernandez-Botran et al. 1986). The murine lymphoma cell line BCL$_1$-3B3 (Brooks et al. 1983) and the human lymphoblastoid cell line, Daudi (Klein et al. 1968), were cultured as described previously (Fernandez-Botran et al. 1989). Small, splenic B cells were enriched by treating suspensions of BDF$_1$ spleen cells with anti-Thy 1.2 antibody (HO.13.4) (Marshak-Rothstein et al. 1979) and baby rabbit complement followed by Percoll density gradient centrifugation (Layton et al. 1985). Stimulated B cells were obtained by culturing enriched B cells for 48 hours with lipopolysaccharide (20 μg/ml) or Sepharose beads coupled to goat anti-mouse immunoglobulin (GAMIg) antibodies (Fernandez-Botran et al. 1989).

Antibodies, lymphokines, and reagents. The monoclonal anti-IL-4 antibody, 11B11 (Ohara and Paul 1985a), was prepared by ammonium sulfate precipitation of hybridoma culture supernatants (SNs). Ascites containing a mouse antibody, TU-27, directed against the p70 subunit of the human IL-2R has been described previously by Takeshita et al. (1989) and was the generous gift of Dr. K. Sugamura, Sendai, Japan. IL-4 was purified from SNs of the T_{H2} cell line, T-286 (Fernandez-Botran et al. 1986), according to the method of Ohara et al. (1985b). Alternatively, IL-4 was used in recombinant form (rIL-4) and was kindly provided by W. Paul (National Institutes of Health, Bethesda, MD) and K. Grabstein (Immunex, Seattle, WA). IL-4 preparations lacked IL-2 and IFN-γ, and their proliferative effect on HT-2 cells could be completely inhibited by anti-IL-4 antibodies. Recombinant human IL-2 was purchased from AMGen (Thousand Oaks, CA). The cross-linking reagents 3,3'-dithiobis (propionic acid hydroxysuccinimide ester) (DTSP) and disuccinimidyl suberate (DSS) were purchased from

Sigma (St. Louis, MO) and Pierce (Rockford, IL), respectively.

Radiolabeled IL-2 and IL-4. [3-^{125}I]iodotyrosyl-rIL-2 (60 μCi/μg) was purchased from Amersham (Arlington Heights, IL). rIL-4 was iodinated with Iodogen (Pierce) and repurified by affinity chromatography on 11B11-Sepharose (Lowenthal et al. 1988). The concentration of the labeled lymphokines was determined by their biological activity in the HT-2 proliferation assay (Fernandez-Botran et al. 1986). The specific activity of the ^{125}I-labeled IL-4 preparation was 2×10^6 to 4×10^6 cpm/pmole.

Cross-linking studies. ^{125}I-labeled IL-2 and ^{125}I-labeled IL-4 were cross-linked to high-affinity IL-2Rs and IL-4Rs, respectively, using the bifunctional cross-linking reagent, DTSP (Fernandez-Botran et al. 1988a, 1989). Briefly, HT-2 or splenic B cells were resuspended at 1×10^7 to 4×10^7 cells/ml in balanced salt solution (BSS)–1% fetal calf serum (FCS) containing either ^{125}I-labeled IL-2 (50 pM) or ^{125}I-labeled IL-4 (10–250 pM) in the presence or absence of a 50- to 100-fold excess of unlabeled lymphokines. After a 60-minute incubation at 4°C, the cells were washed once with phosphate-buffered saline (PBS) and were then resuspended in 1 ml of a 0.5 mM solution of DTSP in PBS and incubated for 30 minutes on ice. The cells were washed three times with BSS–1% FCS and lysed in a buffer consisting of 1% NP-40, 1.5 mM phenylmethylsulfonyl fluoride, 2 mM EDTA in PBS (pH 7.4). The lysates were then subjected to SDS-PAGE. The gels were dried and analyzed by autoradiography and scanning densitometry.

Binding assays. Binding of ^{125}I-labeled IL-2 or ^{125}I-labeled IL-4 to intact cells was determined using centrifugation through an oil cushion to separate bound from free ligand (Fernandez-Botran et al. 1988a). After washing, the cells were resuspended in RPMI 1640 containing 10% FCS at 3×10^5 to 5×10^5 cells/tube (HT-2) or 3×10^6 to 5×10^6 cells/tube (B cells) and incubated with varying concentrations of the labeled lymphokines (1–500 pM) in the presence or absence of a 100-fold molar excess of the respective unlabeled lymphokine in a final volume of 100 μl. After 60 minutes at 4°C, the cells were centrifuged in an Eppendorf microfuge through 0.2 ml of an oil cushion consisting of 45% dibutylphtalate and 55% dioctylphtalate. The tips of the tubes were cut off and counted. Specific binding was determined by subtracting the mean cpm bound in the presence of an excess of unlabeled lymphokine (nonspecific binding) from the mean cpm bound in its absence (total binding). Dissociation constants (K_d) and receptor numbers were estimated from Scatchard analysis of the equilibrium binding data (Scatchard 1949).

Soluble-phase binding assay. Binding of ^{125}I-labeled IL-4 to soluble protein(s) in mouse serum, ascites, or cell culture SNs was determined using gel filtration

through Sephadex G-50 columns to separate free from bound ligand. Briefly, 5–50 μl of sample was incubated with different concentrations of ^{125}I-labeled IL-4 (5–200 pM) in a final volume of 110 μl of RPMI 1640 containing 10% FCS. After 60 minutes at 4°C, the mixtures were applied to 1-ml columns of Sephadex G-50 (medium), previously washed with PBS–10% FCS, and centrifuged at 600g for 90 seconds. The excluded material represented the bound ^{125}I-labeled IL-4, whereas the free ligand was retained by the column. Specific binding was calculated by subtraction of the cpm bound in the presence of a 100-fold molar excess of unlabeled IL-4 (nonspecific binding) from the cpm bound in its absence (total binding).

RESULTS

Cross-linking of ^{125}I-labeled IL-4 to T and B Cells

The different activities of IL-4 on B cells are highly dose-dependent (Severinson et al. 1987; Lebman and Coffman 1988; Snapper et al. 1988), despite the fact that only a single class of IL-4Rs, with a K_d of ~ 50 pM (Nakajima et al. 1987; Ohara and Paul 1987; Park et al. 1987; Lowenthal et al. 1988), has been reported. To further study the structure of IL-4 receptor(s), ^{125}I-labeled IL-4 (100 pM) was bound and cross-linked to T and B cells, and the labeled proteins were analyzed by SDS-PAGE and autoradiography. Under our experimental conditions, the autoradiograms showed the presence of two major bands of ~ 60 kD and ~ 105 kD on resting splenic B cells and bands of ~ 65–75 kD and ~ 105 kD on HT-2 cells (after subtraction of the 18 kD corresponding to IL-4) (Fig. 1). The cross-linking of ^{125}I-labeled IL-4 to both bands was specific, since it could be completely inhibited by the presence of a 50-fold molar excess of unlabeled IL-4 and was not affected by IL-2 (5 nM). Moreover, cross-linking to both bands was dependent on specific binding, since experiments using a human B-cell line, Daudi (which expresses receptors for human IL-4 but does not bind murine IL-4), showed a complete lack of affinity labeling. Interestingly, when ^{125}I-labeled IL-4 was cross-linked to Sepharose-GAMIg-activated B cells or a murine B-lymphoma cell line (BCL$_1$-3B3), the autoradiograms revealed two bands, but the lower M_r band was ~ 10 kD higher than that observed on resting B cells. This size heterogeneity was not dependent on the concentration of ^{125}I-labeled IL-4 used for cross-linking.

Effect of the ^{125}I-labeled IL-4 Concentration on the Cell Surface IL-4-binding Proteins Detected by Cross-linking

Since previous studies had reported the presence of a single protein (60–75 kD) cross-linked to ^{125}I-labeled IL-4 (Ohara and Paul 1987; Park et al. 1987), we questioned whether differences in experimental procedures (IL-4 concentration, cross-linking reagents, etc.)

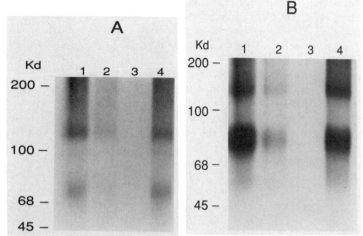

Figure 1. Cross-linking of ^{125}I-labeled IL-4 to splenic B cells (*A*) and HT-2 cells (*B*). Cells were cross-linked with ^{125}I-labeled IL-4 (100 pM) in the absence (lane *1*) or presence of a 5-fold (lane *2*) or a 50-fold (lane *3*) excess un-labeled IL-4 or IL-2 (5 nM) (lane *4*).

resulted in the detection of the larger 105-kD band. Different concentrations of ^{125}I-labeled IL-4 (10–250 pM) were therefore cross-linked to B cells. Such experiments indicated that although the 60–75-kD band was detected at all concentrations of IL-4, the larger 105-kD band was preferentially detected when the higher ^{125}I-labeled IL-4 concentrations were used. When the densities of both bands at each concentration of ^{125}I-labeled IL-4 were quantitated and compared, the ratio of the density of the 105-kD to the 60–75-kD band increased as a function of the concentration of ^{125}I-labeled IL-4, indicating that the detection of the 105-kD band was favored at higher concentrations of IL-4. The cross-linking agent also influenced the ability to detect the 105-kD band. At concentrations of ^{125}I-labeled IL-4 where the labeling of this band was evident, substitution of DTSP for a different cross-linking reagent, DSS, resulted in a marked reduction of the labeling of the 105-kD band.

Effect of IL-4 on the Number and Affinity of IL-2Rs

Previous work from this laboratory demonstrated that IL-4 and IL-2 synergize at inducing the proliferation of activated T_H cell lines (Fernandez-Botran et al. 1988b). On the basis of reports that synergy among a number of hormones (for review, see Zachary and Rozengurt 1985) and hematopoietic growth factors (Walker et al. 1985; Nicola 1987) is accompanied by interactions among their receptors, we hypothesized that interactions between IL-2Rs and IL-4Rs might occur in T cells. To study this hypothesis, we preincubated HT-2 cells with IL-4 and then determined whether the affinity or number of high-affinity (HA) IL-2Rs were affected. Preincubation of HT-2 cells with IL-4 (50 units/ml) at 4°C or 37°C resulted in a partial decrease in the specific binding of ^{125}I-labeled IL-2, especially at the lower concentrations where most of the specific binding is due to HA receptors. Preincubation with unlabeled IL-2 almost completely inhibited subsequent binding of ^{125}I-labeled IL-2. The effect of IL-4 was observed irrespective of the source of IL-4

(i.e., purified or recombinant) and was reversed by the addition of anti-IL-4 antibodies. Furthermore, this phenomenon appeared not to be restricted to T cells, since preincubation of an IL-2R[+]/IL-4R[+] B-lymphoma cell line (BCL$_1$-3B3) also resulted in a partial reduction of the binding of ^{125}I-labeled IL-2. When the binding data were analyzed by Scatchard plots, curvilinear plots were obtained indicating the presence of high- and low-affinity IL-2Rs (Robb et al. 1984). The effect of IL-4 appeared to be due to a partial decrease (~ 45–50%) in the number, but not affinity, of HA IL-2Rs; low-affinity IL-2Rs were not affected. Table 1 summarizes the values for K_d and receptor numbers for untreated cells and cells preincubated with IL-4.

In experiments designed to investigate whether preincubation of HT-2 cells with IL-2 resulted in a decrease in the binding of ^{125}I-labeled IL-4, it was found that this was not the case, suggesting that the effect of IL-4 on HA IL-2Rs is unidirectional (results not shown).

Effect of IL-4 on the Cross-linking of ^{125}I-labeled IL-2 to HA IL-2Rs

HA IL-2Rs have been reported to be composed of at least two different subunits, p55 and p70, both of which can independently bind IL-2 (for review, see Smith 1988). To determine whether the decreased number of HA IL-2Rs observed after preincubation with IL-4 was

Table 1. IL-4 Decreases the Number of High-affinity IL-2Rs on Cells

Cells	Receptor number/cell		% decrease in HA IL-2Rs
	pretreated with		
	medium	IL-4	
HT-2[a]	2810	1680	40.2
HT-2[b]	2670	1646	38.4
BCL$_1$-3B3[a]	1676	955	43.0

A representative experiment of nine that were performed.
[a]4°C.
[b]37°C.

due to preferential interference with one of these subunits, HT-2 cells were preincubated with IL-4 and then cross-linked to ^{125}I-labeled IL-2 under HA conditions. Treatment with IL-4 led to a ~50% decrease in the cross-linking of ^{125}I-labeled IL-2 to both bands (p55 and p70) compared to cells incubated with medium (control) or other cytokines, such as IL-1. In contrast to IL-4, unlabeled IL-2 completely inhibited the cross-linking of ^{125}I-labeled IL-2 to both bands. In addition to the p55 and p70 bands, additional bands of higher M_r (e.g., 105 kD), were also observed in these experiments, confirming the results of other investigators (Saragovi and Malek 1987, 1988; Herrmann and Diamantstein 1987). The cross-linking of ^{125}I-labeled IL-2 to these molecules was also decreased by preincubation of the cells with IL-4. Although the nature of these additional bands is unclear, they may represent additional subunits of the murine HA IL-2R.

Inhibition of the Binding of ^{125}I-labeled IL-4 to Cells by Mouse Ascites

Although the results described above demonstrated an effect of IL-4 on the expression of IL-2Rs, the mechanisms involved remain obscure. One possibility is that receptors for IL-4 and IL-2 may interact through a common subunit or receptor-associated protein. In an attempt to investigate such a possibility, we determined whether antibodies directed against the p70 subunit of the human HA IL-2R (TU-27) (Takeshita et al. 1989) would affect the binding of murine ^{125}I-labeled IL-4 or ^{125}I-labeled IL-2 to their receptors. HT-2 cells were incubated with ^{125}I-labeled IL-4 in the presence and absence of the TU-27 antibody in ascites form or as a purified antibody. The TU-27 ascites profoundly inhibited the binding of ^{125}I-labeled IL-4 to the cells (~80% of specific binding) (Fig. 2), whereas neither the purified TU-27 antibody nor an isotype-matched control IgG$_1$ myeloma protein (MOPC 21) caused significant inhibition. Surprisingly, a control ascites from an IgG$_1$-secreting hybridoma (1B7.11, a mouse anti-DNP

antibody) was comparable to the TU-27 ascites in its ability to inhibit the binding of ^{125}I-labeled IL-4 to cells. These results suggest that a factor present in mouse ascites, and not the purified TU-27 antibody, interferes with the binding of ^{125}I-labeled IL-4 to cells.

Binding of ^{125}I-labeled IL-4 by a Factor in Mouse Serum and Ascites

One possibility to explain the above results was that a factor present in ascites had the ability to bind to IL-4, thereby competing with its binding to membrane IL-4Rs. To test this hypothesis, we developed a soluble-phase binding assay based on size-separation of bound versus free ^{125}I-labeled IL-4. Using this assay, we demonstrated that such an IL-4 binding protein was present not only in ascites, but in mouse serum as well. Moreover, the binding of ^{125}I-labeled IL-4 was specific and saturable (Fig. 3). Binding of ^{125}I-labeled IL-4 to IL-4-BP could be prevented by an excess of unlabeled IL-4, but not by an excess of unlabeled IL-2. Furthermore, the binding of ^{125}I-labeled IL-4 by the IL-4-BP was species-specific, since sera from other species, including rat, rabbit, chicken, and human, did not bind murine IL-4. Cross-linking of ^{125}I-labeled IL-4 to the IL-4-BP showed the latter to have an approximate M_r of 30 kD. Preliminary analyses of sera from different mouse strains have demonstrated that the levels of IL-4-BP in serum from SCID mice are significantly lower than those in serum from other strains ("normal serum"), suggesting that the primary sources of IL-4-BP in vivo might be lymphoid cells. Table 2 summarizes the relative levels of IL-4-BP present in ascites and in normal sera from different mouse strains, sera from immune mice, and sera from control and immunosuppressed animals. Finally, IL-4-BP activity was also detected in culture SNs from mitogen-stimulated T or B cells, albeit at levels lower than those found in normal mouse serum.

DISCUSSION

Cytokines are not restricted in their activity to a particular cell type or a specific function; a single cytokine has the ability to act on a variety of cellular targets

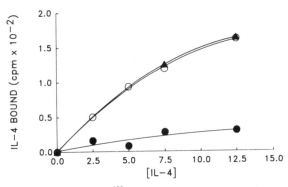

Figure 2. Inhibition of ^{125}I-labeled IL-4 binding to HT-2 cells by TU-27 ascites. HT-2 cells were incubated with different concentrations of ^{125}I-labeled IL-4 in the absence (○) or presence of TU-27 ascites (2 μl/tube) (●) or purified MOPC 21 (IgG$_1$, 10 μg/tube) (▲).

Table 2. Relative Levels of Soluble IL-4-BP in Serum, Ascites, and Tissue Culture Samples

Sample	Relative activity
Normal mouse serum	1.0
Ascitic fluid (hybridoma)	1.8
Normal human serum	0.0
Normal rat serum	0.1
SCID serum	0.2
SN from Con-A-stimulated spleen cells	0.3
SN from LPS-stimulated spleen cells	0.2

IL-4-BP activity was measured using the soluble phase ^{125}I-labeled IL-4-binding assay described in Experimental Procedures. Results are expressed as the ratio of IL-4-BP activity of each sample to that of normal mouse serum (1.0).

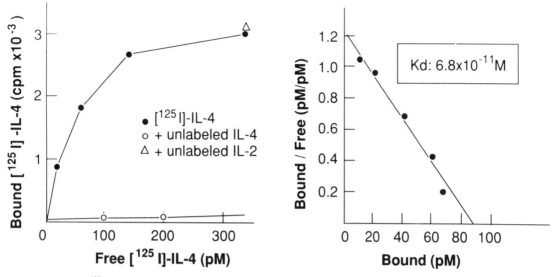

Figure 3. Binding of ^{125}I-labeled IL-4 to an IL-4-BP present in murine ascites. (*Left*) Constant amounts of murine ascites (1B7.11, 5 μl/tube) were incubated with increasing concentrations of ^{125}I-labeled IL-4 in the absence (●) and presence of a 100-fold excess of unlabeled IL-4 (○) or IL-2 (△). (*Right*) Scatchard analysis of binding data shown on left panel.

and to elicit a number of activities (for review, see O'Garra et al. 1988; Vitetta et al. 1989). It is not yet clear, however, how these activities are regulated in vivo. Patterns of synergy or antagonism have been observed among different cytokines (for review, see Sporn and Roberts 1988; Vitetta et al. 1989), and subsets of T_H cells secreting different sets of lymphokines have been described (Mosmann et al. 1986; Bottomly 1988). Taken together, these observations suggest that lymphokine activity must be tightly regulated in vivo, since these molecules mediate many important and diverse effector functions.

Our work has focused on the mechanisms controlling the activity of IL-4 on T and B cells. Evidence presented in this paper suggests that (1) the structure of IL-4 may be more complex than previously reported and that different signals may potentially be elicited at different doses of IL-4; (2) interactions between IL-4 and HA IL-2Rs take place, and some of the activities of IL-4 on T cells and the synergy between IL-2 and IL-4 may result in part from these interactions; and (3) an IL-4-BP in mouse serum may play an important role in the regulation of IL-4 activity in vivo by competing with cellular IL-4Rs for the binding of free IL-4, thus preventing IL-4 from acting on bystander cells.

Experiments performed to study the structure of IL-4Rs by cross-linking different concentrations of ^{125}I-labeled IL-4 to cells showed that, at relatively high concentrations, a protein or protein complex of 105 kD is detected in addition to the previously described 60–75 kD protein (Ohara and Paul 1987; Park et al. 1987). The detection of the larger 105-kD molecule is dependent on the concentration of ^{125}I-labeled IL-4 and the reagent used for cross-linking. In addition, considerable size heterogeneity was observed in the M_r of the smaller 60–75 kD band.

A number of explanations could shed light on the nature of the 105 kD and the 60–75-kD bands: (1) Two

"chains" could be generated by artifactual proteolysis of a larger protein during cross-linking, cell lysis, and electrophoresis; (2) the two chains could be generated by posttranslational processing of a common precursor; (3) the smaller molecule (60–75 kD) could represent the IL-4R, and the 105 kD could be the IL-4R cross-linked to another membrane molecule of ~ 40 kD; (4) the 105 kD could be a separate subunit of the IL-4R involved in binding and/or signaling. Whatever the explanation, the fact that the appearance of the second band was dependent on the concentration of IL-4 raises the possibility that the IL-4R can interact with another molecule(s) on the cell surface, thus having the potential to transmit additional or different signals at different IL-4 concentrations. Thus, stimuli inducing responses characterized by relatively modest levels of IL-4 (e.g., secretion of IgG$_1$) as opposed to high levels of IL-4 (e.g., IgE secretion; Lebman and Coffman 1988; Snapper et al. 1988) might be dependent on the degree to which T_{H2} cells are stimulated by persistent versus nonpersistent antigens and the levels of IL-4 that are secreted as a result.

The synergy between IL-2 and IL-4 (Fernandez-Botran et al. 1988b) could be explained by events taking place intracellularly or at the level or surface receptors. Our results suggest that interactions between IL-2Rs and IL-4Rs might take place. In fact, receptor/receptor interactions have been reported for a number of hormone systems (for review, see Zachary and Rozengurt 1985) and for hematopoietic growth factors (Walker et al. 1985; Nicola 1987). In certain cases, receptor/receptor interactions are manifested by changes in receptor affinity and, in others, by changes in receptor number (down-modulation) (for review, see Zachary and Rozengurt 1985). Interestingly, in our system, the effect of IL-4 on the expression of IL-2Rs was not temperature-dependent, suggesting that an enzymatic process, such as phosphorylation or protein synthesis, is probably not involved. Thus, the effect of IL-4 on IL-2Rs is probably mediated by the binding of IL-4 to IL-4Rs followed by a change in the IL-4R or another membrane molecule that then interacts with HA IL-2Rs. How this interaction occurs is unclear, but it could involve (1) the sharing of a common subunit between IL-4Rs and HA IL-2Rs; (2) direct receptor/receptor interaction; or (3) interaction through a third receptor-associated molecule. It is of interest that "receptor-associated" molecules of 105 kD have been observed in cross-linking experiments involving both IL-2 (Saragovi and Malek 1987, 1988; Hermann and Diamantstein 1987) and IL-4 (Fernandez-Botran et al. 1989). Whether or not this is a common subunit remains to be determined. The availability of antibodies directed against the murine IL-4R should help to clarify this issue.

Experiments performed to investigate the effect of an antibody directed against the human p70 subunit of the human IL-2R (TU-27) (Takeshita et al. 1989) on the binding of ^{125}I-labeled IL-2 and ^{125}I-labeled IL-4 to HT-2 cells, although unable to demonstrate any effect of the TU-27 antibody, revealed the presence of a factor present in mouse and ascites that inhibits the binding of ^{125}I-labeled IL-4 to its membrane receptor. This factor was present not only in the TU-27 ascites, but also in several other samples of ascitic fluid from control hybridomas and serum samples from normal mice.

The binding of IL-4 by this factor (IL-4BP) is specific and saturable. Scatchard analyses revealed that IL-4-BP binds ^{125}I-labeled IL-4 with a K_d similar to that of cellular IL-4Rs (~ 70 pM) (Nakajima et al. 1987; Ohara and Paul 1987; Park et al. 1987; Lowenthal et al. 1988), even though it has a M_r of 30,000. In addition, binding of IL-4 by the IL-4-BP is species-specific. Whether the soluble IL-4-BP represents a secreted form of the IL-4R or whether it is a different protein remains to be determined. However, soluble or secreted forms of receptors are often truncated forms of the surface receptor (Rubin et al. 1985; Treiger et al. 1986; Ikuta et al. 1987; Jacques et al. 1987; Baran et al. 1988). Nonetheless, definitive evidence on the relationship between the IL-4-BP and the IL-4R must await the availability of anti-IL-4R antibodies.

Whatever the relationship of the IL-4-BP to IL-4Rs, the low levels of the former in the serum of SCID mice, compared to sera from other strains, would suggest that lymphoid cells are the main source of IL-4-BP. In this regard, it would also be very important to investigate how stimulation or suppression of the immune system by a variety of agents affects the serum levels of IL-4-BPs.

Soluble IL-2Rs (p55) have been found in SNs of activated murine and human T-cell lines and IL-2R$^+$ tumor cell lines (Rubin et al. 1985; Treiger et al. 1986; Jacques et al. 1987; Baran et al. 1988). However, because of their low affinity for IL-2 (~ 10 nM), their role in immunoregulation is not compelling. Nevertheless, high levels of soluble IL-2Rs have been described in the

sera of AIDS patients, suggesting a possible role in, or a consequence of, immunologically related diseases (Honda et al. 1989). The high affinity of the IL-4-BP for IL-4 and its ability to inhibit binding of IL-4 to cells are very provocative and implicate the IL-4-BP as an immunomodulatory molecule, with the ability to bind free IL-4 in the circulation. This may serve to confine the activity of IL-4 to a local site, thus avoiding effects on other cells. Alternatively, the IL-4-BP could also serve as a "carrier" molecule, delivering IL-4 to sites distant from its secretion.

Taken together, our results suggest that the pleiotropism and multiple actions of cytokines could be due, in part, to events taking place at the receptor level and involving receptor/receptor interactions. In addition, regulation of IL-4 activity in vivo may involve soluble IL-4-binding factors present in the circulation.

ACKNOWLEDGMENTS

We thank Drs. W. Paul (National Institutes of Health) and K. Grabstein (Immunex) for their generous supply of rIL-4. We thank Dr. K. Sugamura (Tohoku University School of Medicine, Sendai, Japan) for his generous gift of TU-27. We also thank Ms. Suzzane Joyner for her expert technical assistance and Ms. Gerry Ann Cheek and Ms. Nelletta Stephens for their valuable secretarial assistance.

REFERENCES

Baran, D., M. Korner, and J. Theze. 1988. Characterization of the soluble murine IL-2R and estimation of its affinity for IL-2. *J. Immunol.* **141:** 539.

Bottomly, K. 1988. A functional dichotomy in CD4$^+$ T lymphocytes. *Immunol. Today* **9:** 268.

Brooks, K., D. Yuan, J.W. Uhr, P.H. Krammer, and E.S. Vitetta. 1983. Lymphokine-induced IgM secretion by clones of neoplastic B cells. *Nature* **302:** 825.

Fernandez-Botran, R., V.M. Sanders, and E.S. Vitetta. 1988a. Interactions between receptors for IL-2 and IL-4 on lines of helper T cells (HT-2) and B lymphoma cells (BCL$_1$). *J. Exp. Med.* **169:** 379.

Fernandez-Botran, R., J.W. Uhr, and E.S. Vitetta. 1989. Cross-linking of interleukin-4 to surface molecules on murine T and B lymphocytes. *Proc. Natl. Acad. Sci.* **86:** 4235.

Fernandez-Botran, R., V.M. Sanders, T.R. Mosmann, and E.S. Vitetta. 1988b. Lymphokine-mediated regulation of the proliferative response of clones of T$_{H1}$ and T$_{H2}$ cells. *J. Exp. Med.* **168:** 543.

Fernandez-Botran, R., V.M. Sanders, K.G. Oliver, Y.W. Chen, P.H. Krammer, J.W. Uhr, and E.S. Vitetta. 1986. Interleukin-4 mediates autocrine growth of helper T cells after antigenic stimulation. *Proc. Natl. Acad. Sci.* **83:** 9689.

Herrmann, T. and T. Diamantstein. 1987. The mouse high affinity IL-2 receptor complex. I. Evidence for a third molecule, the putative γ-chain, associated with the α- and/or β-chain of the receptor. *Immunobiology* **175:** 145.

Honda, M., K. Kitamura, K. Matsuda, Y. Yokota, N. Yamamoto, R. Mitsuyasu, J.-C. Chermann, and T. Tokunaga. 1989. Soluble IL-2 receptor in AIDS. Correlation of its serum level with the classification of HIV-induced diseases and its characterization. *J. Immunol.* **142:** 4248.

kuta, K., M. Takami, C.W. Kim, T. Honjo, T. Miyoshi, Y. Yagaya, T. Kawabe, and J. Yodoi. 1987. Human lymphocyte Fc receptor for IgE: Sequence homology of its cloned cDNA with animal lectins. *Proc. Natl. Acad. Sci.* **84:** 819.

Jacques, Y., B. Le Mauff, F. Boeffard, A. Godard, and J.-P. Soulillou. 1987. A soluble interleukin-2 receptor produced by a normal alloreactive human T cell clone binds interleukin-2 with low affinity. *J. Immunol.* **139:** 2308.

Klein, E., G. Klein, J.S. Nadkarni, J.J. Nadkarni, H. Wigzell, and P. Clifford. 1968. Surface IgM-kappa specificity on a Burkitt lymphoma cell *in vivo* and in derived culture lines. *Can. Res.* **28:** 1300.

Layton, J.E., P.H. Krammer, T. Hamaoka, J.W. Uhr, and E.S. Vitetta. 1985. Small and large B cells respond differently to T cell-derived B cell growth and differentiation factors. *J. Mol. Cell. Immunol.* **2:** 155.

Lebman, D.A. and R.L. Coffman. 1988. Interleukin-4 causes isotype switching to IgE in T cell-stimulated clonal B cell cultures. *J. Exp. Med.* **168:** 853.

Lowenthal, J.W., B.E. Castle, J. Christiansen, J. Schreurs, D. Rennick, N. Arai, Y. Hoy, Y. Takebe, and M. Howard. 1988. Expression of high affinity receptors for murine interleukin-2 (BSF-1) on hemopoietic and nonhemopoietic cells. *J. Immunol.* **140:** 456.

Marshak-Rothstein, A., P. Fink, T. Gridley, D.H. Raulet, M.J. Bevans, and M.L. Gefter. 1979. Properties and applications of monoclonal antibodies directed against determinants on the Thy-1 locus. *J. Immunol.* **122:** 2491.

Mosmann, T.R., H. Cherwinski, M.W. Bond, M.A. Giedlin, and R.L. Coffman. 1986. Two types of murine helper T cell clone. I. Definition according to profiles of lymphokine activities and secreted proteins. *J. Immunol.* **136:** 2348.

Nakajima, K., T. Hirano, K. Koyama, and T. Kishimoto. 1987. Detection of receptors for murine B cell-stimulatory factor-1 (BSF-1): Presence of functional receptors on CBA/N splenic cells. *J. Immunol.* **139:** 774.

Nicola, N.A. 1987. Why do hemopoietic growth factor receptors interact with each other? *Immunol. Today* **8:** 134.

O'Garra, A., S. Umland, T. Defrance, and J. Christiansen. 1988. "B cell factors" are pleiotropic. *Immunol. Today* **9:** 45.

Ohara, J. and W.E. Paul. 1985a. Production of a monoclonal antibody to and molecular characterization of B-cell stimulatory factor-1. *Nature* **315:** 333.

———. 1987. Receptors for B-cell stimulatory factor-1 expressed on cells of haematopoietic lineage. *Nature* **325:** 537.

Ohara, J., S. Lahet, J. Inman, and W.E. Paul. 1985b. Partial purification of murine B cell stimulatory factor (BSF)-1. *J. Immunol.* **135:** 2518.

Park, L.S., D. Friend, K. Grabstein, and D.L. Urdal. 1987. Characterization of the high affinity cell surface receptor for murine B cell-stimulating factor-1. *Proc. Natl. Acad. Sci.* **84:** 1669.

Paul, W.E. 1987. Interleukin 4/B cell stimulatory factor 1: One lymphokine, many functions. *FASEB J.* **1:** 456.

Robb, R.J., W.C. Greene, and C.M. Rusk. 1984. Low and high affinity cellular receptors for interleukin-2. Implications for the level of Tac antigen. *J. Exp. Med.* **160:** 1126.

Rubin, L.A., C.C. Kurman, M.E. Fritz, W.E. Biddison, B. Boutin, R. Yarchoan, and D.L. Nelson. 1985. Soluble interleukin-2 receptors are released from activated human lymphoid cells *in vitro*. *J. Immunol.* **135:** 3172.

Saragovi, H. and T.R. Malek. 1987. The murine interleukin-2 receptor: Irreversible cross-linking of radiolabeled interleukin-2 to high affinity interleukin-2 receptors reveals a noncovalently associated subunit. *J. Immunol.* **139:** 1918.

———. 1988. Direct identification of the murine IL-2 receptor p55-p75 heterodimer in the absence of IL-2. *J. Immunol.* **141:** 476.

Scatchard, G. 1949. The attractions of proteins for small molecules and ions. *Ann. N.Y. Acad. Sci.* **51:** 660.

Severinson, E., T. Naito, H. Tokumoto, D. Fukushima, A. Hirano, K. Hanna, and T. Honjo. 1987. Interleukin-4 (IgG$_1$ induction factor): A multifunctional lymphokine acting also on T cells. *Eur. J. Immunol.* **17:** 67.

Smith, K.A. 1988. The interleukin-2 receptor. *Adv. Immunol.* **42:** 165.

Snapper, C.M., F.D. Finkelman, and W.E. Paul. 1988. Differential regulation of IgG$_1$ and IgE synthesis by interleukin-4. *J. Exp. Med.* **167:** 183.

Sporn, M.B. and A.B. Roberts. 1988. Peptide growth factors are multi-functional. *Nature* **332:** 217.

Takeshita, T., Y. Goto, K. Tada, K. Nagata, H. Asao, and K. Sugamura. 1989. Monoclonal antibody defining a molecule possibly identical to the p75 subunit of interleukin-2 receptor. *J. Exp. Med.* **169:** 1323.

Treiger, B.F., W.J. Leonard, P. Svetlik, L.A. Rubin, D.L. Nelson, and W.C. Greene. 1986. A secreted form of the human interleukin-2 receptor encoded by an "anchor minus" cDNA. *J. Immunol.* **136:** 4099.

Vitetta, E.S., R. Fernandez-Botran, C.D. Myers, and V.M. Sanders. 1989. Cellular interactions in the humoral immune response. *Adv. Immunol.* **45:** 1.

Walker, F., N.A. Nicola, D. Metcalf, and A.W. Burgess. 1985. Hierarchical down-modulation of hemopoietic growth factor receptors. *Cell* **43:** 269.

Watson, J. 1979. Continuous proliferation of murine antigen-specific helper T lymphocytes in culture. *J. Exp. Med.* **150:** 1510.

Zachary, I. and E. Rozengurt. 1985. Modulation of the epidermal growth factor receptor by mitogenic ligands: Effects of bombesin and role of protein kinase C. *Cancer Surv.* **4:** 729.

Interleukin-6 Receptor and a Unique Mechanism of Its Signal Transduction

T. Taga, M. Hibi, Y. Hirata, H. Yawata, S. Natsuka, K. Yasukawa,
T. Totsuka, K. Yamasaki, T. Hirano, and T. Kishimoto
*Division of Immunology, Institute for Molecular and Cellular Biology,
Osaka University, 1-3, Yamada-oka, Suita, Osaka 565, Japan*

Interleukin-6 (IL-6) was originally identified as a T-cell-derived lymphokine that induced a final maturation of B cells into antibody-producing cells; it was called B-cell stimulatory factor 2 (BSF-2) (Hirano et al. 1985). However, molecular cloning of the cDNAs for BSF-2 and several other factors revealed that factors that had previously been called by a variety of names were identical to BSF-2 (Kishimoto and Hirano 1988; Hirano and Kishimoto 1989). The molecules identical with BSF-2 are summarized in Table 1, indicating that IL-6 may have a wide variety of biological functions on various tissues and cells. In fact, the studies with recombinant IL-6 could demonstrate that the activity of IL-6 is not restricted to B-lineage cells, but also affects T cells, hepatocytes, hematopoietic stem cells, nerve cells, plasmacytoma/myelomas, and myeloid leukemia cells. IL-6 has been reported to be involved in (1) induction of immunoglobulin production in activated B cells (Hirano et al. 1986), (2) induction of proliferation of hybridoma/plasmacytoma/myeloma cells (Nordan and Potter 1986; Van Snick et al. 1986, 1987; Van Damme et al. 1987, Kawano et al. 1988), (3) induction of IL-2 production, cell growth, and cytotoxic T-cell differentiation of T cells (Garman et al. 1987; Lotz et al. 1988; Okada et al. 1988; Takai et al. 1988), (4) stimulation of hematopoietic stem cells from G_0 into G_1 stage (Ikebuchi et al. 1987), (5) induction of megakaryocyte maturation (Ishibashi et al. 1989), (6) induction of acute phase response in hepatocytes (Andus et al. 1987; Gauldie et al. 1987), (7) growth inhibition and induction of differentiation of a myeloid leukemia cell line (M1) into macrophages (Miyaura et al. 1988; Shabo et al. 1988), and (8) induction of neural differentiation (Satoh et al. 1988).

In accordance with multifunctional properties of IL-6, the specific receptor for IL-6 (IL-6R) was found to be expressed on a variety of cells (Coulie et al. 1987; Taga et al. 1987). However, the number of the receptor expressed on target cells was only between several hundreds and several thousands as observed in the case of other cytokines. The interaction of IL-6 with its receptor on a B-lymphoblastoid cell line did not induce any known biochemical processes, such as phosphatidylinositol turnover or intracytoplasmic Ca^{++} ion and protein phosphorylations, suggesting the involvement of a certain novel mechanism for signal transduction.

To elucidate how one cytokine can mediate multiple functions, such as growth promotion, growth inhibition, or specific gene expression, we have cloned the cDNA for IL-6R (Yamasaki et al. 1988). The study with cDNA and monoclonal antibodies against the receptor demonstrated that IL-6 triggered the association of IL-6R and the second non-ligand-binding chain that may be involved in signal transduction.

METHODS

Expression cloning of IL-6R. A cDNA library from poly(A)$^+$ RNA of a human NK-like cell line, YT, was constructed utilizing the CDM8 vector (Seed 1987). COS-7 cells were transfected with plasmid DNA by the DEAE-dextran method, and after 2 days' culture, the cells were stained with biotinylated recombinant IL-6 (B-IL-6) and fluorescein-conjugated avidin. Episomal DNA collected from positively sorted cells with the use of a fluorescence-activated cell sorter was amplified in *Escherichia coli* as described previously (Seed 1987) and subjected to a second round of selection. Single colonies were picked up after four rounds of selection, plasmid DNA was individually transfected into COS-7 cells, and pBSF2R.236 was identified.

Preparation of anti-receptor monoclonal antibodies. Insert IL-6R cDNA of pBSF2R.236 was ligated with pZipNeoSV(X)1 (Cepko et al. 1984) at the *Bam*HI site, and pZipNeoIL6R was obtained. A murine T-cell line, CTLL2, and a human T-cell line, Jurkat, both of which did not express IL-6R, were transfected with pZipNeoIL6R, then CTIL6R and JIL6R expressing human IL-6R were obtained. Mice were immunized with CTIL6R, and hybridomas were prepared. A clone, MT18, which could react with JIL6R cells but not with Jurkat cells, was selected. IL-6R was partially purified from a human myeloma cell line, U266, utilizing MT18 monoclonal antibody. Mice were immunized with the partially purified IL-6R, and a hybrid clone that could immunoprecipitate IL-6R was selected and named PM1.

Immunoprecipitation with an anti-receptor monoclonal antibody. Radiolabeled cells (10^7) were suspended in 0.2 ml of digitonin-extraction buffer (1% digitonin, 10 mM triethanolamine [pH 7.8], 0.15 M NaCl, 10 mM iodoacetamide, 1 mM phenylmethylsulfonyl fluoride

Table 1. Molecules Identical with IL-6

B-cell stimulatory factor 2 (Hirano et al. 1986)
Interferon $\beta 2$ (Zilberstein et al. 1986)
26-kD protein (Haegeman et al. 1986)
Hybridoma plasmacytoma growth factor (Van Damme et al. 1987; Van Snick et al. 1988)
Hepatocyte-stimulating factor (Andus et al. 1987; Gauldie et al. 1987)
Cytotoxic T-cell differentiation factor (Okada et al. 1988; Takai et al. 1988)
Macrophage granulocyte inducer protein 2 (Miyaura et al. 1988; Shabo et al. 1988)
Colony-stimulating factor-309 (Ikebuchi et al. 1987)
Thrombopoietin (Ishibashi et al. 1989)

[PMSF]) and rotated for 15 minutes at 4°C. Extracts were centrifuged at 10,000g for 30 minutes and precleared with normal mouse immunoglobulin. IL-6R was immunoprecipitated with 10 μg MT18 and 10 μl protein-A-Sepharose and was subjected to SDS-PAGE after six washes with digitonin-extraction buffer. In some experiments, radiolabeled cells (10^7) were incubated in 0.5 ml of RPMI 1640, 10% fetal calf serum containing 1 μg/ml IL-6 at 37°C for 30 minutes before digitonin-lysis.

Cross-linking of IL-6R. Metabolically labeled U266 cells (10^7) were washed in phosphate-buffered saline (PBS) (pH 7.4) and incubated in 1 ml of 10 mg/ml bovine serum albumin (BSA), RPMI 1640 containing 0.36 mM IL-6 for 1 hour at room temperature. After three washes in ice-cold PBS, the cells were resuspended in 1 ml of PBS (pH 8.3) containing 0.1 mM ethyleneglycol-bis-N-hydroxysuccinimide (EGS) and mixed for 30 minutes at 4°C. Cells were solubilized in 0.2 ml of 0.5% NP-40 in Tris-buffered saline (TBS) (pH 7.4) containing 1 mM PMSF by vortexing for 20 minutes. Extract was centrifuged at 10,000g for 30 minutes, and supernatant was boiled in the presence of 0.5% SDS for 5 minutes. Cross-linked complexes containing IL-6 were immunoprecipitated by 10 μg of affinity-purified rabbit anti-IL-6 antibody (Hirano et al. 1988) and protein-A-Sepharose. Reimmunoprecipitation was performed with the same antibody, and cross-linking bonds in the precipitated complexes were cleaved by hydroxylamine as described previously (Abdella and Smith 1979).

Mutant IL-6R. Mutant IL-6R cDNA encoding amino acid residues 1–403, thus lacking 65 out of 82 intracytoplasmic amino acid residues, was prepared utilizing a Universal Transcription Terminator (Pharmacia) and was named IL6RΔIC. Ψ2 and M1 cells were transfected with IL6RΔIC ligated in pZipNeoSV(X)1 (Cepko et al. 1984), and Ψ2IL6RΔIC and M1IL6RΔIC were obtained. Another mutant IL-6R cDNA encoding amino acids 1–322, thus lacking transmembrane and cytoplasmic domains, was prepared using an in vitro mutagenesis system (Amersham) and was inserted in pSVL vector (Pharmacia). Culture supernatant of COS-7 cells transfected with plasmid by the calcium phosphate method (Wigler et al. 1978), which included soluble IL-6R, was collected on day 2. Mock control was prepared using pSVL vector without the insert.

Cell proliferation assay. M1 and its transformants were seeded in microculture plates (1×10^5 cells/ml, 0.2 ml/well), cultured for 60 hours, and pulsed with [^{3}H]thymidine (1 μCi/well) for another 10 hours. Incorporated radioactivity was measured.

RESULTS AND DISCUSSION

Molecular Cloning of IL-6R

A cDNA library was constructed from poly(A)$^+$ RNA of a human NK-like cell line, YT, with the CDM8 vector (Seed 1987). Plasmid DNA was transfected into monkey COS-7 cells, and the cells were stained with B-IL-6 and fluorescein isothiocyanate-avidin. Cells expressing IL-6R were obtained with a fluorescence-activated cell sorter, resulting in the identification of a candidate plasmid clone, pBSF2R.236. To confirm that this clone contained the cDNA encoding IL-6R, the cDNA was transfected into murine COP cells. More than 10% of the transfected cells expressed IL-6R as measured by B-IL-6 binding. The binding of B-IL-6 was competitively inhibited by excess amounts of rIL-6 but not rIL-1β or rIL-2 (Yamasaki et al. 1988).

JIL6R, a stable transfectant expressing the IL-6R from pBSF2R.236, was established from an IL-6R-negative human T-cell line, Jurkat. As shown in Figure 1, Scatchard plot analysis demonstrated that two classes of IL-6R were expressed on the transfectants: a high-affinity binding site ($K_{d1} \sim 10^{-11}$ M, number of sites per cell [R_1] $\sim 240 \pm 190$) and a low-affinity binding site ($K_{d2} \sim 10^{-9}$ M, $R_2 \sim 12,000 \pm 680$). In the myeloma cell line, U266, the Scatchard plot was also consistent with there being two classes of IL-6R with approximately the same K_d values as the IL-6R of the transfectant cells. The pBSF2R.236 cDNA, therefore, can code for both high- and low-affinity binding sites, although the mechanism that determines the affinity of the IL-6R remains to be elucidated.

The expression of IL-6R mRNA was analyzed by Northern blot analysis. The cDNA probe hybridized to a single species of mRNA of approximately 5000 nucleotides, extracted from the YT cell line. Similar length of IL-6R mRNA was also detected in RNA extracts of the myeloma cell line, U266; the histiocytic leukemia cell line, U937; and the Epstein-Barr-virus-transformed B-cell line, CESS. In fact, these cell lines had been shown to express IL-6R (Taga et al. 1987).

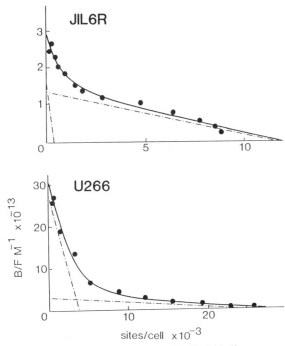

Figure 1. Scatchard analysis of IL-6R. IL-6 binding was assayed in JIL6R and U266 cells using ^{125}I-labeled IL6 (Taga et al. 1987). JIL6R, K_{d1} = 17 ± 14 pM, K_{d2} = 710 ± 110 pM, R_1 = 240 ± 190 sites/cell, R_2 = 12,000 ± 680 sites/cell: U266, K_{d1} = 9.8 ± 2.1 pM, K_{d2} = 740 ± 170 pM, R_1 = 3,000 ± 480 sites/cell, R_2 = 24,000 ± 1,400 sites/cell.

However, the T-cell line, Jurkat, and the Burkitt's lymphoma cell line, BL29, both of which had no detectable IL-6R, had no mRNA that hybridized with the probe. The relatively high concentration of IL-6R mRNA in U266 cells may indicate that IL-6 functions as an autocrine growth factor for myeloma cells (Kawano et al. 1988).

IL-6R Belongs to the Immunoglobulin Superfamily

The nucleotide sequence of the IL-6R cDNA was determined as shown in Figure 2A. There is a single open reading frame, in which the initiator ATG is followed by 467 codons before the termination at triplet TAG. A hydropathy plot of the deduced amino acid sequence showed two major hydrophobic regions, one located between residues 1 and 20, and the other located in the region of residues 359–386. The former is presumably a typical signal peptide and the latter a transmembrane domain. There are six potential N-linked glycosylation sites. The comparison of the deduced amino acid sequence of IL-6R demonstrated the homology with several members of the Ig superfamily (Fig. 2B). The IL-6R sequence between position ~ 20 and 110 fulfills the criteria proposed by Williams and Barclay (1988) for the constant 2 (C2) set of the Ig superfamily. The C2 set includes several adhesion molecules (Arquint et al. 1987; Barthels et al. 1987; Cunningham et al. 1987), the PDGF receptor (Yarden et al. 1986), the CSF-1 receptor (Sherr et al. 1985;

Coussens et al. 1986), the Fcγ receptor (Lewis et al. 1986; Ravetch et al. 1986), and the α1 B-GP (Ishioka et al. 1986). The recently cloned IL-1 receptor was shown to have three Ig-like domains (Sims et al. 1988). Interestingly, the receptors for polypeptide growth factor, such as PDGF, CSF-1, IL-1, and IL-6 could then be grouped in the Ig superfamily.

The IL-6R lacks tyrosine kinase domains, unlike some other growth factor receptors (Ullrich et al. 1984, 1985; Yarden et al. 1986), although IL-6 has been found to be a potent growth factor for myeloma/plasmacytoma cells. The intracytoplasmic portion of IL-6R does not include any unique structure for signal transduction (Yamasaki et al. 1988). The structure of IL-6R is schematically summarized in Figure 3. Recently, the cDNA for a murine homolog of IL-6R was cloned (T. Totsuka et al., in prep.), and its deduced amino acid sequence showed no homology with a human IL-6R in their intracytoplasmic portion, although the extracellular portion was highly homologous between human and mouse. These results strongly suggest that the intracytoplasmic portion of IL-6R may not be responsible for signal transduction, and transduction of the IL-6 signal could be mediated through another molecule associated with the IL-6R.

Regulation of IL-6R Expression

To analyze distribution and regulation of IL-6R expression, monoclonal antibodies against IL-6R were prepared by utilizing a murine transfectant cell line expressing the human IL-6R. Two monoclonal antibodies recognizing different epitopes were prepared. One, PM1, inhibited the binding of ^{125}I-labeled IL-6 to the receptor and blocked the IL-6-dependent growth of a T-lymphoma line, KT3 (Shimizu et al. 1988). PM1 could not bind with IL-6R when it was saturated with IL-6, indicating that this antibody recognizes the IL-6 binding site or its adjacent site on IL-6R. The other, MT18, was not inhibited by IL-6 for its recognition of IL-6R, therefore, this could be used for the detection of IL-6R expressed on normal cells.

To characterize the IL-6R molecule, immunoprecipitation experiments were performed. Both monoclonal antibodies, PM1 and MT18, precipitated a molecule with M_r 80K from a human myeloma cell line, U266. The molecule with the same M_r (80K) was also precipitated from U266 cells by polyclonal antibodies against a synthetic peptide made on the basis of the deduced amino acid sequence corresponding to a part of the cytoplasmic domain of IL-6R. The M_r value of the protein recognized by these antibodies was not in accordance with the molecular weight (50K) calculated from the deduced amino acid sequence, suggesting the posttranslational modification of IL-6R. In fact, enzymatic deglycosylation using N- and O-glycanases converted the 80K form to a 50K product, indicating that IL-6R is a glycoprotein.

The expression of IL-6R on normal B and T cells was examined using two- or three-color immunofluorescent

A

```
-437                                        GGCGGTCCCCTGTTCTCCCCGCTCAGGTGCGGCGCTGTGGCAGGAAGCCACCCCCTCGGTCGGCCGGTGCACGGGGCTGT

-357    TACACCATCCGCTCCGGCTTTCGTAACCGCACCCTGGGACGGCCCAGAGACGCTCCAGCGCGAGTTCCTCAAATGTTTTCCTGCGTTGCCAGGACCGTCCGCCGCTCTGAGTCATGTGC

-238    GAGTGGGAAGTCGCACTGACACTGAGCCGGGCCAGAGGGAGAGGAGCCGAGCGCGGCGCGGGGCCGAGGGACTCGCAGTGTGTGTAGAGAGCCGGGCTCCTGCGGATGGGGGCTGCCCC

-119    CGGGGCCTGAGCCCGCCTGCCCGCCCACCGCCCCGCCCCGCCCCTGCCACCCCTGCCGCCCGGTTCCCATTAGCCTGTCCGCCTCTGCGGGACCATGGAGTGGTAGCCGAGGAGGAAGC
```

```
1      ATG CTG GCC GTC GGC TGC GCG CTG CTG GCT GCC CTG CTG GCC GCG CCG GGA GCG GCG CTG GCC CCA AGG CGC TGC CCT GCG CAG GAG GTG
1      Met Leu Ala Val Gly Cys Ala Leu Leu Ala Ala Leu Leu Ala Ala Pro Gly Ala Ala Leu Ala Pro Arg Arg Cys Pro Ala Gln Glu Val

91     GCA AGA GGC GTG CTG ACC AGT CTG CCA GGA GAC AGC GTG ACT CTG ACC TGC CCG GGA GTA GAG CCG GAA GAC AAT GCC ACT GTT CAC TGG
31     Ala Arg Gly Val Leu Thr Ser Leu Pro Gly Asp Ser Val Thr Leu Thr Cys Pro Gly Val Glu Pro Glu Asp Asn Ala Thr Val His Trp
                                                                                                        *** *** ***

181    GTG CTC AGG AAG CCG GCT GCA GGC TCC CAC CCC AGC AGA TGG GCT GGC ATG GGA AGG AGG CTG CTG CTG AGG AGT CAG CTC CAC GAC
61     Val Leu Arg Lys Pro Ala Ala Gly Ser His Pro Ser Arg Trp Ala Gly Met Gly Arg Arg Leu Leu Leu Arg Ser Gln Leu His Asp

271    TCT GGA AAC TAT TCA TGC TAC CGG GCC GGC CGC CCA GCT GGG ACT GTG CAC TTG CTG GTG GAT GTT CCC CCC GAG GAG CCC CAG CTC TCC
91     Ser Gly Asn Tyr Ser Cys Tyr Arg Ala Gly Arg Pro Ala Gly Thr Val His Leu Leu Val Asp Val Pro Pro Glu Glu Pro Gln Leu Ser
       *** *** ***

361    TGC TTC CGG AAG AGC CCC CTC AGC AAT GTT GTT TGT GAG TGG GGT CCT CGG AGC ACC CCA TCC CTG ACG ACA AAG GCT GTG CTC TTG GTG
121    Cys Phe Arg Lys Ser Pro Leu Ser Asn Val Val Cys Glu Trp Gly Pro Arg Ser Thr Pro Ser Leu Thr Thr Lys Ala Val Leu Leu Val

451    AGG AAG TTT CAG AAC AGT CCG GCC GAA GAC TTC CAG GAG CCG TGC CAG TAT TCC CAG GAG TCC CAG AAG TTC TCC TGC CAG TTA GCA GTC
151    Arg Lys Phe Gln Asn Ser Pro Ala Glu Asp Phe Gln Glu Pro Cys Gln Tyr Ser Gln Glu Ser Gln Lys Phe Ser Cys Gln Leu Ala Val

541    CCG GAG GGA GAC AGC TCT TTC TAC ATA GTG TCC ATG TGC GTC GCC AGT AGT GTC GGG AGC AAG TTC AGC AAA ACT CAA ACC TTT CAG GGT
181    Pro Glu Gly Asp Ser Ser Phe Tyr Ile Val Ser Met Cys Val Ala Ser Ser Val Gly Ser Lys Phe Ser Lys Thr Gln Thr Phe Gln Gly

631    TGT GGA ATC TTG CAG CCT GAT CCG CCT GCC AAC ATC ACA GTC ACT GCC GTG GCC AGA AAC CCC CGC TGG CTC AGT GTC ACC TGG CAA GAC
211    Cys Gly Ile Leu Gln Pro Asp Pro Pro Ala Asn Ile Thr Val Thr Ala Val Ala Arg Asn Pro Arg Trp Leu Ser Val Thr Trp Gln Asp
                                                                       *** *** ***

721    CCC CAC TCC TGG AAC TCA TCT TTC TAC AGA CTA CGG TTT GAG CTC AGA TAT CGG GCT GAA CGG TCA AAG ACA TTC ACA ACA TGG ATG GTC
241    Pro His Ser Trp Asn Ser Ser Phe Tyr Arg Leu Arg Phe Glu Leu Arg Tyr Arg Ala Glu Arg Ser Lys Thr Phe Thr Thr Trp Met Val
                               *** *** ***

811    AAG GAC CTC CAG CAT CAC TGT GTC ATC CAC GAC GCC TGG AGC GGC CTG AGG CAC GTG GTG CAG CTT CGT GCC CAG GAG GAG TTC GGG CAA
271    Lys Asp Leu Gln His His Cys Val Ile His Asp Ala Trp Ser Gly Leu Arg His Val Val Gln Leu Arg Ala Gln Glu Glu Phe Gly Gln

901    GGC GAG TGG AGC GAG TGG AGC CCG GAG GCC ATG GGC ACG CCT TGG ACA GAA TCC AGG AGT CCT CCA GCT GAG AAC GAG GTG TCC ACC CCC
301    Gly Glu Trp Ser Glu Trp Ser Pro Glu Ala Met Gly Thr Pro Trp Thr Glu Ser Arg Ser Pro Pro Ala Glu Asn Glu Val Ser Thr Pro

991    ATG CAG GCA CTT ACT ACT AAT AAA GAC GAT GAT AAT ATT CTC TTC AGA GAT TCT GCA AAT GCG ACA AGC CTC CCA GTG CAA GAT │TCT TCT
331    Met Gln Ala Leu Thr Thr Asn Lys Asp Asp Asp Asn Ile Leu Phe Arg Asp Ser Ala Asn Ala Thr Ser Leu Pro Val Gln Asp │Ser Ser
                                              *** *** ***

1081   TCA GTA CCA CTG CCC ACA TTC CTG GTT GCT GGA GGG AGC CTG GCC TTC GGA ACG CTC CTC TGC ATT GCC ATT GTT CTG│ AGG TTC AAG AAG
361    Ser Val Pro Leu Pro Thr Phe Leu Val Ala Gly Gly Ser Leu Ala Phe Gly Thr Leu Leu Cys Ile Ala Ile Val Leu│ Arg Phe Lys Lys

1171   ACG TGG AAG CTG CGG GCT CTG AAG GAA GGC AAG ACA AGC ATG CAT CCG CCG TAC TCT TTG GGG CAG CTG GTC CCG GAG AGG CCT CGA CCC
391    Thr Trp Lys Leu Arg Ala Leu Lys Glu Gly Lys Thr Ser Met His Pro Pro Tyr Ser Leu Gly Gln Leu Val Pro Glu Arg Pro Arg Pro

1261   ACC CCA GTG CTT GTT CCT CTC ATC TCC CCA CCG GTG TCC CCC AGC AGC CTG GGG TCT GAC AAT ACC TCG AGC CAC AAC CGA CCA GAT GCC
421    Thr Pro Val Leu Val Pro Leu Ile Ser Pro Pro Val Ser Pro Ser Ser Leu Gly Ser Asp Asn Thr Ser Ser His Asn Arg Pro Asp Ala
                                                                                               *** *** ***

1351   AGG GAC CCA CGG AGC CCT TAT GAC ATC AGC AAT ACA GAC TAC TTC TTC CCC AGA TAG CTGGCTGGGTGGCACCAGCAGCCTGGACCCTGTGGATGACAAA
451    Arg Asp Pro Arg Ser Pro Tyr Asp Ile Ser Asn Thr Asp Tyr Phe Phe Pro Arg ---
```

```
1451   ACACAAACGGGCTCAGCAAAAGATGCTTCTCACTGCCATGCCAGCTTATCTCAGGGGTGTGCGGCCTTTGGCTTCACGGAAGAGCCTTGCGGAAGGTTCTACGCCAGGGGAAAATCAGC

1570   CTGCTCCAGCTGTTCAGCTGGTTGAGGTTTCAAACCTCCCTTTCCAAATGCCCAGCTTAAAGGGGTTAGAGTGAACTTGGGCCACTGTGAAGAGAACCATATCAAGACTCTTTGGACAC

1689   TCACACGGACACTCAAAAGCTGGGCAGGTTGGTGGGGGCCTCGGTGTGGAGAAGCGGCTGGCAGCCCACCCCTCAACACCTCTGCACAAGCTGCACCCTCAGGCAGGTGGGATGGATTT

1808   CCAGCCAAAGCCTCCTCCAGCCGCCATGCTCCTGGCCCACTGCATCGTTTCATCTTCCAACTCAAACTCTTAAAAACCCAAGTGCCCTTAGCAAATTCTGTTTTTTCTAGGCCTGGGGACG

1927   GCTTTTTACTTAAACGCCAAGGCCTGGGGGAAGAAGCTCTCTCCTCCCTTTCTTCCCTACAGTTCAAAAACAGCTGAGGGTGAGTGGGTGAATAATACAGTATGTCAGGGCCTGGTCGTT

2046   TTCAACAGAATTATAATTAGTTCCTCATTAGCAGTTTTGCCTAAATGTGAATGATGATCCTAGGCATTTGCTGAATACAGAGGCAACTGCATTGGCTTTGGGTTGCAGGACCTCAGGTG

2165   AGAAGCAGAGGAAGGAGAGGAGAGGGGCACAGGGTCTCTACCATCCCCTGTAGAGTGGGAGCTGAGTGGGGGATCACAGCCTCTGAAAACCAATGTTCTCTCTTCTCCACCTCCCACAA

2284   AGGAGAGCTAGCAGCAGGGAGGGGCTTCTGCCATTTCTGAGATCAAAACGGTTTTACTGCAGCTTTGTTTGTTGTCAGCTGAACCTGGGTAACTAGGGAAGATAATATTAAGGAAGACAA

2403   TGTGAAAAGAAAAATGAGCCTGGCAAGAATGCGTTTAAACTTGGTTTTTAAAAAACTGCTGACTGTTTTCTCTTGAGAGGGTGGAATATCCAATATTCGCTGTGTCAGCATAGAAGTAA

2522   CTTACTTAGGTGTGGGGGAAGCACCATAACTTTGTTTAGCCCAAAACCAAGTCAAGTGAAAAAGGAGGAAGAGAAAAATATTTTCCTGCCAGGCATGGAGGCCCACGCACTTCGGGAG

2641   GTCGAGGCAGGAGGATCACTTGAGTCCAGAAGTTTGAGATCAGCCTGGGCAATGTGA·T·A·A·A·A·CCCCATCTCTACAAAAAGCAT·A·A·A·A·ATTAGCCAAGTGTGGTAGAGTGTGCCTGAAGT

2760   CCCAGATACTTGGGGGGCTGAGGTGGGAGGATCTCTTGAGCCTGGGAGGTCAAGGCTGCAGTGAGCCGAGATTGCACCACTGCACTCCAGCCTGGGGTGACAGAGCAAGTGAGACCCTG

2879   TCTCAAAAAAAAAAAAAAAAAAAAAAAAAAAAAAAAAAAAAAA
```

B

β strand		B'			C		C'		C''			D		E				F	

S---S

```
              *** *       #          * *                                              s*          * *    s s * *
C2-SET        43     50              60                70                              80            90
IL-6 R        VTLTCPGV--EPED-NATVHWVLRKPAAGSH------------------PSRWAGM-------GRRLLLRSVQLHDSGNYSCYRAG
PDGF R  (III) ITIRCIV-MGNDVV---NFQWTYPRMK---SGRLV------------EPVTDYLFGVPS---RIGSILHIPTAELSDSGTYTCNVSV
CSF-1-R (v-fms) AQIVCSA--SNIDV---NFDVSLRHGDTKLTISQQS-----------DFHDNRYQKV-------LTTNLDHVSFQDAGNYSCTATN
Alpha1 B-GP(III) VTLTCQVA--PLSGV--DEQLRRGE-------------------------KEILVPRSSTSP-DRIFFHLNAVALGDGGHYTCRYRL
Fc R    (I)   VTLMCEG--THNPGNS--STQWFHNG----------------------RSIRSQ-------VQASYTEKA-TVNDSGEYRCQMEQ

V-SET
Ig V  kappa   ATLSCRASQSI---SNSYLAWYQQKP-SGSPRLLIYGASTRATGIP-----ARFSGSGSG----TEFTLTISSLQSEDFAVYYCQQYN
Ig V  lambda  VTLTCRSSTGAV--TTSNYANWVQQKP-DHLFTGLIGGTNNRAPGVP-----ARFSGSLIG----NKAALTITGAQTEDEAIYFCALWY
Ig V  heavy   LSLTCTVSGSTF--SNDYYTWVRQPP--GRGLEWIGYVFYHGTSDDTTPLRSRVTMLVDTS--KNQFSLRLSSVTAADTAVVYCARNL
CD4    (I)    VELTCTASQK----KSIQFHWKNSNQI--KILGNQGSFLTK-GPSK---LNDRADSRRSLWD--QGNFPLIIKNLKIEDSDTYICEVED
Poly Ig R (II) VTITCPFTYATR--QLKKSFYKVED------GELVLIIDSSSKEAKDPRYKGRITLQIQST-TAKEFTVTIKHVQLNDAGQYVCQSGS
```

Figure 2. (*See facing page for legend.*)

716

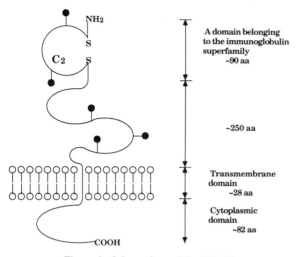

Figure 3. Schematic model of IL-6R.

analysis. Nonstimulated B cells expressed an undetectable amount of IL-6R, regardless of the expression of surface IgD. However, after the stimulation with pokeweed mitogen, IL-6R was observed on IgD-negative B cells with a relatively large size, but subtly on IgD-negative small B cells, and not at all on IgD-positive B cells, as shown in Figure 4. The results indicate that IL-6R is not expressed on resting B cells but is inducible on activated large B cells with an IgD-negative phenotype. This is in agreement with the previous report that IL-6 could induce immunoglobulin production in IgD-negative tonsillar B cells (Kikutani et al. 1986). This also supports the early observation that surface IgD-negative B cells could be led to a final maturation stage to produce immunoglobulins (Kuritani and Cooper 1982). In contrast to B cells, IL-6R was detected on nonstimulated $CD4^+/CD8^-$ as well as $CD4^-/CD8^+$ T cells. The level of IL-6R on both

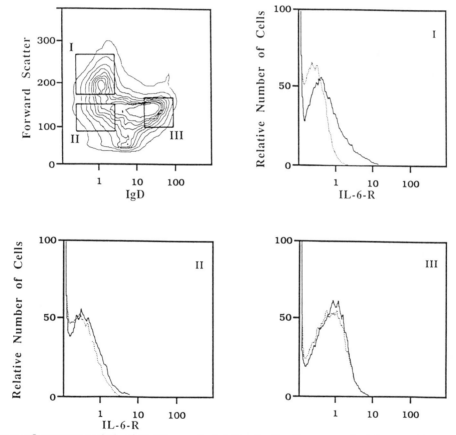

Figure 4. Immunofluorescent analysis of IL-6R on activated B cells. B cells were purified from tonsillar mononuclear cells cultured with pokeweed mitogen for 4 days. Level of surface IgD and forward scatter were expressed in the upper left panel. IgD-negative large (I), IgD-negative small (II), and IgD-positive small (III) cells were analyzed for IL-6R expression using phycocyanine-conjugated MT18 monoclonal antibody. Dotted lines represent unstained controls.

Figure 2. (*A*) Nucleotide sequence and deduced amino acid sequence of IL-6R cDNA. The underlined region is a presumed signal peptide; the box encircles a presumed transmembrane domain; the asterisks show potential N-glycosylation sites; the dots identify a possible poly(A) addition signal. (*B*) Alignment of the IL-6R domain to immunoglobulin superfamily protein domains. (*) Conserved patterns common to the V, C1, and C2 sets: (#) common to the C1 and C2 sets; ($) common to the V and C2 sets (Williams and Barclay 1988). The known locations of β strands in immunoglobulin V domains are marked with bars and capital letters on them. The numbers above the alignment represent positions of amino acids of IL-6R sequence. S---S represents the putative disulfide bond within IL-6R.

T-cell subpopulations was not significantly changed after stimulation with phytohemagglutinin (PHA), although the level of IL-2R expression was greatly increased by PHA stimulation. The difference with regard to the stages at which IL-6R and IL-2R are expressed on T cells may reflect the functional difference of these cytokines: IL-6 acts on T cells at an early stage as an activation factor (Lotz et al. 1988), and IL-2 acts at an activated stage as a growth factor (Smith 1984). The same principle may be applied to B cells: IL-4R and IL-6R are expressed on resting and activated B cells, respectively, with the former acting on B cells at an early stage and the latter at a final maturation stage (Hirano et al. 1984, 1985; Paul and Ohara 1987). Therefore, the functions of various cytokines, although they are pleiotropic, may be controlled by the regulation of the expression of their receptors.

IL-6 Stimulation Triggers the Association of 80K IL-6R and a Second Non-ligand-binding Chain, gp130

To elucidate the possible presence of a signal-transducing molecule associated with IL-6R, the IL-6R molecule was precipitated under nondissociating conditions with a monoclonal anti-IL-6R antibody, MT18. As shown in Figure 5A, MT18 monoclonal antibody precipitated 80K IL-6R from a human plasmacytoma cell line, U266, under mild lysis conditions (1% digitonin buffer). Another polypeptide chain with a M_r of

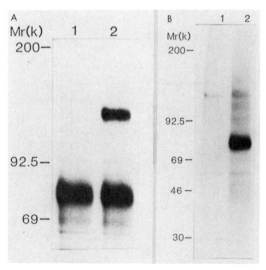

Figure 5. (*A*) IL-6-triggered association of IL-6R and 130K protein. Metabolically labeled U266 cells were incubated with (lane *2*) or without (lane *1*) IL-6 at 37°C for 30 min, and digitonin-lysis was carried out. Immunoprecipitation was performed with MT18 antibody and analyzed on SDS-PAGE under reducing conditions. (*B*) Detection of an IL-6-binding molecule by cross-linking, immunoprecipitation, and cleavage of the cross-linker. Metabolically labeled U266 cells were saturated with (lane *2*) or without (lane *1*) unlabeled IL-6. Cross-linked complexes containing IL-6 were immunoprecipitated with anti-IL-6 antibody, and cross-linking bonds in the complexes were cleaved and analyzed on SDS-PAGE under reducing conditions.

130K was coprecipitated only when the cells were incubated with IL-6 at 37°C for 30 minutes before digitonin-lysis. The result suggests that IL-6 triggered the association of the 80K IL-6R with a cellular 130K molecule. This 130K molecule was further demonstrated to be a glycoprotein by endoglycosidase treatment and thus was called gp130. The association of IL-6R and gp130 could occur when cells were preincubated with IL-6 at 37°C but not at 4°C, although it was previously shown that IL-6 could bind to the receptor at 0°C. The result suggested that the second chain may not be involved in the direct interaction with IL-6. This was confirmed in the experiment shown in Figure 5B. U266 cells were metabolically labeled and saturated with unlabeled IL-6, then cross-linking was performed with a cleavable cross-linker, EGS. Extracted proteins were denatured, and the molecules cross-linked to IL-6 were immunoprecipitated by anti-IL-6 antibody. Intermolecular cross-linking bonds in the immunoprecipitates were cleaved by hydroxylamine, and the samples were analyzed on SDS-PAGE. As shown in Figure 5B, only a protein species with a M_r of about 80K was detected, indicating that the 80K IL-6R was the only molecule involved in the IL-6 binding.

Human 80K IL-6R Can Associate with Murine gp130 and Is Functioning in Murine Cells

Human IL-6R cDNA was transfected to a murine B-lymphoma line, M12, which has no detectable number of IL-6R, and a transformant, M12IL6R, was obtained. A murine gp130 homolog could be coimmunoprecipitated with human IL-6R by monoclonal MT18 antibody when the cells were preincubated with IL-6. Although M12 cells showed no responsiveness to IL-6, M12 IL6R cells responded to IL-6 with a decrease in their growth. The result indicated that M12 cells expressed a murine gp130 homolog but did not bind IL-6 nor respond to IL-6, confirming that gp130 did not have a ligand-binding property by itself.

An Intracytoplasmic Portion of IL-6R Is Not Required for the Association of gp130 and for Signal Transduction

As described previously, an intracytoplasmic portion of IL-6R does not have any unique sequence for signal transduction and is not conserved between human and mouse. This suggests that IL-6R may not be responsible for signal transduction, but an associated chain, gp130, may be involved in transduction of signals. This was confirmed by employing a mutant cDNA of IL-6R that did not have its intracytoplasmic portion (IL6RΔIC). An IL6RΔIC was transfected into a murine Ψ2 cell line or a murine myeloid leukemia cell line, M1, in which IL-6 inhibited its cell growth and induced differentiation into macrophages.

A cDNA of IL-6R or a mutant cDNA, IL6RΔIC, was transfected into Ψ2 cells, and transfectants, Ψ2IL6R and Ψ2IL6RΔIC, were obtained. Anti-IL-6R antibody, MT18, could coprecipitate IL-6R (80K) or the mutant IL-6R lacking its intracytoplasmic portion (75K) with a murine gp130 homolog when transfectants were preincubated with IL-6, indicating that the intracytoplasmic portion of IL-6R was not required for the interaction of IL-6R with a gp130 molecule (Fig. 6A).

M1 cells were transfected with a normal or a deletion-mutated IL-6R cDNA, and both M1 transfectants, M1IL6R and M1IL6RΔIC, expressed 20–46 times higher density of IL-6 binding sites compared to the parental M1 cells. This made the transfectants more sensitive to IL-6. In fact, as shown in Figure 6B, both transfectants, M1IL6R and M1IL6RΔIC, acquired about 70 times higher sensitivity to IL-6 in their growth inhibition, indicating that human IL-6R on murine M1 cells could transduce the IL-6 signal even with a truncated intracytoplasmic region.

Soluble IL-6R Can Associate with gp130 in the Presence of IL-6 and Transduce the IL-6 Signal

The results so far observed indicate that the association of 80K IL-6R and gp130 did not require the intracytoplasmic region of IL-6R and that the signals of IL-6 could be transduced through gp130. To confirm this, we prepared soluble IL-6 receptor without intracytoplasmic and transmembrane portions and asked whether the complex of soluble receptor and IL-6 could bind with gp130 and transduce the signals.

COS-7 cells were transfected with a mutant cDNA, and the culture supernatant containing transiently expressed soluble IL-6R was collected. To confirm that

the soluble IL-6R present in COS-7 cell culture supernatant could bind IL-6, the soluble IL-6R was fixed on anti-IL-6R antibody-coated wells, and ^{125}I-labeled IL-6 was added. The results confirmed that the soluble IL-6R could bind ^{125}I-labeled IL-6. The binding was competitively inhibited by unlabeled IL-6, indicating that the binding was IL-6-specific. To examine whether non-membrane-anchored soluble IL-6R could associate with gp130 in the presence of IL-6, soluble IL-6R was mixed with a surface-iodinated murine B-lymphoma cell line, M12, which did not have IL-6R but expressed a murine gp130 homolog. This was incubated with or without IL-6, then digitonin-lysis and immunoprecipitation with anti-IL-6R antibody, MT18, were carried out. As shown in Figure 7A, gp130 was detected on SDS-PAGE from the cells incubated with soluble IL-6R plus IL-6. The coimmunoprecipitation of gp130 with soluble IL-6R was not observed in the absence of IL-6. Thus, these results confirmed that soluble IL-6R could associate with gp130 in the presence of IL-6.

To ascertain whether the complex of soluble IL-6R and IL-6 could transduce signals through gp130, M1 cells were used in a growth inhibition assay. The cells were incubated with soluble IL-6R or mock control in the presence or absence of varying concentrations of IL-6 for 60 hours and pulsed with [^{3}H]thymidine for 10 hours. As shown in Figure 7B, soluble IL-6R could augment the sensitivity of M1 cells to IL-6 in their growth inhibition compared to mock controls. However, without IL-6, soluble IL-6R did not show any inhibitory effect on M1 cells. The results indicated that the complex of soluble IL-6R and IL-6 could transduce signals by binding with gp130.

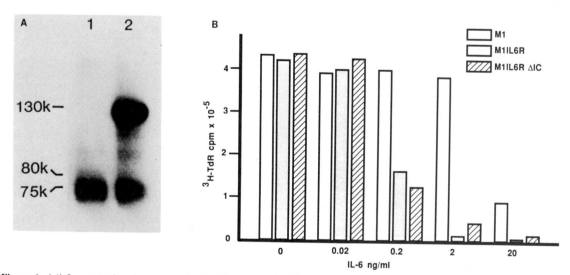

Figure 6. (*A*) Intracytoplasmic portion of IL-6R is not required for the association with gp130. Ψ2IL6RΔIC cells that express mutated IL-6R lacking the intracytoplasmic domain were metabolically labeled and incubated with (lane *2*) or without (lane *1*) IL-6 at 37°C for 30 min. Immunoprecipitation and SDS-PAGE were performed as in Fig. 5A. (*B*) Intracytoplasmic portion is not required for signal transduction. M1, M1IL6R, and M1IL6RΔIC cells were cultured in the presence of indicated concentrations of IL-6 for 60 hr and pulsed with [^{3}H]thymidine for 10 hr. Incorporated radioactivity was measured. Data represent the average of replicates. Errors were within 10%.

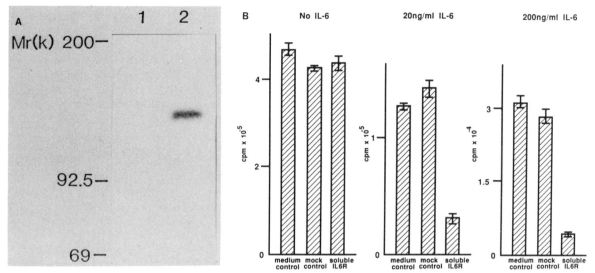

Figure 7. (*A*) Association of soluble IL-6R and gp130 in the presence of IL-6. Surface-iodinated M12 cells were incubated with (lane 2) or without IL-6 (lane 1) at 37°C for 30 min in the presence of COS-7 culture supernatant containing soluble IL-6R. Immunoprecipitation and SDS-PAGE were performed as in Fig. 5A. (*B*) Growth inhibition of M1 cells by soluble IL-6R plus IL-6. M1 cells were cultured with indicated concentrations of IL-6 in the absence (medium control) or presence of 25% COS-7 culture supernatant containing soluble IL-6R or mock control. The same assay was performed as in Fig. 6B. Vertical bars represent S.D.

A Novel Mechanism of the IL-6-mediated Signals: Interaction between a Ligand-binding Chain and a Signal-transducing Chain

We have demonstrated that 80K IL-6R is the only molecule involved in ligand binding and that IL-6R associates with a possible signal transducer, gp130, in the presence of IL-6. These observations indicate that the IL-6R system is composed of two functional chains: a ligand-binding 80K IL-6R and a non-ligand-binding, but signal-transducing, gp130. The binding of IL-6 with IL-6R may induce a certain allosteric change of the receptor molecule at its extracellular portion, which may trigger the association with gp130 as shown schematically in Figure 8. This may be in contrast to the IL-2R system. IL-2R was shown to consist of two membrane polypeptide chains, p55 and p75, both of which have IL-2-binding properties (Sharon et al. 1986; Tsudo et al. 1986; Teshigawara et al. 1987), but only the β chain was shown to mediate the IL-2 signal (Hatakeyama et al. 1987; Robb and Greene 1987).

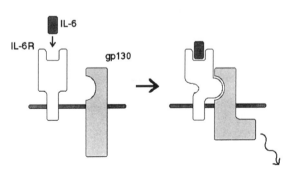

Figure 8. Schematic model of IL-6R and gp130.

ACKNOWLEDGMENTS

This study was supported by a Grant-in-Aid for Specially Promoted Research from the Ministry of Education, Science and Culture. The authors wish to thank Dr. B. Seed and T. Taniguchi for their collaboration in the construction of the cDNA library that was used for the molecular cloning of IL-6R. We thank Ms. M. Harayama and K. Kubota for their secretarial assistance.

REFERENCES

Abdella, P.M. and P.K. Smith. 1979. A new cleavable reagent for cross-linking and reversible immobilization of proteins. *Biochem. Biophys. Res. Commun.* **87:** 734.

Andus, T., T. Geiger, T. Hirano, H. Northoff, U. Ganter, J. Bauer, T. Kishimoto, and P.C. Heinrich. 1987. Recombinant human B cell stimulatory factor 2 (BSF-2/IFNβ2) regulates β-fibrinogen and albumin mRNA levels in Fao-9 cells. *FEBS Lett.* **221:**18.

Arquint, M., J. Roder, L.-S. Chia, J. Down, D. Wilkinson, H. Bayley, P. Braun, and R. Dunn. 1987. Molecular cloning and primary structure of myelin-associated glycoprotein. *Proc. Natl. Acad. Sci.* **84:** 600.

Barthels, D., M.-J. Santoni, W. Wille, C. Ruppert, J.-C. Chaix, M.-R. Hirsch, J.C. Fontecilla-Camps, and C. Goridis. 1987. Isolation and nucleotide sequence of mouse NCAM cDNA that codes for a M_r 79000 polypeptide without a membrane-spanning region. *EMBO J.* **6:** 907.

Cepko, C.L., B.E. Roberts, and R.C. Mulligan. 1984. Construction and applications of a highly transmissible murine retrovirus vector. *Cell* **37:** 1053.

Coulie, P.G., A. Vanhecke, J. Van Damme, S. Cayphas, P. Poupart, L. De Wit, and J. Content. 1987. High affinity sites for human 26-kDa protein (interleukin 6, B-cell stimulatory factor-2, human hybridoma plasmacytoma growth factor, interferon-β 2), different from those of type-1 interferon (α, β) on lymphoblastoid cells. *Eur. J. Immunol.* **17:** 1435.

Coussens, L., C.V. Beveren, D. Smith, E. Chen, R.L. Mitchell, C.M. Isacke, I.M. Verma, and A. Ullrich. 1986. Structural alteration of viral homologue of receptor proto-oncogene *fms* at carboxyl terminus. *Nature* **320:** 277.

Cunningham, B.A., J.J. Hemperly, B.A. Murray, E.A. Prediger, R. Brackenbury, and G.M. Edelman. 1987. Neural cell adhesion molecule: Structure, immunoglobulin-like domains, cell surface modulation, and alternative RNA splicing. *Science.* **236:** 799.

Garman, R.D., K.A. Jacobs, S.C. Clark, and D.H. Raulet. 1987. B-cell-stimulatory factor 2 (β2 interferon) functions as a second signal for interleukin 2 production by mature murine T cells. *Proc. Natl. Acad. Sci.* **84:** 7629.

Gauldie, J., C. Richards, D. Harnish, P. Lansdorp, and H. Baumann. 1987. Interferon β2/B-cell stimulatory factor type 2 shares identity with monocyte-derived hepatocyte-stimulating factor and regulates the major acute phase protein response in liver cells. *Proc. Natl. Acad. Sci.* **84:** 7521.

Haegeman, G., J. Content, G. Volckaert, R. Derynck, J. Tavernier, and W. Fiers. 1986. Structural analysis of the sequence encoding for an inducible 26-kDa protein in human fibroblasts. *Eur. J. Immunol.* **159:** 625.

Hatakeyama, M., T. Doi, T. Kono, M. Maruyama, S. Minamoto, H. Mori, H. Kobayashi, T. Uchiyama, and T. Taniguchi. 1987. Transmembrane signaling of interleukin 2 receptor: Conformation and function of human interleukin 2 receptor (p55)/insulin receptor chimeric molecules. *J. Exp. Med.* **166:** 362.

Hirano, T. and T. Kishimoto. 1989. Interleukin-6 (IL-6). In *Handbook of experimental pharmacology: Peptide growth factors and their receptors* (ed. M.M. Sporn and A.B. Roberts). Springer-Verlag, Berlin. (In press.)

Hirano, T., T. Teranishi, B.H. Lin, and K. Onoue. 1984. Human helper T cell factor(s) IV. Demonstration of a human late-acting B cell differentiation factor acting on *Staphylococcus aureus* Cowan I-stimulated B cells. *J. Immunol.* **133:** 798.

Hirano, T., T. Matsuda, K. Hosoi, A. Okano, H. Matsui, and T. Kishimoto. 1988. Absence of antiviral activity in recombinant B cell stimulatory factor 2 (BSF-2). *Immunol. Lett.* **17:** 41.

Hirano, T., T. Taga, N. Nakano, K. Yasukawa, S. Kashiwamura, K. Shimizu, K. Nakajima, K.H. Pyun, and T. Kishimoto. 1985. Purification to homogeneity and characterization of human B cell differentiation factor (BCDF or BSFp-2). *Proc. Natl. Acad. Sci.* **82:** 5490.

Hirano, T., K. Yasukawa, H. Harada, T. Taga, Y. Watanabe, T. Matsuda, S. Kashiwamura, K. Nakajima, K. Koyama, A. Iwamatu, S. Tsunasawa, F. Sakiyama, H. Matsui, Y. Takahara, T. Taniguchi, and T. Kishimoto. 1986. Complementary DNA for a novel human interleukin (BSF-2) that induces B lymphocytes to produce immunoglobulin. *Nature* **324:** 73.

Ikebuchi, K., G.G. Wong, S.C. Clark, J.N. Ihle, Y. Hirai, and M. Ogawa. 1987. Interleukin-3-dependent proliferation of multipotential hemopoietic progenitors. *Proc. Natl. Acad. Sci.* **84:** 9035.

Ishibashi, T., H. Kimura, T. Uchida, S. Kariyone, P. Friese, and S.A. Burstein. 1989. Human interleukin 6 is a direct promotor of maturation of megakaryocytes in vitro. *Proc. Natl. Acad. Sci.* **86:** 5953.

Ishioka, N., N. Takahashi, and F.W. Putnam. 1986. Amino acid sequence of human plasma α₁B-glycoprotein: Homology to the immunoglobulin supergene family. *Proc. Natl. Acad. Sci.* **83:** 2363.

Kawano, M., T. Hirano, T. Matsuda, T. Taga, Y. Horii, K. Iwato, H. Asaoku, B. Tang, O. Tanabe, H. Tanaka, A. Kuramoto, and T. Kishimoto. 1988. Autocrine generation and essential requirement of BSF-2/IL-6 for human multiple myelomas. *Nature* **332:** 83.

Kikutani, H., H. Nakamura, R. Sata, R. Kimura, K. Yamasaki, R.R. Hardy, and T. Kishimoto. 1986. Delinea-

tion and characterization of human B cell subpopulations at various stages of activation by using a B cell-specific monoclonal antibody. *J. Immunol.* **136:** 4027.

Kishimoto, T. and T. Hirano. 1988. Molecular regulation of B lymphocyte response. *Annu. Rev. Immunol.* **6:** 485.

Kuritani, T. and M.D. Cooper. 1982. Human B cell differentiation II. Pokeweed mitogen-responsive B cells belong to a surface immunoglobulin D-negative subpopulation. *J. Exp. Med.* **155:** 1561.

Lewis, V.A., T. Koch, H. Plutner, and I. Mellman. 1986. A complementary DNA clone for a macrophage-lymphocyte Fc receptor. *Nature* **324:** 372.

Lotz, M., F. Jirik, R. Kabouridis, C. Tsoukas, T. Hirano, and T. Kishimoto. 1988. BSF-2/IL-6 is a costimulant for human thymocytes and T lymphocytes. *J. Exp. Med.* **167:** 1253.

Miyaura, C., K. Onozaki, Y. Akiyama, T. Taniyama, T. Hirano, T. Kishimoto, and T. Suda. 1988. Recombinant human interleukin 6 (B-cell stimulatory factor 2) is a potent inducer of differentiation of mouse myeloid leukemia cells (M1). *FEBS Lett.* **234:** 17.

Nordan, R.P. and M. Potter. 1986. A macrophage-derived factor required by plasmacytomas for survival and proliferation *in vitro*. *Science* **233:** 566.

Okada, M., M. Kitahara, S. Kishimoto, T. Matsuda, T. Hirano, and T. Kishimoto. 1988. BSF-2/IL-6 functions as a killer helper factor in the *in vitro* induction of cytotoxic T cells. *J. Immunol.* **141:** 1543.

Paul, W.E. and J. Ohara. 1987. B-cell stimulatory factor-1/interleukin 4. *Annu. Rev. Immunol.* **5:** 429.

Ravetch, J.V., A.D. Luster, R. Weinshank, J. Kochan, A. Pavlovec, D.A. Portnoy, J. Hulmes, Y.-C.E. Pan, and J.C. Unkeless. 1986. Structural heterogeneity and functional domains of murine immunoglobulin G Fc receptors. *Science.* **234:** 718.

Robb, R.J. and W.C. Greene. 1987. Internalization of interleukin 2 is mediated by the β chain of the high-affinity interleukin 2 receptor. *J. Exp. Med.* **165:** 1201.

Satoh, T., S. Nakamura, T. Taga, T. Matsuda, T. Hirano, T. Kishimoto, and Y. Kaziro. 1988. Induction of neural differentiation in PC12 cells by B cell stimulatory factor 2/interleukin 6. *Mol. Cell. Biol.* **8:** 3546.

Seed, B. 1987. An LFA-3 cDNA encodes a phospholipid-linked membrane protein homologous to its receptor CD2. *Nature* **329:** 840.

Shabo, Y., J. Lotem, M. Rubinstein, M. Revel, S.C. Clark, S.F. Wolf, R. Kamen, and L. Sachs. 1988. The myeloid blood cell differentiation-inducing protein MGI-2A is interleukin 6. *Blood* **72:** 2070.

Sharon, M., R.D. Klausner, B.R. Cullen, R. Chizzonite, and W.J. Leonard. 1986. Novel interleukin-2 receptor subunit detected by cross-linking under high-affinity condition. *Science.* **234:** 859.

Sherr, C.J., C.W. Rettenmier, R. Sacca, M.F. Roussel, A.T. Look, and E.R. Stanley. 1985. The c-*fms* proto-oncogene product is related to the receptor for the mononuclear phagocyte growth factor, CSF-1. *Cell* **41:** 665.

Shimizu, S., T. Hirano, K. Yoshioka, S. Sugai, T. Matsuda, T. Taga, T. Kishimoto, and S. Konda. 1988. Interleukin-6 (B-cell stimulatory factor-2)-dependent growth of a Lennert's lymphoma-derived T-cell line (KT-3). *Blood* **72:** 1826.

Sims, J.E., C.J. March, D. Cosman, M.B. Widmer, H.R. McDonald, C.J. McMahan, C.E. Grubin, J.M. Wignall, J.L. Jackson, S.M. Call, D. Friend, A.R. Alpert, S. Gillis, D.L. Urdal, and S.K. Dower. 1988. cDNA expression cloning of the IL-1 receptor, a member of the immunoglobulin superfamily. *Science* **241:** 585.

Smith, K.A. 1984. Interleukin 2. *Annu. Rev. Immunol.* **2:** 319.

Taga, T., K. Kawanishi, R.R. Hardy, T. Hirano, and T. Kishimoto. 1987. Receptors for B cell stimulatory factor 2 (BSF-2): Quantitation, specificity, distribution and regulation of their expression. *J. Exp. Med.* **166:** 967.

Takai, Y., G.G. Wong, S.C. Clark, S.J. Burakoff, and S.H. Herrmann. 1988. B cell stimulatory factor-2 is involved in the differentiation of cytotoxic T lymphocytes. *J. Immunol.* **140:** 508.

Teshigawara, K., H.-M. Wang, K. Kato, and K.A. Smith. 1987. Interleukin 2 high-affinity receptor expression requires two distinct binding proteins. *J. Exp. Med.* **165:** 223.

Tsudo, M., R.W. Kozak, C.K. Goldman, and T.A. Waldmann. 1986. Demonstration of a non-Tac peptide that binds interleukin 2: A potential participant in a multi-chain interleukin 2 receptor complex. *Proc. Natl. Acad. Sci.* **83:** 9694.

Ullrich, A., J.R. Bell, E.Y. Chen, R. Herrera, L.M. Petruzzelli, T.J. Dull, A. Gray, L. Coussens, Y.-C. Liao, M. Tsubokawa, A. Mason, P.H. Seeburg, C. Grunfeld, O.M. Rosen, and J. Ramachandran. 1985. Human insulin receptor and its relationship to the tyrosine kinase family of oncogenes. *Nature* **313:** 756.

Ullrich, A., L. Coussens, J.S. Hayflick, T.J. Dull, A. Gray, A.W. Tam, J. Lee, Y. Yarden, T.A. Libermann, J. Schlessinger, J. Downward, E.L.V. Mayes, N. Whittle, M.D. Waterfield, and P.H. Seeburg. 1984. Human epidermal growth factor receptor cDNA sequence and aberrant expression of the amplified gene in A431 epidermoid carcinoma cells. *Nature* **309:** 418.

Van Damme, J., G. Opdenakker, R.J. Simpson, M.R. Rubira, S. Cayphas, A. Vink, A. Billiau, and J.V. Snick. 1987. Identification of the human 26-kD protein, interferon $\beta 2$ (IFN$\beta 2$), as a B cell hybridoma/plasmacytoma growth factor induced by interleukin 1 and tumor necrosis factor. *J. Exp. Med.* **165:** 914.

Van Snick, J., A. Vink, S. Cayphas, and C. Uyttenhove. 1987. Interleukin-HP1, a T cell-derived hybridoma growth factor that supports the in vitro growth of murine plasmacytomas. *J. Exp. Med.* **165:** 641.

Van Snick, J., S. Cayphas, J.-P. Szikora, J.-C. Renauld, E. Van Roost, T. Boon, and R.J. Simpson. 1988. cDNA cloning of murine interleukin-HP1: Homology with human interleukin 6. *Eur. J. Immunol.* **18:** 193.

Van Snick, J., S. Cayphas, A. Vink, C. Uyttenhove, P.G. Coulie, M.R. Rubira, and R.J. Simpson. 1986. Purification and NH$_2$-terminal amino acid sequence of a T-cell-derived lymphokine with growth factor activity for B-cell hybridomas. *Proc. Natl. Acad. Sci.* **83:** 9679.

Wigler, M., A. Pellicer, S. Silverstein, and R. Azel. 1978. Biochemical transfer of single-copy eucaryotic genes using total cellular DNA as donor. *Cell* **14:** 725.

Williams, A.F. and A.N. Barclay. 1988. The immunoglobulin superfamily-domains for cell structure recognition. *Annu. Rev. Immunol.* **6:** 381.

Yamasaki, K., T. Taga, Y. Hirata, H. Yawata, Y. Kawanishi, B. Seed, T. Taniguchi, T. Hirano, and T. Kishimoto. 1988. Cloning and expression of human interleukin-6 (BSF-2/IFN$\beta 2$) receptor. *Science* **241:** 825.

Yarden, Y., J.A. Escobedo, W.-J. Kuang, T.L. Yang-Feng, T.O. Daniel, P.M. Tremble, E.Y. Chen, M.E. Ando, R.N. Harkins, U. Francke, V.A. Fried, A. Ullrich, and L.T. Williams. 1986. Structure of the receptor for platelet-derived growth factor helps define a family of closely related growth factor receptors. *Nature* **323:** 226.

Zilberstein, A., R. Ruggieri, J.H. Korn, and M. Revel. 1986. Structure and expression of cDNA and genes for human interferon-β-2, a distinct species inducible by growth-stimulatory cytokines. *EMBO J.* **5:** 2529.

Regulation of the Polyphosphoinositide-specific Phosphodiesterase in B Lymphocytes

G.G.B. Klaus, M.M. Harnett, and K.P. Rigley*

National Institute for Medical Research, Mill Hill, London NW7 1AA, United Kingdom

The biological consequences of the binding of antigen to surface immunoglobulin (sIg) receptors on B lymphocytes has been the subject of considerable debate. In recent years, extensive studies with antibodies directed to sIg receptors (anti-Ig) have shown that cross-linking of these receptors not only induces the activation of virtually all murine B cells, but can induce a substantial fraction of murine B cells to synthesize DNA (for review, see Parker 1980; DeFranco et al. 1982). *Activation* of resting B cells, as judged by increases in cell size and in levels of class II MHC (Ia) antigens, occurs in response to low concentrations of anti-Ig. On the other hand, *commitment* of activated cells to DNA synthesis requires much higher concentrations of antibodies (typically 50–100 μg/ml affinity-purified polyclonal antibodies). It is still a matter of debate how these effects of anti-Ig relate to those occurring in vivo in response to physiological concentrations of relevant antigens. This is especially pertinent to soluble T-dependent protein antigens, which may be rather poor cross-linking agents. However, what has become increasingly evident is that studies with anti-Ig antibodies provide a polyclonal model for B-cell activation by type-2 T-independent (TI-2) antigens. These are typically large polymers, with repeating epitopes, which can cross-link sIg receptors very efficiently. The best evidence for this concept comes from the experiments of Brunswick et al. (1988), who showed that anti-Ig antibodies coupled to long-chain polymers, such as dextran, are mitogenic for B cells at concentrations several orders of magnitude lower than those required for the soluble antibodies.

A variety of studies have now also established that both sIgM and sIgD receptors are typical Ca^{++}-mobilizing receptors. Thus, cross-linking of either isotype with mitogenic antibodies causes the rapid and prolonged hydrolysis of plasma membrane phosphatidylinositol 4,5-bisphosphate (PtdInsP$_2$) by a polyphosphoinositide-specific phosphodiesterase (PPI-PDE), to yield inositol 1,4,5-trisphosphate (InsP$_3$) and 1,2-diacylglycerol (DAG): The former causes the mobilization of intracellular Ca^{++} from stores in the endoplasmic reticulum, whereas the latter induces the activation of the key regulatory enzyme protein kinase C (PKC) (for review, see Cambier et al. 1987; Klaus et

al. 1987). In agreement with results from many diverse cell types, in B lymphocytes, both arms of this branched signaling pathway are important for inducing optimal activation of resting cells. This conclusion is supported by the demonstration that B cells can be induced to proliferate when cultured with a Ca^{++} ionophore, plus a PKC-activating phorbol ester (such as phorbol myristic acetate [PMA] or phorbol dibutyrate [PDB]), but not by either agent alone (Clevers et al. 1985; Klaus et al. 1986).

Recently, it has become clear that many Ca^{++}-mobilizing receptors are coupled to their second-messenger-generating system (the PPI-PDE) by one or more forms of a guanine nucleotide regulatory protein, generically termed G$_p$ (for review, see Cockcroft 1987; Harnett and Klaus 1988c). As we will discuss, this is true of both sIgM and sIgD receptors on B cells. The involvement of G$_p$ in this signaling cascade therefore affords several points of control, which are summarized in Figure 1: (1) at the level of ligand/receptor interaction, since it is evident that optimal signal transduction and B-cell activation via this route only occur following extensive cross-linking of sIg receptors; (2) at the level of sIg interaction with G$_p$ (it is worth emphasizing that the cartoon in Figure 1 does not include accessory molecules that may couple sIg to G$_p$, but that undoubtedly exist [e.g., Hombach et al. 1988]); (3) at the level of G$_p$/PPI-PDE coupling; (4) by direct regulation of the PPI-PDE itself; or (5) by engaging other B-cell receptors, in particular, the Fcγ receptors, which bind aggregated antigen-IgG antibody complexes (Fig. 1b). We will present evidence for the existence of several of these regulatory processes in B cells stimulated with anti-Ig.

EXPERIMENTAL PROCEDURES

Most of the experiments described here have utilized a permeabilized cell system that allows the manipulation of the components of the signaling cascade outlined in Figure 1 (for details, see Harnett and Klaus 1988b). In brief, purified splenic B cells (typically 90–95% sIg$^+$) were labeled with [^{3}H]inositol and permeabilized with streptolysin-O: These cells were equilibrated in Ca^{++} buffers ranging from pCa 7.0 (100 nM) to pCa 3.0 (1 mM). They were then stimulated either with F(ab')$_2$ or intact (IgG) rabbit anti-mouse Fab antibodies, or with monoclonal anti-δ or anti-μ

---

*Present address: Institute of Child Health, 30 Guilford Street, London WC1, United Kingdom.

724 KLAUS, HARNETT, AND RIGLEY

Possible Regulatory Sites in sIg Receptor Signalling

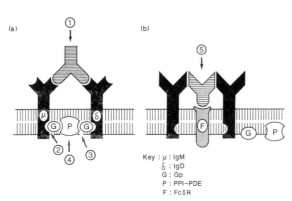

Key : μ : IgM
δ : IgD
G : Gp
P : PPI–PDE
F : FcδR

Figure 1. Possible mechanisms of control in the signaling cascade induced by engaging sIg receptors on B cells. (*a*) B-cell membrane containing sIgM and sIgD receptors. Cross-linking of these activates the guanine-regulatory protein G_p, which in turn activates the PPI-PDE. The cascade can be regulated at the level of ligand-receptor interaction (1), sIg/G_p interaction (2), G_p/PPI-PDE interaction (3), or at the level of the effector enzyme (4). (*b*) Co-ligation of sIg with Fcγ receptors (e.g., by appropriate anti-Ig antibodies or antigen-antibody complexes) can modulate signaling via the antigen receptors. This is further discussed in the text.

antibodies, in the presence or absence of the nonhydrolyzable GTP analog, GTPγS. Released [^{3}H]inositol phosphates were separated by ion-exchange chromatography. In some experiments, cytoplasmic Ca^{++} concentrations ([Ca^{++}]$_i$) were determined spectrofluorometrically in intact cells loaded with the Ca^{++} indicator indo-1 (Bijsterbosch et al. 1986).

Permeabilizing cells uncouple G-protein-linked receptors from their effector enzymes, as a result of the leaching out of endogenous GTP. In these preparations, the G protein can be directly activated by GTPγS: However, optimal activation of G_p, for example, requires the interaction of the G protein with its "excited" receptors (for review, see Cockcroft 1987). In consequence, stimulation with ligand plus GTPγS gives larger (so-called coupled) responses than those to the GTP analog alone. Coupling of receptors to G_p results in activation of the PPI-PDE at [Ca^{++}]$_i$ typically found following receptor stimulation ($\sim$ 1 μM). In addition, the PPI-PDE can be directly activated by supraphysiological concentrations of Ca^{++} ($\sim$ 1 mM) without engaging the receptors.

Evidence for G_p Coupled to sIg Receptor Signaling

In the current series of studies, we initially investigated the effects of GTPγS ± anti-Ig on inositol phosphate release in permeabilized B cells (Harnett and Klaus 1988b). These experiments showed that GTPγS alone induced dose-dependent release of inositol phosphates, thereby indicating that B cells, not surprisingly, contain one or more forms of G_p coupled to the PPI-PDE. A typical coupling experiment is shown in Figure 2. The results demonstrate that the PPI-PDE is virtual-

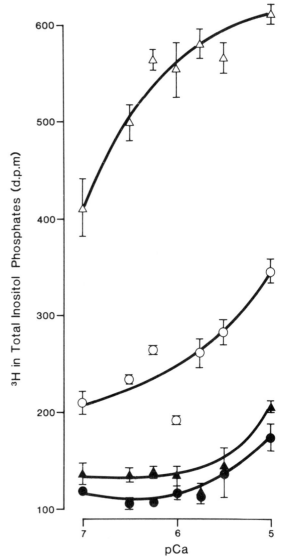

Figure 2. Involvement of G_p in sIg receptor-mediated inositol phospholipid hydrolysis. [^{3}H]Inositol-labeled, permeabilized B cells were equilibrated at the indicated Ca^{++} concentrations and were stimulated with Ca^{++} alone (●), 50 μg/ml F(ab')$_2$ rabbit anti-Ig (▲), 100 μM GTPγS (○), or GTPγS plus anti-Ig (△). Release of total inositol phosphates was determined after 10 min (see Harnett and Klaus 1988b).

ly inactive at resting Ca^{++} levels (pCa 7.0, or 100 nM). Stimulation with Ca^{++} alone induces a minimal response, as does stimulation with anti-Ig alone. GTPγS alone induces a certain level of [^{3}H]inositol phosphate release, which increases in a Ca^{++}-dependent manner. Most significantly, costimulation with anti-Ig plus GTPγS gives a markedly enhanced response, which reaches a plateau at Ca^{++} levels typically found following ligation of sIg in intact cells.

These results formally demonstrate the involvement of an (uncharacterized) form of G_p in sIg-mediated signaling; similar results have been reported in the sIgM$^+$ WEHI-231 B-cell lymphoma (Gold et al. 1987). The above experiments were done with polyclonal anti-

Fab antibodies: Comparable results were obtained with monoclonal anti-δ and anti-μ antibodies, thereby demonstrating that signaling via both sIgM and sIgD receptors is G_p-linked (Harnett and Klaus 1988b).

We wished to characterize the properties of the G protein. It is known that the responses of some G_p-linked receptors in other cell types are inhibited by pertussis toxin, whereas the responses of other Ca^{++}-mobilizing receptors are not affected. Pertussis toxin ADP-ribosylates the α subunits of some G proteins such as G_i, thereby uncoupling the G protein from its receptor (for review, see Milligan 1988). Both our results and those of Gold et al. (1987) indicated clearly that G_p associated with sIg is not a pertussis toxin substrate. Cholera toxin similarly ADP-ribosylates other G proteins, such as G_s: Our experiments showed that pretreatment of B cells with cholera toxin causes a modest ($\sim 30\%$) inhibition of signaling via sIg (Harnett and Klaus 1988b). We believe that this is due to feedback inhibition of $PtdInsP_2$ hydrolysis by cAMP (resulting from the activation of G_s), rather than a reflection of a direct effect of the toxin on the putative G_p.

In these studies, the effects of the toxins on responses elicited by anti-Fab antibodies, or those induced by isotype-specific reagents, were comparable. These results therefore suggested that sIgM and sIgD receptors might be coupled to the same G protein. This question is further addressed below.

Regulation of the PPI-PDE by PKC

PKC has been shown to regulate the polyphosphoinositide signaling pathway at multiple sites in different cell types and receptor systems. It has thus been demonstrated to affect either receptor/G_p (Pfeilschifter and Bauer 1987; Hepler et al. 1988), or G_p/PPI-PDE interaction (Kikuchi et al. 1987; Smith et al. 1987). In B cells, PKC activators such as PMA induce abortive activation (driving cells into the transitional, poised hyper-Ia state termed G_{1T}) on their own (Hawrylowicz et al. 1984; Monroe et al. 1984) and, together with Ca^{++} ionophores, induce a portion of the cells to synthesize DNA (Clevers et al. 1985; Klaus et al. 1986). Paradoxically, PMA and PDB profoundly inhibit anti-Ig-induced B-cell proliferation. This is reflected in their capacity to inhibit both Ca^{++} mobilization and $PtdInsP_2$ hydrolysis induced by these antibodies (Mizuguchi et al. 1986a; Bijsterbosch and Klaus 1987).

We used the permeabilized cell system to investigate the site at which PKC activation inhibits the sIg-induced activation cascade (Harnett and Klaus 1988a). We found that pretreatment of B cells for 10 minutes with PMA inhibits both the basal release of inositol phosphates and the responses to GTPγS on its own, or together with anti-Ig, to a comparable extent. This suggested that PKC activation does not affect sIg/G_p or G_p/PPI-PDE coupling, but rather might affect the activity of the PPI-PDE itself. This possibility was confirmed in the experiments shown in Figure 3. Here the

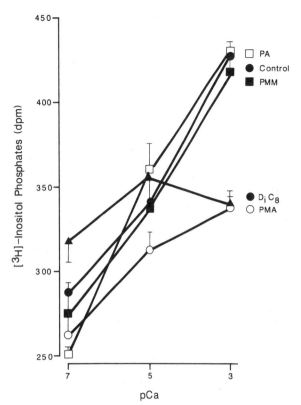

Figure 3. Effects of PKC activators on Ca^{++}-induced activation of the PPI-PDE in B cells. [^{3}H]Inositol-labeled B cells were incubated for 10 min at 37°C with phorbol myristic acetate (PMA), phorbol monoacetate (PA), phorbol monomyristate (PMM) (all at 160 nM), or 160 μM 1.2-dicapryloyl-rac-glycerol (DiC8). They were then permeabilized and stimulated for a further 10 min with the indicated Ca^{++} buffers when release of total inositol phosphates was determined (see Harnett and Klaus 1988a).

PPI-PDE was directly activated by high Ca^{++} concentrations: It can be seen that this response is also inhibited in PMA-pretreated cells. Furthermore, the involvement of PKC in these effects was strengthened by the findings that a synthetic DAG (DiC8) is also active, whereas two phorbol esters that do not stimulate PKC had no effect.

These results indicate that activation of PKC by phorbol esters or DAG leads to inhibition of the PPI-PDE, thereby providing a possible feedback loop to control signaling via sIg receptors. The mechanisms involved are unknown, but the effect may be due to phosphorylation of the PPI-PDE, since this enzyme has been shown to be a PKC substrate in other tissues (Bennett and Crooke 1987).

Regulation of G_p/PPI-PDE Interaction: Receptor Desensitization

A fundamental mystery in B-cell biology is why most resting cells express both sIgM and sIgD receptors. Various suggestions have been put forward to explain this phenomenon, the commonest postulating a possible role for IgD as a maturation marker, rendering developing B cells resistant to tolerization. However, there is no definitive evidence for this concept (for a recent discussion, see Ales-Martinez et al. 1988; Tisch et al. 1988). Certainly, studies with isotype-specific antibodies on normal B cells have indicated that both the biological and early biochemical consequences of engaging sIgM or sIgD are indistinguishable (e.g., Klaus et al. 1985; for review, see DeFranco et al. 1982).

We therefore attempted to find evidence for fine differences in the control of signaling via the two isotypes of sIg. Our earlier results had shown that the effects of pretreating B cells with cholera or pertussis toxins on signaling via the two receptors were identical (Harnett and Klaus 1988b). Similarly, pretreatment with PKC activators caused comparable inhibition of inositol phosphate release caused by either anti-δ or anti-μ (Harnett and Klaus 1988a). These results all pointed to the idea that IgM and IgD receptors share a common form of G_p. Our more recent studies have provided further evidence for this hypothesis (Harnett et al. 1989). First, costimulation of B cells with saturating doses of mitogenic monoclonal anti-μ plus anti-δ antibodies did not induce additive $[Ca^{++}]_i$ increases or inositol phosphate release. Rather, such treatment induced the same responses as the anti-δ alone (this being the more stimulatory of the two antibodies used). The lack of additive responses was not due to a limitation of $PtdInsP_2$ substrate, since stimulation with polyclonal

anti-Ig (which cross-links both classes of sIg indiscriminately) caused a greater response than either anti-isotype (data not shown).

We next analyzed the effects of stimulating B cells sequentially with anti-μ or anti-δ. These experiments revealed a complex and dynamic series of regulatory events, which are illustrated by representative experiments in Figures 4 and 5. First, stimulation via one class of receptor for 60 minutes induces activation of the PPI-PDE, so that the basal levels of inositol phosphate release (Fig. 4) and $[Ca^{++}]_i$ (Fig. 5) of these cells were significantly elevated. Second, the PPI-PDE in these cells was substantially refractory to further stimulation via the heterologous receptors. This was seen in intact cells and in permeabilized cells stimulated with GTPγS with or without the appropriate antibodies (Fig. 4). This refractory state was not due to maximal activation of the PPI-PDE as a result of the primary stimulus, because the activated enzyme could be further stimulated by high Ca^{++} concentrations (data not shown). Rather, it seems to reflect regulation of coupling between G_p and the PPI-PDE. Finally, in cells that had been preincubated with either anti-isotype reagent for 4–8 hours, these regulatory processes had waned. The basal level of PPI-PDE had returned to normal, and the enzyme could again be stimulated via the heterologous receptors. This is illustrated by the $[Ca^{++}]_i$ data in Figure 5, and precisely comparable results were ob-

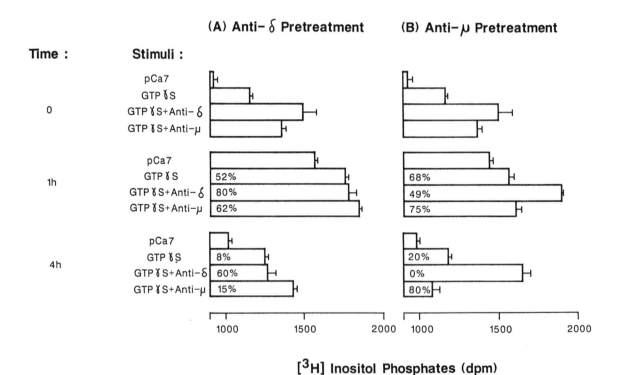

Figure 4. Effects of sequential stimulation of B cells with anti-μ or anti-δ antibodies. B cells were incubated for 1 hr or 4 hr at 37°C with 50 μg/ml of either a monoclonal anti-δ antibody (A) or anti-μ (B), during labeling with [^{3}H]inositol. After washing and permeabilization, the cells were incubated at pCa 7.0 with the indicated stimuli: GTPγS (100 μM), with or without the isotype-specific antibodies (at 50 μg/ml). Release of total inositol phosphates was determined after 10 min. Numbers in the bars represent percentage inhibition of stimulation indices; i.e., stimulated/basal release induced by pCa 7 buffer of the responses of pretreated cells, compared with untreated cells. (Reprinted, with permission, from Harnett et al. 1989.)

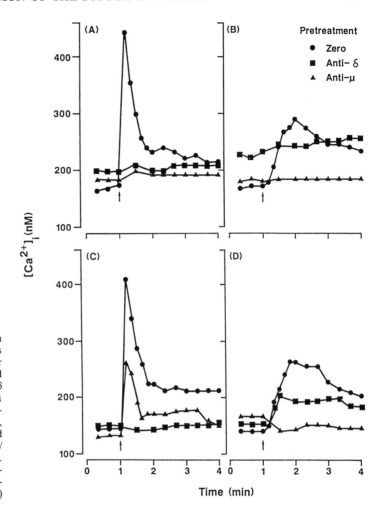

Figure 5. Effects of pretreatment of B cells with anti-μ or anti-δ on subsequent $[Ca^{++}]_i$ increases induced by restimulation of homologous or heterologous receptors. B cells were incubated at 37°C in the presence or absence (●) of anti-δ (■) or anti-μ (▲) (both at 50 μg/ml) for 1 hr (*A* and *B*) or 8 hr (*C* and *D*). During this preincubation period they were loaded with indo-1, washed, loaded into a spectrofluorimeter, and restimulated at the times indicated with 50 μg/ml of anti-δ (*A* and *C*) or anti-μ (*B* and *D*). Fluorescences were converted to $[Ca^{++}]_i$ as described by Bijsterbosch et al. (1986). (Reprinted, with permission, from Harnett et al. 1989.)

tained in inositol phosphate assays. It should be noted that after 4–8 hours of preincubation with anti-δ or anti-μ, the responses of the homologous receptors were still substantially suppressed. The significance of this finding is difficult to assess, because the primary antibody induces modulation and ultimate loss of the receptors from the cell membrane.

We interpret these results as follows. Ligation of one class of sIg induces activation of the PPI-PDE, which may then remain activated even though a substantial proportion of the receptors may have become capped and/or shed from the cell surface. This would therefore provide a feed-forward device to maintain receptor signaling for longer periods and thus provide a continuing stimulus for the progression of activated cells through the cell cycle. The fact that the cells become temporarily refractory to restimulation via the heterologous receptors is further strong evidence that both classes of sIg are controlled by a common form of G_p. This heterologous desensitization operates at the level of G_p/PPI-PDE interaction and could reflect the comodulation of this common G protein with the receptors during patching and capping. This would thereby effectively deprive the heterologous receptors of adequate levels of G_p. Cambier et al. (1988) have

recently described similar heterologous sIg receptor desensitization (measured by lack of Ca^{++} responses and PKC translocation) in B cells. However, in their study, the desensitization persisted for up to 24 hours. Although there are methodological differences between the two studies, we do not have a ready explanation for this apparent discrepancy.

The precise biochemical details involved in these regulatory events remain to be elucidated. However, it is conceivable that PKC activation may again be involved. The existence of a growing number of isozymes of PKC (see, e.g., Yashida et al. 1988) suggests the attractive possibility that different forms of the enzyme may control receptor signaling at different sites.

Modulation of sIg Signaling by Engaging Fc Receptors

All murine B cells carry Fcγ receptors (FcRII), which bind complexed IgG1, IgG2a, and IgG2b antibodies (for review, see Unkeless et al. 1988). There is considerable evidence that the function of these receptors is to modulate B-cell activation. This occurs physiologically via the binding of antigen/antibody complexes, or perhaps anti-idiotypic antibodies, to the

FcR and sIg (for review, see Sinclair and Panaskoltsis 1987). In other words, the FcR on B cells play a central role in feedback inhibition of antibody responses by IgG antibodies, and perhaps also in anti-idiotypic control mechanisms. Rabbit anti-Ig antibodies provide an attractive model for studying the function of the FcR in B-cell activation: Work by a number of groups has clearly demonstrated that intact (IgG) rabbit anti-Ig binds with high affinity to FcRII on mouse B cells. Furthermore, the resulting cross-linking of sIg to the FcR inhibits B-cell activation. Thus, although F(ab')$_2$ fragments of rabbit anti-Ig induce a substantial proportion of mouse B cells to synthesize DNA, the intact antibodies do not: In fact, mixing the intact antibodies with F(ab')$_2$ fragments inhibits their mitogenicity (Phillips and Parker 1983, 1984). More detailed studies showed that the intact antibodies do induce some B-cell activation, but the cells only progress to the hyper-Ia state and not further into cycle (Klaus et al. 1984). These results were puzzling and were only explained when the capacities of the two forms of anti-Ig to induce PtdInsP$_2$ hydrolysis were compared (Bijsterbosch and Klaus 1985; Wilson et al. 1987). These experiments showed that whereas F(ab')$_2$ anti-Ig induces long-lasting activation of the PPI-PDE (as discussed above), the intact antibodies only induced a short-lived release of inositol phosphates, the response being abrogated after about 1 minute. We found that the release of InsP$_3$ during this period was sufficient to induce a near-normal Ca^{++} signal (and presumably abortive activation of PKC), and we postulated that this is sufficient to explain the biological effects of the intact antibodies.

We have recently employed permeabilized B cells to investigate the lesion in the sIg signaling cascade following ligation of the FcR (Rigley et al. 1989a). We reasoned that if engaging the FcR affects the coupling between sIg and G$_p$, then intact anti-Ig should inhibit the coupled response to F(ab')$_2$ anti-Ig plus GTPγS. On the other hand, if it interferes with G$_p$/PPI-PDE coupling, then intact anti-Ig should also inhibit the basal stimulation of the PPI-PDE induced by GTPγS alone. The results of a representative experiment designed to test these possibilities are shown in Figure 6. Here, [^{3}H]inositol-labeled, permeabilized B cells were stimulated at Ca^{++} concentrations ranging from 100 nM to 1 μM with GTPγS, either alone or in the presence of varying combinations of the two forms of anti-Ig. The results show the usual, Ca^{++}-dependent basal stimulation of the PPI-PDE induced by GTPγS alone, and the enhanced response given by F(ab')$_2$ anti-Ig plus the GTP analog. Cells stimulated with intact anti-Ig plus GTPγS gave a small (but reproducible) response over that given by GTPγS alone. Most importantly, incubating B cells with a mixture of intact and F(ab')$_2$ antibodies suppressed the coupled response induced by F(ab')$_2$ anti-Ig down to the residual level given by the intact antibodies plus GTPγS.

These results clearly demonstrate that engaging the FcR uncouples sIg receptors from G$_p$ and does not

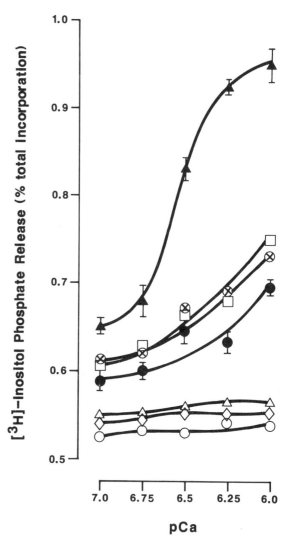

Figure 6. Uncoupling of sIg receptors from G$_p$ by co-cross-linking to the FcR. [^{3}H]Inositol-labeled, permeabilized B cells were equilibrated in the indicated Ca^{++} buffers and were incubated with Ca^{++} alone (○), 50 μg/ml F(ab')$_2$ anti-Ig (△), 150 μg/ml intact anti-Ig (◇), 10 μM GTPγS (●), or with GTPγS in combination with F(ab')$_2$ (▲), intact (⊗), or F(ab')$_2$ plus intact anti-Ig (□). Release of total [^{3}H]inositol phosphates was determined 10 min later. (Reprinted, with permission, from Rigley et al. 1989a.)

affect G$_p$/PPI-PDE coupling or the enzyme itself. Further experiments confirmed the potency of the inhibitory effect: A 0.25:1.0 molar ratio of intact:F(ab')$_2$ antibodies was sufficient to induce 50% of the maximal inhibition of the coupled response (Rigley et al. 1989). The inhibition never exceeded 80%: This presumably reflects the "leakiness" of the system, because it takes a finite period of time for the system to become fully uncoupled (Bijsterbosch and Klaus 1985). In addition, it is possible that individual B cells vary in their susceptibility to FcR-mediated inhibition, perhaps because of differences in the levels of FcR they express.

These results provide a biochemical basis for FcR-mediated inhibition of B-cell activation. Cross-linking of sIg to FcR results in the uncoupling of the antigen receptors from their associated G protein, and in consequence, terminates signaling via sIg. The mechanisms involved in uncoupling are unknown. Earlier studies by Abbas and Unanue (1975) had shown that sIg and FcR are somehow associated in the plane of the B-cell membrane: Since FcR belongs to the Ig-superfamily (Unkeless et al. 1988), this may be due to interactions between complementary domains on the two molecules. It is therefore possible that cross-linking sIg and FcR strengthens the association between the two receptors and that this causes physical dissociation of sIg from G_p.

DISCUSSION

The results of these studies yield further information about the signaling functions of antigen receptors on B cells. It is thus now clear that sIg receptors are classic Ca^{++}-mobilizing receptors and that the signaling cascade involves the participation of an uncharacterized, pertussis-toxin-insensitive guanine nucleotide regulatory protein that controls the activation of the PPI-PDE. As previously mentioned, there is little doubt that anti-Ig stimulation provides a polyclonal model for B-cell activation by TI-2 antigens. All the available evidence points to the concept that the level of PPI-PDE activity plays a pivotal role in determining how far B cells progress through cycle following this mode of activation. This is well-illustrated by the biological effects of intact rabbit anti-Ig, which causes short-lived activation of the PPI-PDE. This is reflected in the abortive activation of resting B cells to the hyper-Ia state termed G_{1T} (Klaus et al. 1984). Our recent studies on the phenotypically immature B cells from CBA/N (*xid*) mice that fail to respond to TI-2 antigens (for review, see Scher 1982) are also in line with this concept. The cells from these mice enlarge and show increased levels of Ia antigens when stimulated with normally mitogenic forms of anti-Ig, but fail to synthesize DNA. Our results indicate that this may be due to a quantitative (and/or qualitative) defect in the PPI-PDE in *xid* B cells (Rigley et al. 1989b). As a result, the level of signaling resulting from sIg cross-linking by anti-Ig (and perhaps by TI-2 antigens) is insufficient to drive the cells further into cycle.

As outlined in Figure 1, the sIg-mediated signaling cascade provides several potential levels of control. Several of these have now been defined, even though the precise biochemical mechanisms involved remain to be elucidated. We have provided evidence that both sIgM and sIgD receptors share a common pool of G_p, and that ligation of one class of sIg causes temporary desensitization of the heterologous receptors (and perhaps of the homologous ones as well). This therefore provides one mechanism for the B cell to control the level of signaling via sIg. Another is a consequence of activation of PKC by DAG produced as a result of $PtdInsP_2$ hydrolysis: This also inhibits signaling, as a result of effects (phosphorylation?) on the PPI-PDE itself. Still a third feedback mechanism is induced by

cross-linking of sIg with FcR, which leads to uncoupling of the antigen receptors from G_p (Fig. 6).

It remains to be seen how the effects induced by anti-Ig relate to the possible influences T-dependent antigens might have on B cells, although there is evidence that hapten-protein conjugates induce inositol phospholipid turnover in purified hapten-binding B cells (Grupp et al. 1987; Myers et al. 1987). Another key question is how the effects of the various lymphokines believed to act on B cells may interact with the signaling cascade resulting from sIg cross-linking. For example, a well-known property of interleukin-4 (IL-4) is its capacity to synergize with anti-Ig to induce resting B cells to synthesize DNA. The signaling pathways utilized by sIg and by IL-4 receptors must therefore interact in some fashion. Yet it is clear that IL-4 does not induce $PtdInsP_2$ hydrolysis or PKC activation (Justement et al. 1986; Mizuguchi et al. 1986b); neither does treatment of B cells with IL-4 detectably modulate the polyphosphoinositide pathway stimulated by anti-Ig (O'Garra et al. 1987).

Clearly, much remains to be learned about details of receptor signaling in B cells. Immediate questions arising from our own work concern the nature of G_p (which has remained notoriously elusive in other cell types) and the mechanism of coupling between sIg and the G protein. Recent evidence suggests that the transmembrane region of sIg is important for signaling (Webb et al. 1989), and this region of the molecule is structurally similar in sIg receptors of different isotypes. There have been various reports of proteins associated with sIg in the B-cell membrane (e.g., Hombach et al. 1988), although there is as yet no definitive evidence for anything approaching the complexity of the CD3 complex in T cells. Nevertheless, it is likely that there are other membrane proteins involved in the signaling cascade, whose precise nature and functions remain to be established.

ACKNOWLEDGMENTS

We are grateful for the invaluable contributions of Mary Holman to these studies. K.R. was supported by a fellowship from the Wellcome Trust.

REFERENCES

Abbas, A.K. and E.R. Unanue. 1975. Interrelationships of surface immunoglobulin and Fc receptors on mouse B lymphocytes. *J. Immunol.* **115:** 1665.

Ales-Martinez, J.E., G.L. Warner, and D.W. Scott. 1988. Immunoglobulins D and M mediate signals that are qualitatively different in B cells with an immature phenotype. *Proc. Natl. Acad. Sci.* **85:** 6919.

Bennett, C.F. and S.T. Crooke. 1987. Purification of a PPI-PLC from guinea pig uterus: Phosphorylation of protein kinase C in vivo. *J. Biol. Chem.* **262:** 13789.

Bijsterbosch, M.K. and G.G.B. Klaus. 1985. Crosslinking of surface Ig and Fc receptors on B lymphocytes inhibits stimulation of inositol phospholipid breakdown via the antigen receptors. *J. Exp. Med.* **162:** 1825.

———. 1987. Tumor-promoting phorbol esters suppress receptor-stimulated inositol phospholipid degradation and Ca^{2+} mobilization in mouse lymphocytes. *Eur. J. Immunol.* **17:** 113.

Bijsterbosch, M.K., K.P. Rigley, and G.G.B. Klaus. 1986. Crosslinking of surface Ig on B lymphocytes induces both intracellular Ca^{2+} release and Ca^{2+} influx: Analysis with indo-1. *Biochem. Biophys. Res. Commun.* **137:** 500.

Brunswick, M., F.D. Finkelman, P.F. Highet, J.K. Inmam, and H.M. Dintzis. 1988. Picogram quantities of anti-Ig antibodies coupled to dextran induce B cell proliferation. *J. Immunol.* **140:** 3364.

Cambier, J.C., Z.Z. Chen, J. Pasternak, J.T. Ransom, V. Sandoval, and H. Pickles. 1988. Ligand-induced desensitization of B cell membrane Ig mediated Ca^{2+} mobilization and protein kinase C translocation. *Proc. Natl. Acad. Sci.* **85:** 6493.

Cambier, J.C., L.B. Justement, M.K. Newell, Z.Z. Chen, L.K. Harris, V. Sandoval, M.J. Klemsz, and J.T. Ransom. 1987. Transmembrane signals and intracellular second messengers in the regulation of quiescent B lymphocyte activation. *Immunol. Rev.* **95:** 37.

Clevers, H.L., J.M.T. Versteegen, T. Logtenberg, F.H.J. Gmelig-Meyling, and R.E. Ballieux. 1985. Synergistic action of A23187 and phorbol ester on human B lymphocyte activation. *J. Immunol.* **135:** 3827.

Cockcroft, S. 1987. Polyphosphoinositide phosphodiesterase: Regulation by a novel guanine nucleotide binding protein, G_p. *Trends Biochem. Sci.* **12:** 75.

DeFranco, A.L., J.T. Kung, and W.E. Paul. 1982. Regulation of growth and proliferation in B cell subpopulations. *Immunol. Rev.* **64:** 161.

Gold, M.R., J.P. Jakway, and A.L. DeFranco. 1987. Involvement of a guanine nucleotide-binding component in membrane IgM-stimulated phosphoinositide breakdown. *J. Immunol.* **139:** 3604.

Grupp, S.H., E.C. Snow, and J.A.K. Harmony. 1987. The phosphatidylinositol response is an early event in physiologically relevant activation of antigen-specific B cells. *Cell. Immunol.* **109:** 181.

Harnett, M.M. and G.G.B. Klaus. 1988a. Protein kinase C activators inhibit the antigen receptor-coupled polyphosphoinositide-specific phosphodiesterase in murine B lymphocytes. *FEBS Lett.* **239:** 281.

———. 1988b. G-protein coupling of antigen receptor-stimulated polyphosphoinositide hydrolysis in B cells. *J. Immunol.* **140:** 3135.

———. 1988c. G-protein regulation of receptor signalling. *Immunol. Today* **9:** 315.

Harnett, M.M., M. Holman, and G.G.B. Klaus. 1989. Regulation of sIgM and IgD-mediated inositol phosphate formation and Ca^{++} mobilization in murine B lymphocytes. *Eur. J. Immunol.* (in press).

Hawrylowicz, C.M., K.D. Keeler, and G.G.B. Klaus. 1984. A comparison of the capacity of anti-Ig antibodies or PMA to activate B cells from CBA/N or normal mice into G1. *Eur. J. Immunol.* **14:** 244.

Hepler, J.R., S. Earp, and T.K. Harden. 1988. Long-term phorbol ester treatment down-regulates protein kinase C and sensitizes the phosphoinositide signalling pathway to hormone and growth factor stimulation. *J. Biol. Chem.* **263:** 7610.

Hombach, J., L. LeClercq, A. Radbruch, K. Rajewsky, and M. Reth. 1988. A novel 34 kD protein co-isolated with the IgM molecule in sIgM-expressing cells. *EMBO J.* **7:** 3451.

Justement, L., Z.Z. Chen, L. Harris, J.T. Ransom, V. Sandoval, C. Smith, D. Rennick, N. Roehm, and J.C. Cambier. 1986. BSF-1 induces membrane protein phosphorylation, but not phosphoinositide metabolism, Ca^{2+} mobilization or membrane depolarization in murine B lymphocytes. *J. Immunol.* **137:** 3664.

Kikuchi, A., K. Ikeda, O. Kozawa, and Y. Takai. 1987. Modes of inhibitory action of protein kinase C in the chemotactic peptide-induced formation of inositol phos-

phates in differentiated HL-60 cells. *J. Biol. Chem.* **262:** 6766.

Klaus, G.G.B., M.K. Bijsterbosch, and R.M.E. Parkhouse. 1985. Activation and proliferation signals in mouse B cells. V. A comparison of the effects of intact and $F(ab')_2$ anti-μ and anti-δ antibodies. *Immunology* **54:** 677.

Klaus, G.G.B., C.M. Hawrylowicz, M. Holman, and K.D. Keeler. 1984. Activation and proliferation signals in mouse B cells. III. Intact (IgG) anti-Ig antibodies activate B cells, but inhibit induction of DNA synthesis. *Immunology* **53:** 693.

Klaus, G.G.B., A. O'Garra, M.K. Bijsterbosch, and M. Holman. 1986. Induction of DNA synthesis in mouse B cells by a combination of Ca^{2+} ionophores and phorbol myristic acetate. *Eur. J. Immunol.* **16:** 92.

Klaus, G.G.B., M.K. Bijsterbosch, A. O'Garra, M.M. Harnett, and K.P. Rigley. 1987. Receptor signalling and crosstalk in B lymphocytes. *Immunol. Rev.* **99:** 19.

Milligan, G. 1988. Techniques used in the identification of pertussis toxin-sensitive G-proteins. *Biochem. J.* **255:** 1.

Mizuguchi, J., M.A. Beaven, J.H. Li, and W.E. Paul. 1986a. Phorbol myristic acetate inhibits anti-IgM mediated signalling in resting B cells. *Proc. Natl. Acad. Sci.* **83:** 4474.

Mizuguchi, J., M.A. Beaven, J. O'Hara, and W.E. Paul. 1986b. BSF-1 action on resting B cells does not require elevation of inositol phospholipid metabolism or increased intracellular Ca^{2+}. *J. Immunol.* **137:** 2215.

Monroe, J.T., J.E. Niedel, and J.C. Cambier. 1984. B cell activation. IV. Induction of cell membrane depolarization and hyper-Ia expression by phorbol esters suggest a role for protein kinase C in mouse B lymphocyte activation. *J. Immunol.* **132:** 1472.

Myers, C.D., M.K. Kriz, T.J. Sullivan, and E.S. Vitetta. 1987. Antigen-induced changes in phospholipid metabolism in antigen-binding B lymphocytes. *J. Immunol.* **138:** 1705.

O'Garra, A., K.P. Rigley, M. Holman, J. McLaughlin, and G.G.B. Klaus. 1987. B cell stimulatory factor-1 reverses Fc receptor mediated inhibition of B lymphocyte activation. *Proc. Natl. Acad. Sci.* **84:** 6254.

Parker, D.C. 1980. Induction and suppression of polyclonal antibody responses by anti-Ig reagents and antigennonspecific helper factor. *Immunol. Rev.* **52:** 115.

Pfeilschifter, J. and C. Bauer. 1987. Different effects of phorbol ester on angiotensin-II and stable GTP analogue-induced activation of the PPI-PDE in membranes isolated from rat renal mesangial cells. *Biochem. J.* **248:** 209.

Phillips, N.E. and D.C. Parker. 1983. Fc-dependent inhibition of mouse B cell activation by whole anti-mu antibodies. *J. Immunol.* **130:** 602.

———. 1984. Crosslinking of B lymphocyte Fc receptors and membrane Ig inhibits anti-Ig-induced blastogenesis. *J. Immunol.* **132:** 627.

Rigley, K.P., M.M. Harnett, and G.G.B. Klaus. 1989a. Co-crosslinking of surface Ig and Fcγ receptors on B lymphocytes uncouples the antigen receptors from their associated G-protein. *Eur. J. Immunol.* **19:** 481.

———. 1989b. Analysis of signalling via surface Ig receptors on B cells from CBA/N mice. *Eur. J. Immunol.* (in press).

Scher, I. 1982. The CBA/N mouse strain: An experimental model illustrating the influence of the X-chromosome on immunity. *Adv. Immunol.* **33:** 2.

Sinclair, N.R. StC. and A. Panaskoltsis. 1987. Immunoregulation by Fc signals. A mechanism for self-nonself discrimination. *Immunol. Today* **8:** 76.

Smith, C.D., R.J. Uhing, and R. Snyderman. 1987. Nucleotide regulatory protein-mediated activation of phospholipase C in human polymorphonuclear leukocytes is disrupted by phorbol esters. *J. Biol. Chem.* **262:** 6121.

Tisch, R., C.M. Roifman, and N. Hozumi. 1988. Functional differences between IgM and IgD expressed on the surface of an immature B cell line. *Proc. Natl. Acad. Sci.* **85:** 6914.

Unkeless, J.C., E. Scigliano, and V.H. Freedman. 1988.

Structure and function of human and murine receptors for IgG. *Annu. Rev. Immunol.* **6:** 251.

Webb, C.F., C. Nakai, and P.W. Tucker. 1989. Immunoglobulin receptor signalling depends on the C-terminus, but not on the H-chain class. *Proc. Natl. Acad. Sci.* **86:** 1977.

Wilson, H.A., D. Greenblatt, C.W. Taylor, J.W. Putney, R.Y.

Tsien, F.D. Finkelman, and T.M. Chused. 1987. The B lymphocyte Ca^{2+} response to anti-Ig is diminished by membrane Ig crosslinkage to the Fc receptor. *J. Immunol.* **138:** 1712.

Yashida, Y., F.L. Huang, H. Nakabayashi, and K.P. Huang. 1988. Tissue distribution and developmental expression of protein kinase C isozymes. *J. Biol. Chem.* **263:** 9868.

Signal Transduction by the Antigen Receptor of B Lymphocytes

A.L. DeFranco, D.M. Page, J.H. Blum, and M.R. Gold

Departments of Microbiology and Immunology and of Biochemistry and Biophysics, and the George Williams Hooper Foundation, University of California, San Francisco, California 94143-0552

The membrane forms of immunoglobulin (mIg) serve as receptors for antigen on B lymphocytes. Following antigen binding, mIg transduces signals, informing components inside the B cell that antigen has been bound. These signals play an important role in the inactivation of immature B cells, a process that contributes to tolerance to self, and in the activation of mature B cells to produce antibodies (Cambier and Ransom 1987; DeFranco 1987). In addition, mIg serves as an endocytotic receptor, promoting internalization of the bound antigen/mIg complex. The internalized antigen is degraded into peptides that form complexes with proteins encoded by class II genes of the major histocompatibility complex (MHC). These complexes go to the cell surface, where they can be recognized as activation signals by antigen-specific helper T cells (Schwartz 1985). The activated helper T cells secrete interleukins that promote B-cell activation and differentiation (Cammisuli et al. 1978; Augustin and Coutinho 1980; Ratcliffe and Julius 1982; DeFranco et al. 1984). Antigen-specific B cells require 1,000 to 10,000-fold less antigen to activate antigen-specific helper T cells than do nonspecific B cells (Rock et al. 1984; Lanzavecchia 1985; Tony et al. 1985). Thus, under limiting antigen conditions, helper T cells would preferentially interact with and activate antigen-specific B cells. In both signal transduction and endocytosis, mIg contributes to responses of only those B cells capable of binding antigen, and thus contributes to the specificity seen in antibody responses.

The importance of membrane forms of Ig as signal transducing receptors for antigens has been demonstrated by examining the effects of antigens or of anti-immunoglobulin antibodies (antireceptor antibodies, used as a surrogate for antigen) on B cells at different developmental stages. Treatment of immature B cells with antigen or anti-Ig results in functional inactivation of the cells, a process referred to as "clonal anergy" (Nossal 1983; Goodnow et al. 1988). Similarly, a subset of B-lymphoma cell lines stop growing in response to anti-Ig, a response that may be analogous to clonal anergy of immature B cells (Ralph 1979; Boyd and Schrader 1981; DeFranco et al. 1982a). In contrast, anti-IgM or anti-IgD induces resting, mature B cells to enter the G_1 phase of the cell cycle (DeFranco et al. 1982b,c). Anti-Ig antibodies also synergize with interleukin-4 to induce B-cell proliferation (Howard et al.

1982). The presence of additional growth and differentiation factors from helper T cells and/or macrophages can trigger further replication and antibody production (Zubler and Kanagawa 1982; Nakanishi et al. 1983). Thus, an antigen-dependent stimulation of B cells can be mimicked by anti-Ig and soluble factors from helper T cells. This view is an oversimplification, however, because different antigens (T-dependent vs. T-independent) may have different additional requirements to stimulate an antibody response. These differences could derive, in part, from differing abilities of various antigens to generate transmembrane signaling by mIg (DeFranco 1987).

mIg Triggers Phosphoinositide Breakdown

The mechanism by which the B-cell antigen receptor transduces the information of antigen binding to the inside of the cell is beginning to be understood. Cross-linking mIg on the surface of the B cell causes hydrolysis of phosphatidylinositol 4,5-bisphosphate ($PtdInsP_2$), yielding inositol 1,4,5-trisphosphate ($InsP_3$), which triggers the release of calcium from internal storage sites, and diacylglycerol (DAG), which activates the protein kinase C (PKC) family of enzymes. A number of studies pointed in this direction (Maino et al. 1975; Coggeshall and Cambier 1984; Monroe et al. 1984) before Bijsterbosch et al. (1985) directly demonstrated the production of $InsP_3$ following addition of anti-Ig to splenic B cells.

The immediate consequences of phosphoinositide breakdown are also well documented in B cells. Anti-Ig causes a rapid rise in intracellular free calcium (Pozzan et al. 1982). The initial calcium rise comes from internal stores of calcium (Pozzan et al. 1982; LaBaer et al. 1986; Ransom et al. 1986), as expected from the fact that most cells have intracellular stores of calcium that are released by $InsP_3$ (Berridge and Irvine 1984). This type of intracellular store is also present in B cells (LaBaer et al. 1986; Ransom et al. 1986). Thus, breakdown of $PtdInsP_2$ generates $InsP_3$, which causes calcium to be released into the cytoplasm. There is also an increase in plasma membrane permeability for calcium, so that extracellular calcium also contributes to the increase in cytoplasmic free calcium (MacDougall et al. 1988). The other second messenger produced upon hydrolysis of $PtdInsP_2$ is DAG, which activates PKC.

Anti-Ig treatment of B cells induces PKC translocation (Chen et al. 1986; Nel et al. 1986), an event thought to reflect activation of the enzyme. Furthermore, anti-Ig induces rapid phosphorylation of many of the same substrates as does phorbol myristic acetate (PMA), an exogenous activator of PKC (Hornbeck and Paul 1986). Thus, anti-Ig induces phosphoinositide breakdown, elevation of cytosolic calcium, and activation of PKC.

Similarly, trinitrophenyl (TNP)-specific B cells have been purified and found to undergo increased phosphatidylinositol labeling in response to TNP-Ficoll (a type-2 T-independent antigen) and in response to TNP-KLH (a soluble protein antigen) (Myers et al. 1987; Grupp et al. 1987). These observations are consistent with the idea that antigens, like anti-Ig, induce breakdown of $PtdInsP_2$ in B cells that can bind these reagents through their antigen receptors.

Since the phosphoinositide second messengers generated in response to anti-Ig or antigen are presumably important for informing the B cell that it has contacted antigen, it is important to know what other factors influence their generation. The B cell Fc receptor (FcRII) has been identified as one such regulator by Bijsterbosch and Klaus (1985). When an intact anti-Ig that binds to FcRII is used, phosphoinositide breakdown is decreased about fivefold compared to that obtained with a $F(ab')_2$ anti-Ig. In addition, anti-Ig-induced signaling is inhibited by about 90% upon activation of PKC with phorbol esters (Mizuguchi et al. 1986, 1987; Gold and DeFranco 1987). This inhibition may reflect a feedback inhibition in which DAG activates PKC, which then inhibits anti-Ig-induced phosphoinositide breakdown. According to this view, the inhibition depends on production of DAG, so the system would be self-limiting, resulting in an intermediate level of phosphoinositide breakdown. Alternatively, other agents (interleukins, etc.) may also influence antigen-induced phosphoinositide breakdown: negatively, by activating PKC and inhibiting phosphoinositide breakdown; or positively, by interfering with the feedback inhibition. It remains to be seen whether these potential sites for regulation are used.

Mechanism of mIgM Signal Transduction

Structural basis of mIgM signal transduction. Membrane IgM differs from secreted IgM in that it is a $\mu_2 L_2$ tetramer. Also, μ_m has an alternative carboxyl terminus consisting of 41 amino acids. These residues include a short, negatively charged linker next to C_H4, a 26-amino-acid putative transmembrane region, which is moderately hydrophobic and lacks charged side chains, and a very short cytoplasmic domain (-Lys-Val-Lys-COOH). Webb et al. (1989) have studied the role of this region in signaling. They transfected genes for a specific IgM idiotype into CH31, a B-lymphoma cell line whose growth is inhibited by anti-IgM. Growth of transfected cells could be inhibited by antibodies against either the endogenous or the transfected mIgMs

expressed on the cell surface. When they replaced the 41 carboxy-terminal amino acids of μ with the analogous region from a class II MHC molecule, growth of transfectants expressing the μ_m-Ia chimeric protein was not inhibited by antibodies against the transfected idiotype. This suggests that the carboxy-terminal 41 amino acids are required for signaling.

We have employed a similar strategy to examine the structural elements of μ involved in phosphoinositide signal transduction. A functionally rearranged μ gene was introduced by electroporation into 2PK3, a transformed B-cell line that expresses mIgG (Lanier et al. 1981). Thus, unlike the system used by Webb et al. (1989), the introduced μ can only form mIgM molecules in which both μ chains are encoded by the transfected gene. As shown in Figure 1, addition of anti-IgM to a mIgM-expressing transfectant of 2PK3 resulted in a clear-cut elevation in the concentration of free cytosolic calcium. Thus, introduced μ is functional for signal transduction in 2PK3 transfectants.

A series of point mutations in the final 40 codons of μ has been created by site-directed mutagenesis. Several of the hydroxyl amino acid residues in the μ transmembrane region were changed to hydrophobic amino acid residues without abolishing the ability to trigger phosphoinositide signaling. A change in the carboxyl terminus from Lys-Val-Lys-COOH to Lys-Arg-COOH also did not abolish signal transduction. This result suggests that the cytoplasmic domain of μ may not be crucial for signal transduction. Additional mutations will be needed to test this issue further. In addition, we

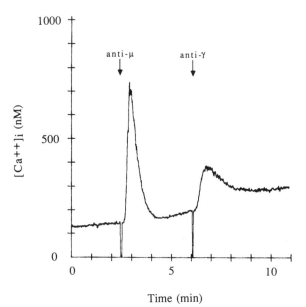

Figure 1. Transfectants of 2PK3 expressing mIgM signal in response to anti-IgM. 2PK3 cells transfected with the μ gene were loaded with the calcium-sensitive dye indo-1, and the fluorescence was monitored at 37°C and converted to intracellular Ca^{++} concentration as described previously (Page and DeFranco 1988). Goat anti-mouse μ and goat anti-mouse γ antibodies were added to final concentrations of 10 μg/ml each.

have introduced insertions of a single amino acid into several positions in the transmembrane region of μ. The possible effect of such mutations on signal transduction capability is not yet clear because these mutated IgMs appear to have much poorer transit to the cell surface (J.H. Blum and A.L. DeFranco, unpubl.). The reason for this defect is currently unknown. In summary, we have not yet localized the structures of μ that are required for signal transduction. This is a promising area, however, since it may help us determine which additional polypeptide(s) interacts with mIgM to mediate signal transduction.

Membrane IgM induces phosphoinositide breakdown via a GTP-dependent signaling component. To characterize the mechanism by which mIg induces $PtdInsP_2$ hydrolysis, we developed an in vitro assay for signaling reactions (Gold et al. 1987). WEHI-231 B-lymphoma cells were incubated with low concentrations of the mild detergent saponin, which were sufficient to permeabilize all of the cells to trypan blue dye. Cellular morphology and receptor activation of adenylyl cyclase were both retained following saponin treatment, demonstrating that membrane structure and function were in part retained.

Phosphoinositide breakdown in these permeabilized cells was assessed by pre-labeling cellular phospholipids with [³H]inositol and following the generation of radiolabeled inositol phosphates (InsPs). InsPs were generated if the permeabilized cells were incubated in the presence of free calcium concentrations of 100 μM or more. Presumably, high levels of calcium ions directly activated the phosphatidylinositol-specific phospholipase C. At more physiological levels of free calcium (100–500 nM), anti-Ig induced $PtdInsP_2$ breakdown in these permeabilized cells. Next, we examined whether there was a requirement for guanine nucleotides as seen in other signaling reactions, such as the hormonal activation of adenylyl cyclase and the rhodopsin-mediated activation of a cGMP phosphodiesterase in the retina (Gilman 1987). Therefore, permeabilized WEHI-231 B cells were incubated in the presence of anti-Ig and various guanine nucleotides (Fig. 2). Anti-Ig induced an increase in InsPs in the absence of added guanine nucleotides. This probably reflects the presence of endogenous GTP (see below). Addition of a nonhydrolyzable derivative of GTP, GTPγS, to the permeabilized cells also caused the production of some InsPs. The combination of anti-Ig and GTPγS was clearly synergistic, however, inducing the release of more InsPs than either alone (Fig. 2A). Other nucleotides and nucleotide analogs were tried in combination with anti-Ig. Only the nonhydrolyzable GTP analogs, GTPγS and GppNHp, synergized with anti-IgM for generation of InsPs. ATPγS was ineffective in this regard, as were GTP, GDP, and GDPβS, an analog of GDP that cannot be phosphorylated to the GTP derivative (Fig. 2B). These results suggested that a GTP-binding component was capable of enhancing $PtdInsP_2$ breakdown in response to anti-Ig.

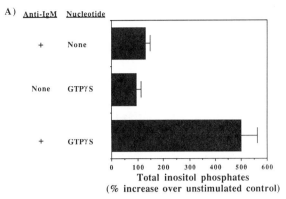

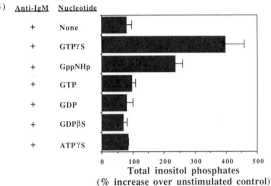

Figure 2. Nonhydrolyzable GTP analogs potentiate signaling by anti-IgM. (*A*) Permeabilized WEHI-231 cells were incubated for 10 min with 10 μg/ml anti-IgM and/or 100 μM GTPγS as indicated. Production of total inositol phosphates was determined and expressed as the percent increase over the unstimulated control (no anti-IgM or GTPγS). The data represent the mean ±S.E.M. for 20 separate experiments. (*B*) Permeabilized WEHI-231 cells were incubated with 10 μg/ml anti-IgM plus 100 μM of the indicated nucleotide. The data are expressed as in *A* and represent the mean ±S.E.M. for 4 independent experiments. Graphs are based on data presented in Gold et al. (1987).

The effects of guanine nucleotides on anti-Ig-induced $PtdInsP_2$ breakdown are similar to what has been reported for hormonal activation of adenylyl cyclase. In this system, a hormone receptor, such as the β-adrenergic receptor, activates a GTP-binding protein (G protein), and the G protein then activates adenylyl cyclase (Gilman 1987). A similar mechanism is used in many signal transduction reactions, with different members of the G-protein family activating different second-messenger-generating enzymes and ion channels. Interaction of an occupied receptor with a G protein causes the G protein to release GDP, allowing it to bind GTP. The G protein then dissociates from the receptor and activates the effector (adenylyl cyclase, etc.). Several seconds later, the G protein hydrolyzes the bound GTP and returns to the inactive GDP form. The G protein with GDP bound is once again available to interact with a receptor and start the cycle again (Gilman 1987).

If a G protein were involved in signaling by mIgM, then various guanine nucleotides should affect this reaction in a predictable way. For example, anti-IgM stimulation of PtdInsP$_2$ breakdown should require the presence of GTP. In addition, it should be enhanced further by addition of a nonhydrolyzable analog of GTP, which would cause the G protein to stimulate phospholipase C continuously, rather than having to recycle. Finally, such events should be inhibited by the presence of GDP, because GDP can compete for the binding of GTP to the G protein that has released its guanine nucleotide.

The second of these conditions, enhancement by nonhydrolyzable analogs of GTP, was observed for anti-Ig-induced phosphoinositide breakdown (Fig. 2). Addition of GTP, however, did not enhance phosphoinositide breakdown. Generation of InsPs was observed in the absence of added guanine nucleotide, and addition of GTP did not increase this response to anti-IgM. One possible explanation for the lack of a GTP effect is that endogenous GTP had not been fully removed from the permeabilized cells and was available to fuel the putative G protein. To test this possibility, GDPβS, a form of GDP that cannot be converted to GTP, was added to the reaction as a competitive inhibitor of binding of the postulated endogenous GTP to the nucleotide binding site on the G protein. GDPβS was able to inhibit anti-Ig-induced production of InsPs in permeabilized WEHI-231 B-lymphoma cells (Table 1). This inhibition was reversed by addition of GTPγS, confirming the competitive nature of the inhibition (data not shown). Thus, inositol phosphate generation seen in the absence of added guanine nucleotide probably depends on endogenous GTP. The protein that utilizes this GTP presumably acts as an intermediary between mIgM and phospholipase C.

Phosphoinositide breakdown in WEHI-231 cells was also found to be activated by AlF$_4^-$ (DeFranco and Gold 1989). This is striking because AlF$_4^-$ binds to several well-studied G proteins and presumably activates them by binding to the GDP-bound G protein in the position that would be occupied by the γ phosphoryl group of GTP (Gilman 1987). Thus, the GTP-binding component involved in signal transduction by mIgM in B cells is likely to be a member of the G-protein family.

As an initial approach to characterizing the nature of the GTP-binding component mediating mIgM signaling, we have examined the effects of two bacterial

Table 1. GDPβS Inhibits Signaling by Anti-IgM

GDPβS (mM)	Total inositol phosphates (cpm)	
	− anti-IgM	+ 10 μg/ml anti-IgM
0	127 ± 38	431 ± 20
0.5	166 ± 2	343 ± 47
1	92 ± 28	289 ± 30
2	121 ± 21	213 ± 58

Permeabilized WEHI-231 cells were incubated for 10 min with or without 10 μg/ml anti-IgM in the presence of the indicated concentrations of GDPβS. In the absence of GDPβS, the production of inositol phosphates in response to 10 μg/ml anti-IgM plus 100 μM GTPγS was 797 ± 15 cpm. A time zero value of 722 cpm was subtracted from all data points. Each data point is the average and range of duplicate points. Table is based on data reported in Gold et al. (1987).

toxins, cholera and pertussis toxins. These toxins modify some G proteins by ADP-ribosylation, resulting in either constitutive activation or inactivation. Anti-IgM-induced phosphoinositide breakdown was not stimulated or inhibited by either cholera toxin or pertussis toxin (Gold et al. 1987). Thus, the GTP-binding protein involved in mIgM signal transduction is not a target for either of these toxins. In contrast, in fibroblasts, platelets, and neutrophils, PtdInsP$_2$ hydrolysis is blocked by pertussis toxin (Brandt et al. 1985; Smith et al. 1985; Paris and Pouyssegur 1986), and in T cells, PtdInsP$_2$ hydrolysis is blocked by cholera toxin (Imboden et al. 1986). Receptor-mediated phosphoinositide breakdown that is insensitive to pertussis toxin and cholera toxin has also been reported in a number of cell types, including liver cells and pituitary cells (Martin et al. 1986; Uhing et al. 1986). In the latter cases, experiments with permeabilized cell or membrane systems indicates the involvement of a GTP-binding signal transducer, as seen in B lymphocytes. Therefore, receptor-mediated PtdInsP$_2$ breakdown appears to be mediated by several G proteins, which can be distinguished on the basis of different susceptibilities to the actions of cholera toxin and pertussis toxin. The G protein mediating mIgM signaling in B cells is of the toxin-insensitive type.

Phorbol esters interfere with G protein–phospholipase C coupling. Although anti-IgM induces phosphoinositide breakdown when added to intact or permeabilized WEHI-231 cells, it fails to do so when added to isolated WEHI-231 membranes. When GTPγS was added to these membranes, however, phosphoinositide breakdown did occur in the absence of anti-IgM. Thus, some change occurred in the membranes during their isolation, and this change made the GTP-binding component bind GTPγS more readily in the absence of an overt receptor stimulus.

The ability of GTPγS to stimulate PtdInsP$_2$ hydrolysis in WEHI-231 membranes isolated in this way provided a means of assessing the functional status of the GTP-binding component that mediates this reaction. As described above, phorbol ester treatment of WEHI-231 cells greatly inhibits anti-IgM-stimulated PtdInsP$_2$ breakdown in intact cells (Gold and DeFranco 1987). Membranes isolated from phorbol-ester-treated cells had a much smaller accumulation of InsPs following stimulation with GTPγS, compared to membranes isolated from untreated cells. The response to AlF$_4^-$ was also inhibited by phorbol ester pretreatment (M.R. Gold and A.L. DeFranco, unpubl.). Thus, the phorbol ester treatment appears to affect either the G protein or the phospholipase C.

Relationship of Phosphoinositide Second Messengers to Growth Regulation Via the Antigen Receptor

Mimicking phosphoinositide second messengers with phorbol esters and calcium ionophores. Anti-IgM triggers PtdInsP$_2$ breakdown in mature, splenic B cells and in the immature B-cell line, WEHI-231. Despite generation of the same second messengers in B cells of different developmental stages, the cells respond to antigen receptor signaling quite differently. Anti-IgM causes mature B cells to enter the G_1 phase of the cell cycle and to proliferate in response to B-cell growth factors (DeFranco 1987). Anti-IgM causes immature B cells to undergo a clonal anergy or clonal deletion response (Nossal 1983). Similarly, WEHI-231 B-lymphoma cells arrest their growth in response to anti-IgM (Ralph 1979; Boyd and Schrader 1981; DeFranco et al. 1982a). Are these disparate biological responses mediated by phosphoinositide second messengers?

One approach to this question is to use pharmacologic agents to mimic the natural second messengers, DAG and calcium. The free concentration of calcium in the cytoplasm of cells can be increased by adding calcium ionophores such as ionomycin or A23187. A major second-messenger function of DAG appears to be the activation of PKC. Cell-permeant DAGs are now available, but they are rapidly metabolized, so continual addition of these components is required to continuously activate PKC. In contrast, the phorbol esters also activate PKC and are metabolized very slowly, such that a single addition of a phorbol ester provides persistent activation of PKC. Thus, two of the phosphoinositide second messengers can be artificially provided to see whether they can induce the relevant biological responses.

The role of phosphoinositide second messengers in mediating the growth-stimulatory response of mature resting B cells to anti-IgM has been analyzed by this mimicking approach. Incubation of mature B cells with calcium ionophore and phorbol ester induces increased expression of class II MHC proteins, entry into the G_1 phase of the cell cycle, and proliferation, either directly, or in combination with interleukin-4 (Clevers et al. 1985; Monroe and Kass 1985; Dugas et al. 1986; Klaus et al. 1986; Paul et al. 1986; Ransom and Cambier 1986; Rothstein et al. 1986; Roifman et al. 1987). Thus, mimicking the phosphoinositide second messengers reproduces many of the effects of anti-IgM. These findings suggest that calcium and DAG play important roles in mediating the response of mature B cells to anti-IgM.

Calcium-depletion experiments also point to the importance of calcium as a second messenger in B cells responding to anti-IgM (Dennis et al. 1987). Removal of extracellular calcium prevented the enhanced expression of class II MHC molecules induced by anti-IgM, but did not prevent enhanced expression induced by bacterial lipopolysaccharide (LPS), a B-cell mitogen that does not elevate intracellular calcium. Thus, calcium was required for the cells to respond to anti-IgM, but not for the cells to respond to LPS. These results suggest that calcium is required for anti-IgM-induced signal transduction events.

Inhibition of WEHI-231 growth by anti-Ig and mimicking reagents. We have taken a similar strategy to assess the roles of calcium and DAG in mediating the anti-IgM-induced growth arrest of WEHI-231 cells. First, the dose of anti-IgM needed to cause growth arrest was determined and compared to the dose response for causing calcium elevation. As little as 100 ng/ml of the Bet 1 monoclonal anti-IgM was sufficient to induce prompt growth arrest. Bet 1 (100 ng/ml) caused the cytoplasmic free calcium to rise slowly to a plateau value slightly less than twofold above the resting value. This rise was complete about 5 minutes after addition of the anti-IgM. In contrast, 5 μg/ml Bet 1 induced the fastest and highest elevation of cytoplasmic free calcium. Lower doses of Bet 1 induced progressively slower and smaller elevations of cytosolic calcium. Interestingly, all doses of anti-IgM that induced growth arrest also caused a similar plateau elevation of cytoplasmic free calcium by 5 minutes of treatment. Thus, the small sustained elevation of calcium correlated better with the biological response, whereas the more dramatic initial elevation of calcium seen in response to 1–5 μg/ml Bet 1 did not (Page and DeFranco 1988).

To elevate intracellular calcium appropriately with a calcium ionophore, it seemed important to mimic the sustained rise in calcium seen with all biologically active doses of anti-IgM. When different doses of ionomycin were added to WEHI-231 cells, 250 nM ionomycin was found to induce a calcium rise that was closest to that induced by 5 μg/ml Bet 1. As with anti-IgM, ionomycin caused cytosolic calcium to rise initially and then return to an intermediate value within a few minutes. Thus, the rise in calcium appears to stimulate the extrusion of calcium and hence a reduction in cytosolic calcium to a value nearer its resting level.

The effect on the growth of WEHI-231 cells of these doses of ionomycin, both by themselves and in combination with various doses of phorbol esters, was examined (Page and DeFranco 1988). Doses of ionomycin up to 250 nM had only modest growth-inhibitory effects on their own, but were effective at inducing growth arrest when combined with low concentrations of phorbol dibutyrate (Table 2). The combination of 175–250 nM ionomycin and 4–7 nM phorbol dibutyrate acted synergistically in inducing growth arrest. Higher levels of phorbol ester did not enhance this growth arrest. Although 100 nM phorbol dibutyrate was nearly as effective on its own as was the combination of ionomycin and lower amounts of phorbol dibutyrate, preliminary data suggest that the amount of activation of PKC by anti-IgM is similar to the amount achieved with quite low doses of phorbol dibutyrate (~4 nM). Thus, the effects of low doses of phorbol dibutyrate are more relevant to the action of anti-IgM-induced signaling.

Although considerable growth inhibition was seen in response to ionomycin and phorbol dibutyrate, in no case were these mimicking agents as efficacious at arresting growth as was anti-IgM. Kinetic analysis of growth arrest revealed that the mimicking reagents were slower at inducing growth arrest than was anti-IgM (Page and DeFranco 1988). Therefore, the combination of ionomycin and phorbol ester was only able to

Table 2. Effect of Phorbol Dibutyrate and Ionomycin on the Proliferation of WEHI-231 Cells

[Phorbol dibutyrate] (nM)	% Growth inhibition[a]			
	[Ionomycin] (nM)			
	0	175	250	500
0	0	24	29	63
2	−4	36	40	71
4	−4	49	66	80
7	10	70	77	83
10	22	68	72	79
20	47	70	72	75
100	72	77	79	n.d.[b]

[a]WEHI-231 cells at 10^5/ml were cultured for 27 hr with 5 μg/ml of the monoclonal anti-IgM Bet 1 or with the indicated concentrations of phorbol 12,13-dibutyrate and ionomycin. [^{3}H]Thymidine was added during the final 3 hr of culture, and incorporation was determined. The ^{3}H incorporation into cells treated with media alone was 112,000 ± 2,000 cpm (mean ± S.E.M.). Results are expressed as % growth inhibition, which is 100% × {1 − (cpm [experimental])/(cpm [media alone])}, and the S.E.M. for each data point was ≤11% of the mean. Cells treated with Bet 1 were 98% inhibited in their growth. Data are taken from Page and DeFranco (1988).

[b]n.d. indicates not determined.

reproduce partially the effect of anti-IgM on the growth of the WEHI-231 immature B-cell line. These results suggest that calcium and DAG are important for mediating the responses of immature B cells to antigen receptor signaling, but that they are not the only relevant second messengers. It is also possible that the pharmacologic agents fail to mimic precisely the anti-IgM-generated second messengers calcium and DAG.

Mutants of WEHI-231 resistant to anti-Ig. There are two main approaches for defining the roles of the phosphoinositide pathway second messengers in mediating the biological effects of antigen receptor signaling. Pharmacologic agents can be used to mimic phosphoinositide pathway second messengers, as described above. The other approach is to interfere with the generation or action of a second messenger and to examine the effect of the biological response. Unfortunately, specific inhibitors of the phosphoinositide pathway are not entirely satisfactory; many are toxic to lymphocytes at inhibitory concentrations. We have been developing a somatic cell genetic approach for removing individual components or limbs of the signaling pathway. Immature B-cell lines such as WEHI-231 are attractive for such an approach, because the growth inhibition provides a straightforward selection for the desired mutants.

Anti-IgM-resistant mutants of WEHI-231 can be readily isolated following mutagenesis and selection. In this way, we isolated over two dozen independent mutants of WEHI-231 that display some resistance to anti-IgM-induced growth arrest (K.A. Fahey and A.L. DeFranco, unpubl.). Many of these are completely or almost completely resistant to growth arrest.

One way in which cells could become resistant to anti-IgM would be to lose expression of mIgM. Two mutants are clearly deficient in this regard: mutant

303.1, which does not express detectable levels of mIgM, and mutant 88.1, which expresses approximately 6% of the normal level. Immunoprecipitation experiments revealed that 303.1 lacks detectable immunoglobulin heavy chains and 88.1 makes both chains but fails to transport them efficiently to the cell surface (L. Matsuuchi, University of California, San Francisco, unpubl.). Several other mutants express three to fivefold less mIgM than do wild-type WEHI-231 cells. Most of the mutants, however, express normal levels of mIgM. Such mutants may be useful for understanding the signaling events by which mIgM regulates cell growth.

We are currently determining which mutants are defective in generation of second messengers and which are defective in their responses to the second messengers. One particularly useful way of addressing this issue is to measure the responses of the mutants to the combination of phorbol ester and calcium ionophore that best mimics anti-Ig-induced second-messenger action in the wild-type cells. If a mutation disrupts signal generation, then one would expect that the response to the combination of phorbol ester and ionophore would be similar to that of the parental WEHI-231 cells. On the other hand, if a mutation interferes with a component involved in responding to either DAG or calcium, then the response to phorbol ester plus ionophore should be greatly reduced. Our preliminary data indicate that some mutants fall into each class. Further experiments will be required to give us greater insight into the nature of the defects in these mutants.

CONCLUSIONS

A great deal is now known about how the antigen receptor on B lymphocytes informs components inside the cell that antigen has been bound. Cross-linking of mIgM by either multivalent antigens or anti-IgM antibodies activates a GTP-binding component, which in turn activates phospholipase C. This enzyme specifically cleaves PtdInsP$_2$, releasing two second messengers, DAG and InsP$_3$. The former compound activates the PKC family of enzymes, whereas the latter compound induces the release of calcium from intracellular storage sites.

Little is known about how these second messengers mediate the divergent biological responses of immature and mature B cells to antigen. Experiments using phorbol esters to activate PKC and calcium ionophores to elevate cytosolic free calcium suggest that these two second messengers play important roles in mediating the early activation events of mature, splenic B cells responding to anti-IgM. Similarly, the combination of phorbol esters and calcium ionophores can partially reproduce the growth-inhibiting effects of anti-IgM on the immature B-lymphoma cell line, WEHI-231. In WEHI-231 cells, the growth arrest mediated by these mimicking reagents is clearly not as rapid as the growth arrest induced by anti-IgM. One possibility is that a third second messenger is involved in the response to anti-IgM. Also important for understanding signal transduction in B cells will be the approach of blocking the actions of individual second messengers, either pharmacologically or by genetic alteration of one of the components of the system. A somatic cell genetic approach is feasible, however, in the immature B-cell lines. Mutants have been isolated, some of which may have defects in the calcium or DAG second-messenger pathway. Further characterization of these mutants will be required to define the locus of the defect. The task of linking early signal transduction events occurring in the first few seconds after antigen binding to the biological responses occurring hours later remains a considerable challenge. Nonetheless, the rapid progress in the last few years in understanding signal transduction events in eukaryotic cells suggests that this goal can be achieved.

ACKNOWLEDGMENTS

This work was supported by grant AI-20038 from the National Institutes of Health. M.R.G. was a fellow of the Arthritis Foundation. D.M.P. was supported in part by a grant from the Lucille P. Markey Charitable Trust and in part by National Institutes of Health training grant 5T32 CA-09270. J.H.B. was supported in part by grants from the Medical Scientist Training Program, the Sussman Endowment Fund, and the Achievement Rewards for College Scientists Foundation.

REFERENCES

Augustin, A. and A. Coutinho. 1980. Specific T helper cells that activate B cells polyclonally. *J. Exp. Med.* **151:** 587.

Berridge, M.J. and R.F. Irvine. 1984. Inositol trisphosphate, a novel second messenger in cellular signal transduction. *Nature* **312:** 315.

Bijsterbosch, M.K. and G.G.B. Klaus. 1985. Crosslinking of surface immunoglobulin and Fc receptors on B lymphocytes inhibits stimulation of inositol phospholipid breakdown via the antigen receptor. *J. Exp. Med.* **162:** 1825.

Bijsterbosch, M.K., C.J. Meade, G.A. Turner, and G.G.B. Klaus. 1985. B lymphocyte receptors and polyphosphoinositide degradation. *Cell* **41:** 999.

Boyd, A.W. and J.S. Schrader. 1981. The regulation of growth and differentiation of a murine B cell lymphoma II. The inhibition of WEHI-231 by anti-immunoglobulin antibodies. *J. Immunol.* **126:** 2466.

Brandt, S.J., R.W. Dougherty, E.G. Lapetina, and J.E. Niedel. 1985. Pertussis toxin inhibits chemotactic peptide-stimulated generation of inositol phosphates and lysosomal enzyme secretion in human leukemic (HL-60) cells. *Proc. Natl. Acad. Sci.* **82:** 3277.

Cambier, J.C. and J.T. Ransom. 1987. Molecular mechanisms of transmembrane signaling in B lymphocytes. *Annu. Rev. Immunol.* **5:** 175.

Cammisuli, S., C. Henry, and L. Wofsy. 1978. Role of membrane receptors in the induction of *in vitro* secondary anti-hapten responses. I. Differentiation of B memory cells to plasma cells is independent of antigen-immunoglobulin receptor interaction. *Eur. J. Immunol.* **8:** 656.

Chen, Z.Z., K.M. Coggeshall, and J.C. Cambier. 1986. Translocation of protein kinase C during membrane immunoglobulin-mediated transmembrane signaling in B lymphocytes. *J. Immunol.* **136:** 2300.

Clevers, H.C., J.M.T. Versteegen, T. Logtenberg, F.H.J.

Gmelig-Meyling, and R.E. Ballieux. 1985. Synergistic action of A23187 and phorbol ester on human B cell activation. *J. Immunol.* **135:** 3827.

Coggeshall, K.M. and J.C. Cambier. 1984. B cell activation. VIII. Membrane immunoglobulins transduce signals via activation of phosphatidylinositol hydrolysis. *J. Immunol.* **133:** 3382.

DeFranco, A.L. 1987. Molecular aspects of B-lymphocyte activation. *Annu. Rev. Cell Biol.* **3:** 143.

DeFranco, A. and M. Gold. 1989. Signal transduction via the B cell antigen receptor: Involvement of a G protein and regulation of signaling. In *Mechanisms of lymphocyte activation and immune regulation* (ed. S. Gupta), vol. 2. Plenum Press, New York. (In press).

DeFranco, A.L., M.M. Davis, and W.E. Paul. 1982a. WEHI-231 as a tumor model for tolerance induction in immature B lymphocytes. In *B and T cell tumors: Biological and clinical aspects* (ed. E.S. Vitetta), p. 445. Academic Press, New York.

DeFranco, A.L., J.T. Kung, and W.E. Paul. 1982b. Regulation of growth and proliferation in B cell subpopulations. *Immunol. Rev.* **64:** 161.

DeFranco, A.L., J.D. Ashwell, R.H. Schwartz, and W.E. Paul. 1984. Polyclonal stimulation of resting B lymphocytes by antigen-activated T lymphocytes. *J. Exp. Med.* **159:** 861.

DeFranco, A.L., E.S. Raveche, R. Asofsky, and W.E. Paul. 1982c. Frequency of B lymphocytes responsive to anti-immunoglobulin. *J. Exp. Med.* **155:** 1523.

Dennis, G., J. Mizuguchi, V. McMillan, F. Finkelman, J. Ohara, and J. Mond. 1987. Comparison of the calcium requirement for the induction and maintenance of B cell class II molecule expression and for B cell proliferation stimulated by mitogens and purified growth factors. *J. Immunol.* **138:** 4307.

Dugas, B., A. Vazquez, B. Klein, J.-F. Delfraissy, M. Rammou, J.-P. Gerard, and P. Galanaud. 1986. Early events in human B cell activation: Metabolic pathways vary according to the first signal used. *Eur. J. Immunol.* **16:** 1609.

Gilman, A.G. 1987. G proteins: Transducers of receptor-generated signals. *Annu. Rev. Biochem.* **56:** 615.

Gold, M.R. and A.L. DeFranco. 1987. Phorbol esters and dioctanoylglycerol block anti-IgM-stimulated phosphoinositide hydrolysis in the murine B cell lymphoma WEHI-231. *J. Immunol.* **138:** 868.

Gold, M.R., J.P. Jakway, and A.L. DeFranco. 1987. Involvement of a guanine nucleotide-binding component in membrane IgM-stimulated phosphoinositide breakdown. *J. Immunol.* **139:** 3604.

Goodnow, C., J. Crosbie, S. Adelstein, T. Lavoie, S. Smith-Gill, R. Brink, H. Pritchard-Briscoe, J. Wotherspoon, R. Loblay, K. Raphael, R. Trent, and A. Basten. 1988. Altered immunoglobulin expression and functional silencing of self-reactive B lymphocytes in transgenic mice. *Nature* **334:** 676.

Grupp, S.A., E.C. Snow, and J.A.K. Harmony. 1987. The phosphatidylinositol response is an early event in the physiologically relevant activation of antigen-specific B lymphocytes. *Cell Immunol.* **109:** 181.

Hornbeck, P. and W.E. Paul. 1986. Anti-immunoglobulin and phorbol esters induce phosphorylation of proteins associated with the plasma membrane and cytoskeleton in murine B lymphocytes. *J. Biol. Chem.* **261:** 14817.

Howard, M., J. Farrar, M. Hilfiker, B. Johnson, K. Takatsu, T. Hamaoka, and W.E. Paul. 1982. Identification of a T cell-derived B cell growth factor distinct from interleukin 2. *J. Exp. Med.* **155:** 914.

Imboden, J.B., D.M. Shoback, G. Pattison, and J.D. Stobo. 1986. Cholera toxin inhibits the T-cell antigen receptor-mediated increases in inositol trisphosphate and cytoplasmic free calcium. *Proc. Natl. Acad. Sci.* **83:** 5673.

Klaus, G.G.B., A. O'Garra, M.K. Bijsterbosch, and M. Holman. 1986. Activation and proliferation signals in mouse B cells. VIII. Induction of DNA synthesis in B cells by a combination of calcium ionophores and phorbol myristate acetate. *Eur. J. Immunol.* **16:** 92.

LaBaer, J., R.Y. Tsien, K.A. Fahey, and A.L. DeFranco. 1986. Stimulation of the antigen receptor of WEHI-231 B lymphoma cells results in a voltage-independent increase in cytoplasmic calcium. *J. Immunol.* **137:** 1836.

Lanier, L.L., N.L. Warner, J.A. Ledbetter, and L.A. Herzenberg. 1981. Quantitative immunofluorescent analysis of surface phenotypes of murine B cell lymphomas and plasmacytomas with monoclonal antibodies. *J. Immunol.* **127:** 1691.

Lanzavecchia, A. 1985. Antigen-specific interaction between T and B cells. *Nature* **314:** 537.

MacDougall, S., S. Grinstein, and E. Gelfand. 1988. Detection of ligand-activated conductive Ca^{2+} channels in human B lymphocytes. *Cell* **54:** 229.

Maino, V.C., M.J. Hayman, and M.J. Crumpton. 1975. Relationship between enhanced turnover of phosphatidylinositol and lymphocyte activation by mitogens. *Biochem. J.* **146:** 247.

Martin, T.F.J., D.O. Lucas, S.M. Bajjalieh, and J.A. Kowalchyk. 1986. Thyrotropin-releasing hormone activates a Ca^{2+}-dependent polyphosphoinositide phosphodiesterase in permeable GH_3 cells. *J. Biol. Chem.* **261:** 2918.

Mizuguchi, J., M.A. Beaven, J. Hu Li, and W.E. Paul. 1986. Phorbol myristate acetate inhibits anti-IgM-mediated signaling in resting B cells. *Proc. Natl. Acad. Sci.* **83:** 4474.

Mizuguchi, J., J. Yong-Yong, H. Nakabayaschi, K.-P. Huang, M.A. Beaven, T. Chused, and W.E. Paul. 1987. Protein kinase C activation blocks anti-IgM-mediated signaling in BAL17 B lymphoma cells. *J. Immunol.* **139:** 1054.

Monroe, J.G. and M.J. Kass. 1985. Molecular events in B cell activation I. Signals required to stimulate G_0 to G_1 transition of resting B lymphocytes. *J. Immunol.* **135:** 1674.

Monroe, J.G., J.E. Niedel, and J.C. Cambier. 1984. B cell activation. IV. Induction of cell membrane depolarization and hyper-I-A expression by phorbol diesters suggests a role for protein kinase C in murine B lymphocyte activation. *J. Immunol.* **132:** 1472.

Myers, C., M. Kriz, T. Sullivan, and E. Vitetta. 1987. Antigen-induced changes in phospholipid metabolism in antigen-binding B lymphocytes. *J. Immunol.* **138:** 1705.

Nakanishi, K., M. Howard, A. Muraguchi, J. Farrar, K. Takatsu, T. Hamaoka, and W.E. Paul. 1983. Soluble factors involved in B cell differentiation: Identification of two distinct T cell-replacing factors (TRF). *J. Immunol.* **130:** 2219.

Nel, A.E., M.W. Wooten, G.E. Landreth, P.J. Goldschmidt-Clermont, H.C. Stevenson, P.J. Miller, and R.M. Galbraith. 1986. Translocation of phospholipid/Ca^{2+}-dependent protein kinase in B-lymphocytes activated by phorbol ester or cross-linkage of membrane immunoglobulin. *Biochem. J.* **233:** 145.

Nossal, G.J.V. 1983. Cellular mechanisms of immunologic tolerance. *Annu. Rev. Immunol.* **1:** 33.

Page, D. and A. DeFranco. 1988. Role of phosphoinositide-derived second messengers in mediating anti-IgM-induced growth arrest of WEHI-231 B lymphoma cells. *J. Immunol.* **140:** 3717.

Paris, S. and J. Pouyssegur. 1986. Pertussis toxin inhibits thrombin-induced activation of phosphoinositide hydrolysis and Na^+/H^+ exchange in hamster fibroblasts. *EMBO J.* **5:** 55.

Paul, W.E., J. Mizuguchi, M. Brown, K. Nakanishi, P. Hornbeck, E. Rabin, and J. Ohara. 1986. Regulation of B-lymphocyte activation, proliferation, and immunoglobulin secretion. *Cell. Immunol.* **99:** 7.

Pozzan, T., P. Arslan, R.Y. Tsien, and T.J. Rink. 1982. Anti-immunoglobulin, cytoplasmic free calcium, and capping in B lymphocytes. *J. Cell Biol.* **94:** 335.

Ralph, P. 1979. Functional subsets of murine and human B lymphocyte cell lines. *Immunol. Rev.* **48:** 107.

Ransom, J.T. and J.C. Cambier. 1986. B cell activation. VII. Independent and synergistic effects of mobilized calcium and diacylglycerol on membrane potential and I-A expression. *J. Immunol.* **136:** 66.

Ransom, J.T., L.K. Harris, and J.C. Cambier. 1986. Anti-Ig induces release of inositol 1,4,5-trisphosphate, which mediates mobilization of intracellular Ca^{++} stores in B lymphocytes. *J. Immunol.* **137:** 708.

Ratcliffe, M. and M. Julius. 1982. H-2-restricted T-B interactions involved in polyspecific B cell responses mediated by soluble antigen. *Eur. J. Immunol.* **12:** 634.

Rock, K.L., B. Benacerraf, and A.K. Abbas. 1984. Antigen presentation by hapten-specific B lymphocytes. I. Role of surface immunoglobulin receptors. *J. Exp. Med.* **160:** 1102.

Roifman, C., S. Benedict, R. Cheung, and E. Gelfand. 1987. Induction of human B cell proliferation and differentiation by the combination of phorbol ester and ionomycin. *Eur. J. Immunol.* **17:** 701.

Rothstein, T.L., T.R. Baeker, R.A. Miller, and D.L. Kolber. 1986. Stimulation of murine B cells by the combination of calcium ionophore plus phorbol ester. *Cell. Immunol.* **102:** 364.

Schwartz, R. 1985. T-lymphocyte recognition of antigen in association with gene products of the major histocompatibility complex. *Annu. Rev. Immunol.* **3:** 237.

Smith, C.D., B.C. Lane, I. Kusaka, M.W. Verghese, and R. Snyderman. 1985. Chemoattractant receptor-induced hydrolysis of phosphatidylinositol 4,5-bisphosphate in human polymorphonuclear leukocyte membranes. *J. Biol. Chem.* **260:** 5875.

Tony, H.-P., N.E. Phillips, and D.C. Parker. 1985. Role of membrane immunoglobulin (Ig) crosslinking in membrane Ig-mediated, major histocompatibility-restricted T cell-B cell cooperation. *J. Exp. Med.* **162:** 1695.

Uhing, R.J., V. Prpic, H. Jiang, and J.H. Exton. 1986. Hormone-stimulated polyphosphoinositide breakdown in rat liver plasma membranes. Roles of guanine nucleotides and calcium. *J. Biol. Chem.* **261:** 2140.

Webb, C.F., C. Nakai, and P.W. Tucker. 1989. Immunoglobulin receptor signaling depends on the carboxyl terminus but not the heavy-chain class. *Proc. Natl. Acad. Sci.* **86:** 1977.

Zubler, R. and O. Kanagawa. 1982. Requirement for three signals in B cell responses. II. Analysis of antigen- and Ia-restricted T helper cell-B cell interaction. *J. Exp. Med.* **156:** 415.

Three B-cell-surface Molecules Associating with Membrane Immunoglobulin

R.M.E. Parkhouse

National Institute for Medical Research, Mill Hill, London NW7 3EL, United Kingdom

The genes coding for antigen receptors on both B and T lymphocytes have now been defined and cloned. Unlike the T cell, where other accessory molecules, such as CD2 (Brown et al. 1989), CD3 (for review, see Moller 1987), CD4, and CD8 (Anderson et al. 1988), have been identified as parts of a functional receptor complex, unequivocal demonstration of similar molecules associating with B-cell-receptor immunoglobulin (Ig) has been slow to accumulate. This is all the more surprising since most B cells simultaneously bear at least two classes of membrane Ig (mIg), IgM and IgD (Abney et al. 1978), with shared $V_H V_L$ domains. Surface, and surface-associated, molecules forming complexes with mIg could play a role in signal transduction (as is thought to occur in the case of the T-cell receptor), antigen processing/presentation, or, as has been postulated (Hombach et al. 1988), in ensuring membrane expression. The present investigation has used biochemical and mIg-comodulation strategies to identify three cell-surface molecules that appear to associate with B-cell mIg.

MATERIALS AND METHODS

Cell suspensions. Spleen cell suspensions were prepared from the Institute's colony of specific pathogen-free CBA × BALB/c female mice, 3–6 months old. The suspension was depleted of T cells by treatment with rat monoclonal antibody (MAb) anti-mouse Thy-1 (NIM-R1) (Chayen and Parkhouse 1982a) and of red cells by ammonium chloride treatment. The small, dense-resting B cells were then recovered from the 85–75% interphase of Percoll gradients (O'Garra et al. 1986).

Surface labeling and coprecipitations. Small, dense resting B cells were labeled with iodine by the lactoperoxidase method and lysed in (1) 1% w/v Nonidet P-40 (NP-40) containing 50 mM iodoacetamide and inhibitors of proteolysis (1 mM phenylmethylsulfonyl fluoride; 1-chloro-4-phenyl-3-L-toluene-P-sulfonamino-butane-2-one [TPCK] [50 μg/ml]; 7-amino-1-chloro-3-L-tosyl-amidoheptan-2-one [TLCK] [25 μg/ml]; aprotinin [Sigma, 100 Kallikrein units/ml [Abney and Parkhouse 1974]), or (2) a similar buffer, but with 1% (w/v) digitonin replacing the NP-40 (Oettgen et al. 1986). Coprecipitation was done by a solid-phase immunoprecipitation technique (SPIT). For direct SPIT assays, flexible PVC microtiter plates were coated over-

night with affinity-purified specific goat anti-mouse K chains, μ chains, δ chains, or normal rabbit Ig (10 μg/1 ml in phosphate-buffered saline [PBS]), prepared as described previously (Chayen and Parkhouse 1982b). For indirect assays, the plates were similarly coated with OX-12 (a mouse MAb anti-rat K chain from A. Williams, University of Oxford), followed by capture of rat monoclonal antibodies to B-cell-surface proteins (8–16 hr, 4°C). Each well then received about 10^6 cpm of ^{125}I surface-labeled, lysed B cells (8–16 hr, 4°C) and was washed with the same solution used for cell lysis, i.e., NP-40 or digitonin. Bound radioactivity was solubilized with 2% (w/v) SDS and then electrophoresed under reducing or nonreducing conditions on 5–20% (w/v) gradient slab gels.

Surface staining and modulation. This was done with purified small, dense B cells (see above). Cells were first reacted (20 min, r.t.) with fluorescein-labeled (FITC), affinity-purified goat anti-mouse Ig (experimentals), or FITC-labeled, affinity-purified goat anti-rabbit Ig (controls) (Southern Biotechnology, Birmingham, Alabama) in PBS containing sodium azide (2 mg/ml) and bovine serum albumin (2 mg/ml) (PBA). Cells were washed twice in RPMI 1640 tissue culture medium with 5% (v/v) fetal calf serum (FCS), resuspended at 2×10^7 to 4×10^7 cells/ml in RPMI 1640/5% FCS and incubated at 37°C for 30 minutes. Under these conditions, the cross-linked mIg in the experimental samples capped and internalized ("modulation"). The cells were washed twice with PBA, treated with 10% (v/v) normal mouse serum (10 min, r.t.), and then stained with rat monoclonal antibodies (20 min, r.t.). The bound rat antibodies were revealed by successive applications of biotin-coupled rat-specific, affinity-purified goat anti-rat Ig and phycoerythrin-coupled streptavidin (PE-SA) (Southern Biotechnology). The biotin anti-rat Ig reagent was diluted in 10% (v/v) normal mouse serum. Samples were analyzed on the Becton Dickinson Facstar plus. For the control samples treated with FITC goat anti-rabbit Ig, the small, dense, viable lymphocytes were selected for analysis of staining with the rat MAb-PE-SA combination. Of these, 95% were B cells as judged by positive staining with FITC-anti-mouse Ig. Analysis of the B cells modulated to surface Ig negativity by treatment with FITC-goat anti-mouse Ig was done by selecting the small, dense, viable, FITC-positive cells for analysis of staining with the rat MAb-PE-SA combination. The rat monoclonal antibodies to mouse lymphocyte glycoproteins used in the study were anti-mouse K chains (OX-20 from A. Williams, University of Oxford), anti-Thy-1 (NIM-R1) (Chayen and Parkhouse 1982a), anti-class I, LFA-1, and μ heavy chains (R.M.E. Parkhouse and A. Rodriguez, unpubl.), anti-class II (NIM-R4) (Andrew and Parkhouse 1986), anti-CDw32 or FcR (24G2, Unkeless et al. 1988), anti-CD23 or FcR low (B3B4, Conrad et al. 1987), JIID, a rat MAb to a 48-kD molecule on B cells, red blood cells, and thymocytes (Symington and Hakamori 1984), and B6G12, an antibody to a 90-kD B-cell-surface protein (R.M.E. Parkhouse and A. Rodriquez, unpubl.).

RESULTS

Association of a 73-kD Dimer with mIg

Surface-labeled B cells were lysed in either NP-40 or digitonin, the latter being a detergent selectively preserving relatively weak non-covalent interactions. Immunoglobulins were immunoselected by the SPIT procedure from both lysates with affinity-purified, polyclonal goat antibodies and analyzed by SDS-PAGE under reducing and nonreducing conditions (Fig. 1). There was no significant background with a control immunoprecipitation using affinity-purified, polyclonal goat anti-rabbit Ig (Fig. 1a). Coprecipitation with anti-mIg, IgM, and IgD yielded the expected μ, δ, and light chains (Fig. 1b,c), μ and light chains (Fig. 1d,e), and δ and light chains (Fig. 1f,g), respectively, and with both detergents (NP-40 and digitonin). An additional pair of bands, M_r values 35K and 38K, was preferentially observed in precipitations from the digitonin lysates (Fig. 1c,e,g). These were absent or present in reduced yields in immunoprecipitates from NP-40 (not detected with IgM; Fig. 1d; reduced yield with IgD, Fig. 1f). Nonreducing analysis of IgM (Fig. 1j) and IgD (Fig. 1i) immunoprecipitated from digitonin lysates yielded a 73-kD component absent in similar SDS-PAGE analysis of material coprecipitated by IgM (Fig. 1h) from an NP-40 lysate. It can therefore be concluded that the 35-kD and 38-kD components associating with mIg in digitonin formed a 73-kD disulfide-linked dimer. Similar coprecipitations conducted with several rat monoclonal antibodies to B-cell-surface components (class I, class II, FcRγ, FcRε, LFA-1) failed to demonstrate any molecular associations preferentially observed in digitonin, as opposed to NP-40, lysates (data not shown).

Cocapping of Two Surface Molecules with mIg

The strategy here was to internalize mIg by pretreatment of B cells with FITC anti-mouse Ig under modulating conditions and then look for changes in staining intensity with a panel of rat antibodies to B-cell-surface proteins.

Treatment of B cells with anti-Ig under modulating conditions (see Materials and Methods) yielded essentially surface Ig-negative cells, as judged by visual in-

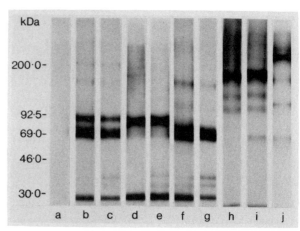

Figure 1. Coprecipitation of a 73-kD heterodimer with sIg. Murine B cells were surface-labeled with ^{125}I and lysed in either digitonin (a, c, e, g, i, j) or NP-40 (b, d, f, h). Coprecipitations were done in both detergents with polyclonal goat anti-mIg (b, c), anti-mouse μ chains (d, e), and anti-mouse δ chains (f, g) and analyzed by SDS-PAGE under reducing conditions. Coprecipitations were also analyzed under nonreducing conditions, and those included in the figure are with anti-mouse δ chains in NP-40 (h) and digitonin (i) and with anti-mouse μ chains in digitonin (j). The level of nonspecific coprecipitation given by a polyclonal goat anti-rabbit Ig was negligible when analyzed under reducing (a) or nonreducing (not shown) conditions. The position of the molecular-weight markers is indicated. For details, see Materials and Methods.

spection and the reduction of staining with a rat monoclonal antibody to mouse μ chains (Fig. 2d, dashed line). Similar treatment of B cells with an unrelated antibody (FITC-goat anti-rabbit Ig) failed to affect the subsequent staining with the panel of rat monoclonal antibodies, for example, the anti-μ chains (Fig. 2d, solid line). As expected, negative controls with medium (Fig. 2b) or an unrelated monoclonal antibody (anti-mouse Thy-1) (Fig. 2c) simply yielded unstained cells. The anti-Ig-modulated mIg-negative cells can, however, be recognized as B cells on the cell sorter by virtue of their internally located FITC-goat anti-mouse Ig, and so, in the case of the anti-Ig-modulated sample, these positively identified B cells were examined for subsequent staining with the rat MAb-PE-SA combinations. Following this experimental protocol, modulation of mIg failed to affect staining with antibodies to mouse class I and LFA-1 (data not shown), class II (Fig. 2e), FcR-γ (Fig. 2f), and FcR-ε (Fig. 2g), but a significant reduction was observed with MAbs J11D (Fig. 2h) and B6G12 (Fig. 2i).

DISCUSSION

The possible association of the B-cell antigen receptor (mIg) with other membrane or membrane-associated molecules is still a relatively unexplored area. Such association, however, could conceivably play a critical role in the generation of second signals following interaction with antigen, or in subcellular

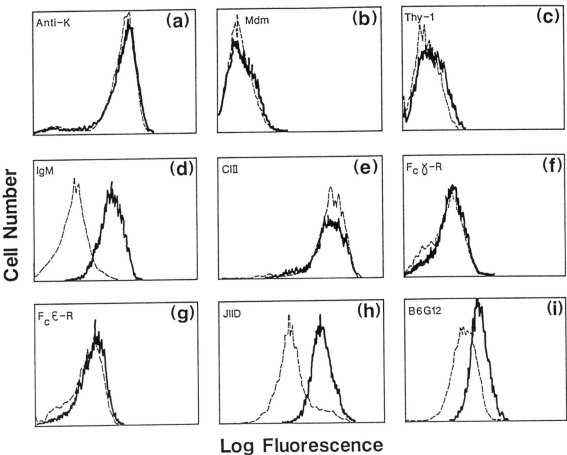

Figure 2. Cocapping of two B-cell-surface molecules with mIg. Murine B cells were capped and modulated with FITC-goat anti-Ig, counterstained with rat MAbs-biotin goat anti-rat Ig-PE-SA. The modulated B cells (i.e., FITC-positive small lympho-cytes) were examined for PE staining in the cell sorter (dashed line). Control B cells were treated with FITC-goat anti-rabbit Ig and then similarly stained with the rat MAb systems (solid lines). Rat MAbs were anti-mouse, Thy-1 (c), μ heavy chains (d), class II (e), FcRγ (f), FcRϵ (g), and rat MAbs J11D (h) and B6G12 (i). The negative control is given by tissue culture medium (b). For details, see Materials and Methods. In panel a, staining with rat MAb OX-20 (anti-mouse K chain) was done after control (goat anti-rabbit Ig) modulation (solid line) and without control or anti-mIg modulation (dashed line).

traffic to (membrane representation) and from (antigen presentation) the cell surface. Three arguments in par-ticular raise this possibility: the simultaneous presence of two Ig classes, usually IgM and IgD, on single resting B cells (Abney et al. 1978); the conserved nature of the transmembrane mIg domain, both between different species and between different Ig classes (Early et al. 1980; Rabbits et al. 1981; Bernstein et al. 1984); and the absence of a cytoplasmic mIg domain potentially capable of generating a second message. It is therefore logical to postulate a necessity for mIg-associating molecules, as indeed has been done (Tyler et al. 1982; Yamawaki-Kataoka et al. 1982).

Two experimental approaches have been pursued to identify molecules associating with mIg on B cells. The first, a biochemical procedure that relies on immuno-precipitation from digitonin lysates of surface-iodinated B cells, has been successfully used to directly demon-strate weak noncovalent interactions between certain T-cell-surface glycoproteins (see Oettgen et al. 1986; Brown et al. 1989). Following the same protocol, but with purified resting B cells, we have now identified an

mIg-associated 73-kD heterodimer composed of disul-fide-linked 35-kD and 38-kD components. This differs from the IgM-associating 68-kD homodimer of a μ-chain-transfected plasmacytoma (Hombach et al. 1988), not only in its structure, but also in the fact that it appears to associate with IgD as well as IgM. Further-more, the 73-kD heterodimer is easily detected in ly-sates of ^{125}I-surface-labeled resting B cells, whereas the 68-kD plasmacytoma homodimer was poorly labeled by ^{125}I-labeled lactoperoxidase (Hombach et al. 1988). Whether the latter is indeed synthesized by resting B cells, therefore, has not yet been addressed by the direct experiment of biosynthetic labeling and copre-cipitation from digitonin cell lysates. The function of the 73-kD heterodimer has yet to be determined, but its capacity to interact with both mIgD and mIgM does suggest a possible role as a component of a mIg re-ceptor complex functioning in B-cell activation. As has recently been reviewed (Klaus et al., this volume), both IgD and mIgM similarly operate via the polyphos-phoinositide-specific phosphodiesterase pathway dur-ing B-cell activation. Finally, both the 73-kD heterodimer and the 68-kD homodimer are structurally distinct from other molecules that have been previously described as associating with mIg, but through the use of different experimental protocols (Rosenspire and Choi 1982; Koch and Haustein 1983; Newell et al. 1987; Gupta and Ward 1988).

The second approach for detecting molecules associating with mIg in B-cell membranes was based on a conventional cocapping protocol. In this case, mIg was capped with anti-Ig, and the resulting Ig-negative ("modulated") cells were then screened with a panel of monoclonal antibodies. Most antibodies tested (anti-class I, -class II, -LFA-1, -FcR-γ, -FcR-ϵ) reacted equally well with control and modulated B cells. With two monoclonal antibodies, however, there was a significant reduction in surface representation following anti-Ig-induced modulation of mIg. One of these was a MAb (B6G12) reactive with a 90-kD surface component, as yet lacking correlation with existing CD markers. The other (J11D), recognizes a carbohydrate-rich glycoprotein found on murine B cells, red cells, and thymocytes (Symington and Hakamori 1984), which may be integrated into membranes either via a defined transmembrane domain or via a phosphoinositol linkage (C. Kinnon, unpubl.). The observed reduction of cell-surface expression of a B-cell-surface marker following anti-Ig-induced modulation could be due to cocapping and consequent internalization with mIg. An alternative possibility is release from the surface, perhaps due to anti-Ig-induced enzyme action. The latter perhaps might be inherently more attractive in the case of phosphoinositol-linked membrane molecules, such as the phosphoinositol-linked molecular target of the J11D antibody.

In summary, three membrane molecules have been identified that appear to associate with mIg on small, resting B cells. Their functions in the physiology of these cells remain to be explained.

ACKNOWLEDGMENTS

It is a pleasure to thank Graham Preece and Nick Clark for their expert assistance.

REFERENCES

Abney, E.R. and R.M.E. Parkhouse. 1974. A candidate for immunoglobulin D present on murine B lymphocytes. *Nature* 252: 600.

Abney, E.R., M.D. Cooper, J.F. Kearney, A.R. Lawton, and R.M.E. Parkhouse. 1978. Sequential expression of immunoglobulin on developing mouse B lymphocytes: A systematic survey which suggests a model for the generation of immunoglobulin isotype diversity. *J. Immunol.* 120: 2041.

Anderson, P., C. Morimoto, J.B. Breitmeyer, and S.F. Schlossman. 1988. Regulatory interactions between membranes of the immunoglobulin superfamily. *Immunol. Today* 9: 199.

Andrew, E.M. and R.M.E. Parkhouse. 1986. Immune induction of Ia antigens in activated T cells and in kidney epithelial cells in mice. *Immunology* 58: 603.

Bernstein, K.E., C.B. Alexander, E.P. Reddy, and R.E. Mage. 1984. Complete sequence of a cloned cDNA encoding rabbit secreted μ-chain of V_Ha2 allotype: Comparisons with V_Ha1 and membrane μ sequences. *J. Immunol.* 132: 490.

Brown, M.H., D.A. Cantrell, G. Brattsand, M.J. Crumpton, and M. Gullberg. 1989. The CD2 antigen associates with the T-cell antigen receptor CD3 antigen complex on the surface of human T lymphocytes. *Nature* 339: 551.

Chayen, A. and R.M.E. Parkhouse. 1982a. Preparation and properties of a cytotoxic monoclonal anti-mouse Thy-1 antibody. *J. Immunol. Methods* 49: 17.

———. 1982b. B cell subpopulations in the mouse: Analysis with monoclonal antibodies NIM-R2 and NIM-R3. *Eur. R. Immunol.* 12: 725.

Conrad, D.H., T.J. Waldschmidt, W.T. Lee, M. Rao, A.D. Keegan, R.J. Noelle, R.G. Lynch, and M.R Kehry. 1987. Effect of B cell stimulatory factor-1 (interleukin 4) on Fcϵ and Fcγ receptor expression on murine B lymphocytes and B cell lines. *J. Immunol.* 139: 2290.

Early, P., J. Rogers, M. Davis, K. Calame, M. Bond, R. Wall, and L. Hood. 1980. Two mRNAs can be produced from a single immunoglobulin μ gene by alternative RNA processing pathways. *Cell* 20: 313.

Gupta, S.K. and B.A. Woda. 1988. Ligand-induced association of surface immunoglobulin with the detergent insoluble cytoskeleton may involve actinin. *J. Immunol.* 140: 176.

Hombach, J., L. Leclercq, A. Radbruch, K. Rajewsky, and M. Reth. 1988. A novel 34-kd protein co-isolated with the IgM molecule in surface IgM-expressing cells. *EMBO J.* 7: 3451.

Koch, N. and D. Haustein. 1983. Association of surface IgM with two membrane proteins on murine B lymphocytes detected by chemical crosslinking. *Mol. Immunol.* 20: 33.

Moller, G., ed. 1987. *Immunological reviews: Activation antigens and signal transduction in lymphocyte activation.* Munksgaard, Copenhagen.

Newell, M.K., L.B. Justement, J.H. Freed, and J.C. Cambier. 1987. Phosphorylation of a mIg associated protein complex. *Fed. Proc.* 46: 1203.

Oettgen, H.C., C.L. Pettey, W.L. Maloy, and C. Terhorst. 1986. A T3-like protein complex associated with the antigen receptor on murine T cells. *Nature* 320: 272.

O'Garra, A., D.J. Warren, M. Holman, A.M. Popham, C.J. Sanderson, and G.G.B. Klaus. 1986. Interleukin 4 (B cell growth factor II/esoinophil differentiation factor) is a mitogen and differentiation factor for preactivated murine B lymphocytes. *Proc. Natl. Acad. Sci.* 83: 5228.

Rabbits, T.H., A. Forster, and C.P. Milstein. 1981. Human immunoglobulin heavy chain genes: Evolutionary comparisons of $C\mu$, $C\delta$, and $C\gamma$ genes and associated switch sequences. *Nucleic Acids Res.* 9: 4509.

Rosenspire, A.J. and Y.S. Choi. 1982. Relation between actin-associated proteins and membrane immunoglobulin in B-cells. *Mol. Immunol.* 19: 1515.

Symington, F.W. and S.-I. Hakamori. 1984. Hematopoietic subpopulations express cross-reactive, lineage-specific molecules detected by monoclonal antibody. *Mol. Immunol.* 21: 507.

Tyler, B.M., A.F. Cowman, S.D. Gerondakis, J.M. Adams, and O. Bernard. 1982. mRNA for surface immunoglobulin γ chains encodes a highly conserved transmembrane sequence and a 28-residue intracellular domain. *Proc. Natl. Acad. Sci.* 79: 2008.

Unkeless, J.C., E. Scigliano, and V.H. Freedman. 1988. Structure and function of human and murine receptors for IgG. *Annu. Rev. Immunol.* 6: 251.

Yamawaki-Kataoka, Y., S. Nakai, T. Miyata, and T. Honjo. 1982. Nucleotide sequences of gene segments encoding membrane domains of immunoglobulin γ chains. *Proc. Natl. Acad. Sci.* 79: 2623.

Signal Transduction through Interleukin-5 Receptors

K. Takatsu, N. Yamaguchi, Y. Hitoshi, E. Sonoda,
S. Mita, and A. Tominaga

Department of Biology, Institute for Medical Immunology, Kumamoto University
Medical School, 2-2-1 Honjo, Kumamoto 860, Japan

The B-cell response to an antigen is regulated by helper T cells specific for the same antigenic molecule. Helper T cells recognize antigen in the context of class II major histocompatibility complex (MHC) molecules on accessory cells and/or B cells and secrete B-cell stimulatory factors (BSFs), which can induce B-cell growth and differentiation (for review, see Howard and Paul 1983; Kishimoto 1985; Takatsu 1988).

A decade ago, we identified one of the BSFs that acts as T-cell-replacing factor (TRF) in the cell-free supernatants (Sup) of T cells from *Mycobacterium tuberculosis* (Tbc)-primed mice that had been stimulated with purified protein derivative (PPD)-presenting cells (Takatsu et al. 1980a), and established a TRF-producing T-cell hybridoma B151K12 (B151) by means of fusion between Tbc-primed T cells and murine thymoma BW5147 (Takatsu et al. 1980b; Takatsu and Hamaoka 1982). TRF activity was initially assessed by using T-cell-depleted dinitrophenyl–keyhole limpet hemocyanin (DNP-KLH)-primed splenic B cells as differentiation-inducing activity to anti-DNP IgG antibody-secreting cells. Then, murine chronic B-cell leukemia BCL_1 cells were shown to differentiate into IgM-secreting cells in response to B151-Sup, which possess TRF activity. The molecule responsible for TRF activity was purified to homogeneity from B151-Sup and was found to be an acidic glycoprotein with M_r of 50,000–60,000 on gel permeation. Then a monoclonal antibody against this molecule was developed (Harada et al. 1987b). We thus found that the TRF-active molecule also shows activity for B-cell growth factor II (BCGFII) (Harada et al. 1985; Swain and Dutton 1982). It has also been shown that the TRF molecule increases in the expression of IL-2 receptors on B cells and synergizes with IL-2 for Ig production (Harada et al. 1987a; Loughnan et al. 1987; Nakanishi et al. 1988). Furthermore, the TRF molecule was found to play an important role in the antigen-specific and polyclonal IgM-production through MHC-linked as well as factor-mediated T/B-cell interaction (Rasmussen et al. 1988).

The recent molecular cloning of complementary DNA encoding the TRF molecule has confirmed that TRF is a novel lymphokine and is reponsible for both growth and differentiation of B cells (Kinashi et al. 1986; Azuma et al. 1987). Because of the diverse activities and targets of TRF (see below), this lymphokine is now accepted as interleukin-5 (IL-5). Natural as well as recombinant murine IL-5 has been shown to be a biological mediator active in a variety of lymphoid and nonlymphoid functions, although IL-5 was believed to be active exclusively on B cells (Takatsu et al. 1988). IL-5 increases in the expression of IL-2 receptors on antigen-stimulated thymocytes, resulting in the generation of cytotoxic T cells in the presence of IL-2 (killer-helper activity) (Takatsu et al. 1987). IL-5 also affects hematopoietic precursor cells for proliferation and terminal differentiation into eosinophils (eosinophil differentiation factor, EDF) (Sanderson et al. 1988; Yamaguchi et al. 1988a; Yokota et al. 1988) and acts on mature eosinophils for their activation (Yamaguchi et al. 1988b).

The biologically active form of IL-5 having an apparent M_r of 45,000–50,000 is a homodimer of M_r 25,000–30,000 (Tominaga et al. 1988). Since the IL-5 monomer does not show any biological activity, dimer formation is obligatory for the expression of biological activity (T. Takahashi et al., unpubl.). Deglycosylated IL-5 is biologically active and has an M_r of 25,000–30,000, and its monomer has an M_r of 12,000–14,000 (A. Tominaga et al., in prep.), suggesting that the N-linked carbohydrate moiety is not essential for the biological activity of IL-5. IL-5 mRNA is constitutively expressed in B151 cells and is detectable in the phorbol-12-myristate-acetate (PMA) or Con-A-stimulated T-cell lines and PPD-stimulated Tbc-primed cells (Tominaga et al. 1988). The genomic organization of IL-5 has also been determined. Murine and human IL-5 genes have four exons and three introns with similar organizations (Tanabe et al. 1987; Takahashi et al. 1988).

The availability of purified recombinant IL-5 enabled us to measure the binding of IL-5 to its cell-surface receptor. It has been shown that IL-5 acts on target cells via a specific receptor and that there are two classes (high- and low-affinity) of IL-5-binding sites on IL-5-responsive cells (Mita et al. 1988). Furthermore, cross-linking studies of radiolabeled IL-5 with the use of a murine IL-5-dependent early B-cell line (T88-M) yielded two cross-linked complexes with M_r values of 92,500 and 160,000 (Mita et al. 1989).

In this paper, we present two topics: In the first part, we discuss in some detail recent findings concerning IL-5-induced IgA production; in the second part, we describe molecular and functional properties of murine IL-5 receptors.

INDUCTION OF IgA PRODUCTION BY IL-5

It has recently been reported that IL-5 induces IgA production of lipopolysaccharide (LPS)-stimulated splenic B cells (IgA-enhancing factor) (Coffman et al. 1988; Harriman et al. 1988; Beagley et al. 1989). We reported that IL-5 induces secondary anti-DNP IgA production of DNP-primed, surface IgA-positive (sIgA⁺) B cells (Matsumoto et al. 1989). It is still controversial, however, whether IL-5 is a class-switching factor from μ- to α-chain or a maturation factor for sIgA⁺ B cells. To clarify the mechanisms of IgA induction by IL-5, we examined effects of other cytokines, namely transforming growth factor-beta (TGF-β) on IgA production. TGF-β is synthesized and secreted by a variety of cells and is reported to affect the immune system, including inhibition of lymphocyte proliferation, antibody production, and natural killer (NK) cell function (Sporn et al. 1986). However, it is not known whether TGF-β affects the expression of particular Ig-isotype expression in the immune system.

Experimental Procedures

Mice. BALB/c mice were purchased from Japan SLC Inc., and were maintained in the Laboratory Animal Facility of Kumamoto University.

Reagents. TB13 rat IgG₁ monoclonal antibodies against mouse IL-5, rabbit anti-mouse IgA and anti-IgG₁ antibodies, horseradish peroxidase (HRPO)-coupled anti-IgA and IgG₁ antibodies, goat anti-mouse IgM and HRPO-anti-mouse IgM antibodies, and purified goat anti-mouse IgA antibody have been described previously (Harada et al. 1987b; Matsumoto et al. 1989; Sonoda et al. 1989). Human recombinant TGF-β1 was a gift from Genentech, Inc. (South San Francisco, CA). IL-5 was purified as described previously (Mita et al. 1988).

Antibody production in vitro. Surface IgA-negative (sIgA⁻) B cells were fractionated from T-cell-depleted B cells by the panning method. Unfractionated B cells and sIgA⁻ B cells ($1 \times 10^5/0.2$ ml/well) were cultured in a 96-well microplate in the presence of 10 μg/ml LPS as described previously (Matsumoto et al. 1989). Re-

combinant cytokines were added 24 hours after the commencement of the culture. For enzyme-linked immunosorbent assay (ELISA), cells were cultured for 7 days and Sup were collected. ELISA assays were carried out as described previously (Sonoda et al. 1989).

Results and Discussion

Mechanisms of IL-5- and TGF-β-induced IgA production by LPS-stimulated B cells. When LPS-stimulated unfractionated B cells were cultured with IL-5, polyclonal IgA secretion as well as polyclonal IgM and IgG₁ secretion were enhanced (Table 1). Addition of TGF-β alone also augmented IgA production, whereas IgM and IgG₁ production were relatively inhibited. Addition of both IL-5 and TGF-β caused striking enhancement of IgA production. Then we analyzed the time-course of addition of IL-5 and TGF-β for examining their effects on IgA production. Simultaneous addition of TGF-β and IL-5 induced maximal IgA production. Addition of IL-5 on day 2 or 3 from the onset of culture also augmented TGF-β-induced IgA production. In contrast, addition of TGF-β on day 2 or 3 showed no enhancing effect on IL-5-induced IgA production (data not shown). These results indicate that IL-5 induces IgA, IgM, and IgG₁ production, whereas TGF-β selectively enhances IgA production; and that TGF-β exerts its activity on the early period and IL-5 is required for the late period of the culture, suggesting that IL-5- and TGF-β-induced IgA production may be governed by different mechanisms.

Compared with the responses of unfractionated B cells and sIgA⁻ B cells, IL-5 acts predominantly on unfractionated B cells that include both sIgA⁺ and sIgA⁻ B cells, but not on purified sIgA⁻ B cells for IgA production. However, TGF-β acts on sIgA⁻ B cells as well as unfractionated B cells for IgA production (Table 1). Addition of both IL-5 and TGF-β also caused striking enhancement of IgA production from sIgA⁻ B cells. Therefore, these results suggest that IL-5 and TGF-β have different roles in the induction of IgA production. IL-5 may be a maturation factor for already committed Ig class-switching B cells such as sIgM⁺, sIgG₁⁺, and sIgA⁺ B cells. On the other hand, TGF-β may be one of class-switching factors, exclusive-

Table 1. Effects of IL-5 and/or TGF-β on Ig Production by LPS-stimulated B Cells

Stimulant	Unfractionated B cells (ng/ml)			sIgA⁻ B cells (ng/ml)		
	IgM	IgG₁	IgA	IgM	IgG₁	IgA
Medium	25,000	640	84	17,200	640	<20
IL-5 (4 ng/ml)	56,000	740	440	19,200	720	52
TGF-β (1 ng/ml)	11,800	120	448	7,300	98	690
IL-5 (4 ng/ml) + TGF-β (1 ng/ml)	24,400	76	1,580	11,300	184	1,320
Medium: LPS (−)	1,160	<20	<20	2,760	<20	<20

Unfractionated B cells or sIgA⁻ B cells were cultured with LPS (10 μg/ml) for 7 days. IL-5 and/or TGF-β were added on day 1. After the culture, IgA levels in supernatants were titrated by ELISA assay. Results were expressed as mean value of triplicate cultures.

ly from sIgA⁻ to sIgA⁺ B cells, and may also induce maturation of sIgA⁺ B cells. Thus, it is interesting to explore the mechanisms of Ig secretion by means of IL-5 and TGF-β. Especially induction of IgA secretion by IL-5 and/or TGF-β has taken into consideration the involvement of IL-5 and TGF-β in mucosal immunity.

IL-5 RECEPTOR: STRUCTURE AND FUNCTION

Since IL-5 acts on different target cells, resulting in the induction of diverse biological activities, it is important to clarify the molecular characteristics of IL-5 receptor (IL-5R) and the functionally IL-5-responsive cells in vivo. In this paper, we describe the characterization of the murine IL-5R and IL-5R-positive cells with the use of monoclonal antibodies (MAbs) that we developed.

Experimental Procedures

Reagents and cell lines. Preparation of [³⁵S] methionine-labeled deglycosylated IL-5 (M_r 26,000) and establishment of the IL-5-dependent early B-cell line (T88-M) have been described previously (Mita et al. 1988; Tominaga et al. 1989).

Production of monoclonal antibody. Hybridomas were established by means of fusions between rat spleen cells that had been immunized with membrane-enriched fractions of T88-M cells and mouse myeloma cells (N. Yamaguchi et al., in prep.). Hybridoma Sup were assayed by two different methods using T88-M cells, i.e., by competitive inhibition assay of ³⁵S-labeled IL-5 binding and of IL-5-dependent proliferation. Two positive clones (H7 and T21) and one negative clone (Y2) were selected for further evaluation.

FACS analysis. Cells were stained with FITC-coupled monoclonal antibodies to CD 5 (Ly-1) and IgM or with biotinylated H7 followed by phycoerythrin-conjugated streptavidin (PE-Av) and were analyzed on a FACScan. To analyze T-cell-depleted peritoneal populations, the cells that gave high obtuse scatter signals were excluded by gating out.

SDS-PAGE analysis. For cross-linking experiments, cells were incubated with ³⁵S-labeled deglycosylated IL-5 and subsequently cross-linked with disuccinimidyl tartarate (DST). After washing, cells were lysed with lysis buffer containing 1% Triton X-100 and a mixture of proteinase inhibitors. Lysates were analyzed by SDS-PAGE and autoradiography (Mita et al. 1989). For immunoprecipitation experiments, cells were radioiodinated by the glucose oxidase-lactoperoxidase method. Cells were then lysed with lysis buffer containing 0.5% 3-([3-cholamidopropyl] dimethyl-ammonio)-1-propane sulfate (CHAPS) and a mixture of proteinase inhibitors. Lysate was analyzed by SDS-PAGE and autoradiography (N. Yamaguchi et al., in prep.).

Results and Discussion

³⁵S-labeled IL-5/IL-5R complexes detectable by cross-linking. Since purified IL-5 displays high heterogeneity in M_r because of differential glycosylation, we prepared ³⁵S-labeled deglycosylated IL-5 to estimate the precise M_r of IL-5-binding proteins by cross-linking studies. This IL-5 preparation is biologically active and manifests relatively homogeneous in M_r. M_r of deglycosylated IL-5 preparation could be precisely determined at 26,000 and 13,000 under nonreducing and reducing conditions, respectively (data not shown). As shown in Figure 1, two major cross-linked complexes with ³⁵S-labeled deglycosylated IL-5 at approximate M_r of 81,000 (a major species) and 140,000 (a minor species) were detected on T88-M cells under nonreducing conditions (Fig. 1A). Under reducing conditions, M_r 72,000 and 150,000 cross-linked complexes were detected (Fig. 1B), and both bands disappeared in the presence of excess amounts of unlabeled IL-5 (Fig. 1C). After subtraction of M_r of deglycosylated IL-5, M_r of IL-5-binding proteins are estimated to be 55,000 and 114,000; and 59,000 and 137,000 under nonreducing and reducing conditions, respectively. Molecular sizes of cross-linked complexes mentioned in this paper are different from those described in our previous reports (Mita et al. 1989). This may come from the difference in IL-5 preparations.

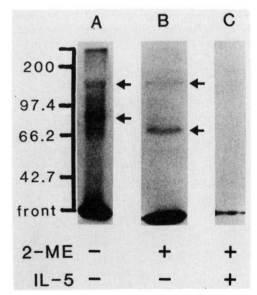

Figure 1. Autoradiograph of cross-linking of ³⁵S-labeled IL-5-binding protein. T88-M cells were incubated with ³⁵S-labeled deglycosylated IL-5 and cross-linked with DST. After several washings, cells were lysed with 1% Triton X-100, and the lysate was analyzed with SDS-PAGE under nonreducing (*A*) or reducing (*B* and *C*) conditions. In lane *C*, unlabeled IL-5 was added before cross-linking. Autoradiography was made after electrophoresis. Molecular mass markers are shown in kD.

Identification of IL-5R in T88-M cell lysates. To identify IL-5-binding molecules more directly, surface-radioiodinated T88-M cells were extracted with CHAPS, cell extracts were reacted with IL-5-coupled beads, and eluates were analyzed by SDS-PAGE under reducing conditions. A band with an apparent M_r of 60,000 was observed in the eluate from IL-5-coupled beads (Fig. 2, lane A) in contrast to the eluate from control beads (lane B). The M_r of IL-5-binding protein seems to be similar to that of a major species estimated by cross-linking studies as shown in Figure 1.

Production and characterization of monoclonal antibodies to T88-M cells. We selected two MAbs, H7 and T21, which could competitively block both high-affinity and low-affinity binding of ^{35}S-labeled IL-5 to T88-M cells. In cytofluorometric analysis, the antigens recognized by H7 and by T21 were detected on T88-M, BCL$_1$-B20, and MOPC104E cells, which were shown to display binding sites for IL-5 on the cell surface. In contrast, reactivities of these MAbs were not observed to X5563 (myeloma), FDC-P1 (IL-3-dependent line), or MTH (IL-2-dependent line), which express undetectable levels of IL-5-binding site. When T88-M cells were preincubated with an approximately tenfold molar excess of unlabeled IL-5 prior to staining with H7 or T21, the binding of H7 or T21 was dramatically inhibited (data not shown). Thus, H7 and T21 appear to define a surface antigen exclusively on IL-5-responsive cells.

H7 (IgG$_{2a}$) and T21 (IgG$_1$) MAbs inhibited IL-5-induced [3H]thymidine incorporation by T88-M cells at minimum 50 pM, whereas irrelevant MAb Y2, which binds to T88-M cells, had no significant effect at a concentration up to 100 nM. In agreement with these data, H7 as well as T21 inhibited IL-5-induced proliferation of other murine IL-5-responsive B-cell lines (BCL$_1$, J-87, and T-88), and H7 or T21 MAb itself did not have any stimulatory effects on [3H]thymidine incorporation. H7 and T21 MAbs showed no significant inhibitory effects even at 500 nM on IL-2, IL-3, or IL-4 activities. Neither H7 nor T21 inhibited DNA synthesis on Con-A-activated T cells and of LPS-stimulated B cells. Thus, the inhibitory effects of T21 or H7 are restricted to IL-5-mediated events. Collectively, we conclude that both H7 and T21 MAbs are reactive with an epitope identical to or near the binding site for IL-5 on IL-5R.

H7-positive peritoneal B cells respond to IL-5 in a high frequency. We examined the direct cell binding of MAb to normal lymphoid cells by FACS analysis. Splenic B cells from unstimulated mice expressed a significant number of H7 and T21 antigens, and their numbers were increased two- to threefold by culturing the cells for 48 hours with IL-5 or LPS (data not shown). Intriguingly, almost all of the T-cell-depleted sIgM$^+$ B cells from the peritoneal cavity reacted with H7 MAb (Fig. 3A). Approximately 67% of total H7$^+$ cells were also CD5 (Ly-1)$^+$ (Fig. 3B). Some of them (~25%) were H7$^+$ and CD5$^-$. We then tested for IL-5-responsiveness of peritoneal and splenic B cells by IgM secretion. As shown in Table 2, peritoneal B cells responded to IL-5 for their polyclonal IgM production, and four times as many IgM plaque-forming cells (pfc) were detected as were observed in splenic B cells, of which responses were completely inhibited by H7 and T21 MAbs. Limiting dilution analysis revealed that approximately 1 out of 15 peritoneal B cells responded to IL-5 for IgM-producing cells, whereas 1 out of 900 splenic B cells responded to IL-5 for 2-day culture.

The use of MAbs has generally directed toward defining subpopulations of B cells. In this context, results of the expression of H7 antigen on peritoneal B cells are somehow interesting. H7$^+$ peritoneal B cells, consisting of both CD5$^+$ and CD5$^-$ B-cell populations, respond well to IL-5 for IgM production. The frequency of peritoneal B cells that respond to IL-5 are approximately 60-fold higher than that of splenic B cells. Taking account of the fact that proportions of H7$^+$ B cells in peritoneal B cells are higher than those of splenic B cells, H7-positivity correlates with IL-5 responsiveness. Herzenberg et al. (1986) demonstrated that CD5$^+$ B cells are self-replenishing, reside in the peritoneal cavity, and produce autoantibodies. Although we have not yet tested whether H7$^+$ peritoneal B cells produce autoantibody, it will become quite important to examine the development and function of IL-5R$^+$ peritoneal B cells.

Large proportions (>60%) of bone marrow cells (gated for myeloid cells) were stained with T21 MAb, but few (<5%), if any, stained with H7 MAb (data not shown). They also showed weak responsiveness to IL-5 for DNA synthesis. This may suggest that T21 antigen

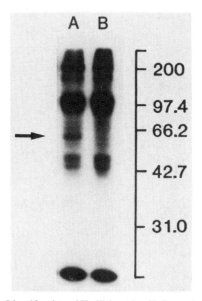

Figure 2. Identification of IL-5R by using IL-5-coupled beads. Eluate from IL-5-coupled beads (lane *A*) and from control beads (lane *B*) after adsorption of extracts prepared from ^{125}I-labeled T88-M cells were analyzed by SDS-PAGE under reducing conditions and autoradiography. Molecular mass markers are shown in kD.

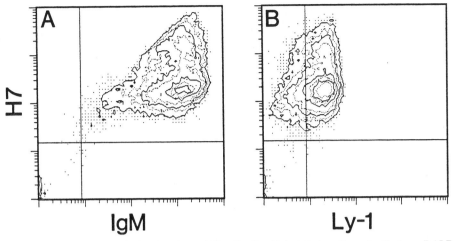

Figure 3. Dual color flow cytometry analysis of peritoneal B cells. T-cell-depleted peritoneal cells from BALB/c mice were stained first with FITC-labeled MAb to CD5 (Ly-1), IgM, or biotinylated H7, followed by PE-Av. (*A*) H7 vs. sIgM or (*B*) H7 vs. CD5 (Ly-1) by using FACScan. Relative fluorescence intensity was expressed by logarithmic amplification.

Table 2. Peritoneal B Cells Give Rise to IgM-producing Cells in Response to IL-5

IL-5 (pg/ml)	Antibody (μg/ml)	Polyclonal IgM pfc response	
		peritoneal B cells	splenic B cells
0	0	225	120
400	0	1190	290
400	H7 5	260	110
400	T21 5	242	96

Peritoneal B cells (1×10^5) or splenic B cells were cultured for 3 days in the presence or in the absence of IL-5. Antibody was added on day 0. After the culture, numbers of IgM pfc were enumerated. Results are expressed as mean pfc of triplicate cultures.

on bone marrow may not be a functional IL-5 receptor and may be somewhat different from that on IL-5-responding T88-M cells or peritoneal B cells.

Molecular characterization of IL-5R. When the extracts from radioiodinated T88-M cells or MOPC104E cells were immunoprecipitated and analyzed with SDS-PAGE under reducing conditions, precipitates with H7 (Fig. 4, lanes B and E) and T21 (lanes C and F) showed a major band with M_r 60,000 and a minor band with M_r 45,000. Precipitates with control antibody showed a minor band with M_r 45,000 (Fig. 4, lanes A and D). However, we did not detect a major band with M_r 60,000 with the use of X5563 (lanes H and I). When T88-M cells were preincubated with unlabeled IL-5 (20 μM), followed by immunoprecipitation with H7, the precipitation of M_r 60,000 component was inhibited (data not shown), indicating that at least one of the IL-5R components is the protein with M_r 60,000. Furthermore, the molecule with M_r 60,000 defined by H7 could be digested with N-glycanase to yield a protein band of approximately M_r 55,000 (data not shown). No apparent major bands of higher M_r under nonreducing conditions were detected, suggesting that the IL-5R does not appear to be covalently linked to other proteins with intermolecular disulfide bridges. However, IL-5R appears to have a compact conformation that is stabilized by intramolecular disulfide bridges because the receptor molecule migrated somewhat faster in nonreducing conditions as compared with reducing

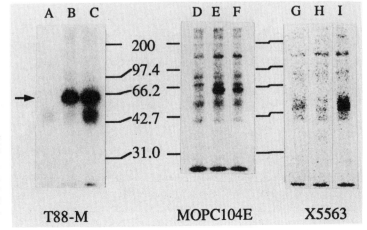

Figure 4. SDS-PAGE and autoradiography of immunoprecipitation of T88-M, MOPC104E, or X5563 cells by H7 (lanes *B*, *E*, and *H*), T21 (lanes *C*, *F*, and *I*), or control IgG (lanes *A*, *D*, and *G*). The proteins adsorbed to antibody-coupled beads were eluted with SDS and were analyzed by SDS-PAGE under reducing conditions. Molecular mass markers are shown in kD.

conditions (data not shown). Recently, Rolink et al. (1989) reported the production of the rat anti-mouse IL-5R MAbs R52.120 and R52.625. Our anti-IL-5R MAbs H7 and T21 seem to recognize different molecules from these recognized by their monoclonal antibodies by two lines of evidence. First, MAbs R52.120 and R52.625 react with 10–15% myeloid cells in the bone marrow, and 10–14% in the peritoneum of adult mice. MAb H7 does not react with bone marrow cells and binds 85–90% peritoneal B cells. Second, MAbs R52.120 and R52.625 precipitate three proteins with M_r 46,000, 130,000, and 140,000. We need more experiments to ascertain relationships of molecules recognized by our monoclonal antibodies and theirs.

The availability of monoclonal antibody against IL-5R will allow many interesting studies to be done in the future. These include biochemical and physiologic characterization of the entire IL-5R and evaluation of the synthesis of the IL-5R at the biochemical and molecular levels. Additional studies will include evaluation of the role of IL-5 in IL-5-driven proliferation in every aspect of B-cell function, including differentiation and maturation of B-cell memory. It will be of great interest to examine the role of the IL-5R molecule in transducing IL-5 signals. Although the identity of an additional protein that appears to be involved in the formation of functional high-affinity receptor remains unclear, it is important to purify sufficient quantities of the receptor by utilizing an immunoaffinity column with H7 or T21. Finally, evaluation of the expression of the IL-5R in various disease states may allow further understanding of the true role of IL-5 in murine B-cell physiology.

CONCLUDING REMARKS

IL-5 is a glycoprotein with a molecular mass of 50,000–60,000 that is produced and secreted by T cells upon stimulation with antigens and mitogens. IL-5 induces at least IgM, IgG$_1$, and IgA production by activated B cells. IL-5-induced IgA production by LPS-stimulated B cells is enhanced by TGF-β, which itself induces IgA-production by LPS-stimulated sIgA$^-$ B cells. IL-5 triggers its targets through specific receptors that consist of two binding sites (high-affinity and low-affinity). The IL-5R molecule recognized by MAb H7 and T21 is a glycoprotein whose M_r is approximately 60,000. More than 90% of sIgM$^+$ B cells from peritoneum are IL-5R$^+$, and 67% of them are also CD5 (Ly-1)$^+$. IL-5-induced IgM production of peritoneal B cells was inhibited by anti-IL-5R monoclonal antibodies, indicating that IL-5R-bearing B cells may consist of a subpopulation of B cells.

ACKNOWLEDGMENTS

We express our deep appreciation to our colleagues for sharing their data and ideas. We thank the many collaborators and generous individuals who have supplied us with reagents, and we thank Drs. K. Ishizaka and K. Onoue for their encouragement and thoughtful suggestions throughout this study. Support was provided in part by a Grant-in-Aid from the Japanese Ministry of Education, Culture, and Science; by Special Coordination Funds for promoting science and technology from the Science and Technology Agency; by a grant from the Osaka Foundation for Promotion of Clinical Immunology; and by a Grant-in-Aid from Tokyo Biochemical Research Foundation.

REFERENCES

Azuma, C., T. Tanabe, M. Konishi, T. Kinashi, T. Noma, F. Matsuda, Y. Yaoita, K. Takatsu, L. Hammerstrom, C.I. Smith, E. Severinson, and T. Honjo. 1987. Cloning of cDNA for human T cell-replacing factor (interleukin 5) and comparison with mouse homologue. *Nucleic Acids Res.* **14:** 9149.

Beagley, K.W., J.H. Eldridge, H. Kiyono, M.P. Everson, W.J. Koopman, T. Honjo, and J.R. McGhee. 1989. Recombinant murine IL-5 induces high rate synthesis in cycling IgA-positive Peyer's patch B cells. *J. Immunol.* **141:** 2035.

Coffman, R., B. Seymour, D. Hiraki, J. Christiansen, B. Shrader, H. Cherwinsky, H. Savelkoul, F. Finkelman, M. Bond, and T. Mosmann. 1988. The role of T cell products in mouse B cell differentiation and isotype regulation. *Immunol. Rev.* **102:** 5.

Harada, N., Y. Kikuchi, A. Tominaga, S. Takaki, and K. Takatsu. 1985. BCGFII activity on activated B cells of a purified murine T cell-replacing factor (TRF) from a T cell hybridoma (B151K12). *J. Immunol.* **134:** 3944.

Harada, N., M. Matsumoto, N. Koyama, A. Shimizu, T. Honjo, A. Tominaga, and K. Takatsu. 1987a. T cell-replacing factor/IL-5 induces not only B-cell growth and differentiation, but also increased expression of IL-2 receptor on activator B cells. *Immunol. Lett.* **15:** 205.

Harada, N., T. Takahashi, M. Matsumoto, T. Kinashi, J. Ohara, Y. Kikuchi, N. Koyama, E. Severinson, Y. Yaoita, T. Honjo, N. Yamaguchi, A. Tominaga, and K. Takatsu. 1987b. Production of a monoclonal antibody useful in the molecular characterization of murine T cell-replacing factor (TRF) and B cell growth factor II (BCGF II). *Proc. Natl. Acad. Sci.* **84:** 4581.

Harriman, G.R., D.Y. Kunimoto, J.F. Elliott, V. Paetkau, and W. Strober. 1988. The role of IL-5 in IgA B cell differentiation. *J. Immunol.* **140:** 3033.

Herzenberg, L.A., A.M. Stall, P.L. Lalor, C. Sidman, W.A. Moore, D.R. Parks, and L.A. Herzenberg. 1986. The Ly-1 B cell lineage. *Immunol. Rev.* **93:** 81.

Howard, M. and W.E. Paul. 1983. Regulation of B-cell growth and differentiation by soluble factors. *Annu. Rev. Immunol.* **1:** 307.

Kinashi, T., N. Harada, E. Severinson, T. Tanabe, P. Sideras, M. Konishi, C. Azuma, A. Tominaga, S. Bergstedt-Lindqvist, M. Takahashi, F. Matsuda, Y. Yaoita, K. Takatsu, and T. Honjo. 1986. Cloning of complementary DNA encoding T cell-replacing factor and identity with B cell-growth factor II. *Nature* **324:** 70.

Kishimoto, T. 1985. Factors affecting B cell growth and differentiation. *Annu. Rev. Immunol.* **3:** 133.

Loughnan, M.S., K. Takatsu, N. Harada, and G.J.V. Nossal. 1987. T cell-replacing factor (IL-5) induces expression of IL-2-R on murine B cells. *Proc. Natl. Acad. Sci.* **84:** 5399.

Matsumoto, R., M. Matsumoto, S. Mita, Y. Hitoshi, M. Ando, S. Araki, N. Yamaguchi, A. Tominaga, and K. Takatsu. 1989. Interleukin 5 induces maturation but not class-switching of surface IgA-positive B cells into IgA-secreting cells. *Immunology* **66:** 32.

Mita, S., N. Harada, S. Naomi, Y. Hitoshi, K. Sakamoto, M. Akagi, A. Tominaga, and K. Takatsu. 1988. Receptors for

T cell-replacing factor (TRF)/interleukin 5 (IL-5). Quantitation, specificity, and its implications. *J. Exp. Med.* **168:** 863.

Mita, S., A. Tominaga, Y. Hitoshi, K. Sakamoto, T. Honjo, M. Akagi, N. Yamaguchi, A. Tominaga, and K. Takatsu. 1989. Characterization of high-affinity receptors for interleukin 5 (IL-5) on IL-5 dependent cell lines. *Proc. Natl. Acad. Sci.* **86:** 2311.

Nakanishi, K., T. Yoshimoto, Y. Katoh, S. Ono, K. Matsui, K. Hiroishi, T. Noma, T. Honjo, K. Takatsu, K. Higashino, and T. Hamaoka. 1988. Both B151-TRF1 and interleukin 5 regulate immunoglobulin secretion and IL 2 receptor expression on a cloned B lymphoma line. *J. Immunol.* **140:** 1168.

Rasmussen, R., K. Takatsu, N. Harada, T. Takahashi, and K. Bottomly. 1988. T cell-dependent hapten-specific and polyclonal B cell responses require release of interleukin 5. *J. Immunol.* **140:** 705.

Rolink, A.G., F. Melchers, and R. Palacios. 1989. Monoclonal antibodies reactive with the mouse interleukin 5 receptor. *J. Exp. Med.* **169:** 1693.

Sanderson, C.J., H.D. Campbell, and I.G. Young. 1988. Molecular and cellular biology of eosinophils differentiation factor (IL-5) and its effect on human and mouse B cells. *Immunol. Rev.* **102:** 29.

Sonoda, E., R. Matsumoto, H. Hitoshi, M. Sugimoto, S. Araki, A. Tominaga, N. Yamaguchi, and K. Takatsu. 1989. Transforming growth factor-beta (TGF-β) induces IgA production and acts additively with IL-5 for IgA production. *J. Exp. Med.* (in press).

Sporn, M.B., A.B. Roberts, L.M. Wakefield, and R.K. Associan. 1986. Transforming growth factor-β: Biological function and chemical structure. *Science* **233:** 532.

Swain, S.L. and R.W. Dutton. 1982. Production of a B cell growth-promoting activity, (DL)BCGF, from a cloned T cell line and its assay on the BCL$_1$ B cell tumor. *J. Exp. Med.* **156:** 1821.

Takahashi, M., M.C. Yoshida, H. Satoh, J. Hilgers, Y. Yaoita, and T. Honjo. 1988. Chromosomal mapping of the mouse IL-4 and human IL-5 genes. *Genomics* **4:** 3256.

Takatsu, K. 1988. B cell growth and differentiation factors. *Proc. Soc. Exp. Biol. Med.* **188:** 243.

Takatsu, K. and T. Hamaoka. 1982. DBA/2Ha mice as a model of an X-linked immunodeficiency which is defective in the expression of TRF-acceptor site(s) on B lymphocytes. *Immunol. Rev.* **64:** 25.

Takatsu, K., A. Tominaga, and T. Hamaoka. 1980a. Antigen-induced T cell-replacing factor (TRF). I. Functional characterization of a TRF-producing helper T cell subset and genetic studies on TRF production. *J. Immunol.* **124:** 2424.

Takatsu, K., K. Tanaka, A. Tominaga, Y. Kumahara, and T. Hamaoka. 1980b. Antigen-induced T cell-replacing factor (TRF). III. Establishment of T cell hybrid clone continuously producing TRF and functional analysis of released TRF. *J. Immunol.* **125:** 2646.

Takatsu, K., Y. Kikuchi, T. Takahashi, T. Honjo, M. Matsumoto, N. Harada, N. Yamaguchi, and A. Tominaga. 1987. Interleukin 5, a T cell derived B cell differentiation factor also induces cytotoxic T lymphocytes. *Proc. Natl. Acad. Sci.* **84:** 4234.

Takatsu, K., A. Tominaga, N. Harada, S. Mita, M. Matsumoto, Y. Kikuchi, T. Takahashi, and N. Yamaguchi. 1988. T cell-replacing factor (TRF)/interleukin 5 (IL-5): Molecular and functional properties. *Immunol. Rev.* **102:** 107.

Tanabe, T., M. Konishi, T. Migita, T. Noma, and T. Honjo. 1987. Molecular cloning and structure of the human interleukin-5 gene. *J. Biol. Chem.* **262:** 16580.

Tominaga, A., M. Matsumoto, N. Harada, T. Takahashi, Y. Kikuchi, and K. Takatsu. 1988. Molecular properties and regulation of mRNA expression for murine T cell-replacing factor (TRF)/IL-5. *J. Immunol.* **140:** 1175.

Tominaga, A., S. Mita, Y. Kikuchi, Y. Hitoshi, K. Takatsu, S.-I. Nishikawa, and M. Ogawa. 1989. Establishment of IL-5 dependent early B cell lines by long-term bone marrow cultures. *Growth Factors* **1:** 135.

Yamaguchi, Y., T. Suda, M. Eguchi, Y. Miura, N. Harada, A. Tominaga, and K. Takatsu. 1988a. Purified interleukin 5 (IL-5) supports the terminal differentiation and of murine eosinophilic precursors. *J. Exp. Med.* **163:** 46.

Yamaguchi, Y., Y. Hayashi, Y. Sugama, Y. Miura, T. Kasahara, S. Kitamura, M. Torisu, S. Mita, A. Tominaga, K. Takatsu, and T. Suda. 1988b. Highly purified murine interleukin 5 (IL-5) stimulates eosinophil function and prolongs in vitro survival: IL5 as an eosinophil chemotactic factor. *J. Exp. Med.* **167:** 1737.

Yokota, T., N. Arai, J. de Vries, H. Spits, J. Banchereau, A. Zlotnik, D. Rennick, M. Howard, Y. Takebe, S. Miyatake, F. Lee, and K. Arai. 1988. Molecular biology of interleukin 4 and interleukin 5 and biology of their products that stimulate B cells, T cells, and hematopoietic cells. *Immunol. Rev.* **102:** 137.

Structure and Regulation of the Leukocyte Adhesion Receptor LFA-1 and Its Counterreceptors, ICAM-1 and ICAM-2

M.L. Dustin, J. Garcia-Aguilar, M.L. Hibbs, R.S. Larson, S.A. Stacker, D.E. Staunton, A.J. Wardlaw, and T.A. Springer

Center for Blood Research, Boston, Massachusetts 02115; Committee on Cell and Developmental Biology and Department of Pathology, Harvard Medical School, Boston, Massachusetts 02115

Immune responses hinge on appropriate interactions between T lymphocytes and antigen-presenting cells (APC) or target cells. Although immunological specificity is mediated by antigen receptors (Bjorkman et al. 1987), antigen-specific cytotoxicity and helper-T-lymphocyte responses require lymphocyte function associated-1 (LFA-1) and other "accessory molecules" (Springer et al. 1987). LFA-1 mediates adhesion between lymphocytes and other cells and, in the process, may inform the cell of its environment via signal transduction mechanisms (Springer et al. 1987; van Noesel et al. 1988), as do other integrins (Menko and Boettinger 1987). Therefore, we will refer to LFA-1 as an adhesion receptor. LFA-1 mediates adhesion by binding to cell-surface molecules on other cells that include ICAM-1 and ICAM-2 (Marlin and Springer 1987; Makgoba et al. 1988b; Staunton et al. 1989a). We will refer to these ligand molecules as counterreceptors, based on the idea that they may also be capable of transducing signals.

In the first part of this paper, we present an overview of recent work on LFA-1 and ICAM structure. In the second part, we present data that address another key problem: How is the LFA-1/ICAM mechanism regulated in interactions of T lymphocytes with other cells? The interaction of lymphocyte adhesion receptors and their counterreceptors has no intrinsic immunological specificity. This raises the question of how adhesion mechanisms function within the context of the immune response; that is, how is T-lymphocyte adhesion regulated? ICAM-1 expression is regulated by cytokines and differentiation with changes occurring over a period of several hours to days (Clark et al. 1986; Dustin et al. 1986). Increasing ICAM-1 expression at sites of inflammation is a powerful mechanism for increasing the potential for interaction of local cells with T lymphocytes. However, these changes are too slow to account for the kinetics of antigen-specific cytolytic T-lymphocyte interactions with target cells in which contact is followed by a brief period of strong adhesion and then detachment from the target cell (Martz 1977; Poenie et al. 1987); we will refer to the latter process as de-adhesion. A clue to a more dynamic mode of regulation was provided by the observation of phorbol-ester-stimulated aggregation of lymphocytes.

Phorbol-ester-stimulated aggregation occurs within 1 hour, is blocked by LFA-1 monoclonal antibody (MAb) and ICAM-1 MAb, but is not accompanied by a change in LFA-1 or ICAM-1 expression (Patarroyo et al. 1985; Rothlein and Springer 1986b; Rothlein et al. 1986). Here, we have further examined phorbol ester stimulation of adhesion in such a way that it was possible to determine whether LFA-1 or ICAM activity is regulated. These observations were extended to examine the effects of stimulation through the T-cell antigen receptor (TCR). Our results show that LFA-1 avidity for ICAM-1 is profoundly increased by phorbol-ester- or TCR-mediated stimulation. The TCR-stimulated increase in avidity is transient, suggesting a mechanism for de-adhesion after execution of TCR-triggered regulatory or effector functions. On the basis of these observations and previous studies that have shown that LFA-1 requires energy for function (Marlin and Springer 1987), we propose that the TCR acts as a switch controlling use of cellular energy to convert LFA-1 from a low-avidity to a high-avidity state.

METHODS

Monoclonal antibodies. The following monoclonal antibodies were used as ascites or purified IgG: TS2/4 (native LFA-1α, IgG1), TS1/18 (native LFA-1β, IgG1), TS1/22 (native or denatured LFA-1α, IgG1) (Sanchez-Madrid et al. 1983), RR1/1 (ICAM-1, IgG1) (Rothlein et al. 1986), OKT3 (CD3, IgG2a) (Kung et al. 1979), and Leu4 (CD3, IgG1, a generous gift from R. Evans) (Evans et al. 1981).

LFA-1 α and β cDNAs. cDNAs have been described previously (Kishimoto et al. 1987; Larson et al. 1989). Amino acid residue numbering is for the mature protein.

RNase mapping and identification of leukocyte adhesion deficiency (LAD) mutations. The location of mutations in β subunits of LAD patients 2 and 14 were determined by forming hybrids of patient RNA with a radiolabeled antisense cDNA probe and digesting the hybrids with RNase A and RNase T1 (A.J. Wardlaw et al., in prep.). This method is sensitive to single mismatches. cDNA libraries prepared with antisense β

oligonucleotides as primers for reverse transcriptase were generated from patient RNA, and clones were isolated using the normal β subunit cDNA as a probe. Dideoxy sequencing of patient cDNAs was used to identify mutations, the locations of which were revealed by RNase mapping (A.J. Wardlaw et al., in prep.). The mutations were introduced into the normal β cDNA in pCDM8 by subcloning of fragments from the mutant β subunit or by site-directed mutagenesis. Sequencing was used to confirm that these were the only mutations.

Oligonucleotide-directed mutations. Point mutations of cDNA inserts were generated in the CDM8 vector according to the method of Kunkel (1985).

Genomic cloning of ICAM-2. A human genomic library (5×10^5 colonies) in the cosmid vector pWE15 (kindly donated by G.A. Evans, Salk Institute, La Jolla, California) on nitrocellulose filters was probed with the human ICAM-2 cDNA by standard methods (J. Garcia-Aguilar and T.A. Springer, in prep.). Three identical 40-kb cosmid clones were obtained. The ICAM-2 gene was in a 9-kb *Sma* fragment that was subcloned into pGEM-7 and sequenced using oligonucleotide-primed dideoxy sequencing.

Transfections. COS cells were transfected with cDNA clones in the CDM8 vector using a standard DEAE-dextran transfection method (Aruffo and Seed 1987). Transient expression was examined by indirect immunofluorescence flow cytometry on day 3 or 4. Patient and control B-lymphoblastoid cell lines (B-LCL) were transfected by electroporation with the β-subunit cDNA in an episomally replicating vector containing an Epstein-Barr virus (EBV) origin of replication and a hygromycin-resistance marker constructed by fusing parts of CDM8 and p205118a (kindly provided by B. Seed, Massachusetts General Hospital, Boston, Massachusetts) (M.L. Hibbs et al., in prep.). Cells were grown in 200 μg/ml hygromycin for 6 weeks to obtain stable lines expressing transfected β subunit.

Adhesion receptor purification. ICAM-1 was immunoaffinity purified from spleens of patients with hairy cell leukemia or from JY B-LCL (Marlin and Springer 1987). LFA-1 was immunoaffinity purified from SKW3 T-lymphoma lysates using the TS2/4 LFA-1 MAb and elution at pH 11.5 in the presence of 2 mM MgCl$_2$ (Dustin and Springer 1989). Monoclonal antibodies were coupled to Sepharose as described previously (March et al. 1974). SKW3 lysates, immunoaffinity isolates, and eluted material were prepared as described previously (Kürzinger and Springer 1982). In batch experiments (described in Fig. 2, lanes 1–10), LFA-1 bound to TS2/4-Sepharose was treated for 30 minutes at 4°C with elution buffer (50 mM triethylamine [pH 11.5], 0.15 M NaCl, 1% octylglucoside [OG] detergent with or without divalent cations). Material remaining bound to the beads was eluted with SDS and subjected to SDS-PAGE. The neutralized pH 11.5

eluates were subjected to a second round of immunoaffinity isolation with anti-β-Sepharose, and the bound material was also eluted with SDS and subjected to SDS-PAGE (Laemmli 1970).

Adhesion receptor reconstitution and binding assays. Purified proteins in 1% OG detergent were combined with phospholipids and liposomes formed by dialysis as described previously (Brian and McConnell 1984). Glass-supported planar membranes were formed on 5-mm coverslips glued to the bottom of 96-well microplates. Alternatively, purified LFA-1 and ICAM-1 in 1% OG were adsorbed to polystyrene microtiter plate wells by addition of 5 μl of the detergent-solubilized protein to 45 μl of 25 mM Tris (pH 8.0), 0.15 M NaCl, 2 mM MgCl$_2$ (TSM). After a 16-hour incubation at 4°C, the plates were incubated for 1 hour at room temperature in 1% BSA/TSM and then washed with assay media. The amount of protein bound was quantitated by radiometric assay with directly iodinated monoclonal antibody at 10 μCi/μg. Binding assays were performed in RPMI 1640, 10% fetal bovine serum (FBS), 25 mM HEPES (pH 7.4) (assay media). Cells labeled with Na$_2^{51}$CrO$_4$ ($\sim 5 \times 10^4$) were pretreated with blocking monoclonal antibody and then centrifuged onto adhesion-molecule-coated surfaces at 10g for 5 minutes and then washed after 5–15 minutes as specified. Alternatively, cells were allowed to settle at 1g for 1 hour before washing. Washing consisted of aspirating media to 50 μl (glass-supported planar membranes) or completely (plastic-adsorbed protein) and adding 200 μl of fresh media eight (planar membranes) or three (plastic-adsorbed protein) times. Resting T cells were isolated from whole blood by plastic adherence and nylon wool filtration and were used within 24 hours of drawing blood. In binding assays, resting T lymphocytes were washed by flicking media from the plates eight times with 100 μl added between each wash. Flicking was more effective for thoroughly removing unbound peripheral blood lymphocytes (PBL-T), which were more difficult to remove by aspiration due to their small size. It was also quicker, allowing more careful kinetic analysis (see below). Since COS cells bind to plastic under standard conditions, different conditions were used to measure binding of transfected COS cells. Binding assays were performed using phosphate-buffered saline (PBS) buffer with 5% FBS, 2 mM MgCl$_2$, and 0.025% NaN$_3$ for 60 minutes at 24°C, followed by four washes using a 26 ga. needle (ICAM-1 transfectants) or an 18 ga. needle (LFA-1 transfectants) for aspiration. The smaller needle used with ICAM-1 transfectants results in slower aspiration and lower shear force.

Conjugate formation assays. Resting T lymphocytes purified as above were labeled with sulfofluorescein diacetate, and LFA-1$^-$ B-LCL were labeled with hydroethidine as described previously (Luce et al. 1985). Resting T lymphocytes were pretreated with CD3 MAb at 4°C and washed. Resting T lymphocytes and B-LCL were mixed at a 1:2 ratio with the appropriate monoclonal antibody or anti-Ig added and allowed to settle for 1 hour at 4°C or centrifuged for 5 minutes at 10g at 24°C before they were incubated 5 minutes at 37°C. The pellets were resuspended by vortexing and analyzed on a Coulter Epics V using filters and data collection modes described previously (Luce et al. 1985).

RESULTS

Leukocyte Adhesion Receptors

Elucidation of the primary structure of LFA-1 and ICAMs has linked these molecules to two adhesion receptor families and a large body of existing knowledge about the function of other members of these families. LFA-1 is a noncovalent heterodimer with an α subunit (CD11a) of 180 kD and a β subunit (CD18) of 95 kD. LFA-1 shares its β subunit polypeptide with two other cell-surface heterodimers, Mac-1 (CD11b) and p150,95 (CD11c). All of these molecules are implicated in adhesion. Elucidation of the primary structure of the β subunit led to the definition of a new adhesion receptor family based on sequence comparison to a previously published chicken fibronectin receptor subunit (Tamkun et al. 1986; Kishimoto et al. 1987). This group is now referred to as the integrin family, after the important concept that these molecules integrate the outside (extracellular matrix and other cells) and inside (cytoskeleton) of cells (Hynes 1987). Currently, three subfamilies are characterized by their distinctive β subunits: β_1, the VLA or fibronectin receptor subfamily; β_2, the leukocyte integrin subfamily that includes LFA-1; and β_3, the IIbIIIa/vitronectin receptor subfamily (Hynes 1987). This organization may require revision on the basis of the recent identification of additional β subunits that associate with previously known α subunits (Cheresh et al. 1989; Kajiji et al. 1989). There is indirect evidence that the concept of cytoskeletal integration may apply to LFA-1 (Kupfer and Singer 1989). Lymphocyte utilization of adhesion receptors that are shared with virtually all other cells in the body suggests that generation of form in the immune system has much in common with morphogenesis in other multicellular systems.

LFA-1 Structure: β Subunit

The primary structure of the β_2 subunit was of particular interest for two reasons: (1) It is shared between all three leukocyte adhesion receptors and (2) it is defective in LAD, a disease characterized by absence of all three leukocyte integrins and by recurrent life-threatening bacterial infections (Anderson and Springer 1987). It was subsequently found that the β subunits are more highly conserved than the α subunits both between species and between subfamilies. The most striking aspect of this conservation is the perfect alignment of the 56 cysteine residues between β subunits (Kishimoto et al. 1987). The concentration of cysteine residues in 4 repeats between residues 449 and 628 (Fig. 1) suggests a relatively rigid structure in terms of mechanical flexibility.

The most highly conserved region among β_1, β_2, and β_3 (53–63% identity) is between residues 100 and 341. Three LAD mutations, in which the β_2 subunit is synthesized but fails to associate with α subunits, fall into this region, suggesting that it is important for $\alpha\beta$ subunit association. The first LAD mutation characterized was caused by a point mutation in a splice-acceptor site resulting in aberrant splicing out of an exon and deletion of residues 310–339 (Kishimoto et al. 1989). We have characterized mutations in two other LAD patients that result in single amino acid substitutions (A.J. Wardlaw, in prep.). Mutations detected by RNase mapping and sequencing of indicated regions in patient cDNA clones cause substitution of glycine 147 to arginine (G147R) in patient 2 and leucine 127 to proline (L127P) in one allele from patient 14 (Fig. 1). Studies on other integrins implicate this highly conserved region of the β subunit in ligand binding. Peptides containing the sequence RGD act as ligand analogs for several integrins (although not for LFA-1). Cross-link-

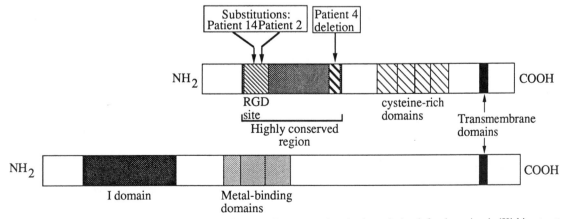

Figure 1. Schematic of LFA-1 α and β subunits. Regions are drawn to scale using boundaries defined previously (Kishimoto et al. 1987, 1989; Larson et al. 1989). The "RGD site" is the smallest gp IIbIIIa peptide to which an RGD peptide was cross-linked (D'Souza et al. 1988) and is highly homologous to the indicated region of the LFA-1 β subunit.

ing of photoaffinity analogs of RGD peptides to a platelet fibrinogen receptor (gpIIbIIIa), followed by isolation and sequencing of labeled fragments (D'Souza et al. 1988), suggests that the highly conserved region (residues 109–171) has a role in ligand binding (Fig. 1). Combination of data about different integrins thus suggests that the ligand-binding region may be one of close association between α and β.

LFA-1 Structure: α Subunit

Although the β subunit is implicated in binding to ligand by the RGD peptide cross-linking studies just mentioned and antibody-blocking experiments, it is clear that different α subunits impart different ligand-binding specificities when associated with the same β subunit. cDNA cloning of LFA-1α (α_L) (Larson et al. 1989) and a number of other α subunits shows that these proteins are structurally related transmembrane proteins (Fig. 1). A striking feature of integrin α subunits including LFA-1 is the presence of either three or four putative divalent cation binding sites that are similar to Ca^{++}/Mg^{++} binding sequences in calmodulin, troponin C, and parvalbumin. Notably, LFA-1 function is dependent on divalent cations, primarily Mg^{++} (Rothlein and Springer 1986). LFA-1, the other leukocyte integrins, and the collagen receptor VLA-2 all have a 200-amino-acid inserted domain (I domain) toward the amino-terminal end of the α subunit (Fig. 1) that is strikingly homologous to the three A domains of von Willebrand factor, two domains of cartilage matrix protein, and a single domain in the complement components C2 and factor B (Corbi et al. 1988; Pytela 1988; Larson et al. 1989; Takada and Hemler 1989). The A1 and A2 domains of von Willebrand factor have been shown to be functional domains in binding of heparin, collagen, and platelet glycoprotein Ib (Girma et al. 1987). The presence of I domains in the leukocyte integrins and VLA-2, but not in four other integrins, suggests that integrins containing the I domain may have more complex ligand recognition, incorporating recognition elements of the I domains as well as recognition elements common to all integrins.

Purification of LFA-1 in Functional Form

We made use of putative divalent cation-binding sites in the α subunit of LFA-1 to purify it in a functionally active form. LFA-1 α and β subunits dissociate under previously described elution conditions (Kürzinger and Springer 1982; Larson et al. 1989) and, as such, are inactive in adhesion assays (M.L. Dustin and T.A. Springer, unpubl.). To test the ability of divalent cations to stabilize LFA-1 subunit interactions, Mg^{++} or Ca^{++} were included in the pH 11.5 buffer used to elute LFA-1 from MAb-Sepharose. This yielded intact $\alpha\beta$ complexes as shown by coprecipitation of the α and β subunits using either β-chain-specific monoclonal antibody (Fig. 2, lanes 6 and 7) or α-chain-specific monoclonal antibody (Fig. 2, lanes 9 and 10). The subunits

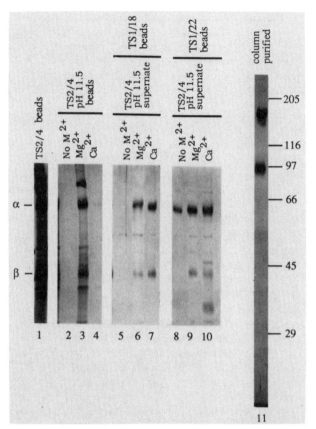

Figure 2. Divalent cation requirements for elution of intact LFA-1 from TS2/4 MAb-Sepharose and SDS-PAGE of purified LFA-1. TS2/4 beads with bound LFA-1 (lane *1*) or material remaining bound to beads after treatment at pH 11.5 in the presence of indicated divalent cation (lanes *2–4*); material re-isolated from neutralized pH 11.5 eluates with TS1/18 MAb (lanes *5–7*) or TS1/22 MAb (lanes *8–10*). Purified LFA-1 (1 μg) (lane *11*). Proteins were heated to 100°C with reducing sample buffer and run on SDS-7%-PAGE. Lanes *1–10* and lane *11* were from different gels.

were dissociated in the absence of divalent cations, resulting in precipitation of only the α subunit alone with α-chain-specific monoclonal antibody and no precipitation with β-chain-specific monoclonal antibody (Fig. 2, lanes 5 and 8). We should point out that removal of divalent cations from LFA-1 solubilized in Triton X-100 at pH 7–8 does not result in dissociation, since intact LFA-1 is readily obtained from cell detergent lysates prepared with EDTA (Sanchez-Madrid et al. 1983). Apart from providing a method for purifying intact LFA-1, these experiments provide the first evidence that divalent cations bind to LFA-1.

Intact LFA-1 purified as described above was tested for cell binding. LFA-1 was reconstituted into unilaminar liposomes at different lipid:protein ratios, and glass-supported planar membranes were formed that had a range of LFA-1 densities. L428 Reed-Sternberg cells and SKW3 T-lymphoma cells bound to these membranes in an LFA-1 density-dependent manner (Fig. 3). This binding was blocked efficiently by LFA-1 monoclonal antibody. Prior cell–cell adhesion studies

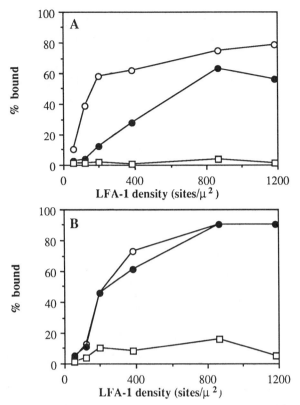

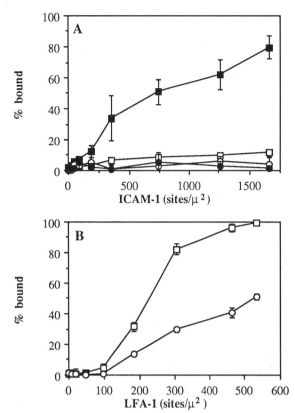

Figure 3. Binding of L428 (*A*) or SKW3 (*B*) cells to LFA-1 in planar membranes. Binding of ^{51}Cr-labeled SKW3 or L428 cells was measured by incubating cells on LFA-1 planar membranes with the indicated density of LFA-1 for 60 min at 37°C and then washing eight times by aspiration. Cells were incubated in the presence of 50 μg/ml control IgG (○), ICAM-1 MAb (●), or LFA-1 MAb (□).

Figure 4. Binding of JY cells to LFA-1 or ICAM-1 adsorbed to plastic at 37°C or 4°C. Binding of ^{51}Cr-labeled JY cells was measured by centrifuging (10*g* for 5 min) cells onto the bottom of microtiter wells coated with the indicated density of purified LFA-1 or ICAM-1 at 4°C and incubating for 10 min at 37°C (squares) or 4°C (circles). Similar results were obtained if cells were allowed to settle for 1 hr at 4°C. Binding to LFA-1 was performed in the presence (filled symbols) and absence (open symbols) of 50 μg/ml ICAM-1 MAb. Binding to ICAM-1 was performed in the presence (filled symbols) or absence (open symbols) of 50 ng/ml PMA. Cells were pretreated with PMA for 30 minutes at 37°C prior to cooling to 4°C for centrifugation. This was required to obtain efficient binding of cells to ICAM-1.

indicated the presence of LFA-1 counterreceptors besides ICAM-1 on several hematopoietic cell lines and endothelial cells. These studies showed that L428 cells have both ICAM-1-dependent and -independent components, whereas SKW3 has only the ICAM-1-independent component (Makgoba et al. 1988a; Rothlein et al. 1986). The ICAM-1 on L428 is only required for binding when LFA-1 is at a relatively low density as indicated by blocking with ICAM-1 monoclonal antibody; at higher LFA-1 density, the other LFA-1 counterreceptor(s) is sufficient for efficient binding. In contrast, binding of SKW3 to LFA-1 is not blocked by ICAM-1 monoclonal antibody at any LFA-1 density, suggesting that ICAM-1 is not involved in this binding. These experiments confirmed the presence of an LFA-1 counterreceptor distinct from ICAM-1 and provided a powerful approach to its functional cloning (see below).

Adhesion mechanisms are susceptible to inhibition at low temperatures; this can indicate a requirement for membrane fluidity (lateral mobility) or metabolic energy. As described previously (Marlin and Springer 1987), binding of JY cells to ICAM-1 substrates is temperature-sensitive with no adhesion observed at 4°C, even when cells are pretreated with phorbol esters

at 37°C (Fig. 4A). However, there is significant binding of JY cells to LFA-1 substrates at 4°C (50% reduced compared to 37°C) (Fig. 4B). The relative contributions of ICAM-1 and other ICAMs to low-temperature binding could not be determined without antibodies to other ICAMs. These reciprocal experiments show that the temperature sensitivity of the LFA-1/ICAM mechanism is due to cell-surface LFA-1. The loss of function of cell-surface LFA-1 at low temperature must be related to a cellular property, since purified LFA-1 can bind cell-surface ICAM-1 at 4°C. Furthermore, purified LFA-1 binds to purified ICAM-1 equally well at 4°C and 37°C (Dustin and Springer 1989).

Expression of Recombinant LFA-1

An important approach to understanding LFA-1 structure/function relationships is to express recombinant LFA-1 molecules in animal cells. When LFA-1 α and β subunits were transfected into COS cells, the chains were assembled properly, and LFA-1 was expressed on the cell surface (not shown) (R.S. Larson et al., in prep.). LFA-1 expressed in COS cells was functional, based on binding of transfected COS cells to ICAM-1 substrates (R.S. Larson et al., in prep.). Transfection of the α subunit alone did not lead to expression of α chain, as would be expected from the LAD patients who lack β_2 and fail to express α. However, transfection of β_2 alone did result in expression of small amounts of human β_2 epitopes. Whether α subunits normally associated with β_1 can complement expression or whether β_2 can be expressed on its own is unknown. The COS cell system was used to express β_2 cDNAs containing the mutations found in LAD patients 2 and 14 (A.J. Wardlaw et al., in prep.). Coexpression in COS cells of the α subunit and β_2 subunit with the L149P mutation led to weak expression of α chain and two β_2 chain epitopes but no expression of the TS1/18 β_2 chain epitope, which requires subunit association, and no detectable ICAM-1-binding activity (not shown). The expression results are consistent with the phenotype of patient 14, who had a moderate deficiency that resulted from two mutant alleles, only one of which has been sequenced. There was no expression in COS cells of α or β epitopes when β subunit with the G169R mutation was cotransfected with the α subunit (not shown). Reversion of these mutant cDNAs to wild type by site-directed mutagenesis restored expression in COS cells. These results confirmed that the changes found in LAD cDNAs can account for the LAD phenotype.

Wild-type β subunit cDNA expressed in EBV-transformed B-LCL derived from LAD patients using an episomally replicating EBV-based vector rescued expression of the LFA-1 complex (Table 1) (M.L. Hibbs et al., in prep.). The LFA-1 was functional, since these cells showed strong phorbol-ester-stimulated adhesion to ICAM-1-coated plates (Table 1 and see below). The ability to rescue LFA-1 expression in LAD patient-derived cell lines provides conclusive evidence that the defect is in the β_2 subunit, a model for future gene therapy, and a powerful system in which to analyze the function of in vitro mutagenized β subunits.

ICAM-1

ICAM-1 is a single-chain glycoprotein of about 90 kD with a deglycosylated size of 55 kD. The identity of ICAM-1 as an LFA-1 counterreceptor was proven by binding of LFA-1$^+$ cells to purified ICAM-1 with

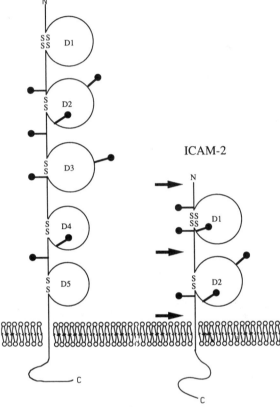

Figure 5. Schematic representation of ICAM-1 and ICAM-2. Loop motifs represent Ig-like domains. The number of SS pairs in each loop represents the number of predicted disulfide bridges between cysteine residues/domain. Domains 4 and 5 of ICAM-1 are missing a β strand present in the other domains. The arrows indicate the positions of exon boundaries determined by genomic cloning of ICAM-2. Each Ig domain is in a single exon.

Table 1. Transfection of LAD Patient B-lymphoblastoid Cells with β Subunit cDNA Restores LFA-1 Surface Expression and Function

LFA-1 Expression (mean fluorescence)		Binding to ICAM-1 substrates (%)	
		Expt. 1	Expt. 2
Control	82	48 ± 2	78 ± 2
Patient 2	1	1.3 ± 0.1	
Patient 2 + β	53	30 ± 2	
Patient 12	0		2.8 ± 0.5
Patient 12 + β	44		31 ± 3

LFA-1 expression was determined by indirect staining and immunofluorescence flow cytometry. The mean fluorescence is given in linear units. Binding of chromium-labeled cells to LFA-1 adsorbed to plastic was performed as in Methods.

specific inhibition by LFA-1 monoclonal antibody (Marlin and Springer 1987). ICAM-1 is a member of the immunoglobulin superfamily and was the first member of this family to be shown to interact with an integrin (Simmons et al. 1988; Staunton et al. 1988). As shown by Greve et al. (1989) and confirmed by Staunton et al. (1989b), ICAM-1 also is the receptor for the major group of rhinoviruses, which are responsible for about 50% of common colds. Coordinate effects of ICAM-1 monoclonal antibody on LFA-1 binding and rhinovirus binding suggest similar interaction sites (Staunton et al. 1989b). Deletion studies were undertaken to localize the LFA-1 and rhinovirus-14 binding sites of ICAM-1 to the smallest region this approach would allow. Sequence homologies predict that ICAM-1 is folded into 5 Ig-like domains (Fig. 5). ICAM-1 with 1 or 2 domains deleted by oligonucleotide-directed mutagenesis was expressed in COS cells (D.E. Staunton et al., in prep.). ICAM-1 constructs with domain 3 or domains 4 + 5 deleted are well expressed, based on

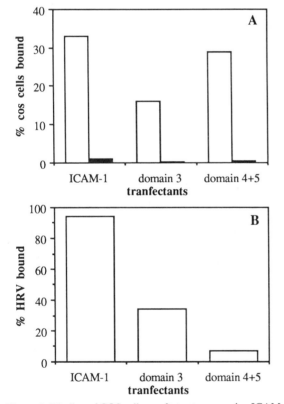

Figure 6. Binding of COS cell transfectants expressing ICAM-1 and ICAM-1 deletion mutants to LFA-1 on plastic. Forms of ICAM-1 with deletions between residues 185 and 284 (domain 3⁻) and residues 284 and 489 (domain 4 + 5⁻) were generated by oligonucleotide-directed mutagenesis. (*A*) Binding of ^{51}Cr-labeled cells was measured in the presence (filled bars) and absence (open bars) of 10 μg/ml ICAM-1 MAb. (*B*) Binding of ^{35}S-labeled rhinovirus 14 (HRV) was performed as described previously (Staunton et al. 1989b). COS cell and rhinovirus binding is normalized for variations in COS cell expression of ICAM-1 forms using mean linear fluorescence intensity determined by indirect immunofluorescence flow cytometry with the RR1/1 MAb.

immunofluorescence, and are functional in binding to LFA-1 and rhinovirus 14 (Fig. 6). The low rhinovirus-14 binding to the ICAM-1 domain 4 + 5 deletion may be due to decreased distance of the binding domains from the cell membrane, leading to greater steric hindrance from the glycocalyx. However, this binding is significant, suggesting that this construct does retain the binding site for the rhinovirus 14. On the basis of these data, the LFA-1 and rhinovirus-14 binding site on ICAM-1 binding site can be localized to domain 1 and/or 2.

Identification of ICAM-2

Recently, a second LFA-1 counterreceptor, ICAM-2, has been cloned using functional screening in COS cells (Staunton et al. 1989a). A cDNA was isolated that conferred on COS cells the ability to bind to purified LFA-1 coated on petri dishes in the presence of ICAM-1 monoclonal antibody. ICAM-2 is smaller than ICAM-1 with two predicted Ig-domains that are 34% homologous to the two most amino-terminal domains of ICAM-1 (Fig. 5). Although ICAM-1 and ICAM-2 might appear to account for all of the functional data on LFA-1 counterreceptors, the existence of other counterreceptors cannot be ruled out. The ability of ICAM-2 to bind LFA-1 while having only two Ig-like domains is consistent with mapping of the LFA-1-binding site of ICAM-1 to domains 1 and 2. Genomic cloning of ICAM-2 (J. Garcia-Aguilar and T.A. Springer, in prep.) shows that each of the predicted Ig-like domains of ICAM-2 is encoded in a separate exon (Fig. 5), as has been found for most other members of the Ig superfamily. Other members, such as NCAM, have two exons per domain.

Regulation of the LFA-1/ICAM-1 Adhesion Pathway

Understanding regulation of the LFA-1/ICAM adhesion mechanism is crucial to understanding how adhesion receptors can participate in antigen-specific interactions in the immune system. Early experiments with peritoneal exudate cytotoxic T lymphocytes (CTL) demonstrated a fivefold preference of CTL to bind to specific antigen-expressing targets rather than to an identical cell type not expressing the appropriate antigen (Berke and Levey 1972). Prior to knowledge of adhesion receptors, it was suggested that this adhesion was mediated by the TCR binding to specific antigen on target cells. Generation of function-blocking monoclonal antibody to CTL led to discovery of the "accessory molecules" LFA-1 and Lyt-2, which were proposed to act with antigen receptors to mediate adhesion (Springer et al. 1982). It was subsequently speculated that LFA-1 might be involved in a TCR-regulated "adhesion strengthening" step (Martz et al. 1983). However, this speculation received little acceptance because no experimental evidence in support of it was obtained. Quite the opposite idea became accepted—that interaction mediated by LFA-1 preceded antigen recognition based on studies using cloned human CTL, which showed that these cells adhere strongly to a wide range of target cell types regardless of antigen recognition (Shaw et al. 1986; Spits et al. 1987). These results are at odds with the numerous results obtained with murine CTL (Martz 1987). We believe that this discrepancy may be related to the manner in which the human CTL were maintained in vitro or the time period after restimulation at which they were used. Both murine and human CTL are able to recycle (kill multiple targets); they must be able to "de-adhere" from targets. Therefore, we examined the possibility that the LFA-1/ICAM adhesion mechanism could be involved in antigen-specific adhesion and de-adhesion.

We became interested in the question of LFA-1 regulation when it was observed by us and other investigators that phorbol-ester-stimulated leukocyte homotypic adhesion was dependent on LFA-1 (Patarroyo et al. 1985; Rothlein and Springer 1986). The first issue we addressed was whether LFA-1 avidity, ICAM avidity, or some general cellular property, such as ability to spread on substrates, was modulated by phorbol ester activation. An ideal system in which to study this question is binding of cells that express both LFA-1 and ICAMs to purified LFA-1 or purified ICAM-1 on inert surfaces. These reciprocal studies allowed the effects of phorbol esters or other stimuli on single cell-surface adhesion receptors to be determined. The SKW3 T lymphoma, the JY B-LCL, and resting T cells adhere to ICAM-1-coated substrates very poorly, if at all (Fig. 7A,C). In contrast, binding of the same cells to LFA-1 is highly efficient (Fig. 7B,D), as was observed in the planar membrane system. This result alone suggests a difference in the nature of cell-surface ICAM-1 and LFA-1: The former is constitutively active on most cells, whereas the latter is not. Addition of phorbol ester resulted in a dramatic increase in adhesion of all three cell types to ICAM-1, but no change or a twofold shift in the concentration dependence of binding to LFA-1. This result clearly demonstrates that the activity of cell-surface LFA-1 is profoundly regulated by phorbol esters, but the activity of cell-surface ICAMs is not. The shift in the LFA-1 density-dependence of binding of JY or SKW3 cells in the presence of phorbol myristic acetate (PMA) was correlated with increased spreading, which may be related to a nonspecific effect of PMA on cell deformability. It is also clear that ICAMs expressed on SKW3 or resting T cells (ICAM-2?) as well as ICAM-1 expressed on JY cells do not show avidity regulation, but it is not known at this point whether cell-surface LFA-1 avidity for ICAM-2 is regulated as it is for ICAM-1. Purified ICAM-2 will be required for these studies.

TCR Regulation of LFA-1 Avidity

Is regulation of cell-surface LFA-1 avidity physiologically relevant to antigen-specific T lymphocyte cell–cell interactions? The ability of TCR ligation to trigger increased LFA-1 avidity was tested. TCR cross-linking on resting T cells with mouse CD3 monoclonal antibody and anti-mouse Ig is required to obtain a rapid increase in phosphatidylinositol (PtdIns) turnover and intracellular Ca^{++} (Lerner et al. 1988). Resting T cells were used, since they had low basal adhesion to ICAM-1 and are clearly a relevant model for cells taking part in the initiation of immune responses. CD3 monoclonal antibody of the IgG subclass alone had no effect on adhesion to ICAM-1, but addition of anti-Ig caused a dramatic increase in T-cell adhesion to ICAM-1 (Fig. 7C). In contrast, there was no effect of TCR cross-linking on binding to LFA-1 (Fig. 7D). This process had specificity for CD3, since cross-linking a CD5 monoclonal antibody, which bound to the same number of sites per cell, induced only a twofold increase in binding (not shown). The TCR-triggered adhesion to ICAM-1 was completely blocked by LFA-1 monoclonal antibody or ICAM-1 monoclonal antibody (not shown).

Does the effect of TCR cross-linking on LFA-1 avidity occur through direct communication or signaling pathways? TCR-mediated signaling, including PtdIns-turnover and tyrosine phosphorylation, are blocked by elevation of cytoplasmic cAMP prior to receptor cross-linking (Kaibuchi et al. 1982; Klausner et al. 1987; Lerner et al. 1988). Treatment of resting T cells with the cell-permeable cAMP analog, dibutyryl cAMP (dbcAMP), prior to TCR cross-linking strongly inhibited stimulation of binding to ICAM-1 substrates. A similar effect was seen with the adenylate cyclase activator forskolin (25 μM) in combination with the phosphodiesterase inhibitor IBMX (0.5 mM) (not shown). However, dbcAMP or forskolin/IBMX had no effect on PMA-stimulated adhesion (Fig. 7C), indicating that inhibition of the TCR-stimulated adhesion was not due to toxicity. This suggests that the TCR effect on LFA-1 occurs via cytosolic second messengers and that LFA-1 is a transducer of signals from the cytosol to the extracellular space; i.e., inside-out signaling.

The kinetics of the TCR-stimulated increase in LFA-1 avidity was examined with the hope that its reversal could provide a mechanism for the de-adhesion of antigen-specific T lymphocytes. Strikingly, when anti-Ig was added to CD3 monoclonal-antibody-treated resting T cells in suspension and variable amounts of time were allowed to elapse before centrifuging cells onto ICAM-1 substrates, adhesion to ICAM-1 peaked at 10 minutes and decreased to basal levels by 30 minutes (Fig. 7E). In contrast, cells treated with PMA in suspension remained in the high LFA-1 avidity state for at least 40 minutes. There was no change in LFA-1 density at 0, 5, or 30 minutes after cross-linking as determined with fluorescein isothiocyanate (FITC)-LFA-1 monoclonal antibody and immunofluorescence flow cytometry (not shown). Furthermore, cells treated with CD3 monoclonal antibody and anti-Ig for 30 minutes and then treated with phorbol ester again adhered efficiently to ICAM-1, suggesting that 30 minutes after TCR cross-linking, the adhesion machinery was still intact but was no longer activated (not shown).

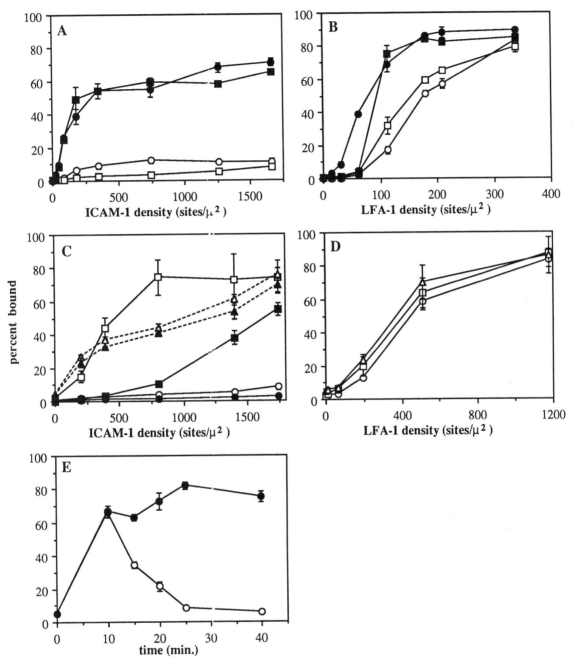

Figure 7. Effect of activation on binding of lymphocytes to ICAM-1 or LFA-1. Binding of JY cells (circles) or SKW3 cells (squares) to ICAM-1 (*A*) or LFA-1 (*B*) on plastic at indicated density in the absence (open symbol) or presence (filled symbol) of 50 ng/ml PMA. Resting T-lymphocyte binding to ICAM-1 (*C*) or LFA-1 (*D*) with no addition (circles), 50 ng/ml PMA (triangles), or mouse CD3 MAb and anti-mouse IgG (squares) all in the absence (open symbols) or presence (filled symbols) of 1 mM dbcAMP. (*E*) Kinetics of PMA or CD3 MAb-stimulated binding to ICAM-1 (1000 sites/μ^2). PMA or anti-mouse IgG was added to untreated or CD3 MAb-pretreated cells in suspension, respectively, and the cells were centrifuged onto the plate at the indicated period of time. Included in the time shown is the 5-min centrifugation and 6-min incubation on the ICAM-1 substrate.

Does TCR cross-linking have a similar effect on cell–cell adhesion in the presence of other adhesion pathways? Furthermore, are other adhesion mechanisms regulated by the TCR? These are important questions, since the interaction of cloned CTL with target cells is not only dependent on the LFA-1/ICAM mechanism, but also on the CD2/LFA-3 adhesion mechan-

ism. Conjugate formation between resting T lymphocytes and LFA-1⁻ B-LCL was determined by two-color fluorescence flow cytometry (Luce et al. 1985). In this system, a low level of spontaneous conjugate formation was observed (Fig. 8) in contrast to the high level (40–80%) observed with cloned CTL adhering to B-LCL targets. The efficiency of conjugate formation was

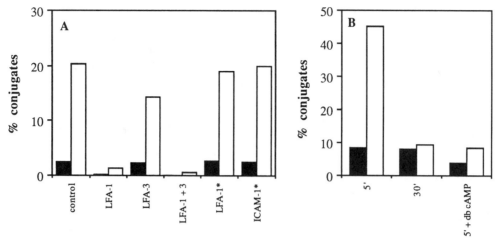

Figure 8. Conjugate formation between resting T lymphocytes and B-LCL. (*A*) Resting T lymphocytes labeled with sulfofluorescein diacetate were preincubated without (filled bars) or with (open bars) OKT3 CD3 MAb at 4°C and washed three times. Pretreated T lymphocytes (1.7×10^6) were allowed to co-sediment with hydroethidine-labeled B-LCL (3.3×10^6) in 50 μl for 1 hr at 4°C in the presence of 5 μg/ml anti-mouse IgG2a and the indicated IgG1 MAb. The pellet was incubated at 37°C for 6 min, resuspended by vortexing, and analyzed by fluorescence flow cytometry. (*B*) Similar to above, except T and B cells were co-centrifuged 20g for 5 min at 24°C. Resting T cells were pretreated 30 min at 37°C with anti-mouse IgG2a or 15 min at 24°C with 1 mM dbcAMP where indicated. The centrifugation was needed to allow kinetic study and study of dbcAMP effect under conditions used for binding to purified adhesion receptors.

dramatically increased by cross-linking the TCR, and the stimulated adhesion was completely inhibited by LFA-1 monoclonal antibody but only partially inhibited by CD2 or LFA-3 monoclonal antibody (Fig. 8A), and showed the same transience as adhesion to substrate with basal adhesion 30 minutes after cross-linking (Fig. 8B). TCR-stimulated cell–cell adhesion was also inhibited by dbcAMP. Thus, regulation of LFA-1 avidity is distinct from regulation of CD2 (Selvaraj et al. 1987). Furthermore, these results show that the LFA-1 adhesion mechanism has a prominent role in regulating interactions with targets expressing both ICAM-1 and LFA-3.

DISCUSSION

The current model for structure of LFA-1 and other integrins is not highly refined, but homologies, analysis of mutations affecting subunit association, and chemical cross-linking studies with RGD peptides point to potentially important regions of α and β subunits. The most striking features of the α subunit are the I domain and the putative divalent cation repeats. The I domain may be a relatively independent folding unit, based on its appearance in many different contexts. It is attractive to speculate that the I domain may have a critical role in binding to counterreceptors; this is consistent with the ligand-binding role of the homologous "A" domains in vWF. However, the general requirement for divalent cations in all integrin-mediated interaction suggests that the putative metal-binding repeats may have an important role in binding or in maintaining an active conformation of other sites (Hynes 1987). Direct binding of divalent cations to two other integrins has been demonstrated previously (Gailit and Ruoslahti

1988). The most direct evidence for the function of putative divalent cation-binding sites in LFA-1 is the ability of Mg^{++} and Ca^{++} to stabilize LFA-1 subunit interactions at high pH (this paper and M.L. Dustin and T.A. Springer, in prep.). This explains the Mg^{++} requirement of LFA-1/ICAM interaction. The identification of two point mutations that can cause the LAD phenotype in a highly conserved region of the β subunit suggests that the region of β implicated in RGD binding by photoaffinity labeling (D'Souza et al. 1988) may also be a critical region of the β subunit for contact with α. This is consistent with α and β coming together to form a binding pocket, the conformation of which may be profoundly affected by divalent cations bound to the α subunit. The conformation of this hypothetical pocket could also be a target for regulation of LFA-1 avidity by phorbol esters or TCR signaling. Systems to express in vitro mutated α and β subunits are available to test these hypotheses.

ICAM-1 structure is more easily modeled, since ICAM-1 is homologous to immunoglobulins, for which high-resolution crystal structures are available. The deletion studies suggest that the minimal unit for expression and function comprises the two amino-terminal Ig-like domains. This is supported by the two-domain structure of ICAM-2.

We have succeeded in resolving LFA-1- and ICAM-mediated adhesion and have strong evidence that LFA-1 avidity for ICAM-1 is regulated. Adhesion of lymphocytes to purified ICAM-1 adsorbed to plastic was dramatically increased by phorbol ester treatment, whereas adhesion of the same cell types to purified LFA-1 on plastic was slightly affected by phorbol ester treatment, the most dramatic effect being an increase in cell spreading. A role of LFA-1 avidity regulation in antigen-specific interactions was revealed by TCR cross-linking, which increases LFA-1 avidity without affecting cell-surface ICAMs or CD2, the latter in a cell–cell adhesion system. The TCR stimulation of LFA-1 avidity appeared to be mediated by intracellular signals, since it was blocked by dbcAMP or agents that increase cytoplasmic cAMP by endogenous mechanisms. A striking characteristic of the TCR-stimulated increase in LFA-1 avidity is that it peaks at 5–10 minutes after cross-linking and returns to basal levels by 30 minutes. This transience is consistent with the ability of T lymphocytes to de-adhere from antigen-presenting cells or target cells expressing specific antigens. The kinetics of the increase and subsequent decrease in LFA-1 avidity is very similar to the kinetics of CTL/ target interactions (Martz 1977; Poenie et al. 1987). The kinetics of LFA-1 avidity changes and adhesion may be influenced by the extent of TCR cross-linking and the density of ICAMs. In this regard, lymphokines generated by T cells are potent up-regulators of ICAM-1 on several cell types (Dustin et al. 1988) and such that products of T-cell activation could influence adhesion kinetics over the course of an immune response.

Regulation of LFA-1 avidity by the TCR provides a mechanism for adhesion molecule function within the context of specific immune recognition. We would propose that LFA-1 is in a low-avidity state or inactive on resting T lymphocytes. When T lymphocytes encounter antigen-expressing target cells, ligation of the TCR results in conversion of LFA-1 to a high-avidity state leading to strong adhesion. A subsequent change in a second-messenger profile may cause the return of LFA-1 to the low-avidity state allowing de-adhesion.

The mechanism by which LFA-1 avidity is regulated by PMA or the TCR is not known but should be attacked from many angles in the next few years. A change in LFA-1 conformation or redistribution in the membrane seems most likely. A striking property of cell-surface LFA-1-dependent adhesion is the requirement for elevated temperature and energy, which is not seen for cell-surface ICAMs (above and not shown). We propose that the conversion of LFA-1 from the low- to high-avidity states triggered by the TCR requires input of metabolic energy. Phosphorylation of the cytoplasmic domain of LFA-1, or of another protein with which it interacts, may be the switch regulated by the TCR. The energy input, utilized to drive the equilibrium between adherence and nonadherence toward adherence, may be analogous to the energy used to drive an otherwise unfavorable biochemical reaction. Avidity regulation is not unique to LFA-1. Another well-characterized example is the integrin gpIIbIIIa on platelets, which does not bind fibrinogen on inactivated platelets but shows high-affinity binding (29–45 mM K_d) after treatment of platelets with ADP (Di Minno et al. 1983). Another potential example of transient avidity regulation is stimulation of Mac-1-dependent binding of neutrophils to bind iC3b opsonized erythrocytes, endothelial cells, or each other by PMA or chemotactic

peptides, which has similar kinetics to the increase in LFA-1 avidity reported here (Wright and Meyer 1986; Buyon et al. 1988; Lo et al. 1989). However, these experiments are less well controlled than those described here, since stimulation of neutrophil aggregation may also involve up-regulation of the counterreceptor, which is not defined. Mac-1 is present in an intracellular pool in monocytes and granulocytes, which may be up-regulated or exchanged with cell-surface Mac-1 (there is no intracellular pool of LFA-1 in lymphocytes), and PMA has drastic effects on monocytes and granulocytes, resulting in strong activation of the respiratory burst, degranulation, vacuolation, and proteolytic removal of surface proteins (Wright and Meyer 1986; Huizinga et al. 1988). Phorbol esters induce transient effects in neutrophils while producing sustained effects in lymphocytes; it is possible that transience in neutrophils reflects mechanisms different from those defined here. Mac-1 has been shown to cluster in the plane of the membrane upon stimulation with kinetics similar to those of iC3b binding (Detmers et al. 1987). One possible mechanism for avidity increase and clusterings for integrins is interactions with cytoskeletal proteins such as talin (Burridge and Connell 1983). In fact, talin has been shown to colocalize with LFA-1 to sites of adhesion in antigen-specific helper T-lymphocyte interactions with B cells, suggesting that this putative interaction may be regulated by the TCR (Kupfer and Singer 1989). However, this redistribution has not been correlated with a change in LFA-1 avidity or the efficiency of adhesion. It is intriguing that talin/LFA-1 co-redistribution was more sensitive to antigen dose than the reorientation of the Golgi apparatus and microtubule organizing center, which are associated with directed lymphokine secretion by helper T cells and lethal hit delivery by CTL.

We have defined the primary structure of the adhesion receptor LFA-1 and its counterreceptors ICAM-1 and ICAM-2. We also present a mechanism by which these molecules can be used to dynamically regulate lymphocyte adhesion. The inside-out signaling through LFA-1 may be a general capability of integrins and could be of general importance in regulating cell–cell and cell–matrix interactions during development or tissue remodeling. TCR stimulation of T lymphocytes led to a temporal gradient of LFA-1 activity. The same mechanisms acting at different parts of a cell could generate spatial gradients of adhesion receptor avidity. In the model studied here, the TCR was ligated all over the cell with a soluble monoclonal antibody, whereas in the physiological interactions, TCR would be engaged only at the site of cell contact, and avidity enhancement might only apply to LFA-1 molecules in or recruited to that area, generating a spatial gradient of LFA-1 avidity. Intrinsic or chemotactic factor-driven spatial gradients of integrin avidity from high at the leading edge of a cell to low at the trailing edge could provide a means for de-adhesion at the trailing edge (Bretscher 1988) and could drive cell migration.

REFERENCES

Anderson, D.C. and T.A. Springer. 1987. Leukocyte adhesion deficiency: An inherited defect in the Mac-1, LFA-1, and p150,95 glycoproteins. *Annu. Rev. Med.* **38:** 175.

Aruffo, A. and B. Seed. 1987. Molecular cloning of a CD28 cDNA by a high efficiency COS cell expression system. *Proc. Natl. Acad. Sci.* **84:** 8573.

Berke, G. and R.H. Levey. 1972. Cellular immunoabsorbents in transplantation immunity. Specific in vitro deletion and recovery of mouse lymphoid cells sensitized against allogeneic tumors. *J. Exp. Med.* **135:** 972.

Bjorkman, P.J., M.A. Saper, B. Samraoui, W.S. Bennett, J.L. Strominger, and D.C. Wiley. 1987. The foreign antigen binding site and T cell recognition regions of class I histocompatibility antigens. *Nature* **329:** 512.

Bretscher, M.S. 1988. Fibroblasts on the move. *J. Cell Biol.* **106:** 235.

Brian, A.A. and H.M. McConnell. 1984. Allogeneic stimulation of cytotoxic T cells by supported planar membranes. *Proc. Natl. Acad. Sci.* **81:** 6159.

Burridge, K. and L.J. Connell. 1983. A new protein of cell adhesion plaques and ruffling membranes. *J. Cell Biol.* **97:** 359.

Buyon, J.P., S.B. Abramson, M.R. Philips, S.G. Slade, G.D. Ross, G. Weissman, and R.J. Winchester. 1988. Dissociation between increased surface expression of Gp165/95 and homotypic neutrophil aggregation. *J. Immunol.* **140:** 3156.

Cheresh, D.A., J.W. Smith, H.M. Cooper, and V. Quaranta. 1989. A novel vitronectin receptor integrin ($\alpha_v \beta_x$) is responsible for distinct adhesive properties of carcinoma cells. *Cell* **57:** 59.

Clark, E.A., J.A. Ledbetter, R.C. Holly, P.A. Dinndorf, and G. Shu. 1986. Polypeptides on human B lymphocytes associated with cell activation. *Hum. Immunol.* **16:** 100.

Corbi, A.L., T.K. Kishimoto, L.J. Miller, and T.A. Springer. 1988. The human leukocyte adhesion glycoprotein Mac-1 (complement receptor type 3, CD11b) α subunit: Cloning, primary structure, and relation to the integrins, von Willebrand factor and factor B. *J. Biol. Chem.* **263:** 12403.

Detmers, P.A., S.D. Wright, E. Olsen, B. Kimball, and Z.A. Cohn. 1987. Aggregation of complement receptors on human neutrophils in the absence of ligand. *J. Cell Biol.* **105:** 1137.

DiMinno, G., P. Thiagarajan, B. Perussia, J. Martinez, S. Shapiro, G. Trinchieri, and S. Murphy. 1983. Exposure of platelet fibrinogen-binding sites by collagen, arachidonic acid, and ADP: Inhibition by a monoclonal antibody to the glycoprotein IIb-IIIa complex. *Blood* **61:** 140.

D'Souza, S.E., M.H. Ginsberg, T.A. Burke, S.C.-T. Lam, and E.F. Plow. 1988. Localization of an Arg-Gly-Asp recognition site within an integrin adhesion receptor. *Science* **242:** 91.

Dustin, M.L. and T.A. Springer. 1989. Linkage between antigen receptors and the adhesion molecule LFA-1 regulates lymphocyte adhesion and deadhesion. *Nature* (in press).

Dustin, M.L., D.E. Staunton, and T.A. Springer. 1988. Supergene families meet in the immune system. *Immunol. Today* **9:** 213.

Dustin, M.L., R. Rothlein, A.K. Bhan, C.A. Dinarello, and T.A. Springer. 1986. Induction of IL-1 and interferon, tissue distribution, biochemistry, and function of a natural adherence molecule (ICAM-1). *J. Immunol.* **137:** 245.

Evans, R.L., D.W. Wall, C.D. Platsoucas, F.P. Siegal, S.M. Fikrig, C.M. Testa, and R.A. Good. 1981. Thymus-dependent membrane antigens in man: Inhibition of cell-mediated lympholysis by monoclonal antibodies to TH2 antigen. *Proc. Natl. Acad. Sci.* **78:** 544.

Gailit, J. and E. Ruoslahti. 1988. Regulation of the fibronectin receptor affinity by divalent cations. *J. Biol. Chem.* **263:** 12927.

Girma, J.-P., D. Meyer, C.L. Verweij, H. Pannekoek, and J.J. Sixma. 1987. Structure-function relationship of human von Willebrand factor. *Blood* **70:** 605.

Greve, J.M., G. Davis, A.M. Meyer, C.P. Forte, S.C. Yost, C.W. Marlor, M.E. Kamarck, and A. McClelland. 1989. The major human rhinovirus receptor is ICAM-1. *Cell* **56:** 839.

Huizinga, T.W.J., C.E. Van Der Schoot, C. Jost, R. Klaassen, M. Kleijer, A.E.G.K. Von dem Borne, D. Roos, and P.A.T. Tetteroo. 1988. The PI-linked receptor FcRIII is released on stimulation of neutrophils. *Nature* **333:** 667.

Hynes, R.O. 1987. Integrins: A family of cell surface receptors. *Cell* **48:** 549.

Kaibuchi, K., Y. Takai, Y. Ogawa, S. Kimura, Y. Nishizuka, T. Nakamura, A. Tomomura, and A. Ichihara. 1982. Inhibitory action of adenosine 3',5'-monophosphate on phosphatidylinositol turnover: Difference in tissue response. *Biochem. Biophys. Res. Commun.* **104:** 105.

Kajiji, S., R.N. Tamura, and V. Quaranta. 1989. A novel integrin (alpha E beta 4) from human epithelial cells suggests a fourth family of integrin adhesion receptors. *EMBO J.* **8:** 673.

Kishimoto, T.K., K. O'Connor, and T.A. Springer. 1989. Leukocyte adhesion deficiency: Aberrant splicing of a conserved integrin sequence causes a moderate deficiency phenotype. *J. Biol. Chem.* **264:** 3588.

Kishimoto, T.K., K. O'Connor, A. Lee, T.M. Roberts, and T.A. Springer. 1987. Cloning of the beta subunit of the leukocyte adhesion proteins: Homology to an extracellular matrix receptor defines a novel supergene family. *Cell* **48:** 681.

Klausner, R.D., J.J. O'Shea, H. Luong, P. Ross, J.A. Bluestone, and L.E. Samelson. 1987. T cell receptor tyrosine phosphorylation. Variable coupling for different activating ligands. *J. Biol. Chem.* **262:** 12654.

Kürzinger, K. and T.A. Springer. 1982. Purification and structural characterization of LFA-1, a lymphocyte function-associated antigen, and Mac-1, a related macrophage differentiation antigen. *J. Biol. Chem.* **257:** 12412.

Kung, P.C., G. Goldstein, E.L. Reinherz, and S.F. Schlossman. 1979. Monoclonal antibodies defining distinctive human T cell surface antigens. *Science* **206:** 347.

Kunkel, T.A. 1985. Rapid and efficient site-specific mutagenesis without phenotypic selection. *Proc. Natl. Acad. Sci.* **82:** 488.

Kupfer, A. and S.J. Singer. 1989. Cell biology of cytotoxic and helper T cell functions. Immunofluorescence microscopic studies of single cells and cell couples. *Annu. Rev. Immunol.* **7:** 309.

Laemmli, U.K. 1970. Cleavage of structural proteins during the assembly of the head of bacteriophage T4. *Nature* **227:** 680.

Larson, R.S., A.L. Corbi, L. Berman, and T.A. Springer. 1989. Primary structure of the LFA-1 α subunit: An integrin with an embedded domain defining a protein superfamily. *J. Cell Biol.* **108:** 703.

Lerner, A., B. Jacobson, and R.A. Miller. 1988. Cyclic AMP concentrations modulate both calcium flux and hydrolysis of phosphatidylinositol phosphates in mouse T lymphocytes. *J. Immunol.* **140:** 936.

Lo, S.K., P.A. Detmers, S.M. Levin, and S.D. Wright. 1989. Transient adhesion of neutrophils to endothelium. *J. Exp. Med.* **169:** 1779.

Luce, G.G., S.O. Sharrow, S. Shaw, and P.M. Gallop. 1985. Enumeration of cytotoxic cell-target cell conjugates by flow cytometry using internal fluorescent stains. *BioTechniques* **3:** 270.

Makgoba, M.W., M.E. Sandes, G.E.G. Luce, E.A. Gugel, M.L. Dustin, T.A. Springer, and S. Shaw. 1988a. Functional evidence that intercellular adhesion molecule-1 (ICAM-1) is a ligand for LFA-1 in cytotoxic T cell recognition. *Eur. J. Immunol.* **18:** 637.

Makgoba, M.W., M.E. Sanders, G.E.G. Luce, M.L. Dustin, T.A. Springer, E.A. Clark, P. Mannoni, and S. Shaw.

1988b. ICAM-1: Definition by multiple antibodies of a ligand for LFA-1 dependent adhesion of B, T and myeloid cell. *Nature* **331:** 86.

March, S.C., I. Parikh, and P. Cuatrecasas. 1974. A simplified method for cyanogen bromide activation of agarose for affinity chromatography. *Anal. Biochem.* **60:** 149.

Marlin, S.D. and T.A. Springer. 1987. Purified intercellular adhesion molecule-1 (ICAM-1) is a ligand for lymphocyte function-associated antigen 1 (LFA-1). *Cell* **51:** 813.

Martz, E. 1977. Mechanism of specific tumor cell lysis by alloimmune T-lymphocytes: Resolution and characterization of discrete steps in the cellular interaction. *Contemp. Top. Immunobiol.* **7:** 301.

———. 1987. LFA-1 and other accessory molecules functioning in adhesions of T and B lymphocytes. *Hum. Immunol.* **18:** 3.

Martz, E., W. Heagy, and S.H. Gromkowski. 1983. The mechanism of CTL-mediated killing: Monoclonal antibody analysis of the roles of killer and target cell membrane proteins. *Immunol. Rev.* **72:** 73.

Menko, A.S. and D. Boettinger. 1987. Occupation of the extracellular matrix receptor, integrin, is a control point for myogenic differentiation. *Cell* **51:** 51.

Patarroyo, M., P.G. Beatty, J.W. Fabre, and C.G. Gahmberg. 1985. Identification of a cell surface protein complex mediating phorbol ester-induced adhesion (binding) among human mononuclear leukocytes. *Scand. J. Immunol.* **22:** 171.

Poenie, M., R.Y. Tsien, and A. Schmitt-Verhulst. 1987. Sequential activation and lethal hit measured by $[Ca^{++}]_i$ in individual cytolytic T cells and targets. *EMBO J.* **6:** 2223.

Pytela, R. 1988. Amino acid sequence of the murine Mac-1 alpha chain reveals homology with the integrin family and an additional domain related to von Willebrand factor. *EMBO J.* **7:** 1371.

Rothlein, R. and T.A. Springer. 1986. The requirement for lymphocyte function-associated antigen 1 in homotypic leukocyte adhesion stimulated by phorbol ester. *J. Exp. Med.* **163:** 1132.

Rothlein, R., M.L. Dustin, S.D. Marlin, and T.A. Springer. 1986. A human intercellular adhesion molecule (ICAM-1) distinct from LFA-1. *J. Immunol.* **137:** 1270.

Sanchez-Madrid, F., J. Nagy, E. Robbins, P. Simon, and T.A. Springer. 1983. A human leukocyte differentiation antigen family with distinct alpha subunits and a common beta subunit: The lymphocyte function-associated antigen (LFA-1), the C3bi complement receptor (OKM1/Mac-1), and the p150,95 molecule. *J. Exp. Med.* **158:** 1785.

Selvaraj, P., M.L. Dustin, R. Silber, M.G. Low, and T.A. Springer. 1987. Deficiency of lymphocyte function-associated antigen-3 (LFA-3) in paroxysmal nocturnal

hemoglobinuria: Functional correlates and evidence for a phosphatidylinositol membrane anchor. *J. Exp. Med.* **166:** 1011.

Shaw, S., G.E.G. Luce, R. Quinones, R.E. Gress, T.A. Springer, and M.E. Sanders. 1986. Two antigen-independent adhesion pathways used by human cytotoxic T cell clones. *Nature* **323:** 262.

Simmons, D., M.W. Makgoba, and B. Seed. 1988. ICAM, an adhesion ligand of LFA-1, is homologous to the neural cell adhesion molecule NCAM. *Nature* **331:** 624.

Spits, H., W. van Schooten, H. Keizer, G. van Seventer, M. Van de Rijn, C. Terhorst, and J.E. de Vries. 1986. Alloantigen recognition is preceded by nonspecific adhesion of cytotoxic T cells and target cells. *Science* **232:** 403.

Springer, T.A., M.L. Dustin, T.K. Kishimoto, and S.D. Marlin. 1987. The lymphocyte function-associated LFA-1, CD2, and LFA-3 molecules: Cell adhesion receptors of the immune system. *Annu. Rev. Immunol.* **5:** 223.

Springer, T.A., D. Davignon, M.K. Ho, K. Kürzinger, E. Martz, and F. Sanchez-Madrid. 1982. LFA-1 and Lyt-2,3, molecules associated with T lymphocyte-mediated killing; and Mac-1, an LFA-1 homologue associated with complement receptor function. *Immunol. Rev.* **68:** 111.

Staunton, D.E., M.L. Dustin, and T.A. Springer. 1989a. Functional cloning of ICAM-2, a cell adhesion ligand for LFA-1 homologous to ICAM-1. *Nature* **339:** 61.

Staunton, D.E., S.D. Marlin, C. Stratowa, M.L. Dustin, and T.A. Springer. 1988. Primary structure of intercellular adhesion molecule 1 (ICAM-1) demonstrates interaction between members of the immunoglobulin and integrin supergene families. *Cell* **52:** 925.

Staunton, D.E., V.J. Merluzzi, R. Rothlein, R. Barton, S.D. Marlin, and T.A. Springer. 1989b. A cell adhesion molecule, ICAM-1, is the major surface receptor for rhinoviruses. *Cell* **56:** 849.

Takada, Y. and M.E. Hemler. 1989. The primary structure of VLA-2/collagen receptor/α-2 subunit (GPIa): Homology to other integrins and presence of possible collagen-binding domain. *J. Cell Biol.* **109:** 397.

Tamkun, J.W., D.W. DeSimone, D. Fonda, R.S. Patel, C. Buck, A.F. Horwitz, and R.O. Hynes. 1986. Structure of integrin, a glycoprotein involved in the transmembrane linkage between fibronectin and actin. *Cell* **46:** 271.

van Noesel, C., F. Miedema, M. Brouwer, M.A. deRie, L.A. Aarden, and R.A.W. Van Lier. 1988. Regulatory properties of LFA-1 α and β chains in human T-lymphocyte activation. *Nature* **333:** 850.

Wright, S.D. and B.C. Meyer. 1986. Phorbol esters cause sequential activation and deactivation of complement receptors on polymorphonuclear leukocytes. *J. Immunol.* **136:** 1759.

Transcriptionally Defective Retroviruses Containing *lacZ* for the In Situ Detection of Endogenous Genes and Developmentally Regulated Chromatin

W.G. KERR, G.P. NOLAN, A.T. SERAFINI, AND L.A. HERZENBERG

Department of Genetics, Stanford University, Stanford, California 94305

Previously, we demonstrated that expression of transduced *Escherichia coli lacZ* can be detected in individual mammalian cells with a fluorescence-activated cell sorter (Nolan et al. 1988), a technique referred to as FACS-GAL. This fluorogenic assay permits the quantitative measurement of *E. coli* β-galactosidase (β-Gal) in individual viable cells. This technique also permits rare cells expressing β-Gal to be isolated utilizing the sorting capacity of the FACS. We have taken advantage of this feature to isolate β-Gal-expressing cells where the *lacZ* gene is under the control of endogenous transcription control elements. To permit the isolation of such cells, we have developed systems for delivering a reporter gene, *E. coli lacZ*, into the genome of mammalian cells in such a way that its expression is dependent on endogenous transcription control elements. We have stably introduced *lacZ* into the genome of mammalian cell lines by infection with *lacZ* gene search retroviruses, as well as by transfection with a splice acceptor/*lacZ* construct, AcLac. Each *lacZ* gene search virus we have developed requires that the flanking cellular sequences complement some transcriptional deficiency of the provirus for β-Gal to be expressed by the infected cell. The *lacZ* gene search viruses consist of an enhancer element search virus, Enhsr1, a promoter search virus, Prosr1, and a gene search virus containing a splice acceptor/*lacZ* fusion, Gensr1.

By studying the expression of *lacZ* derived by infection with either Enhsr1 or Prosr1, we demonstrate that individual β-Gal-expressing clones have very different distributions of activity, both qualitatively and quantitatively. We demonstrate that these broad ranges of *lacZ* expression seen in many individual clones represent a controlled variation in expression that is probably cyclical. Since expression in these clones is dependent on endogenous transcription elements, this may also be a common feature of cellular genes. As further proof of the endogenous control, we have been able to identify Enhsr1 clones where *lacZ* expression is regulated in a differentiation-stage-dependent manner. These Enhsr1 clones were derived from infections of a differentiation-inducible pre-B-cell line, 70Z/3, demonstrating the presence of multiple stage-specific enhancers involved in the differentiation of B-lineage cells.

Introduction of a splice acceptor/*lacZ* construct either by transfection of the AcLac construct or by infection with the AcLac virus into mammalian cells results in transcriptional and translational fusion of *lacZ* to endogenous genes and their protein products and thus provides the most pristine in situ measurement of endogenous transcriptional control we have developed. As with Enhsr1 and Prosr1, we find that distributions of β-Gal activity differ both qualitatively and quantitatively between individual clones. Since these proteins retain the enzymatic activity of bacterial β-Gal while also exhibiting the mammalian characteristic of subcellular localization, we propose that this represents a model for molecular evolution of multidomain, multifunctional proteins via exon shuffling. Moreover, the high frequency of success in generating in vivo gene fusions by introduction of the AcLac neo-exon into the genome strongly supports exon shuffling as a mechanism for generating novel protein structures in molecular evolution. Finally, we have used a retrovirus containing the splice acceptor/*lacZ* (Gensr1) to obtain gene fusions that are differentially regulated in B-lineage cell lines.

METHODS

FACS-GAL assay and immunofluorescence. FACS-GAL assay has been described previously (Nolan et al. 1988; Nolan 1989). For two-color analysis by FACS-GAL and immunofluorescence, 70Z/3 cells were first hypotonically loaded with fluorescein-di-galactoside (FDG) (from Molecular Probes, Junction City, Oregon) as described previously, brought back to isotonicity at 4°C, and pelleted. The pellet was resuspended in 100 μl of cold staining medium containing 10 μg/ml biotinylated monoclonal anti-Igκ. After incubation on ice for 15 minutes, the cells were washed three times with 2 ml of ice-cold staining medium and pelleted at 4°C. After the third pelleting, cells were resuspended in 100 μl of Texas Red (from Molecular Probes) complexed avidin (Vector Laboratories, Burlingame, California) and incubated on ice for 15 minutes. Cells were washed three times as before and resuspended in 100 μl of staining medium containing 1 μg/ml propidium iodide (to mark dead cells). In some experiments, where indicated, phenylethylthiogalactosidase (PETG), a strong, hydrophobic competitive inhibitor of β-Gal, was added to a concentration of 1 mM to stop hydrolysis of FDG to fluorescein (Nolan 1989). Single-color FACS analyses are presented as graphs (density 100%). Dual-color FACS analyses are presented as dual-color contour plots, 5% probability.

Infection of cells by Enhsr1, Prosr1, and Gensr1 viruses. 70Z/3 cells were infected by cocultivation for 16–18 hours with the Ψ2 lines producing Enhsr1 (Ψ2/E2) or Prosr1 (Ψ2/P10) in the presence of 2 μg/ml polybrene. The Enhsr1 or Prosr1 producer cell lines were irradiated with 3000 rads of γ-radiation prior to cocultivation with 70Z/3 to prevent further cell division by the producer cell line. *Gensr1* infections were done by cocultivation of 70Z/3 cells with the ecotropic producer line Ψ2/A36 or, in the case of NFS-5.3, with the amphotropic producer, PA/A8. Nearly confluent monolayers of *Gensr1* producers were UV-irradiated for 30–40 seconds in a sterile tissue culture cabinet prior to cocultivation with 70Z/3 or NFS-5.3 cells in the presence of 2 μg/ml polybrene. All LPS treatments were done at a concentration of 10 μg/ml (Difco, *S. typhosa* 0901 Westphal). IL-4 inductions were done at 20 units/ml (a kind gift from A. O'Garra and M. Howard, DNAX, Palo Alto, California).

Indolyl galactoside (X-Gal) histochemistry. Cells were fixed in 4% paraformaldehyde in phosphate-buffered saline. Cells were stained with the histochemical dye 5-bromo-4-chloro-indolyl-galactoside (Sigma) for a period of either 3 hours or overnight at 37°C, the length of staining prior to photography depending on the activity of the individual 293/AcLac clone. Cells were photographed using a Zeiss D7082 microscope (courtesy of H. Blau, Stanford University).

Immunoprecipitation and SDS-PAGE analysis of 293/AcLac β-Gal fusion proteins. Approximately 10^7 cells of each 293 AcLac clone were preincubated in 1 ml of methionine-deficient RPMI 1640 with 10% fetal calf serum for 1 hour. The cells were then pulsed with 400 μCi [^{35}S]methionine and 80 μCi [^{35}S]cysteine for 4 hours. The cells were then pelleted and lysed in 1 ml of 1% Nonidet P-40, 0.15 M NaCl, 50 mM Tris (pH 7.5), and 1 mM phenylmethylsulfonyl fluoride. The cell lysates were preadsorbed by the addition of 10 μg of anti-HLA and Pansorbin (Calbiochem, San Diego, California). For the final precipitation, 10 μg of monoclonal anti-β-Gal (Promega, Madison, Wisconsin) was added to the lysates with precipitation being achieved by addition of Pansorbin. Immunoprecipitated proteins were resolved after reduction by electrophoresis on a 7.5% SDS-polyacrylamide gel and visualized by autoradiography.

AcLac construct and transfection into 293 cells. The 125-bp splice acceptor of the Moloney leukemia virus *env* gene (derived from a *Bam*HI, *Kpn*I digest of pZip-NeoSV[X]) (Cepko et al. 1984) was fused to the 5' terminus of the *lacZ* gene by direct replacement of the cytomegalovirus promoter and *lacZ* initiator codon (removed by *Kpn*I, *Bam*HI digestion) of pON405 (kindly provided by E. Mocarski, Stanford University). The resulting plasmid is called pAcLac. An approximately 4.2-kb fragment containing the splice acceptor/*lacZ* followed by the SV40 poly(A) site was isolated from a *Bam*HI, *Hin*dIII digest of pAcLac. This fragment was cotransfected with SV2neo (Southern and Berg 1982) at a fivefold molar excess into 293 cells by a CaPO$_4$ precipitation procedure (Graham et al. 1980).

Construction of transcriptionally defective retroviruses containing lacZ. The *lacZ*-containing plasmid, pON405 (a kind gift from B. Manning and E. Mocarski, Stanford University), was digested with *Dra*I, and a 3.5-kb fragment containing *lacZ* was isolated. *Bam*HI linkers were ligated onto this 3.5-kb *Dra*I fragment, and the ligation was digested with *Bam*HI and *Sal*I. The digest was separated on a 1% low-melting agarose gel, and the 3.2-kb *Bam*HI-*Sal*I fragment was isolated. This *lacZ*-containing *Bam*HI-*Sal*I fragment was ligated to a purified 6.5-kb *Xho*I-*Bam*HI fragment generated by digestion of either plasmid, pJrEnh- or pJrPro- (a kind gift from H. Stuehlmann, Stanford University and Brad Guild, MIT). After transformation into JM109 on X-Gal-containing LB plates, blue colonies were selected for further analysis to confirm the correct orientation of *lacZ*. Construction of the AcLac-containing retrovirus and isolation of *Gensr1* ecotropic and amphotropic producer lines will be described in a subsequent manuscript.

RESULTS

Expression of Transduced *lacZ* Is Controlled by Endogenous Transcription Control Elements

We have demonstrated previously that expression of transduced *lacZ* can be detected in viable mammalian cells with a fluorescence-activated cell sorter (Nolan et al. 1988; Nolan 1989), a technique referred to as FACS-GAL. The retrovirus used in this earlier study had *lacZ* under the control of an internal promoter, the SV40 late promoter; however, expression varied among independent clones containing different integration sites, suggesting that endogenous transcription control elements were influencing the expression of *lacZ* (Nolan 1989). To more accurately assess the control of introduced reporter genes by endogenous transcription control elements, we have constructed self-inactivating (SIN) retroviruses containing *lacZ*. These retroviruses will deliver *lacZ* into the chromatin of a target cell after the removal of the Moloney 72-bp enhancer element (enhancer-search, Enhsr1) or after removal of the entire Moloney transcription control region (promoter-search, Prosr1) (illustrated for Enhsr1 in Fig. 1). This can be accomplished because the U3 of the 3' long terminal repeat (LTR) serves as the template for reverse transcription of the U3 region in both 3' and 5' LTRs (Varmus et al. 1982). Thus, if a

Enhsr1

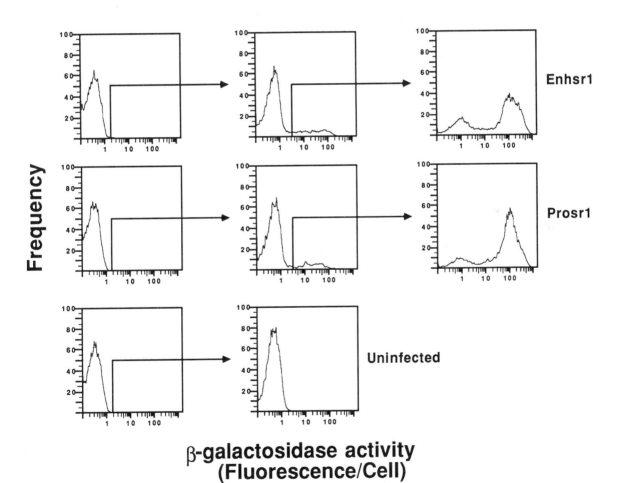

Figure 1. Schematic depiction of Enhsr1 and model for *lacZ* expression. This figure depicts how a *lacZ*-encoding provirus that lacks the Moloney leukemia virus enhancer region (stippled box) would be generated from the Enhsr1 construct. The provirus generated from Enhsr1 will lack the viral enhancer region (stippled box) but will still retain CAAT and TATA box motifs (hatched box). This defective proviral transcriptional unit can be activated by an enhancer element (stippled oval) in the flanking, endogenous chromatin. Thus, with Enhsr1, viral integrations near endogenous enhancer elements will result in *lacZ* expression.

β-galactosidase activity
(Fluorescence/Cell)

Figure 2. FACS enrichment of *lacZ*-expressing cells. Following cocultivation of 70Z/3 cells with the Ψ2 Prosr1 and Enhsr1 producer cell lines (see Methods), the 70Z/3 cells expressing *lacZ* were enriched by sorting based on their fluorescence due to cleavage of FDG to fluorescein. After expansion for 1 week, the cells were again stained by the FACS-GAL technique, reanalyzed, and again sorted for fluorescein-positive cells. This secondary sorted population was reanalyzed by FACS-GAL after 1 week of expansion in culture. Uninfected 70Z/3 cells were also stained and sorted by FACS-GAL. Cleavage was allowed to proceed for 2 hr, and false-positive cells were sorted. After expansion for 1 week in culture, the cells were stained and analyzed by FACS-GAL as before. We saw no increase in false-positive cells.

deletion is introduced into the 3' U3 in the initial retroviral construct, this deletion will be transmitted to both LTRs of the provirus following infection and integration (Yu et al. 1986). Since our constructs contain no internal promoter or other known regulatory elements, *lacZ* expression is dependent on readthrough transcription from an endogenous promoter with Prosr1 or *cis*-activation of the promoter in the viral LTR by a proximal enhancer element with Enhsr1 (Kerr et al. 1989).

Figure 2 shows that rare *lacZ*-expressing cells can be sorted by FACS-GAL following cocultivation of 70Z/3 cells with the Enhsr1 and Prosr1 virus producer lines. The initial percentage of *lacZ*⁺ cells following infection is quite low, as would be expected for these transcriptionally defective retroviruses. In fact, only infection with Enhsr1 gives percentages of positive cells significantly greater than the background frequency of false positives seen in uninfected cells. However, these rare *lacZ*⁺ cells can be sorted under sterile conditions by FACS-GAL and cultured, and a subsequent sort can be done to achieve a high degree of enrichment. Data in Figure 2 show that the initial percentage of *lacZ*⁺ cells following infection (Enhsr1: 0.5–0.6%, Prosr1: 0.1–0.2%) is enriched after two rounds of sorting and culture to 70–90% *lacZ*⁺ cells among the 70Z/3 cells. Thus, infection with either Enhsr1 or Prosr1, followed by sorting for *lacZ*⁺ cells via FACS-GAL, allows one to obtain a population of cells with random integrations of the *lacZ* reporter gene either under the control of nearby endogenous enhancer elements (Enhsr1) or downstream from active, endogenous promoters (Prosr1). In all uninfected mammalian cell lines examined, there is a low frequency of cells that are positive when loaded with FDG and analyzed by FACS-GAL, even though they express no *E. coli lacZ* gene. The positive phenotype of these cells is not heritable, since a sort of these rare positives from uninfected 70Z/3 by FACS-GAL sorting shows no enrichment; therefore, the phenotype of these rare cells is not stable.

The population of *lacZ*⁺ 70Z/3 cells obtained by FACS-GAL sorting contains many cells with independent integrations of *lacZ* at different sites in the genome, since individual clones derived from these pools have different characteristic patterns of *lacZ* expression. Figure 3 shows some representative *lacZ* expression patterns of fluorescence per cell for different clones derived from infections with Enhsr1 and Prosr1. These patterns of expression remain reproducible after repeated reculture and reanalysis, implying that they are stably transmitted to daughter cells following cell division (data not shown). This stability of expression was tested further by sorting low, medium, and high expressing cells from individual Enhsr1 clones and reexamining their pattern of expression after 1 week of culture. An example is shown in Figure 4. Each sort, when regrown, recapitulates the distribution of *lacZ* activity shown by the parent clone. The data in Figure 4 suggest that the broad *lacZ* expression patterns we see by FACS-GAL represent a controlled variation in transcription which, we suggest, is cyclical. Expression of many eukaryotic genes may also be under such cyclical control.

The ability of *lacZ* to be regulated in a differentiation-stage-dependent manner in individual Enhsr1-infected clones of 70Z/3 further demonstrates endogenous control of *lacZ* expression in integrations derived from Enhsr1. The pre-B-cell line, 70Z/3, differentiates in vitro to an IgMκ-expressing B cell after 24 hours of culture in lipopolysaccharide (LPS)-containing medium (Paige et al. 1978). One of the Enhsr1 clones, 7e17-17, shows nearly complete repression of *lacZ* expression after 24 hours of culture in medium with LPS (Fig. 5a), whereas other clones examined were either unresponsive to LPS treatment or showed only minor variations in expression (Kerr et al. 1989). To demonstrate that 7e17-17 cells had differentiated from pre-B to the B-cell stage while repressing *lacZ*, the cells were analyzed simultaneously for β-Gal activity as well as for IgMκ expression on the cell surface. In response to LPS, 7e17-17 cells acquire ex-

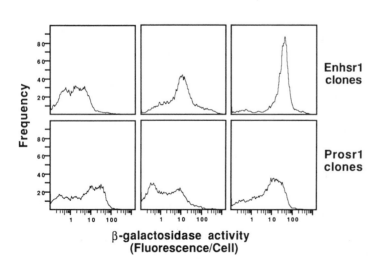

Figure 3. *lacZ*-expressing clones exhibit different patterns of activity. Cells of the individual Enhsr1 and Prosr1 clones were loaded hypotonically with FDG and analyzed by FACS after 2 hr of enzymatic cleavage at 4°C.

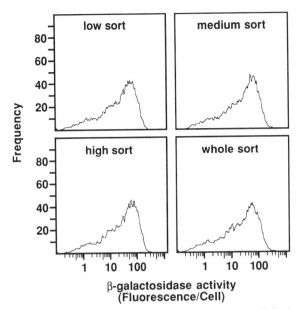

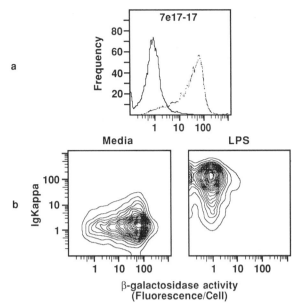

Figure 4. Stability of *lacZ* expression pattern in Enhsr1 clones. The Enhsr1 clone, 7e15, was stained and analyzed by FACS-GAL with enzymatic cleavage being halted at 1 hour by bringing the cells to 1 mM PETG. 50,000 cells were sorted from the 5–10, 45–50, and 90–95 percentiles of the 7e15 distribution (low, medium, and high, respectively). 50,000 cells from the whole, ungated distribution were also sorted. The sorted cells were grown for 1 week and reanalyzed by FACS-GAL as before.

Figure 5. Regulation of *lacZ* and κ light-chain expression following LPS induction of the Enhsr1 clone, 7e17-17 cells. Equal numbers of 7e17-17 cells were cultured either in normal media or in media containing 10 μg/ml of LPS for 24 hr. The cells were then stained as described above and analyzed on the FACS. (*a*) Graphs representing β-Gal activity of 7e17-17 cells after 24 hr in LPS-containing media (solid line) or in normal media (broken line). (*b*) Dual parameter FACS analysis of κ light-chain expression (Texas Red) vs. β-Gal (fluorescein) in 7e17-17 cells cultured in normal media or in LPS-containing media.

pression of surface IgMκ expression while β-Gal is repressed (Fig. 5b). Therefore, LPS either simultaneously transmits positive and negative regulatory signals to a differentiating pre-B cell or initiates a cascade of events that result in both positive and negative regulation of genes in the nucleus of the pre-B cell. Induction of κ light-chain expression via NF-κB is one well-documented effect of LPS on 70Z/3 cells (Sen and Baltimore 1986a,b). However, the repression of *lacZ* expression in 7e17-17 cells suggests that LPS can act to repress the transcription of a locus or loci expressed at the pre-B-cell stage of B-lineage differentiation. We believe this to be the first indication that LPS can play a negative regulatory role in the gene expression of B-lineage cells.

If Enhsr1 is integrated in a region of chromatin near a B-cell stage-specific enhancer in 70Z/3, *lacZ* expression would be induced by LPS. To increase our chances of finding integrations of Enhsr1 near enhancers active in the B-cell stage and not in the pre-B-cell stage, we infected cells in the presence of LPS and kept them in LPS up until cloning of *lacZ*⁺ cells by FACS-GAL sorting. Analysis of 230 clones derived from two different infections revealed several 70Z/3 clones with Enhsr1 integrations in chromatin regions where transcription is induced by LPS. Two examples, clones 7e129-3 and 7e131-3, show induction of *lacZ* expression following culture of the cells in LPS for a period of 24 hours (Fig. 6). Interestingly, only a portion of the cells within the clone appear to undergo an induction of *lacZ*

expression by LPS, despite the fact that all the cells have expressed surface IgMκ (demonstrated for 7e129-3 and 7e131-3, Fig. 6). DNA cell-cycle analysis of these Enhsr1 clones indicates that no stage of the cell cycle is specifically correlated with *lacZ* expression in these clones (W. Kerr et al., in prep.). Thus, there may be B-cell stage-specific enhancers that do not *cis*-activate constitutively during this stage of differentiation but rather can be considered "fluctuating" enhancers. The gene products such enhancers regulate may require only a transitory period of transcription to achieve the level of expression necessary for proper B-cell function. These fluctuating enhancers may be a necessary requirement for the rapid changes in phenotype that occur during the antigen-dependent phase of B-cell differentiation.

In Vivo Mammalian Gene Fusions with a Splice Acceptor *lacZ* Neo-exon

To improve the accuracy of measuring transcriptional control of endogenous genes in situ, we have developed a system in which transcriptional and translational fusion with the endogenous gene and its protein product are both required for *lacZ* expression. To accomplish this, we constructed AcLac, a *lacZ* artificial exon (neo-exon), by replacing the 5′ terminus and

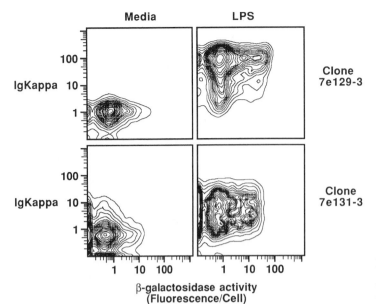

Media   LPS

IgKappa 100 / 10 / 1   Clone
                                                       7e129-3

IgKappa 100 / 10 / 1   Clone
                                                       7e131-3

        1 10 100   1 10 100

β-galactosidase activity
   (Fluorescence/Cell)

Figure 6. B-cell stage-specific expression of *lacZ* in the Enhsr1 clones, 7e129-3 and 7e131-3. Cells were cultured, stained, and analyzed similarly to 7e17-17 cells in Fig. 5.

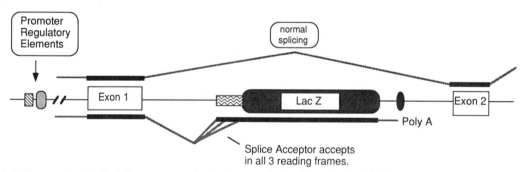

```
        I      II   III              IV  A↓                    B↓              C↓
AACTTCCCTGACCCTGACATGACAAGAGTTACTAACAGC  CCC TCT CTC CAA GCT CAC TTA CAG
                                         Pro Ser Leu Gln Ala His Leu Gln

GCT CTC TAC TTA GTC CAG CAC GAA GTC TGG AGA CCT CTG GCG GCA GCC TAC CAA
Ala Leu Tyr Leu Val Gln His Glu Val Trp Arg Pro Leu Ala Ala Ala Tyr Gln

GAA CAA CTG GAC CGA CCG GTG GTA CCG GTG GGT GAA GAC CAG AAA
Glu Gln Leu Asp Arg Pro Val Val Pro Val Gly Glu Asp Gln Lys ---> lacZ
```

Figure 7. Splice acceptor/*lacZ*, AcLac, construct for in situ transcriptional/translational fusion to endogenous genes. The upper half of the figure is the sequence of the *env* splice acceptor/*lacZ* construct prior to transfection showing the four consensus lariat branch points (solid bars, I–IV) and the three potential consensus splice acceptor intron/exon boundaries (arrows, A–C). The potential branch site-acceptor site pairs are I with A, II with A or B, III with A or B, and IV with C (Mann and Baltimore 1985; Lazo et al. 1987). Splice donation from an upstream exon to one of the three potential splice acceptor sites will fuse to the acceptor-*lacZ* sequence shown. The translated peptide sequence of the splice acceptor *lacZ* region is shown. The lower half of the figure is a schematic representation of a model fusion of *lacZ* to an upstream exon mediated by the MLV *env* splice acceptor. The endogenous promoter/regulatory elements drive transcription. The normal splicing pattern of the gene is depicted. Introduction of the splice acceptor/*lacZ* construct into an intron of an endogenous gene leads to interruption of normal splicing and direct transcriptional/translational fusion to the *lacZ* gene (only one of the three potential transcriptional fusions can lead to translation of a *lacZ* fusion protein). The polyadenylation signal is provided by the introduced construct.

initiator codon of *lacZ* with the Moloney *env* gene splice acceptor (Mann and Baltimore 1985; Lazo et al. 1987) (see Fig. 7). Following introduction of AcLac into cells, generation of enzymatically active β-Gal requires the following: (1) integration of the *lacZ* neo-exon into an intron of a gene, (2) interruption of the normal splicing of this gene by splicing of the *lacZ* neo-exon to an upstream exon resulting in transcriptional fusion of *lacZ* to the endogenous transcript, (3) initiation of translation at the AUG of the endogenous transcript with translational elongation into the coding frame of *lacZ*, and (4) folding of the β-Gal "domain" during assembly of this new multidomain protein in a manner that permits association into enzymatically active tetramers. Since AcLac is completely dependent on cellular sequences for expression of β-Gal, successful integrations should more accurately reflect the transcriptional control of the endogenous gene relative to Enhsr1 and Prosr1.

We believe that generation of β-Gal expression via introduction of AcLac into the genome mimics exon shuffling that is proposed to take place in the molecular evolution of multidomain proteins (Blake 1978; Gilbert 1978). The basic tenet of these theories is that eukaryotic genes are collections of exons that were brought together by recombination within intron sequences. There are numerous examples of genes that have arisen via duplication and diversification of a single exon (e.g., Ig superfamily) (Gilbert 1985; Gilbert et al. 1986). The evolution of genes derived from several different ancestral exons is less common, but the LDL receptor is one notable example (Sudhof et al. 1985). A corollary of this hypothesis is that the individual domains encoded by exons represent integrally folded protein units (Blake 1978). This would permit evolution of multidomain proteins with multiple functions to occur at a higher probability.

We introduced the AcLac neo-exon into the chromatin of a human embryo kidney cell line, 293, by transfection. After selecting for stable transfectants with G418, we sorted a population of *lacZ*[+] cells from the pool of G418-resistant 293 transfectants. Following expansion of this *lacZ*[+] pool of 293 cells, individual *lacZ*[+] cells were cloned by FACS-GAL. Analysis of these individual clones by FACS-GAL showed patterns of expression that were unique to individual clones (Fig. 8), indicating that *lacZ* expression is under the control of different endogenous transcription elements. We find that expression can vary quite significantly within an individual clone, indicating that our original observations with Enhsr1 and Prosr1 were not an artifact introduced by the presence of Moloney viral sequences. This controlled variation in expression may

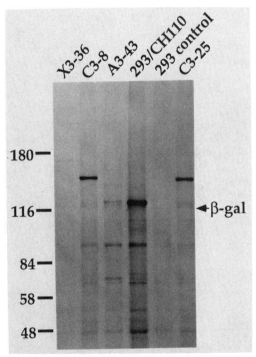

Figure 9. Clonal variation in molecular weight of splice acceptor/*lacZ* in vivo gene fusions. Immunoprecipitation analysis of β-Gal fusion proteins in four representative AcLac/293 clones (X3-36, C3-8, A3-43, C3-25) show different apparent molecular weights greater than that of *E. coli* β-Gal (revealed by Coomassie staining; indicated by an arrow). Purified *E. coli* β-Gal (Sigma) (5.5 µg) was added to the labeled cell lysate of 293 cells (*293 control*), and immunoprecipitated as described above. As a further control, 293 cells stably expressing CH110 (*trpA-lacZ* fusion protein) (Hall et al. 1983) were also analyzed by immunoprecipitation analysis (*293/CH110*). Migration of molecular-weight standards is indicated at the left.

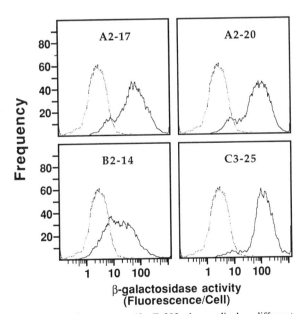

Figure 8. Splice acceptor/*lacZ* 293 clones display different patterns of β-Gal expression when analyzed by FACS-GAL. A suspension of each 293/AcLac clone was loaded hypotonically with FDG at 37°C. At 1 min, 2 ml of ice-cold isotonic medium was added to stop hypotonic loading. At 5 min, the cell suspension was brought to 1 mM PETG. The cells were kept on ice until analysis by FACS. The solid lines represent fluorescence per cell for the indicated AcLac/293 clone, and the dotted lines represent the parent line, 293, treated in a similar fashion.

thus be reflective of the transcriptional control of many cellular genes.

To confirm that β-Gal activity in the 293 AcLac clones was derived by transcriptional and translational fusion with an endogenous gene, we biosynthetically labeled 293/AcLac clones, immunoprecipitated with a monoclonal anti-β-Gal, and analyzed these immuno-precipitates by SDS-PAGE. In Figure 9, we show the results of this analysis for four representative clones, which indicate that the β-Gal in these clones is of a higher apparent molecular weight than *E. coli* β-Gal or a *trpA-lacZ* fusion protein (CH110). The increased apparent molecular weight of β-Gal expressed by these cells indicates that it results from transcriptional and translational fusions with endogenous upstream exons in transcriptionally active genes.

Histological analysis of the X-Gal precipitates resulting from β-Gal activity in these 293/AcLac clones revealed that β-Gal activity is confined to discrete cellular and subcellular locations in each clone (see Fig. 10). Thus, in addition to the AcLac neo-exon forming novel multidomain proteins that have retained the enzymatic activity of β-Gal, these proteins retain functional targeting domains of the endogenous protein.

These clones have been readily isolated by FACS-GAL from three independent transfections of AcLac into 293 cells where the initial percentage of positive cells was about 1% in all three transfections (data not shown). Thus, the AcLac neo-exon can be seeded into the genome of a mammalian cell and generate enzymatically active fusion proteins with endogenous mammalian proteins that retain the subcellular localization determined by upstream encoded, endogenous

protein domains. Although the mechanism for molecular evolution of multidomain proteins cannot be directly studied, the introduction of the AcLac neo-exon into the genome of a cell provides a model system for molecular evolution of novel protein structures. Our ability to readily isolate novel multidomain proteins with AcLac provides examples of exon shuffling similar to what occurs in molecular evolution of multifunctional, multidomain proteins composed of different ancestral exons.

Transduced AcLac Forms Gene Fusions in B-lineage Cell Lines

We have inserted the AcLac construct into the same transcriptionally defective retrovirus construct that was used to construct Prosr1 (manuscript in prep.). If integration of the provirus containing AcLac is in an intron of an endogenous gene in the proper transcriptional orientation, β-Gal should be expressed from the integrated provirus in the same manner as transfection of AcLac was in 293 cells. Integration of the provirus derived from this retroviral construct will place *lacZ* in the chromatin of a cell without the known Moloney transcription control elements being present, and, thus, expression of *lacZ* should mimic the transcriptional regulation at this locus.

In Figure 11, we demonstrate the endogenous control of *lacZ* in clones derived from infection of the pre-B cell lines, 70Z/3 and NFS5.3. We demonstrate endogenous control of expression in these clones because they are differentially regulated. In the case of the 70Z/3 clones, 7a65 and 7a135, the expression of

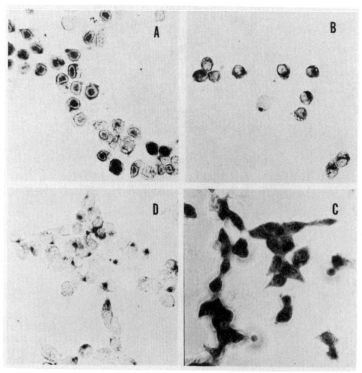

Figure 10. Subcellular localization of β-Gal with splice acceptor/*lacZ* in vivo gene fusions. (*A*) Nuclear localized β-Gal; (*B*) cytoplasmic β-Gal; (*C*) diffuse, whole cell β-Gal; (*D*) perinuclear localized β-Gal.

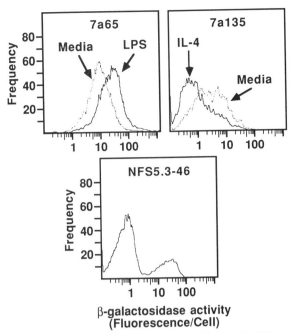

Figure 11. Differential expression of *lacZ* in pre-B-cell lines infected with Gensr1. LPS (7a65) and IL-4 (7a135) treatment of cells is described above. All clones were hypotonically loaded with FDG with enzymatic cleavage halted at 2 hr by bringing the cells to 1 mM PETG. The cells were then analyzed by FACS.

lacZ is modified by treatment of the cells with immuno-modulators (IL-4, LPS). *lacZ* expression undergoes a threefold induction in 7a65 with LPS and is partially repressed in 7a135 by IL-4. In NFS5.3-46, the expression of *lacZ* fluctuates within the clone. That variation may be linked to cell-cycle events is presently under investigation.

DISCUSSION

We have demonstrated that the genome of a mammalian cell can be seeded with transcriptionally defective, *lacZ*-encoding retroviruses to isolate cells expressing *lacZ* under the control of endogenous transcription control elements. This goal was made feasible by the recently developed FACS-GAL technique, which permits rare cells expressing *lacZ* to be sorted from a population that is primarily negative (Nolan et al. 1988; Kerr et al. 1989). With the combination of the *lacZ* gene search retroviruses and FACS-GAL, we can study, in individual viable cells, the transcriptional control of a gene in its native context, thus permitting transcriptional control to be appreciated as a cell distribution rather than as a mean of this distribution (e.g., CAT assay, RNA assay).

Utilizing different *lacZ* gene search retroviruses (Enhsr1, Prosr1, and Gensr1) that have different requirements for *lacZ* expression, we have consistently found that the distribution of β-Gal activity differs both quantitatively and qualitatively among either Enhsr1, Prosr1, or Gensr1 clones, attesting to their transcrip-

tional control by cellular sequences flanking the provirus containing *lacZ*. The unique distributions we see are inherited by daughter cells, since the patterns are stable with continuous culture as well as in subclones. The wide variation in β-Gal activity we see in cells of a single clone appears to be controlled, since cells of either low, medium, or high β-Gal activity within the distribution of the clone recapitulate the distribution of the parental cells. The most likely explanation for the variation of β-Gal activity in these clones is fluctuations in the transcription rate of the reporter gene, *lacZ*. If this variation is indeed determined at the transcriptional level, our results would suggest that this is a common feature in the transcriptional control of cellular genes.

Convincing evidence for the endogenous control of *lacZ* is the identification of Enhsr1 clones where *lacZ* expression is dependent on the differentiation stage of 70Z/3 cells. We have identified an Enhsr1 clone (7e17-17) where *lacZ* is repressed when 70Z/3 cells differentiate to the B-cell stage under the influence of LPS. In addition, we have also found Enhsr1 clones (7e129-3, 7e131-3) where LPS-induced differentiation causes induction of *lacZ* expression; however, only a portion of the cells within these clones express *lacZ* while in LPS. We suggest that this B-cell stage enhancer has an on/off or fluctuating expression pattern, even though the 70Z/3 cells are all at the B-cell stage of differentiation. One could envision such fluctuating enhancers as being responsible for the regulation of genes that are expressed at the B-cell stage, which are later down-regulated if the cell encounters its antigen during the antigen-dependent phase of B-cell differentiation (e.g., Ia expression).

We were also able to obtain endogenously controlled expression of *lacZ* through transfection with a splice acceptor/*lacZ* neo-exon, AcLac, or by infection with a retrovirus containing AcLac, Gensr1. Since expression of *lacZ* in these clones is derived by both transcriptional and translational fusion with an endogenous gene, we believe that these in situ gene fusions with the *lacZ* reporter gene offer a more accurate measurement of endogenous transcriptional control. As with Enhsr1 and Prosr1 clones, we find that AcLac and Gensr1 clones have unique and characteristic distributions of β-Gal activity, reflecting the transcriptional regulation of the loci where they have integrated. We have also found that certain Gensr1 clones differentially regulate expression of *lacZ*, suggesting that Gensr1 will allow us to tag genes expressed at different stages in lymphoid differentiation.

We believe that, in addition to acting as an in situ measure of transcription, the expression of β-Gal following the introduction of the AcLac neo-exon into the genome mimics events that take place in the exon-shuffling model of molecular evolution. Because these in vivo gene fusions with *lacZ* retain features of both the introduced AcLac neo-exon (enzymatic activity) and the endogenous exon (subcellular targeting), we believe these experiments demonstrate that exon shuffling is a valid mechanism for evolution of novel multidomain protein structures. The high frequency with which we were able to obtain β-Gal expression in three independent transfections with the AcLac neo-exon suggests that these transfections may provide a model system for examining the requirements for successful and aberrant exon-shuffling events.

The development of the *lacZ* gene search retroviruses and the FACS-GAL assay come at a time when the *E. coli* gene, *lacZ*, is being used in a variety of systems to study developmentally regulated gene expression in higher eukaryotes (O'Kane and Gehring 1987; Allen et al. 1988; Gossler et al. 1989). The *lacZ* gene search viruses offer an efficient means to introduce *lacZ* into the genome of mammalian cells, and FACS-GAL permits the rare cells expressing *lacZ* to be isolated following infection. The combination of these two techniques provides a novel means to identify and study transcriptionally active regions of the mammalian genome and, thus, will facilitate the study of mammalian gene expression.

ACKNOWLEDGMENTS

We thank Dr. Leonore Herzenberg (Stanford University) for helpful discussion. We also thank Bruce Blakeley, Dr. Simon Hughes, and Dr. Helen Blau for assistance with microscopy and photography. In addition, we thank C.M. Tarlinton, G. Jager, C. Rattazzi, and J. Johnsen for expert technical assistance. W.G.K. was supported by the National Institutes of Health training program in immunology, AI-07290. This work was supported by NIH grant CA-42509.

REFERENCES

Allen, N.D., D.G. Can, S.C. Barton, S. Hettle, and M.A. Surami. 1988. Transgenes as probes for active chromosomal domains in mouse development. *Nature* 333: 852.

Blake, C.C.F. 1978. Do genes-in-pieces imply proteins-in-pieces? *Nature* 273: 267.

Cepko, C.A., B.E. Roberts, and R.C. Mulligan. 1984. Construction and applications of a highly transmissible murine retrovirus shuttle vector. *Cell* 37: 1053.

Gilbert, W. 1978. Why genes in pieces? *Nature* 271: 501.

———. 1985. Genes-in-pieces revisited. *Science* 228: 823.

Gilbert, W., M. Marchionni, and G. McKnight. 1986. On the antiquity of introns. *Cell* 46: 151.

Gossler, A., A.L. Joyner, J. Rossant, and W.C. Skarnes. 1989. Mouse embryonic stem cells and reporter constructs to detect developmentally regulated genes. *Science* 244: 463.

Graham, F.L., J. Smiley, W.C. Russell, and R. Nairn. 1977. Characteristics of a human cell line transformed by DNA from human adenovirus type 5. *J. Gen. Virol.* 36: 59.

Graham, F.L., S. Bacchetti, and R. McKinnon. 1980. Transformation of mammalian cells with DNA using the calcium technique. In *Introduction of macromolecules into viable mammalian cells* (ed. R. Baserga et al.), p. 3. Alan R. Liss, New York.

Hall, C.V., P.E. Jacob, G.M. Ringold, and F.J. Lee. 1983. Expression and regulation of *Escherichia coli lacZ* gene fusions in mammalian cells. *Mol. Appl. Genet.* 2: 101.

Kerr, W.G., G.P. Nolan, and L.A. Herzenberg. 1989. *In situ* detection of transcriptionally active chromatin and genetic regulatory elements in individual viable mammalian cells. *Immunology* (in press).

Lazo, P.A., V. Prasad, and P.N. Tsichlis. 1987. Splice acceptor site for the *env* message of Moloney murine leukemia virus. *J. Virol.* 61: 2038.

Mann, R. and D. Baltimore. 1985. Varying the position of a retrovirus packaging sequence results in the encapsidation of both unspliced and spliced RNAs. *J. Virol.* 54: 401.

Nolan, G.P.J. 1989. "Individual cell gene regulation studies and *in situ* detection of transcriptionally active chromatin using fluorescence-activated cell sorting with a viable cell fluorographic assay." Ph.D. thesis. Stanford University.

Nolan, G.P., S. Fiering, J.F. Nicolas, and L.A. Herzenberg. 1988. Fluorescence-activated cell analysis and sorting of viable mammalian cells based on β-D-galactosidase activity after transduction of *Escherichia coli lacZ*. *Proc. Natl. Acad. Sci.* 85: 2603.

O'Kane, C.J. and W.H. Gehring. 1987. Detection *in situ* of genomic regulatory elements in *Drosophila*. *Proc. Natl. Acad. Sci.* 84: 9123.

Paige, C.J., P.W. Kincade, and P. Ralph. 1978. Murine B cell leukemia with inducible surface immunoglobulin expression. *Science* 121: 641.

Sen, R. and D. Baltimore. 1986a. Multiple nuclear factors interact with the immunoglobulin enhancer sequences. *Cell* 46: 705.

———. 1986b. Inducibility of κ immunoglobulin enhancer-binding protein NF-κB by a post-translational mechanism. *Cell* 47: 921.

Southern, P. and P. Berg. 1982. A new dominant hybrid selective marker for higher eukaryotic cells. *J. Mol. Appl. Genet.* 1: 327.

Sudhof, T.C., J.L. Goldstein, M.S. Brown, and D.W. Russell. 1985. The LDL receptor gene: A mosaic of exons shared with different proteins. *Science* 228: 815.

Varmus, H.E. 1982. Form and function of retroviral proviruses. *Science* 216: 812.

Yu, S.F., T. von Ruden, P.W. Kantoff, C. Garber, M. Sieberg, U. Ruther, W.F. Anderson, E.F. Wagner, and E. Gilboa. 1986. Self-inactivating retroviral vectors designed for transfer of whole genes into mammalian cells. *Proc. Natl. Acad. Sci.* 83: 3194.

Induction of Tolerance by Embryonic Thymic Epithelial Grafts in Birds and Mammals

N.M. Le Douarin, C. Corbel, C. Martin, M. Coltey, and J. Salaün

Institut d'Embryologie Cellulaire et Moléculaire
du CNRS et du Collège de France, 94736 Nogent-sur-Marne Cedex, France

The thymus plays a decisive role in the ontogeny of T lymphocytes. Hematopoietic cells (HCs) homing to this organ follow two differentiation pathways: one leading to thymocytes and mature T cells that are exported to the periphery, where they carry out cell-mediated immunity, and the other giving rise to macrophages and dendritic cells, residing mainly in the thymic medulla, where they form a sessile stroma, the renewal of which has not been well documented so far. Development of functional T cells in the thymus involves extensive proliferation of T-cell precursors and the acquisition by the differentiating thymocytes of various specific phenotypic markers and the functional reactivities characteristic of mature T cells (Bevan et al. 1976; Teh et al. 1977; Stutman 1978; Zinkernagel and Doherty 1979; Scollay et al. 1984; Kingston et al. 1985; Rothenberg and Lugo 1985; Davis and Bjorkman 1988). It is generally considered that the repertoire of mature T cells is selected during this intrathymic phase of T-cell development (Sprent et al. 1988); however, the cellular and molecular mechanisms responsible for this thymic selection are still poorly understood. In particular, the respective contribution of the two stromal components of the thymus epithelium and dendritic cells to these processes is controversial. It has been proposed (for review, see Sprent et al. 1988) that tolerance and hence clonal deletion of autoreactive clones, is induced by the hematopoietically derived dendritic cells of the medulla, whereas major histocompatibility complex (MHC) restriction would be selected in contact with epithelial cells.

With the aim of investigating whether the epithelial component of the thymus plays a role in tolerance induction during ontogeny, we have devised an experimental system in which the thymic rudiment can be manipulated (i.e., removed or grafted) when it is still in a purely epithelial state, before its seeding by HCs. This can be done in the avian embryo, a model particularly appropriate to study certain aspects of the ontogeny of the immune system because it is available for experimentation in the egg during the entire period of development. Moreover, it is possible to construct chimeric tissues and chimeric animals composed of two closely related species of birds, the chick and the Japanese quail. The cells belonging to each species in these chimeras can be recognized by means of the structure of their interphase nucleus; a large amount of constitutive heterochromatin is associated with the nucleolus in all the embryonic and adult cell types of the quail (Le Douarin 1969, 1973).

We have taken advantage of these characteristics to devise experiments in which foreign tissue was introduced into the embryo early in development, before its immune system had started to develop. The question raised concerned the immunological status of the graft after birth, when the host's immune function has reached maturity.

The foreign tissue was either a limb bud or the anlage of the bursa of Fabricius, on the one hand, and the thymus rudiment, on the other hand. We were able to demonstrate that severe and acute rejection occurred after birth, in xenogeneic combinations where a limb bud or a bursa from a quail was grafted into a chick embryo. However, full tolerance could be induced when the thymic epithelial rudiment from the same donor was grafted together with the other organ.

Basically similar results were obtained in experiments performed in mice where, given the impossibility of operating on the embryo at the appropriate stage, we used athymic nude mice as recipients for thymic epithelium grafts.

RESULTS

Immune Rejection after Birth of a Quail Limb Bud Grafted into a Chick Embryo at Embryonic Day 4 (E4)

The graft performed, as indicated in Figure 1a, was done on 242 embryos; 30 chickens hatched. In most cases, the grafted wing was well developed and mobile, as in Figure 1b. In others, it was somewhat shortened. Pigmentation of the quail wing was often seen but not invariably so, depending on whether or not the quail limb bud had been colonized at the time of operation by melanoblasts originating from the neural crest. The latter reach the anterior limb bud at stage 15–18 of Zacchei (1961), about the time of its removal from the quail donor.

During the first postnatal week, the growth of the grafted wing was comparable to that of a normal age-matched quail. Signs of immune rejection started during either the first or the second postnatal week with edema, and the rejection immediately became acute, with suppuration followed by necrosis and, finally, autoamputation of the wing in all cases (Fig. 2). During

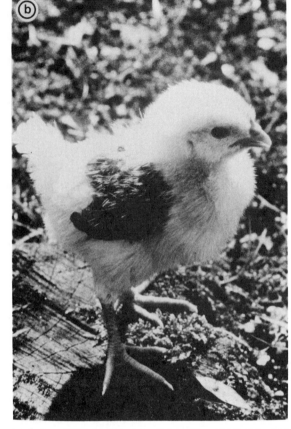

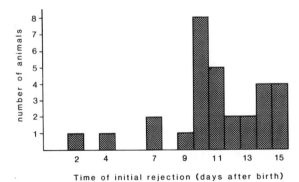

Figure 1. Xenogeneic quail-to-chick wing chimeras. (*a*) Experimental design of limb-bud transplantation. The right limb bud of an E3.5 quail embryo is substituted for its counterpart in an E4 chick recipient. (*b*) Nine-day chick carrying a quail limb. The limb is well developed and healthy.

the acute phase of the immune response, the animal stopped growing, usually without losing weight. Growth then began again, and the chimeras' weight reached approximately the value of age-matched normal chickens.

During rejection, the host developed a humoral response involving antibodies directed against common quail antigens that could be detected by immunocytochemistry on cultured quail embryonic fibroblasts.

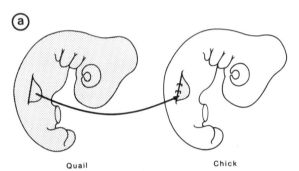

Figure 2. Time of appearance after birth of acute rejection in xenogeneic grafts of the wing from E3.5 quail to E4 chick embryos. (Reprinted, with permission, from Ohki et al. 1987.)

The antibodies against quail cell-surface antigens became detectable in the serum of the chimeras 1–18 days after the appearance of the first signs of rejection. This suggests that the cellular and humoral responses to the graft occur independently, a conclusion that was further supported by early bursectomy of the recipient embryos; in three chick host embryos, the anlage of the bursa of Fabricius (the site of B-cell differentiation in birds) was surgically removed at E5 (Belo et al. 1985), 1 day after implantation of the quail wing bud. Such animals cannot develop antibody response to injected antigens (Corbel et al. 1987); however, they rejected the wing acutely at postnatal days 10, 11, and 12 (P10, P11, and P19), respectively.

It is important to note that the quail limb rudiment just begins to receive vascular buds at the time of grafting, as can be seen in Figure 3, after staining the vascular endothelium with the monoclonal antibody (MAb) QH1, which (like MB1, Péault et al. 1983) recognizes an antigenic determinant expressed by quail, and not chick, endothelial and blood cells (Pardanaud et al. 1987). However, as shown by Pardanaud et al. (1989) and also confirmed by us (results not shown), not only do these few donor endothelial buds fail to expand, but they virtually disappear after grafting and are replaced by recipient-derived vasculariza-

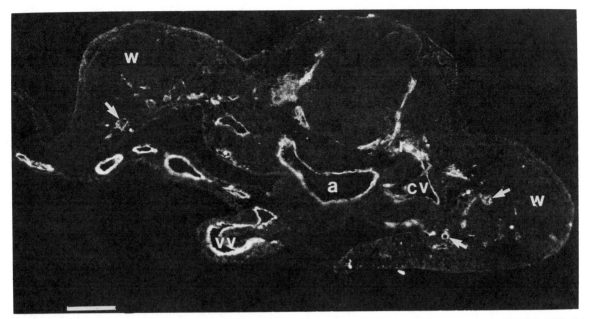

Figure 3. Cross section at the wing-bud level of a quail embryo at stage 17 of Zacchei (1961) immunostained with MAb QH1. (a) Aorta; (cv) cardinal vein; (vv) vitelline vein; (w) wing bud. Bar, 100 μm. Vessel endothelial cells show an immunoreactivity with MAb QH1. Some vascular profiles are present at the base of the limb bud (arrows), whereas the distal part is negative. (Reprinted, with permission, from Pardanaud et al. 1989).

tion. Besides blood vessels and blood cells, the quail limb also receives nerves and their lining Schwann cells, of neural crest origin, from the chick host.

Graft of a Quail Bursa of Fabricius into a Chick Embryo at E4.5-5

It has been established previously that the bursa of Fabricius becomes colonized via a single influx of HCs that takes place between E7 and E11 in the quail and between E8 and E14 in the chick (Fig. 4a; Houssaint et al. 1976). We devised a surgical method to remove the bursa prior to its colonization by HCs at E4.5–E5 (Belo et al. 1985). Of 252 chick embryos bursectomized at

E5, 24 (9.5%) survived up to E19 and 14 (6%) overcame the hatching crisis. Eight survived long enough for their humoral function to be studied. Although they were not totally devoid of B cells (Table 1), they were unable to mount an immune response against any of the antigens that they received (Table 2) (Corbel et al. 1987).

E4.5–5 bursectomized chickens ($n = 382$) received an in situ graft of a bursal rudiment from an E4.5 quail, and 23 (7%) of these quail-to-chick bursal chimeras were able to hatch. Colonization of the quail bursa by chick HCs followed the quail timing, showing once more that the colonized organ, and not the colonizing HCs, is the decisive component of the system for HCs

Table 1. B Lymphocytes in Peripheral Organs of E5-bursectomized Chicks

Chickens	Peripheral blood[a]		Spleen[a]	
	IgM[+]	B-L[+]	IgM[+]	B-L[+]
Bursectomized bird				
BuX 007	<0.1	11.0	dead	dead
BuX 353	0.5	0	n.d.	n.d.
BuX 020	<0.1	n.d.[c]	dead	dead
BuX 014	0.8	n.d	0.4	n.d.
BuX 021	<0.1	5.4	1.4	6.6
BuX 012	1.9	n.d.	n.d.	n.d.
BuX 009	0.7	2.7	0.8	7.9
BuX 222	<0.1	3.5	0.2	20.4
BuX 221	<0.1	10.9	<0.1	10.7
Controls[b]				
$\bar{X} \pm$ S.D.	19.0 ± 1.1	21.5 ± 1.4	23.4 ± 5.5	28.0 ± 6.2

[a] Percentages of cells expressing surface IgM and B-L antigen were determined by immunofluorescence analysis.
[b] ($\bar{X}$) Values for controls are means from four normal birds ±S.D.
[c] (n.d.) Not done.
(BuX *n*) A particular bursectomized chick (Corbel et al. 1987).

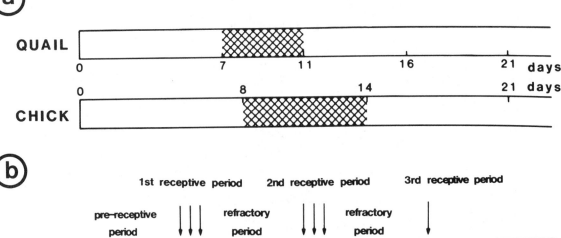

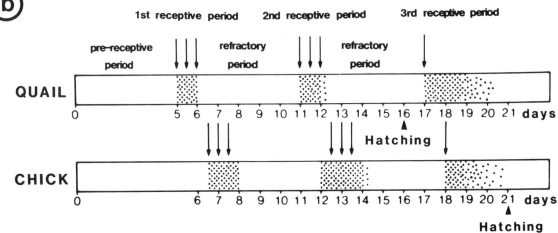

Figure 4. Colonization of bursal (*a*) and thymic (*b*) epitheliomesenchymal rudiments by HCs in quail and chick embryos (Le Douarin and Jotereau 1973, 1975; Houssaint et al. 1976; Coltey et al. 1987).

homing into the primary lymphoid organs (see Le Douarin 1978; Le Douarin et al. 1984).

Graft of a quail bursa resulted in the restoration of B-cell humoral function of the bursectomized chickens. In addition to the fact that the quail-to-chick bursal chimeras possessed virtually normal levels of peripheral

B cells, they were also able to mount specific humoral responses against foreign antigens (Table 3).

The postnatal evolution of such xenogeneic bursal grafts was, however, comparable to that of the limb-bud grafts, i.e., they were also acutely rejected. However, the exact postnatal day at which rejection of the

Table 2. Immune Response of Bursectomized Chicks

	No stimulation (IgG)	First stimulation		Second stimulation		Third stimulation	
		IgG	aHGG	IgG	aHGG	IgG	aHGG
BuX							
840	1.0	1.7	0	1.65	0	1.3	0
353	0.4	0.7	0	3.3	0	4.9	0
012	0.75	1.2	0	1.5	0	dead	dead
021	0.2	0.08	0	0.3	0	n.d.	0
222	0.4	0.4	0	0.4	0	0.15	0
009*	0	0	0	0	0	0	0
007*	0	0	0	0	0	0	0
221*	0	0	0	0	0	0	0
Controls							
$\bar{X}$	2.7	5.2	246	6.0	438	8.2	666
±S.D.	0.25	2.2	256	2.4	278	3.5	838

Concentrations of serum IgG (mg/ml) and anti-human gamma globulin (HGG) antibodies (μg/ml) were quantified by enzyme-linked immunosorbent assay (ELISA). (n.d.) Not determined; (*) animals in which production of IgM was checked by SDS-PAGE and immuno-blotting.

Table 3. Immune Response of Bursal Chimeras

Chimera	No stimulation (IgG)	First stimulation		Second stimulation		Third stimulation	
		IgG	aHGG	IgG	aHGG	IgG	aHGG
416	0.8	0.85	0	2.6	17	6.0	8
070	5.4	6.3	60	12.6	270	18.0	480
067	2.9	4.9	60	6.3	840	5.8	780
846	3.6	2.8	36	3.1	90	5.4	160
354	5.8	9.0	285	9.9	315	dead	dead
837	3.7	6.3	4	7.8	14	7.8	32
016	3.0	5.7	33	5.3	700	dead	dead
$\bar{X}$	3.6	5.1	68	6.8	320	8.6	292
S.D.	1.7	2.6	98	3.6	330	5.3	331

Chicks bursectomized and grafted with a quail bursal rudiment at E5 were immunized at 5–6 weeks of age. Concentrations of total serum IgG (mg/ml) and anti-human gamma globulin (HGG) antibodies (μg/ml) were determined by ELISA at weekly intervals.

bursal stroma began was more difficult to assess, for obvious reasons. From the results indicated in Table 4, one can assume that the host's immune attack on the quail bursa began during the second week post-hatching, in some cases, and that rejection was completed in all birds within the second month of life.

Induction of Tolerance of the Xenogeneic Quail Limb Bud or Bursa of Fabricius by Thymic Epithelial Implants

Thymus development has been investigated previously in quail and chick embryos, and the timing of their seeding by HCs has been established precisely (for review, see Le Douarin 1978; Le Douarin et al. 1984). The thymic primordium is the first hematopoietic organ to be colonized by HCs during ontogeny. Moreover, colonization proceeds according to a cyclic periodicity separated by phases during which the thymus is not receptive for HCs (Fig. 4b).

During this work, we noticed that the epitheliomesenchymal rudiment of the quail thymus introduced into a chick embryo at E3 was seeded by chick HCs and yielded an apparently normal thymus that appeared healthy even several weeks after birth of the chick host (unpublished observation mentioned in Ohki et al. 1987). This suggested that the thymic epithelium could escape the immune surveillance of the host even in a xenogeneic association. In view of the paramount role recognized for the thymus in self/nonself-discrimination, it was tempting to investigate whether the epitheliomesenchymal thymus rudiment from the quail

Table 4. Time at Which Rejection of the Quail Bursa Was Observed in Quail-to-Chick Bursal Chimeras

Age of sacrifice (days)	No. of chimeras with rejection/ no. of cases studied
5	0/2
6	0/1
10	3/5
21	1/2
42	3/3
63	5/5
91	1/1

donor of the wing was capable of inducing a state of tolerance such that the quail wing was tolerated more or less permanently.

The experiment designed to test this hypothesis was as follows: The limb bud from E3.5 to E4 quail was grafted on the chick recipient as before. About 12–20 hours later, the thymic epithelial rudiments arising from the third and fourth pharyngeal pouches were removed as completely as possible from the chick host embryo (Martin 1983) and thereafter replaced by their counterpart from the donor of the quail wing (for technical details, see Ohki et al. 1987).

At that stage, neither the quail nor the chick thymic primordia has yet been colonized by HCs, and when transplanted heterospecifically, the lymphocytes, dendritic cells, and macrophages that they subsequently contain are derived from the host (Le Douarin and Jotereau 1973, 1975; Guillemot et al. 1984; Le Douarin et al. 1984). Consequently, no precursor cells of the monocytic or lymphocytic lineages were included in the thymic epithelial transplant.

Of the 291 chick embryos subjected to this operation, 16 hatched and survived in a healthy state. In all of these birds, the grafted wing remained in good condition for a longer period than that of the control chimeras, which had not been grafted with quail thymus (Fig. 5).

One animal (ADC 60), which never exhibited any signs of rejection, was sacrificed at the age of 483 days (16 months). During the first 2 weeks after birth, the grafted quail wing had grown at a rate close to that of an age-matched quail. However, its growth subsequently decreased, leading to a smaller wing in the adult than in the adult quail control. Because the grafted wing was not pigmented in this bird, two biopsies were performed at 154 and 283 days. After sacrifice, the whole wing was also processed for histology. Skin, connective tissues, muscles, and bones of the quail type were identified on the basis of the structure of their nuclei. No sign of inflammation was present. A blood sample was taken from this animal before sacrifice. No antibodies against common quail antigens could be detected by the immunocytochemical test on cultured fibroblasts (Fig. 5). Three injections of human gamma

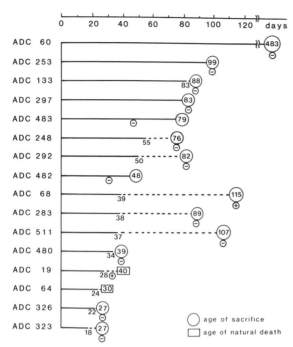

Figure 5. Xenogeneic grafts of the wing bud (E4) and thymic epithelial primordia (E5) from quail to chick embryos. (Solid line) Maintenance of the wing in a healthy state after birth; (dashed line) wing with signs of rejection; (− and +) the result and timing of the test for the anti-quail humoral reaction detected by immunocytochemistry on cultured quail fibroblast. (Reprinted, with permission, from Ohki et al. 1987.)

Table 5. Tolerance of the Grafted Bursa in Thymobursal Chimeras

No. of operated embryos	No. of hatched embryos	Chimeras sacrificed between 47 and 83 days	
		rejected BF	tolerated BF
150	14 (9.3%)	1 (12.5%)	7 (87.5%)

(BF) Bursa of Fabricius.

In both experimental series, the thymuses were analyzed for chimerism using either quail- or chick-specific anti-B-L MAbs TAC1 and TAP1, respectively (Guillemot et al. 1984) or the Feulgen staining procedure for DNA, which allows quail and chick cells to be distinguished (Le Douarin 1969, 1973). In the chimeric thymuses, MAb TAC1 reacted with the epithelial cells of the cortex, whereas the medullary dendritic cells of hematopoietic origin expressed chicken class II antigens as revealed by MAb TAP1 (Fig. 6). Analysis of the thymic lobes developing in both the limb-thymus and the thymobursal quail-to-chick chimeras revealed that the thymic epithelial anlage of the chick recipient had not been completely removed, with the exception of two animals. The thymic lobes developing in the chimeras were therefore constituted either of quail or of chick epithelial cells but only rarely of a mixture of both. In all cases, the thymic lobes containing quail epithelial cells had been populated by chick HCs. No quail HCs were ever detected in these thymuses, either by Feulgen stain or by anti-MB1 monoclonal antibody. Tolerance of either the quail wing or the quail bursa was induced in all cases where at least one third of the total volume of the thymus was made up of quail epithelial cells (Ohki et al. 1988; Belo et al. 1989). It must be noted that the physiological postnatal regression of the thymus takes place at different times in quail and chick: at ~2 months in the former and 7 months in the latter (Ohki et al. 1988). Tolerance of the wing persists after the quail thymic lobes have undergone regression and when the chick lobes seem to be still able to produce peripheral T cells.

globulins were performed at weekly intervals from 6 months of age. One week after each injection, the antibody response was measured and was found to be similar to that of control chickens.

Similarly, no rejection of the wing was observed in four other birds (ADC 253, ADC 297, ADC 482, and ADC 483) (Fig. 5). In ADC 133, a slight edema appeared on the wing at 83 days. None of these six birds produced antibodies directed against common quail antigens. ADC 19 and ADC 68, in which rejection of the wing began at P28 and P39, respectively, were the only chimeras of this group to produce antibodies to quail antigens. However, no antibodies were detected in other birds (ADC 323 and ADC 326) in which rejection appeared earlier, showing once more that cell-mediated and humoral immune responses are dissociated.

Skin grafts from B4 or B12 strains were performed (at 86 days in ADC 253, 73 days in ADC 297, and 6.5 months in ADC 60) and were promptly rejected. Concanavalin A (Con A) stimulation of circulating T cells, carried out on the birds that did not reject the wing, led to normal proliferative responses.

Similar results were obtained for grafts of quail bursa of Fabricius. When the epitheliomesenchymal thymic rudiment from the bursa quail donor was also implanted at E4.5, no immune attack of the quail bursa stroma was observed (Table 5) (Belo et al. 1989).

Effect of the Thymic Epithelium in Tolerance Induction in Mammals

In view of the results obtained in birds, it was of interest to determine whether a role of the epithelial component of the thymus in self/nonself-discrimination could also be demonstrated in mammals. Because the mammalian embryo is not easily available for microsurgery at the early stages of thymic ontogeny, we used the athymic nude mouse, in which a thymic epithelial rudiment is introduced during the early postnatal days under the skin of the dorsal aspect of the neck.

In the mouse, thymus development proceeds from the endoderm of the third branchial pouch, which starts to grow and be colonized by HCs from E11 onward. The fact that the presumptive thymic rudiment is devoid of HCs and unable to develop into a lymphoid

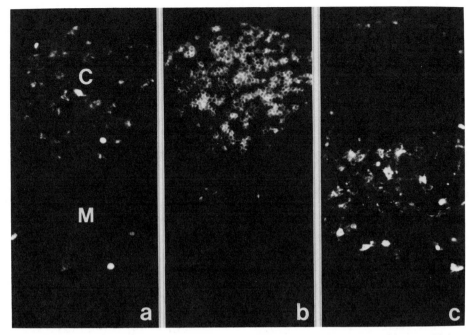

Figure 6. Immunocytochemical analysis of chimerism in the grafted thymus from a thymo-bursal chimera at 80 days. Consecutive sections were stained with quail anti-B-L MAb (TAC1) (*a*); MAb T10 A6, specific for avian thymocytes (Houssaint et al. 1985) (*b*); chick anti-B-L MAb (TAP1) (*c*). (C) Cortex; (M) medulla. (Reprinted, with permission, from Corbel et al. 1989.)

thymus at E10 if it is cultured in the absence of a source of HCs has been fully documented in the past (Metcalf and Moore 1971; Fontaine-Pérus et al. 1981; Good et al. 1983; Salaün et al. 1986). The graft experiments were carried out as indicated in Figure 7.

BALB/c (H-2^d) nude mice were grafted between the day of birth and P13 with 10–15 third branchial arch regions removed from E10 mice of either C3H (H-2^k) or BALB/c euthymic embryos, according to the experimental series.

Restoration of T-cell function was observed in iso- and allogeneically grafted mice. Of 50 newborn mice grafted with BALB/c E10 thymic rudiments, 12 were reconstituted successfully. This was readily apparent at ~3 months of age by the fact that the mice did not lose weight and remained healthy, in contrast to their unreconstituted littermates.

At 4–5 months of age, these animals received a syngeneic and an allogeneic skin graft (Fig. 7). Rejection of the allogeneic skin occurred between 15 and 28 days after implantation (mean value, 18 ± 1.4 days), but the syngeneic skin was accepted in all cases. In normal euthymic BALB/c mice of our colony C3H or C57BL/6, skin grafts were rejected at times ranging from 12 to 15 days.

The 12 mice were sacrificed at 7–10 months of age for T-cell function tests. The neck region was dissected and transplants were removed and treated for histological examination. Microscopic observation showed well-differentiated thymuses and, in some cases, various tissues that had developed from branchial arch mesenchyme and endoderm (cartilage, parathyroid). Spleen and lymph nodes were aseptically removed for in vitro tests. Lymphocytes from the engrafted nude mice were able to react against allogeneic stimulator cells, whereas nontransplanted nude mice were unresponsive.

In the mixed lymphocyte reaction (MLR), the stimulation index varied from 1.53 to 10.23 for spleen or lymph node cells, with a mean value for the 12 mice tested of 3.55 ± 0.63 (for spleen cells). Con A stimulation was significantly higher than in nu/nu mice that had not been grafted.

Cytotoxicity against C3H and C57BL/6 splenocytes was significant in all cases. Particularly high responses were obtained in three of the six mice tested. Nongrafted nude mice failed to generate specific alloreactive cytotoxic T cells. The percentage of Thy-1-2 splenocytes varied from 27% to 33% in the 12 reconstituted mice, a number close to that found in euthymic BALB/c mice (35–38%) and, in any case, much higher than in nonengrafted nude BALB/c mice (3–10%) (Khazaal et al. 1989).

The fully allogeneic thymic epithelium has the same potential to reconstitute the T-cell compartment of athymic nude mice and to induce tolerance for skin grafts of the thymic MHC haplotype. Eighty four BALB/c (H-2^d) nude mice were grafted with thymic rudiments from C3H (H-2^k) E10 embryos. Sixty seven of these mice died before 5 months, which corresponds to the life span of nongrafted nu/nu control mice, but the remaining 17 animals were in good health. Tail skin grafts of recipient (BALB/c), donor (C3H), and third-party (C57BL/6) types were performed on 15 of these mice. Rejection of the C57BL/6 skin occurred after

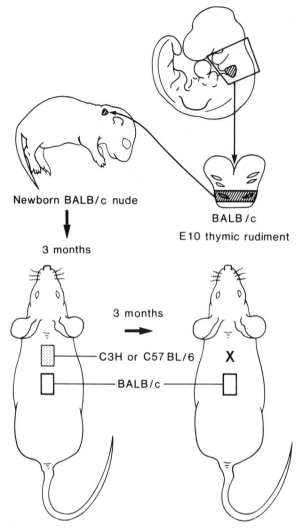

Newborn BALB/c nude

BALB/c
E10 thymic rudiment

3 months

3 months

C3H or C57BL/6

BALB/c

X

Figure 7. Summary of graft experiments. The third branchial pouch removed from a 10-day euthymic BALB/c embryo is grafted under the skin of a newborn BALB/c nude mouse. At 3 months, this nude recipient received two skin grafts: one from a euthymic adult BALB/c mouse and another from a euthymic allogeneic adult C3H or C57BL/6 mouse. (Reprinted, with permission, from Khazaal et al. 1989.)

9–30 days, in all cases. Syngeneic BALB/c skin grafts and skin grafts of thymic epithelium donor haplotype were tolerated in all cases.

Thirteen of these mice were sacrificed 3–5 months after grafting the skin. They were from 9 to 12 months old and in good health. Well-developed thymuses were recovered, as in the case of syngeneic grafts.

We compared the ability of splenic T lymphocytes of nude mice reconstituted with syngeneic or allogeneic thymus epithelium with normal euthymic BALB/c mice to develop in vitro responses against BALB/c, C3H, and third-party MHC mismatched targets. The majority (9/13) of tolerant nude mice showed a readily detectable response, indicating that donor H-2-reactive T cells are not only deleted in those animals, but they are functionally competent to divide (Table 6). In the same way, they showed a killing activity against C3H cells comparable to that displayed against C57BL/6 cells. Four others were fully tolerant (J. Salaün et al., in prep.).

DISCUSSION AND CONCLUSIONS

The possibility of constructing avian chimeras between quail and chick embryos, in which cells of each species can be identified easily, provided the impetus for a series of studies performed in our laboratory on cell migrations and cell interactions during embryogenesis (see, e.g., Le Douarin 1982; Le Douarin and MacLaren 1984). Most of these studies were carried out entirely in embryos and therefore did not encompass the postnatal period. Several years ago, however, we decided to follow up the fate of chickens in which part of the neural epithelium (hence, of the central and peripheral nervous system) had been replaced by their quail counterpart. Such birds are able to hatch and have a sensorimotor behavior compatible with fairly long-term survival because they remain healthy for several weeks to several months after birth (Kinutani and Le Douarin 1985; Kinutani et al. 1986, 1989). However, in virtually all cases, peripheral and

Table 6. Mixed Lymphocyte Reaction

Responder cells		Stimulator cells		
		BALB/c	C3H	C57BL/6
Tolerant (4/13)	BALB/c Nu + Tep 1	8733	35,269[a]	35,219[a]
	BALB/c	4521	48,487	32,356
Non-tolerant (9/13)	BALB/c Nu + Tep 2	3116	17,270[a]	16,236[a]
	BALB/c	8587	30,267	26,882
	BALB/c Nu + Tep 3	4875	6,889[b]	11,236[a]
	BALB/c	5478	17,191	16,051

(Typical responses)

Incorporation of ^{3}HTdR (mean cpm for three replicates).
[a] Significant at 99% (F-test).
[b] Not significant (F-test).

central nervous tissues are subsequently subjected to immune rejection from the host, a phenomenon that manifests itself by the development of a neurological syndrome with the anatopathological characteristics of encephalomyelitis and neuritis. We thought that the absence (or very weak) expression of class I MHC antigens by neural cells could be the prime reason for the long delay before the onset of the host's immune attack. This was substantiated by the fact that grafting either a limb bud or a bursa of Fabricius rudiment during embryogenesis led to rejection of the quail organ within 2 or 3 weeks of hatching. The only quail tissue expressing both class I and class II antigens and not arousing the host's immune response was the epitheliomesenchymal rudiments of the thymus (Ohki et al. 1987). Such tolerance to thymic grafts has already been reported in mice and chickens for allogeneic combinations (Ready et al. 1984; Jordan et al. 1985; Houssaint et al. 1986; von Boehmer and Hafen 1986).

It was therefore of interest to test whether thymic epithelial implants of the same MHC haplotype as the grafted organ (limb or BF) would be able to prevent its rejection in the embryonic graft systems just described. Because the birds (quail or chick) used in these experiments were from outbred flocks, both the thymic and limb or bursal implants were taken from the same donor. A partial thymectomy was carried out in the recipient prior to thymic grafts. This led to the development of a chimeric thymus in which some lobes had an epithelial network of quail origin, and others developed from the remaining anlage of the chick host. Tolerance of either bursa or wing was observed, provided that at least about one third of the thymus contained quail epithelial cells. This duality in the type of epithelial cells present in the thymic lobes raises the problem of the mechanism through which tolerance is induced. If one excludes the unlikely possibility that T cells differentiated in chick lobes can recirculate in quail lobes, it must be assumed that tissue graft tolerance can exist even if only a subset of T cells have been subjected to quail antigens during their intrathymic phase of differentiation and then tolerized. These tolerant quail T cells would therefore be able to prevent the chicken thymus-derived lymphocytes to be activated by the peripheral quail antigens of either the limb or the bursa.

Moreover, it is clear that even when grafted into a chick, the quail thymus undergoes physiological regression ~5 months earlier than its chick counterpart. Therefore, in thymic quail-to-chick chimeras, the quail thymic lobes are already regressed, whereas the chick lobes are still in a functional state. During this postnatal period, however, tolerance of the quail organ is still maintained.

Due to the fact that the animals used in these studies were outbred, further studies such as skin grafts in adults and in vitro tests of reactivity of host lymphocytes to donor cells were not feasible. In contrast, this was possible in the system in which athymic nude BALB/c mice were used as recipients for E10, allogeneic thymic epithelial grafts. Our findings in this model demonstrate that thymic epithelium from fully allogeneic donors, uncontaminated by HCs, induces tolerance to major and minor histocompatibility antigens, as shown by the permanent tolerance of skin grafts from the thymus donor. In these chimeras, where no thymic epithelium of the host is present, one must assume that tolerance to self-antigens is brought about by the hematopoietically derived stroma cells (dendritic cells and macrophages) of the thymus. Despite possessing a thymus with an allogeneic epithelial component, these mice did not exhibit any detectable immune disorder during their life spans. As already determined by other investigators, using a slightly different experimental design in which nude mice were engrafted with older thymuses depleted of HCs by various means (Hong et al. 1979; von Boehmer and Schubiger 1984; Jenski and Hong 1985; Jordan et al. 1985; Schuurman et al. 1986, 1987; Furukawa et al. 1988; Jenski et al. 1988; Jenski and Miller 1988), T lymphocytes of such chimeras can be activated by MHC products of the thymic epithelial type. Although such split tolerance did not always occur (4 out of 13 mice were fully tolerant, in MLR, cytotoxicity, and skin graft tests) in our experiments, it was found in a majority of cases. Several hypotheses may be proposed to account for the lack of correlation between in vivo and in vitro tolerance. First, tolerance to skin graft may not apply to other tissues; experiments are in progress to study in vivo tolerance to other cell types. Alternatively, cells reactive to MHC of the donor type may be subjected in some way to a suppressive mechanism in vivo. A number of groups have reported in vitro reactivities toward syngeneic target cells, which may represent the equivalent, in normal individuals, of those found in tolerized animals.

ACKNOWLEDGMENTS

We thank B. Henri and Y. Rantier for the illustrations and E. Bourson for typing the manuscript. This work was supported by the Centre National de la Recherche Scientifique, the Institut National de la Santé et de la Recherche Médicale, and by grants from the Fondation pour la Recherche Médicale Française and the Ligue Nationale Française contre le Cancer.

REFERENCES

Belo, M., C. Corbel, C. Martin, and N.M. Le Douarin. 1989. Thymic epithelium tolerizes chickens to embryonic grafts of quail bursa of Fabricius. *Int. Immunol.* **1**: 105.

Belo, M., C. Martin, C. Corbel, and N.M. Le Douarin. 1985. A novel method to bursectomize avian embryos and obtain quail-chick bursal chimeras. I. Immunocytochemical analysis of such chimeras by using species-specific monoclonal antibodies. *J. Immunol.* **135**: 3785.

Bevan, M.J., R.E. Langman, and M. Cohn. 1976. H-2 antigen-specific cytotoxic T cells induced by concanavalin A: Estimation of their relative frequency. *Eur. J. Immunol.* **6**: 150.

Coltey, M., F.V. Jotereau, and N.M. Le Douarin. 1987. Evidence for a cyclic renewal of lymphocyte precursor cells in the embryonic chick thymus. *Cell Differ.* **22:** 71.

Corbel, C., M. Belo, C. Martin, and N.M. Le Douarin. 1987. A novel method to bursectomize avian embryos and obtain quail-chick bursal chimeras. II. Immune response of bursectomized chicks and chimeras and post-natal rejection of the grafted quail bursas. *J. Immunol.* **138:** 2813.

———. 1989. Grafts of the bursal primordium in quail→ chick chimeras are tolerated after implantation of thymic epithelium. *Prog. Clin. Biol. Res.* **307:** 31.

Davis, M.M. and P.J. Bjorkman. 1988. T-cell antigen receptor genes and T-cell recognition. *Nature* **334:** 395.

Fontaine-Pérus, J.C., F.M. Calman, C. Kaplan, and N.M. Le Douarin. 1981. Seeding of the 10-day mouse thymic rudiment by lymphocyte precursors in vitro. *J. Immunol.* **126:** 2310.

Furukawa, F., S. Ikehara, R.A. Good, T. Nakamura, S. Inoue, H. Tanaka, S. Inamura, and Y. Hamashima. 1988. Immunological status of nude mice engrafted with allogeneic or syngeneic thymuses. *Thymus* **12:** 11.

Good, M.F., K.W. Pyke, and G.J.V. Nossal. 1983. Functional clonal deletion of cytotoxic T-lymphocyte precursors in chimeric thymus produced in vitro from embryonic anlagen. *Proc. Natl. Acad. Sci.* **80:** 3045.

Guillemot, F.P., P.D. Oliver, B.M. Péault, and N.M. Le Douarin. 1984. Cells expression Ia-antigens in the avian thymus. *J. Exp. Med.* **160:** 1803.

Hong, R., H. Schulte-Wissermann, E. Jarrett-Toth, S.D. Horowitz, D.D. Manning. 1979. Transplantation of cultured thymic fragments. II. Results in nude mice. *J. Exp. Med.* **149:** 398.

Houssaint, E., M. Belo, and N.M. Le Douarin. 1976. Investigations on cell lineage and tissue interactions in the developing bursa of Fabricius through interspecific chimeras. *Dev. Biol.* **53:** 250.

Houssaint, E., E. Diez, and F.V. Jotereau. 1985. Tissue distribution and ontogenic appearance of a chicken T lymphocyte differentiation marker. *Eur. J. Immunol.* **15:** 305.

Houssaint, E., A. Torano, and J. Ivanyi. 1986. Split tolerance induced by chick embryo thymic epithelium allografted to embryonic recipients. *J. Immunol.* **136:** 3155.

Jenski, L.J. and B.A. Miller. 1988. Thymic influence on the lymphocyte self MHC repertoire. II. Cytotoxic T-lymphocyte precursors. *Thymus* **11:** 151.

Jenski, J., M.L. Belloni, and B.A. Miller. 1988. Thymic influence on the T lymphocyte self MHC repertoire. I. Helper T lymphocyte precursors. *Thymus* **11:** 135.

Jordan, R.K., J.H. Robinson, N.A. Hopkinson, K.C. House, and A.L. Bentley. 1985. Thymic epithelium and the induction of transplantation tolerance in nude mice. *Nature* **314:** 454.

Khazaal, I., J. Salaün, M. Coltey, F. Calman, and N.M. Le Douarin. 1989. Restoration of T-cell function in nude mice by grafting the epitheliomesenchymal thymic rudiment from 10 day-old euthymic embryos. *Cell Differ.* **26:** 211.

Kingston, R., E.J. Jenkinson, and J.J.T. Owen. 1985. A single stem cell can recognize an embryonic thymus, producing phenotypically distinct T-cell populations. *Nature* **308:** 738.

Kinutani, M. and N.M. Le Douarin. 1985. Avian spinal cord chimeras. I. Hatching ability and post hatching survival in homo- and heterospecific chimeras. *Dev. Biol.* **111:**243.

Kinutani, M., M. Coltey, and N.M. Le Douarin. 1986. Postnatal development of a demyelinating disease in spinal cord chimaeras. *Cell* **45:** 307.

Kinutani, M., K. Tan, J. Desaki, M. Coltey, K. Kitaoka, Y. Nagano, Y. Takashima, and N.M. Le Douarin. 1989. Avian spinal cord chimeras. Further studies on the neurological syndrome affecting the chimeras after birth. *Cell Differ.* **26:** 145.

Le Douarin, N.M. 1969. Particularités du noyau chez la Caille japonaise (Coturnix coturnix japonica). Utilisation de ses particularités comme "marquage biologique" dans des re-cherches sur les interactions tissulaires et les migrations cellulaires au cours de l'ontogenése. *Bull. Biol. Fr. Belg.* **103:** 435.

———. 1973. A biological cell labeling technique and its use in experimental embryology. *Dev. Biol.* **30:** 217.

———. 1978. Ontogeny of hematopoietic organs studied in avian embryo interspecific chimeras. *Cold Spring Harbor Conf. Cell Proliferation* **5:** 5.

———, ed. 1982. *The neural crest.* Cambridge University Press, Cambridge, England.

Le Douarin, N.M. and F.V. Jotereau. 1973. Origin and renewal of lymphocytes in avian embryo thymuses studied in interspecific combinations. *Nat. New Biol.* **246:** 25.

———. 1975. Origin of haematopoietic stem cells in the embryonic bursa of Fabricius and bone-marrow studied through interspecific chimaeras. *J. Exp. Med.* **142:** 17.

Le Douarin, N.M. and A. MacLaren, eds. 1984. *Chimeras in developmental biology.* Academic Press, London.

Le Douarin, N.M., F. Dieterlen-Liévre, and P.D. Oliver. 1984. Ontogeny of primary lymphoid organs and lymphoid stem cells. *Am J. Anat.* **170:** 261.

Martin, C.S. 1983. Total thymectomy in the early chick embryo. *Arch. Anat. Microsc.* **72:** 107.

Metcalf, D. and M.A.S. Moore, eds. 1971. *Haemopoietic cells.* Elsevier, North-Holland, Amsterdam.

Ohki, H., C. Martin, M. Coltey, and N.M. Le Douarin. 1988. Implants of quail thymic epithelium generate permanent tolerance in embryonically constructed quail/chick chimeras. *Development* **104:** 619.

Ohki, H., C. Martin, C. Corbel, M. Coltey, and N.M. Le Douarin. 1987. Tolerance induced by thymic epithelial grafts in birds. *Science* **237:** 1032.

Pardanaud, L., F. Yassine, and F. Dieterlen-Liévre. 1989. Relationship between vasculogenesis, angiogenesis and haemopoiesis during avian ontogeny. *Development* **105:** 473.

Pardanaud, L., C. Altmann, P. Kitos, F. Dieterlen-Liévre, and C.A. Buck. 1987. Vasculogenesis in the early quail blastodisc as studied with a monoclonal antibody recognizing endothelial cells. *Development* **100:** 339.

Péault, B.M., J.P. Thiery, and N.M. Le Douarin. 1983. Surface marker for the hemopoietic and endothelial cell lineages in the quail that is defined by a monoclonal antibody. *Proc. Natl. Acad. Sci.* **80:** 2976.

Ready, A.R., E.J. Jenkinson, R. Kingston, and J.J.T. Owen. 1984. Successful transplantation across major histocompatibility barrier of deoxyguanosine-treated embryonic thymus expressing class II antigens. *Nature* **310:** 231.

Rothenberg, E. and J.P. Lugo. 1985. Differentiation and cell division in the mammalian thymus. *Dev. Biol.* **112:** 1.

Salaün, J., F. Calman, M. Coltey, and N.M. Le Douarin. 1986. Construction of chimeric thymuses in the mouse fetus by in utero surgery. *Eur. J. Immunol.* **16:** 523.

Scollay, E., P. Bartlett, and K. Shortman. 1984. T cell development in the adult murine thymus: Changes in the expression of the surface antigens Ly 2, L3T4 and B2A2 during development from early precursor cells to emigrants. *Immunol. Rev.* **82:** 79.

Schuurman, H.J., L.M.B. Vaessen, R. Broekhuizen, C.J.W. Brandt, M.C. Holewijn, J.G. Vos, and J. Rozing. 1987. Implantation of cultured thymic fragments in congenitally athymic (nude) rats. *Scand. J. Immunol.* **26:** 129.

Schuurman, H.J., L.M.B. Vaessen, J.G. Vos, A. Hertogh, J.G.N. Geertzema, C.J.W. Brandt, and J. Rozing. 1986. Implantation of cultured thymic fragments in congenitally athymic (nude) rats: Ignorance of thymic epithelial haplotype in generation of alloreactivity. *J. Immunol.* **137:** 2440.

Sprent, J., D. Lo, E.K. Gao, and Y. Ron. 1988. T cell selection in the thymus. *Immunol. Rev.* **101:** 173.

Stutman, O. 1978. Intrathymic and extrathymic T cell maturation. *Immunol. Rev.* **42:** 138.

Teh, H.S., E. Harley, R.A. Phillips, and R.G. Miller. 1977.

Quantitative studies on the precursors of cytotoxic lymphocytes. I. Characterization of a clonal assay and determination of the size of clones derived from single precursors. *J. Immunol.* **118:** 1049.

von Boehmer, H. and K. Hafen. 1986. Minor but not major histocompatibility antigens of thymus epithelium tolerize precursors of cytolytic T cells. *Nature* **320:** 636.

von Boehmer, H. and K. Schubiger. 1948. Thymocytes appear to ignore class I major histocompatibility complex antigens expressed on thymus epithelial cells. *Eur. J. Immunol.* **14:** 1048.

Zacchei, A.M. 1961. Lo sviluppo embrionale della quaglia giapponese (Coturnix coturnix japonica T.e S.). *Arch. Ital. Anat. Embryol.* **66:** 36.

Zinkernagel, R.M. and P.C. Doherty. 1979. MHC-restricted cytotoxic T cell: Studies on the biological role of polymorphic major transplantation antigens determining T cell restriction-specificity, function and responsiveness. *Adv. Immunol.* **27:** 51.

T-cell Tolerance to H-2 Molecules: Role of the Thymus

J. Sprent, E.-K. Gao, and S.R. Webb

Department of Immunology, Research Institute of Scripps Clinic, La Jolla, California 92037

Although it has long been known that T cells arise in the thymus (Miller and Osoba 1967), the mechanisms controlling the differentiation of thymocytes into mature T cells are still only partly understood. The prevailing view at present is that the thymus has two main functions: (1) From a very large pool of precursor cells, the thymus selects a subset of T cells that is tailored to recognize antigen in the extrathymic environment, and (2) the thymus maintains self-tolerance by destroying T cells that display overt autoreactivity. This paper deals with the mechanisms involved in self-tolerance induction and the range of cell types that participate in this process. Before discussing tolerance, however, it is useful to dwell briefly on positive selection, i.e., the process used to generate the postthymic repertoire of T cells.

Positive Selection

Studies on bone marrow chimeras (von Boehmer and Sprent 1976; Bevan 1977) and thymus-grafted mice (Fink and Bevan 1978; Zinkernagel et al. 1978) have provided compelling evidence that the pattern of major histocompatibility complex (MHC)-restricted specificity displayed by mature extrathymic T cells is determined in the thymus during T-cell ontogeny. These studies strongly suggest that for mature T cells to display MHC-restricted specificity to self-MHC molecules, the T cells must encounter these particular MHC molecules on a radio-resistant component of the thymus (Fink and Bevan 1978; Zinkernagel et al. 1978), probably on epithelial cells in the cortex (Lo and Sprent 1986). Direct support for this concept of *positive selection* of T cells in the thymus has come from recent work on T-cell receptor (TCR) transgenic mice (Kisielow et al. 1988a; Sha et al. 1988).

In discussing the mechanism of positive selection, it is essential to consider the paradox that very few thymocytes are selected for export to the secondary lymphoid organs, despite the large size of the thymus. For example, the maximal release of T cells from the thymus in young mice is only 1×10^6 to 2×10^6 per day (for review, see Scollay and Shortman 1985). Bearing in mind that the thymus of young mice contains 1×10^8 to 2×10^8 cells, nearly all of which have a rapid turnover, it is inescapable that the vast majority of thymocytes die in situ. How can one explain this strange

phenomenon? At one time, it was argued that the rapid turnover of thymocytes reflected an anti-self-proliferative response. This response facilitated somatic hypermutation of TCR molecules and resulted in a proportion of T cells acquiring the requisite form of covert MHC-restricted specificity displayed by mature postthymic T cells. This line of reasoning is now untenable because there is little, if any, convincing evidence for somatic mutation of TCR molecules. Furthermore, the rapid turnover of thymocytes appears to be restricted to TCR⁻ cells: Once TCR molecules appear on the cell surface, division ceases and the cell enters interphase (Parkin et al. 1988).

At face value, the simplest explanation for the wide-scale death of cells in the thymus is that cell death is a reflection of self-tolerance induction. The main problem with this notion is that it is difficult to imagine that the vast majority of thymocytes could be autoreactive. It is also hard to envisage why such cells would be conserved during evolution.

The explanation favored for the massive death of cells in the thymus is based on the assumption that the specificity range of TCR molecules expressed on early thymocytes is enormous and can encompass all of the alleles of each of the MHC molecules of the species as a whole. Thus, if a species expresses 100 different MHC haplotypes, the thymus of each individual member of that species will produce 100 different subsets of thymocytes, some with specificity for strain *a* MHC, some for strain *b* MHC, etc. At the level of a single individual, however, only a tiny fraction of this large pool of precursor cells would be useful in the postthymic environment. Thus, a strain *a* mouse needs to generate *a*-restricted T cells but does not want, for example, *b*- or *c*-restricted cells. How does this individual discard the T cells it does not need? The simplest explanation is that thymocytes are programmed to destroy themselves, and the only way thymocytes can avoid self-destruction is to receive a protective ("do not die") signal from epithelial cells. Delivery of this protective signal is restricted to potentially useful T cells, i.e., to T cells that have binding specificity for the self-MHC molecules expressed on thymic epithelium. Thus, in a strain *a* individual, binding to epithelial cells is restricted to the *a*-restricted subset of thymocytes. These cells receive a signal that counteracts programmed cell death, and the cells survive for export to the periphery. All other T cells—T cells with, for example, b- or c-restricted specificity—fail to receive a protective signal and undergo autodestruction.

This ad hoc model accommodates most of the available facts on thymocyte differentiation, but it clearly poses many complex questions, particularly the *nature* of the putative protective signal provided by epithelial cells. The key obstacle in addressing this issue experimentally is that at present, positive selection can only be studied at the level of the intact thymus. Real progress in understanding the mechanism of positive selection will probably depend on being able to reproduce thymocyte maturation in cultures containing dissociated suspensions of purified epithelial cells plus defined populations of stem cells.

Negative Selection

Because postthymic T cells remain in interphase for prolonged periods and move continuously through tissues containing high concentrations of MHC molecules, it follows that in the absence of antigen, the specificity of T cells for self-MHC molecules is below the threshold required for cell triggering. T cells thus display self-tolerance. Although it has long been argued that self-MHC tolerance reflects clonal deletion of cells with overt autoreactivity, the entry into the literature of T-suppressor cells, the "autologous mixed-lymphocyte reaction (MLR)," etc., stimulated attempts to seek *direct* evidence for the concept of clonal deletion as a mechanism of tolerance. Formal proof for clonal deletion has come from the recent finding that intrathymic expression of H-2 I-E molecules in mice results in selective destruction of a subset of T cells, i.e., T cells expressing $V_\beta 17a$ TCR molecules (Kappler et al. 1987). These T cells are destroyed in situ in the thymus, presumably because $V_\beta 17a$ TCR molecules happen to express strong reactivity to I-E molecules. Significantly, the deletion of $V_\beta 17a^+$ T cells in the thymus is prominent only at the level of cells expressing a high density of TCR molecules, which suggests that deletion occurs at a relatively late stage of thymocyte maturation.

Although the notion that clonal deletion of auto-MHC-reactive T cells takes place in the thymus is now well accepted, detailed information on the mechanisms of tolerance is still quite sparse. In particular, there is still considerable debate on which cell types control tolerance induction.

One of the most useful models for addressing this question is to allow T cells to differentiate in an MHC-different thymus and then examine the level of tolerance to the allo-MHC molecules of the graft. Initial studies with this system showed that T cells from congenitally athymic nude mice given H-2-different neonatal thymus grafts manifested surprisingly little tolerance to the donor strain in vitro (Zinkernagel et al. 1980). Thus, culturing T cells from these mice with stimulator cells of donor origin generated strong cyto-toxic T lymphocyte (CTL) activity against graft-type target cells. Such lack of tolerance was conspicuous only at many months postgrafting, which led investigators to postulate that tolerance is not controlled by an endogenous component of the thymus but by a population of bone-marrow-derived cells with a relatively short lifespan.

Direct support for this idea came from studies with fetal thymuses cultured with deoxyguanosine (dGuo) in vitro (Jenkinson et al. 1982); this treatment destroys lymphohematopoietic cells but leaves the epithelial component of the thymus apparently intact. The notable result with this technique is that both for thymus-grafted mice and for thymic organ cultures maintained in vitro, T cells differentiating in dGuo-treated H-2-different fetal thymuses retain strong responsiveness to graft-type H-2 determinants (von Boehmer and Schubiger 1984; Jenkinson et al. 1985). This finding applies to primary mixed-lymphocyte reactions (MLRs) (an assay for T-cell proliferation), as well as to CTL generation. With the subsequent observation that the tolerogenicity of dGuo-treated thymuses can be restored by addition of small numbers of purified graft-type dendritic cells (Matzinger and Guerder 1989), most groups have assumed that tolerance induction is controlled largely or, perhaps, entirely by bone-marrow-derived cells, especially dendritic cells. Because dendritic cells reside in the thymic medulla and are rare in the cortex, the suggestion was put forward that positive and negative selection are strictly compartmentalized, with positive selection taking place in the cortex and negative selection (tolerance) occurring in the medulla (Lo et al. 1986). In the case of negative selection, this scenario obviously hinges on the assumption that tolerance is controlled exclusively by dendritic cells or related bone-marrow-derived cells. In fact, recent evidence suggests that this assumption is invalid and that several different cell types, including T cells and epithelial cells, can contribute to tolerance induction, depending on the assay system used.

Tolerogenicity of T cells. The notion that tolerance occurs solely in the medulla has clearly been challenged by experiments with TCR transgenic mice (Kisielow et al. 1988b; Sha et al. 1988). These studies indicate that tolerance of T cells to H-2 class I molecules in the thymus occurs in the cortex at a very early stage of differentiation, i.e., at or before the stage when thymocytes begin to express CD4 and CD8 accessory molecules. This finding contrasts with the studies on $V_\beta 17a$ expression, where the presence of I-E molecules in the thymus deletes $V_\beta 17a^+$ mature thymocytes (medullary cells expressing either CD4 or CD8 molecules but not both) but causes only minimal deletion of immature $V_\beta 17a^+$ thymocytes (cortical cells expressing both CD4 and CD8 molecules) (Kappler et al. 1987). In speculating on why tolerance induction occurs at a later stage of differentiation for $V_\beta 17a$ T cells than for the T cells generated in the above TCR transgenic lines, it should be noted that the tolerogens in the two systems are quite different: $V_\beta 17a$ T cells are deleted by H-2 class II (I-E) molecules, whereas tolerance in the transgenic lines is directed to class I molecules. Tolerance induction at the level of immature thymocytes might thus apply only to class-I-reactive cells, with tolerance of class-II-reactive cells taking place largely or solely in the medulla. This issue will be discussed later.

One explanation for the early induction of tolerance to class I molecules is that thymocytes, themselves, are tolerogenic. Because H-2 expression by thymocytes is largely limited to class I molecules, the tolerogenicity of thymocytes would presumably be directed exclusively to class-I-reactive T cells. Direct support for this notion has come from the finding that intrathymic transfer of purified CD4⁻ CD8⁻ thymic stem cells into an H-2-different thymus leads to tolerance induction to self (donor)-class I molecules but not to self-class II molecules (Shimonkevitz and Bevan 1988).

Tolerogenicity of thymic epithelial cells. Despite the evidence from studies on T cells differentiating in dGuo-treated thymuses, other data are difficult to reconcile with the notion that thymic epithelial cells are completely nontolerogenic. Thus, there are a number of reports that T cells differentiating in allogeneic thymuses depleted of lymphohematopoietic cells show at least partial tolerance to thymus-type MHC molecules (Good et al. 1983; Flajnik et al. 1985; Jordan et al. 1985; Houssaint et al. 1986; Le Douarin, this volume). Likewise, transgenic mice in which I-E molecules appear to be expressed selectively in thymic epithelial cells show considerable tolerance to transgenic I-E molecules (Widera et al. 1987; Marrack et al. 1988).

Because of the confusion in the literature, we have recently been reinvestigating the role of thymic epithelial cells in tolerance induction. A summary of our recent data on two different experimental systems is given below. The data are still incomplete and have yet to be published.

Tolerance in nude mice given dGuo-treated fetal thymus grafts. The approach used here is to take day-14 fetal thymuses from $(B6 \times DBA/2)F_1$ ($H-2^b \times H-2^d$) embryos and culture the thymuses with dGuo for 5 days in vitro, using established techniques (Jenkinson et al. 1982; von Boehmer and Schubiger 1984). The dGuo-treated thymuses are grafted under the kidney capsule of B6 nude mice. To guard against incomplete removal of lymphohematopoietic cells by the dGuo treatment, the thymus-grafted mice are left for 2–4 months and then given whole-body irradiation plus Thy-1-marked B6.PL ($H-2^b$, Thy-1.1) T-depleted bone marrow cells. The new wave of T cells generated in the thymus-grafted mice is isolated by selecting for Thy-1.1⁺ T cells. Purified T cells or T-cell subsets are then cultured in vitro with B10.D2 spleen stimulator cells, i.e., cells expressing graft-type $H-2^d$ determinants. The results obtained to date are summarized in Table 1.

In accordance with the findings of other workers (von Boehmer and Schubiger 1984), culturing T cells from the thymus-grafted mice with B10.D2 stimulators plus concanavalin A (Con A) supernatant generates strong CTL activity to B10.D2 target cells (Con A blasts). Likewise, strong proliferative responses occur when purified CD8⁺ cells from the thymus-grafted mice are cultured with B10.D2 stimulators in the presence of recombinant IL-2 (rIL-2). According to these parameters, there is no evidence that T-cell differentiation in the dGuo-treated thymus grafts leads to tolerance induction; however, very different results are observed when T cells are cultured in the absence of added lymphokines. Thus, whereas purified CD8⁺ cells from normal B6 mice respond well to B10.D2 stimulators, with or without addition of IL-2, CD8⁺ cells from the thymus-grafted mice give virtually no response to B10.D2 in the absence of added IL-2. These data refer to CD8⁺ cells. Somewhat different results are observed with CD4⁺ cells. When mature CD4⁺ cells are prepared from spleen or lymph nodes of the thymus-grafted mice, primary MLRs to B10.D2 stimulators are

Table 1. T-cell Function in B6 Nude Mice Grafted with dGuo-treated Thymuses Taken from $(B6 \times DBA/2)F_1$ Embryos: Split Tolerance to Graft-type ($H-2^d$) Stimulators

Assay	Responder cells ± lymphokines cultured with B10.D2 stimulators	Response to B10.D2($H-2^d$) by T cells from — normal B6	B6 nude mice with dGuo-treated $H-2^d$ thymus grafts
CML[a]	spleen T + Con A s/n	+ + + +	+ + + +
MLR	lymph node CD8⁺ + rIL-2	+ + + +	+ + + +
MLR	lymph node CD8⁺	+ + + +	±[b]
MLR	lymph node CD4⁺	+ + + +	+ +
MLR	thymus CD4⁺(CD8⁻)	+ + + +	±[b]

Summary of data on tolerance induction in T cells differentiating in adult B6 ($H-2^b$) nude mice grafted with day-14 $(B6 \times DBA/2)F_1$ ($H-2^b \times H-2^d$) fetal thymuses cultured for 5 days in vitro with 1.4 mM dGuo. As discussed in the text, the thymus-grafted mice were left for a period of 2–4 months to allow disappearance of any APCs that might have survived the dGuo treatment. The mice were then irradiated (800 rads) and reconstituted with B6 Thy-1.1 bone marrow cells. The Thy-1.1⁺ T cells differentiating in the thymus-grafted mice were then tested in vitro for responsiveness to thymic-type $H-2^d$ stimulator cells.

[a]Cell-mediated lympholysis.
[b]These responses were virtually undetectable.

reduced by ~70% relative to the response of normal B6 CD4$^+$ cells. Tolerance of CD4$^+$ cells is therefore considerable, but not complete. Interestingly, this partial tolerance of CD4$^+$ cells applies only to extrathymic cells. Thus, the mature component of CD4$^+$ (CD8$^-$) cells isolated from the thymus graft, itself, displays near *complete* unresponsiveness to B10.D2 stimulators; responses to third-party H-2 differences remain high.

How can one explain these confusing findings? In the case of the CD8$^+$ subset of T cells, the data suggest that these H-2 class-I-reactive cells manifest a subtle form of tolerance: Reactivity to graft-type H-2 determinants is high (implying a lack of clonal deletion) but is apparently restricted to helper-dependent cells, i.e., to cells that function only in the presence of exogenous lymphokines. Therefore, the implication is that contact of early CD8$^+$ cells with thymic epithelial cells somehow prevents the production of helper-independent CD8$^+$ cells, i.e., cells that can synthesize their own growth factors. Speculating on how the thymus results in this change of phenotype is difficult because the essential difference between helper-dependent and helper-independent CD8$^+$ cells is unclear. The possibility favored currently is that helper-independent cells are simply a minor subset of CD8$^+$ cells expressing high-affinity TCRs. Because of their high affinity, these helper-independent cells can be tolerized (deleted) through contact with thymic epithelium. The vast majority of alloreactive CD8$^+$ cells are probably helper-dependent cells, i.e., cells that depend heavily on exogenous help provided either by the helper-independent subset of CD8$^+$ cells or by CD4$^+$ cells. In contrast to helper-independent CD8$^+$ cells, we envisage that the affinity of helper-dependent CD8$^+$ cells is quite low, i.e., too low for the cells to be tolerized by thymic epithelium.

The notion that thymic epithelium can selectively tolerize high-affinity T cells could also explain the partial tolerance seen for lymph node CD4$^+$ cells. Thus, the nontolerant component of lymph node CD4$^+$ cells from dGuo-thymus grafted mice might represent a discrete subset of low-affinity cells. The obvious problem with this line of reasoning is that there are no direct assays for measuring TCR affinity at present, either for CD4$^+$ or for CD8$^+$ cells. Moreover, the argument that thymic epithelium spares low-affinity cells selectively fails to explain why tolerance is apparently complete at the level of thymocytes (at least for CD4$^+$ cells) but is only partial for extrathymic T cells. Before discussing this paradox, it is first useful to consider the main features of tolerance induction in a quite different model.

Tolerance in parent → F$_1$ bone marrow chimeras. Studies carried out on bone marrow chimeras a number of years ago showed that T cells developing in heavily irradiated F$_1$ mice reconstituted with a mixture of bone marrow cells taken from both parental strains led to a state of complete tolerance induction (von Boehmer and Sprent 1976). Thus, the T cells that developed from each population of parental strain stem cells exhibited total unresponsiveness to the opposite parental strain. The completeness of tolerance induction was considered to reflect the fact that immature T cells in the double chimeras encountered H-2 determinants of the opposite parental strain on macrophages (MΦ) and dendritic cells, i.e., cells with strong antigen-presenting cell (APC) function. If these cells were essential for tolerance induction, it was reasoned that reconstituting irradiated F$_1$ mice with bone marrow cells of only one parental strain would not lead to tolerance. The heavy dose of irradiation would destroy the bone-marrow-derived cells of the host rapidly, with the result that newly generated donor-derived T cells would fail to encounter host-type APCs and would therefore not be tolerized. The results verified this prediction only partially. Thus, the donor T cells from the chimeras did elicit significant primary MLRs to host-type H-2 determinants, but this response was considerably reduced relative to the response of normal parental strain T cells (Sprent et al. 1975). Moreover, there was complete tolerance to the host for CTL activity.

These findings raised the possibility that tolerance is not controlled solely by bone-marrow-derived cells. Alternatively, the dose of irradiation (900 rads) used to prepare the chimeras might not have been sufficient to cause total removal of host bone-marrow-derived cells. To attempt to distinguish between these two possibilities, we have recently been examining tolerance induction in parent → F$_1$ chimeras prepared with very heavy irradiation, i.e., 1300 rads. When examined at 4 months postirradiation, these chimeras contain no detectable host-type APCs, i.e., cells able to stimulate primary MLRs by normal parental strain T cells. Likewise, frozen sections of spleen, lymph nodes, and skin of the chimeras reveal a virtual absence of cells expressing a high density of host class II (Ia) molecules (high Ia expression being a characteristic feature of cells with APC function).

Despite the apparent absence of host-type APCs, the T cells generated in these supralethally irradiated parent → F$_1$ chimeras show a considerable degree of tolerance to the host (Table 2). In the case of CD8$^+$ cells, tolerance is virtually complete. These cells show total unresponsiveness to host-type APCs in vitro, even in the presence of added lymphokines, and fail to differentiate into host-specific CTLs. This finding clearly contrasts with the minimal tolerance of CD8$^+$ cells seen in thymus-grafted nude mice (see above). In this respect, it should be emphasized that it is still uncertain whether the tolerance of CD8$^+$ cells in parent → F$_1$ chimeras is induced within the thymus or in the post-thymic environment. The possibility that tolerance is induced extrathymically deserves serious consideration, because virtually all cells in the body, including nonhematopoietic cells, express appreciable levels of class I molecules. In contrast, class II molecules are expressed at only a very low level on nonhematopoietic cells. The crucial question, which we have yet to ad-

Table 2. Features of Tolerance Induction in Parent→F$_1$ Chimeras Prepared with Double Irradiation (1300 rads + 1000 rads)

Cells tested	Response to host-type H-2 determinants
Lymph node CD8$^+$	complete specific unresponsiveness to host-type APC ± added lymphokines
CD4$^+$	50–70% specific reduction in MLR to host-type APCs; residual MLR is unusually susceptible to inhibition with anti-Ia antibody, suggesting that the response is controlled by low-affinity cells 60–80% reduction of V$_\beta$11$^+$ cells in I-E→I-E$^+$ combinations transfer of cells to further host-type F$_1$ mice leads to proliferation but fails to cause lethal GVHD
Thymus CD4$^+$(CD8$^-$)	>95% selective reduction of MLR to host-type APCs; deletion of V$_\beta$11$^+$ cells is no more marked than in lymph nodes.

The data summarize findings on (B6 × CBA)F$_1$ (H-2^b × H-2^k) mice exposed to 1300 rads and reconstituted with T-depleted B6 or CBA bone marrow cells. The mice were left for 4–6 months and given a second dose of irradiation (1000 rads) and more parent-strain bone marrow cells. Lymph nodes and thymocytes were removed from the host 2–3 months later. To ensure that the T cells studied were derived from the second dose of bone marrow cells, Thy-1.1$^+$ bone marrow was used for secondary reconstitution of B6→F$_1$ chimeras.

dress, is whether tolerance of CD8$^+$ cells in parent→F$_1$ chimeras is evident *within* the thymus.

Like CD8$^+$ cells, the CD4$^+$ cells in heavily irradiated parent→F$_1$ chimeras exhibit strong tolerance to host-type APCs. According to some parameters, the tolerance of CD4$^+$ cells is virtually complete. Thus, whereas even very small doses of normal parental strain CD4$^+$ cells cause lethal graft-versus-host disease (GVHD) in irradiated F$_1$ hosts, transfer of large doses of CD4$^+$ cells from the chimeras to further irradiated host-type F$_1$ mice causes no mortality. The tolerance of CD4$^+$ cells appears to reflect clonal deletion, because in I-E→I-E$^+$ combinations, the CD4$^+$ cells in the chimeras show a 60–80% reduction in the proportion of V$_\beta$11$^+$ cells. (Like V$_\beta$17a$^+$ T cells, V$_\beta$11$^+$ T cells are selectively deleted in I-E$^+$ strains [Bill et al. 1989].) The possibility that tolerance in the chimeras reflects incomplete elimination of host-type APCs seems unlikely because various procedures designed to ensure "complete" removal of these cells fail to abrogate tolerance induction. These procedures include conditioning the chimeras with repeated injection of anti-host-Ia monoclonal antibody and subjecting the chimeras to a second dose of irradiation (1000 rads) several months after the initial dose.

Although parent→F$_1$ chimeras seem to be completely devoid of cells with anti-host effector function, lymph node CD4$^+$ cells from the chimeras do manifest the potential to mount proliferative responses to host-type APCs in vitro. Similar proliferative responses occur when the chimera CD4$^+$ cells are exposed to host-type APCs in vivo, i.e., by transferring T cells from the chimeras into further irradiated host-type F$_1$ mice. The proliferative response of the chimera lymph node CD4$^+$ cells to host-type APCs in vitro has two characteristics. First, the response tends to be quite low, i.e., two- to fourfold lower than the response given by a comparable number of normal parental strain CD4$^+$ cells; this reduction in the potency of the chimera cells parallels the 70–80% clonal deletion of V$_\beta$11$^+$ cells. Second, the anti-host response by the chimera CD4$^+$ cells is unusually sensitive to inhibition by anti-host-Ia antibody. This finding suggests that the response is mediated by low-affinity cells.

Because the lymph node CD4$^+$ cells from parent→F$_1$ chimeras appear to be devoid of cells with anti-host effector function (e.g., cells able to elicit lethal GVHD), the proliferative responses to host-type APCs can be viewed as a sterile MLR. As discussed above, we favor the notion that this residual responsiveness to the host is mediated by a small subset of low-affinity cells, high-affinity cells having been deleted during ontogeny. Are these cells deleted in the thymus or in the postthymic environment? To address this question, we studied tolerance induction in parent→F$_1$ chimeras given parental-strain thymus grafts. Thymectomized (a × b)F$_1$ mice were exposed to heavy irradiation (1300 rads) and reconstituted with parent a bone marrow cells. The chimeras were left for several months to allow disappearance of host-type APCs and were then grafted with an irradiated parental-strain a thymus. The notable finding here was that the strain a CD4$^+$ cells differentiating in the strain a thymus grafts did not exhibit tolerance to host strain b H-2 determinants. The CD4$^+$ cells from the thymus-grafted mice showed no deletion of V$_\beta$11$^+$ cells and gave strong proliferative responses to strain b APCs in vitro. This finding applied not only to lymph node CD4$^+$ cells, but also to CD4$^+$-enriched cells prepared from the thymus grafts. The anti-b MLR of both CD4$^+$ populations was as high as that for CD4$^+$ cells taken from normal strain a mice. The lack of tolerance seen for thymectomized chimeras given parent *a* thymus contrasted with strong tolerance induction in control chimeras grafted with a host-type $(a \times b)F_1$ thymus.

The above data suggest, at least for MLR and $V_\beta 11$ expression, that the tolerance of $CD4^+$ cells in parent $\rightarrow F_1$ chimeras is not induced in the postthymic environment. By exclusion, it would follow that tolerance is induced intrathymically. In this respect, the striking finding is that the mature component of $CD4^+$ ($CD8^-$) thymocytes from the chimeras gives virtually no response to host-type APCs in vitro but responds well to third-party APCs. For $CD4^+$ cells, the tolerance seen in parent $\rightarrow F_1$ chimeras thus has close similarities with the tolerance developing in nude mice given dGuo-treated thymus grafts (see above). In both models the tolerance of $CD4^+$ cells is extensive (although not complete) for lymph node $CD4^+$ cells but near absolute for mature $CD4^+$ cells obtained from thymus. Because the thymus in each model is devoid of endogenous APCs, tolerance presumably reflects contact with thymic epithelial cells per se (although a contribution from some other radio-resistant stromal component of the thymus cannot be excluded). To account for the higher level of tolerance seen within the thymus as compared to that in postthymic T cells, our working hypothesis is that thymic epithelial cells can induce two different types of unresponsiveness, i.e., clonal deletion and anergy.

The paucity of $V_\beta 11^+$ $CD4^+$ cells in $I-E^- \rightarrow I-E^+$ chimeras implies that clonal deletion is the major mechanism of tolerance induction mediated by thymic epithelium. This form of tolerance applies to T cells with potential effector function (cells able to mediate GVHD, etc.) and also includes the bulk of cells participating in primary MLR. The only $CD4^+$ cells that evade clonal deletion by thymic epithelium appear to be the cells that give low sterile proliferative responses, i.e., responses not associated with production of effector function. The simplest explanation for the failure to tolerize these cells is that the affinity of the cells for the H-2 molecules on thymic epithelium is quite low, i.e., too low for the production of the signals that lead to clonal deletion. Why, then, is tolerance of $CD4^+$ cells more marked within the thymus than in the extrathymic tissues? In considering this paradox, it should be stressed that the deletion of $V_\beta 11^+$ $CD4^+$ cells in parent $\rightarrow F_1$ chimeras is no more marked in thymus than in lymph nodes. The thymocytes from the chimeras thus appear to be in a refractory state. To explain this phenomenon, it is suggested that in addition to causing clonal deletion, thymic epithelium is capable of down-regulating T cells, especially low-affinity T cells. The affected T cells are not destroyed but are rendered temporarily anergic. This state persists while the cells remain in the thymus but wanes rapidly when the cells escape to the extrathymic environment. An alternative possibility is that the down-regulation signal from thymic epithelium temporarily heightens the susceptibility of T cells to tolerance induction mediated by other cell types, e.g., APCs.

Either mechanism could account for the profound unresponsiveness of thymocytes to APCs in vitro.

Why are thymic epithelial cells less tolerogenic than bone-marrow-derived cells? Although the data in the two model systems discussed above suggest that thymic epithelium is capable of deleting subsets of $CD4^+$ and $CD8^+$ cells and can induce a form of anergy in other cells, full tolerance induction clearly requires the presence of thymic APCs. Why thymic epithelial cells cause only partial elimination of T cells is a matter for speculation. As discussed above, we favor the idea that clonal deletion mediated by epithelial cells is restricted to high-affinity T cells, perhaps because the density of H-2 molecules or various accessory molecules is lower on epithelial cells than on APCs. According to this scheme, epithelial cells are intrinsically less capable than APCs of delivering tolerogenic signals to T cells.

The alternative viewpoint is that thymic epithelial cells and thymic APCs display different sets of self-peptides on their H-2 molecules (Marrack et al. 1988). Thymic epithelial cells might express a smaller range of self-peptides and thus be incapable of eliminating T cells with specificity for unique peptides expressed only on APCs and not on epithelial cells. The anti-host MLR by $CD4^+$ cells from parent $\rightarrow F_1$ chimeras could then be viewed as a response to unique peptides on APCs, i.e., to peptides not encountered during ontogeny in the thymus. The main problem with this line of reasoning is that it fails to explain why the $CD4^+$ cells mediating the anti-host MLR are conspicuously devoid of effector function. In our view, it is much easier to regard the anti-host MLR as simply a response of low-affinity cells.

The evidence that thymic epithelial cells can control two diametrically opposite functions, positive and negative selection, prompts the question whether these two functions operate in the same compartment of the thymus. The most obvious possibility is that positive and negative selection both occur in the cortex, i.e., through contact with the dense network of cortical epithelial cells. It should be emphasized, however, that epithelial cells are demonstrable in the medulla as well as in the cortex. Epithelial cells are difficult to visualize in the medulla of the normal thymus because of the dense accumulation of Ia^+ $M\Phi$/dendritic cells in this region. However, Ia^+ epithelial cells are easily detected in the medulla of parent $\rightarrow F_1$ chimeras, i.e., where the Ia^+ $M\Phi$/dendritic cells are all of donor origin. Although the function of medullary epithelial cells is unknown, it is quite possible that these cells play a significant role in tolerance induction. Indeed, the tolerogenicity of thymic epithelium might be solely restricted to these cells. Hence, one cannot exclude the scheme considered earlier where T-cell selection is strictly compartmentalized, with positive selection occurring in the cortex and tolerance induction being limited to the medulla or the cortico-medullary junction. (As discussed previously, this idea is applicable only to $CD4^+$ cells, because tolerance of $CD8^+$ cells can probably be induced in the cortex through contact with class I molecules on thymocytes.)

At present, there is no direct evidence on which particular type of epithelium has tolerogenic properties. Resolving this question will probably depend on devising methods for causing selective stimulation of one type of thymic epithelium or preparing transgenic lines in which H-2 genes are expressed selectively in only one compartment of the thymus.

Are Mature T Cells Susceptible to Tolerance Induction?

Recent studies on transgenic lines in which foreign H-2 molecules are expressed selectively in various extrathymic tissues (Lo et al. 1988; Markmann et al. 1988; Morahan et al. 1989) have focused new attention on the long-standing issue of whether mature T cells are susceptible to tolerance induction. The results obtained to date with these transgenic models indicate that expression of foreign H-2 molecules in such tissues as the pancreas does cause various forms of tolerance, although tolerance is generally not complete. The mechanism of tolerance induction in these models, however, is far from clear. Perhaps the most interesting possibility is that tolerance is a consequence of T cells recognizing antigen displayed selectively on cell types that lack typical APC function. Thus, whereas antigens expressed on APCs are immunogenic for mature T cells, antigens presented by cell types that lack APC function, e.g., pancreatic β cells, lead to down-regulation of T cells. A considerable amount of recent evidence is consistent with this idea (Jenkins et al. 1988; Markmann et al. 1988).

A crude but simple approach for examining postthymic tolerance of T is to transfer mature T cells into H-2-different irradiated mice and test whether the donor T cells eventually show tolerance to the host. This approach might seem impractical because the recipients would be expected to die from GVHD. In practice, one can avoid the problem of lethal GVHD by using the following adoptive transfer system.

Studies with H-2 mutant strains of mice have shown that under certain conditions, isolated class I or class II

H-2 differences are each capable of eliciting a high incidence of lethal GVHD (Sprent et al. 1986). $CD8^+$ cells account for GVHD directed to class I differences, whereas $CD4^+$ cells cause anti-class II GVHD. This H-2 class specificity of $CD4^+$ and $CD8^+$ cells for GVHD induction appears to be near absolute. Thus, with transfer of B6 T-cell subsets to irradiated class-I-different $(B6 \times bm1)F_1$ mice, $CD8^+$ cells elicit 90–100% mortality, whereas $CD4^+$ cells cause no mortality. Conversely, only $CD4^+$ cells produce mortality in class-II-different $(B6 \times bm12)F_1$ hosts. The striking finding for each of these strain combinations is that transfer of very large doses of donor $CD4^+$ cells provides marked protection against lethal GVHD (Sprent et al. 1988; J. Sprent and M. Schaefer, unpubl.). Thus, the severe mortality seen in irradiated $(B6 \times bm1)F_1$ mice given small doses of B6 $CD8^+$ cells can be greatly reduced or abolished by coinjecting large numbers ($\geq 2 \times 10^7$) of B6 $CD4^+$ cells. Similarly, the heavy mortality seen in irradiated $(B6 \times bm12)F_1$ recipients of B6 $CD4^+$ cells only occurs when $CD4^+$ cells are transferred in small doses (10^5 to 10^6). With transfer of large doses of $CD4^+$ cells, mortality rates decrease paradoxically to a low level. Why bulk populations of $CD4^+$ cells provide protection against lethal GVHD is still unclear. Because lethal GVHD is low in mice kept under germ-free conditions (Pollard et al. 1976), the most likely explanation for the protective effects of $CD4^+$ cells is that these cells provide the host with "instant" cellular immunity and thereby enable the recipients to repel pathogens. In the absence of infection, the hosts develop only sublethal GVHD.

Like purified populations of $CD4^+$ cells, transfer of bulk populations of unseparated spleen cells (but not $CD4^-$ spleen) provides excellent protection against lethal GVHD. Thus, both for $(B6 \times bm1)F_1$ and $(B6 \times bm12)F_1$ recipients, transfer of 10^8 unseparated B6 spleen cells to hosts exposed to heavy irradiation generally leads to only very limited mortality. What happens to the donor T cells in these hosts (Table 3)?

For the B6 → bm1 combination, the recipients generally survive with no obvious symptoms of GVHD for 1 year or more posttransfer. When killed and autopsied, however, the mice show considerable atrophy of the

Table 3. Fate of B6 T-cell Subsets Transferred to Heavily Irradiated Mice Expressing Class I or Class II H-2 Differences

Hosts given 1000 rads plus 10^8 unseparated B6 spleen cells	Immune status of hosts at 6–12 months post-transfer
$(B6 \times bm1)F_1$ (class I difference)	severe atrophy of lymphoid tissues suggestive of a persistent GVH reaction donor $CD8^+$ cells generate strong anti-host CTL activity in vitro in the presence of exogenous lymphokines
$(B6 \times bm12)F_1$ (class II difference)	no pathology of lymphoid organs donor $CD4^+$ cells generate high MLR to host-type APCs in vitro but fail to cause lethal GVHD upon transfer to irradiated host-type mice

lymphoid organs. The spleens are small and fibrotic and lymph nodes are difficult to find, which suggests that the donor B6 CD8$^+$ cells caused severe irreversible tissue damage. The key question is whether the host-reactive component of donor T cells persists in these hosts or eventually becomes tolerant. The striking finding is that culturing spleen T cells from these mice with host-type APCs plus Con A supernatant in vitro generates a high level of anti-host CTL activity. According to this parameter, even at >1 year posttransfer, the donor CD8$^+$ cells show no tolerance to the host. In future studies, we plan to examine other parameters for host responsiveness, including skin graft rejection and production of lethal GVHD.

The consequences of transferring B6 spleen cells to class-II-different irradiated (B6 × bm12)F$_1$ hosts are somewhat different. With this class-II-incompatible strain combination, the recipients typically go through a severe crisis at ~2 weeks posttransfer and develop prominent splenomegaly. Most of the mice recover rapidly, however, and remain in excellent health for 1 year or more. When killed and autopsied, these long-term recipients show remarkably little evidence of GVHD. In particular, the spleen and lymph nodes appear to be normal in terms of size, content of lymphocyte subsets, and histology. Nevertheless, the CD4$^+$ cells recovered from the spleen and lymph nodes of these mice give strong MLRs to host-type APCs in vitro. In fact, the magnitude of this response is very similar to that of normal B6 CD4$^+$ cells. However, despite the conspicuous lack of tolerance seen in MLRs, transfer of CD4$^+$ cells from B6→bm12 spleen chimeras into further irradiated (B6 × bm12)F$_1$ hosts does not cause lethal GVHD.

In considering these findings, it is important to point out that B6→bm12 spleen chimeras show a rapid elimination of host APCs soon after reconstitution. The disappearance of host APCs presumably removes the main stimulus for the GVH reaction and thereby allows most of the host-reactive CD4$^+$ cells to revert to a resting state. This would account for the absence of lymphoid hypertrophy or signs of GVHD in the long-term survivors. Why, then, do the CD4$^+$ cells fail to cause GVHD on further transfer? There are at least two possibilities: First, the long-term residence of the donor CD4$^+$ cells in the chimeras might have led to selective tolerance of a subset of cells with GVHD-inducing properties. The alternative possibility is that the CD4$^+$ cells were not tolerized (deleted) but simply switched their phenotype. Thus, the initial contact of the donor CD4$^+$ cells with host APC might have induced an irreversible change in the properties of the cells, i.e., a change sufficient to allow the cells to retain their proliferate potential when subsequently exposed to host APCs in vitro but not to produce GVHD on further transfer. Some support for this second idea has come from a recent experiment in which B6→bm12 spleen chimeras were injected with normal B6 CD4$^+$ cells at 9 months postreconstitution, i.e., at a stage long after the host APCs had disappeared. (The injected

CD4$^+$ cells carried a Thy-1 marker for identification, and the hosts were given light irradiation.) The significant finding was that the CD4$^+$ cells recovered from the mice 1 month later *did* cause lethal GVHD upon further transfer. Under these conditions, the CD4$^+$ cells thus showed no evidence of tolerance induction.

The data on the two types of long-term spleen chimeras described above are still incomplete, and various other assays for anti-host reactivity need to be examined. Nevertheless, the existing data suggest that it is surprisingly difficult to induce more than minor degrees of tolerance in mature T cells. Despite the evidence that partial unresponsiveness of mature T cells *can* be induced under certain circumstances, e.g., in H-2 transgenic mice (see above), it would seem fair to state that fully mature T cells in the postthymic environment are far more refractory to tolerance induction than immature T cells in the thymus. Under normal physiological conditions, therefore, it would seem likely that tolerance to self-antigens takes place largely and perhaps exclusively in the thymus. The critical question is whether a subsidiary mechanism for tolerance induction operates when postthymic T cells encounter self-antigens that are normally sequestered, e.g., brain and thyroid antigens that are released as the result of trauma. This issue has yet to be resolved.

ACKNOWLEDGMENTS

This work was supported by grants CA-38355, AI-21487, and CA-25803 from the U.S. Public Health Service. The typing skills of Ms. Barbara Marchand are gratefully acknowledged.

REFERENCES

Bevan, M.J. 1977. In a radiation chimaera, host H-2 antigens determine immune responsiveness of donor cytotoxic cells. *Nature* 269: 417.

Bill, J., O. Kanagawa, D.L. Woodland, and E. Palmer. 1989. The MHC molecule I-E is necessary but not sufficient for the clonal deletion of V$_\beta$11-bearing T cells. *J. Exp. Med.* 169: 1405.

Fink, P.J. and M.J. Bevan. 1978. H-2 antigens of the thymus determine lymphocyte specificity. *J. Exp. Med.* 148: 766.

Flajnik, M.F., L. du Pasquier, and N. Cohen. 1985. Immune responses of thymus/lymphocyte embryonic chimeras: Studies on tolerance and major histocompatibility complex restriction in *Xenopus*. *Eur. J. Immunol.* 15: 540.

Good, M.F., K.W. Pyke, and G.J.V. Nossal. 1983. Functional clonal deletion of cytotoxic T-lymphocyte precursors in chimeric thymus produced in vitro from embryonic *anlagen*. *Proc. Natl. Acad. Sci.* 80: 3045.

Houssaint, E., A. Torano, and J. Ivanyi. 1986. Split tolerance induced by chick embryo thymic epithelium allografted to embryonic recipients. *J. Immunol.* 136: 3155.

Jenkins, M.K., J.D. Ashwell, and R.H. Schwartz. 1988. Allogeneic non-T spleen cells restore the responsiveness of normal T cell clones stimulated with antigen and chemically modified antigen-presenting cells. *J. Immunol.* 140: 3324.

Jenkinson, E.J., L.L. Franchi, R. Kingston, and J.J.T. Owen. 1982. Effect of deoxyguanosine on lymphopoiesis in the developing thymus rudiment in vitro: Application in the production of chimeric thymus rudiments. *Eur. J. Immunol.* **12**: 583.

Jenkinson, E.J., P. Jhittay, R. Kingston, and J.J.T. Owen. 1985. Studies on the role of the thymic environment in the induction of tolerance to MHC antigens. *Transplantation* **39**: 331.

Jordan, R.K., J.H. Robinson, N.A. Hopkinson, K.C. House, A.L. Bentley. 1985. Thymic epithelium and the induction of transplantation tolerance in nude mice. *Nature* **314**: 454.

Kappler, J.W., N. Roehm, and P. Marrack. 1987. T cell tolerance by clonal elimination in the thymus. *Cell* **49**: 273.

Kisielow, P., H.S. Teh, H. Bluthmann, and H. von Boehmer. 1988a. Positive selection of antigen-specific T cells in thymus by restricting MHC molecules. *Nature* **335**: 730.

Kisielow, P., H. Bluthmann, U.D. Staerz, M. Steinmetz, and H. von Boehmer. 1988b. Tolerance in T-cell-receptor transgenic mice involves deletion of non-mature CD4$^+$8$^+$ thymocytes. *Nature* **333**: 742.

Lo, D. and J. Sprent. 1986. Identity of cells that imprint H-2-restricted T-cell specificity in the thymus. *Nature* **318**: 672.

Lo, D., Y. Ron, and J. Sprent. 1986. Induction of MHC-restricted specificity and tolerance in the thymus. *Immunol. Res.* **5**: 221.

Lo, D., L.C. Burkly, G. Widera, C. Cowing, R.A. Flavell, R.D. Palmiter, and R.L. Brinster. 1988. Diabetes and tolerance in transgenic mice expressing class II MHC molecules in pancreatic beta cells. *Cell* **53**: 159.

Markmann, J., D. Lo, A. Naji, R.D. Palmiter, R.L. Brinster, and E. Heber-Katz. 1988. Antigen presenting function of class II MHC expressing pancreatic beta cells. *Nature* **336**: 476.

Marrack, P., D. Lo, R. Brinster, R. Palmiter, L. Burkly, R.A. Flavell, and J. Kappler. 1988. The effect of thymus environment on T cell development and tolerance. *Cell* **53**: 627.

Matzinger, P. and S. Guerder. 1989. Does T-cell tolerance require a dedicated antigen-presenting cell? *Nature* **338**: 74.

Miller, J.F.A.P. and D. Osoba. 1967. Current concepts of the immunological function of the thymus. *Physiol. Rev.* **47**: 437.

Morahan, G., J. Allison, and J.F.A.P. Miller. 1989. Tolerance of class I histocompatibility antigens expressed extrathymically. *Nature* **339**: 622.

Parkin, I.G., J.J.T. Owen, and E.J. Jenkinson. 1988. Proliferation of thymocytes in relation to T-cell receptor β-chain expression. *Immunology* **64**: 97.

Pollard, M., L.F. Chang, and K.K. Srivastava. 1976. The role of microflora in development of graft-versus-host disease. *Transplant Proc.* **8**: 533.

Scollay, R. and K. Shortman. 1985. Cell traffic in the adult thymus: Cell entry and exit, cell birth and death. In *Recognition and regulation in cell-mediated immunity* (ed. J.D. Watson and J. Marbrook), p. 3. Marcel Dekker, New York.

Sha, W.C., C.A. Nelson, R.D. Newberry, D.M. Kranz, J.H. Russell, and D.Y. Loh. 1988. Positive and negative selection of an antigen receptor on T cells in transgenic mice. *Nature* **336**: 73.

Shimonkevitz, R.P. and M.J. Bevan. 1988. Split tolerance induced by the intrathymic adoptive transfer of thymocyte stem cells. *J. Exp. Med.* **168**: 143.

Sprent, J., H. von Boehmer, and M. Nabholz. 1975. Association of immunity and tolerance in irradiated F$_1$ hybrid mice reconstituted with bone marrow lymphocytes from one parental strain. *J. Exp. Med.* **142**: 321.

Sprent, J., M. Schaefer, E.-K. Gao, and R. Korngold. 1988. Role of T cell subsets in lethal graft-versus-host disease (GVHD) directed to class I versus class II H-2 differences. I. L3T4$^+$ cells can either augment or retard GVHD elicited by Lyt-2$^+$ cells in class-I-different hosts. *J. Exp. Med.* **167**: 556.

Sprent, J., M. Schaefer, D. Lo, and R. Korngold. 1986. Properties of purified T cell subsets. II. In vivo responses to class I vs. class II H-2 differences. *J. Exp. Med.* **163**: 998.

von Boehmer, H. and K. Schubiger. 1984. Thymocytes appear to ignore class I major histocompatibility complex antigens expressed on thymus epithelial cells. *Eur. J. Immunol.* **14**: 1048.

von Boehmer, H. and J. Sprent. 1976. T cell function in bone marrow chimeras: Absence of host-reactive T cells and cooperation of helper T cells across allogeneic barriers. *Transplant. Rev.* **29**: 3.

Widera, G., L.C. Burkly, C.A. Pinkert, E.C. Bottger, C. Cowing, R.D. Palmiter, R.L. Brinster, and R.A. Flavell. 1987. Transgenic mice selectively lacking MHC class II (I-E) antigen expression on B cells: An in vivo approach to investigate Ia gene function. *Cell* **51**: 175.

Zinkernagel, R.M., G.M. Callahan, J. Klein, and G. Dennert. 1978. Cytotoxic T cells learn specificity for self H-2 during differentiation in the thymus. *Nature* **271**: 251.

Zinkernagel, R.M., A. Althage, E. Waterfield, B. Kindred, R.M. Welsh, G. Callahan, and P. Pincetl. 1980. Restriction specificities, alloreactivity, and allotolerance expressed by T cells from nude mice reconstituted with H-2-complete or -incomplete thymus grafts. *J. Exp. Med.* **151**: 376.

Activation versus Tolerance: A Decision Made by T Helper Cells

S. Guerder and P. Matzinger*

Basel Institute of Immunology, 4058 Basel, Switzerland

Twenty years ago, Peter Bretscher and Mel Cohn proposed the "two signal hypothesis" for lymphocyte activation, which dealt with the ongoing need to maintain self-tolerance in the face of B-cell hypermutation (Bretscher and Cohn 1970). They suggested that a B cell must receive two consecutive signals in order to be activated: Signal 1 from the antigen and Signal 2 from a second cell specific for the same antigen, e.g., a T helper cell (Cohn 1989). Under this model, a B cell that mutates and becomes autoreactive would find itself alone and unable to receive Signal 2, except in those exceedingly rare circumstances where an autoreactive T helper cell arises at the same time and in the same place. Thus, a newly autoreactive B cell, receiving only Signal 1 from the autoantigen, would not respond. The model also went one step farther; to prevent accumulation of autoreactive cells with time, it suggested that interaction with antigen alone (Signal 1) in the absence of Signal 2 should be an obligatorily tolerogenic event, stopping autoreactive mutants as soon as they appeared. Although this model was originally proposed to explain activation of B cells, its principles are also valid for T cells, and we show here that mature cytotoxic T lymphocytes (CTLs) do indeed follow the same rules.

Test System

Like B cells, CTLs need help (Pilarski 1977; Keene and Forman 1982; Raulet and Bevan 1982). Although the source and nature of this help have not always been easy to demonstrate (von Boehmer et al. 1984; Buller et al. 1987), one clear-cut example is seen in the CTL response to the histocompatibility antigen Qa-1, a response analogous to a hapten-carrier response in B cells. The "hapten" is the histocompatibility antigen Qa-1^b, and the "carrier" can be a minor histocompatibility (H) antigen such as H-Y. Keene and Forman showed that B6-Tla^a mice (which carry the Qa-1^a allele) (Flaherty and Rinchik 1980; Jenkins et al. 1983) can be immunized to C57BL/6 (B6; Qa-1^b) only if the immunizing cells also carry a helper antigen such as H-Y, and that both antigens must be presented on the same cell, a form of hapten-carrier linkage (Keene and Forman 1982). Figure 1 shows an example. Female B6-Tla^a mice make exceedingly weak in vitro primary CTL responses against Qa-1^b (Fig. 1a), and the response is

not improved by prior priming in vivo with cells bearing only Qa-1^b (Fig. 1b). However, Figure 1 shows that the mice are able to generate perfectly good responses provided they are primed in vivo with cells bearing Qa-1^b associated with the male antigen H-Y (Fig. 1c) or with the minor H antigens found on BALB.B (Fig. 1d).

The helper effect of the H-Y antigen is not simply due to a modification of the Qa-1 molecule itself. First, no helper antigens are required for boosting in vitro (Keene and Forman 1982). Second, CTLs specific for Qa-1^b lyse B6 male and female targets equally well, and third, male B6-Tla^a mice (which are tolerant of H-Y) cannot be primed to Qa-1^b by an injection of B6 male cells (data not shown). This supports the suggestion of Keene and Forman that the priming effect is actually due to the activation of H-Y-specific T helper cells which can assist the CTL precursors specific for Qa-1.

Recognition of Qa-1 Is Tolerogenic in the Absence of a Helper Determinant

Having confirmed that an injection of cells bearing only Qa-1^b differences was not an immunogenic procedure, we asked whether such an encounter with Signal 1 would have any effect at all. Would CTL precursors specific for Qa-1^b be rendered tolerant or would the antigen be essentially transparent to the immune system, leaving it untouched—neither primed nor tolerized?

Figure 2 shows that the immune system does not ignore cells bearing Qa-1^b alone. As seen before, an unprimed mouse does not respond to Qa-1^b (Fig. 2a), whereas mice primed with Qa-1^b plus H-Y (Fig. 2b) or Qa-1^b plus BALB minor antigens (Fig. 2c) respond well. Figure 2d shows that an injection of cells bearing Qa-1 in the absence of a helper determinant drives the recipient into an antigen-specific nonresponsive state. Mice injected with cells bearing Qa-1^b are unable to respond later to an injection of cells bearing Qa-1^b plus H-Y. The response cannot be rescued by adding T-cell helper factors to the in vitro culture in the form of concanavalin A supernatants (not shown) or by adding more helper determinants in the second injection, since the 29 minor histocompatibility antigens of BALB.B (Bailey and Mobraaten 1969) fail to supply enough help to generate a response to Qa-1 (Fig. 2e). In both cases, the unresponsiveness is specific only for Qa-1^b and does not interfere with responses to H-Y or the

---

*Present address: National Institutes of Health, Building 4, Room 111, Bethesda, Maryland 20892.

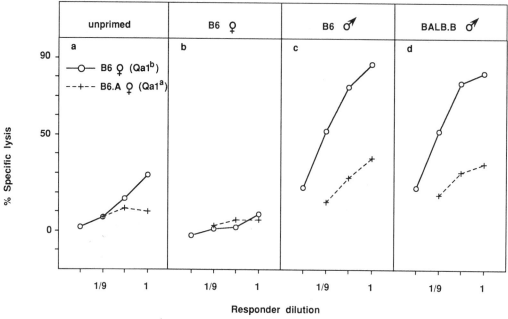

Figure 1. Characteristics of the anti-Qa-1[b] response in B6-Tla[a] mice. B6-Tla[a] (B6.A) female mice were left unprimed (*a*) or primed with 10[7] spleen cells from B6 female mice (*b*), B6 male mice (*c*), or BALB.B male mice (*d*). Two weeks later, 4×10^6 spleen cells were cultured with 2×10^6 irradiated (3200 rads) B6 female spleen stimulator cells. After 5 days, the killing activity of the cultures was tested against B6 female (○) or B6.A female (×) 2-day Con A blasts labeled previously for 2 hr with ⁵¹Cr. The percentage of specific lysis is calculated as follows: (experimental release − spontaneous release/detergent release − spontaneous release) × 100. Responder dilution is calculated from the number of responder cells originally cultured. The highest point corresponds to an effector:target ratio of 133:1.

BALB minors. Thus, CTL precursors are driven into a state of unresponsiveness when they encounter Qa-1 in the absence of a carrier antigen.

Tolerance Can Also Occur in the Presence of the Helper Determinant

If the induced state of unresponsiveness is truly due to a lack of Signal 2 from T helper cells, rather than a direct effect of carrier-free Qa-1, animals depleted of T helper cells should invariably become unresponsive when immunized with Qa-1, regardless of the presence or absence of a carrier molecule. We tested this by eliminating CD4⁺ cells before immunizing mice with cells bearing various combinations of Qa-1 plus carrier antigens. The recipient B6-Tla[a] female mice were injected twice, 24 hours apart, with a synergistic pair of monoclonal antibodies to CD4 and then with B6 female (Qa-1[b] alone) or B6 male (Qa-1[b] + H-Y) cells. Thus, the CTL precursors were allowed to encounter the Qa-1[b] antigen in its fully immunogenic form but in the absence of any CD4⁺ T helpers capable of delivering Signal 2. Nine weeks later, after the CD4⁺ T-cell population had been replenished, we injected the animals again. If any CTL had survived the first encounter with Signal 1 alone, they should respond to the immunization now given in the presence of Signal 2.

Figure 3 shows that temporarily removing T helper cells does not by itself abrogate immune responsiveness to Qa-1; mice treated with αCD4 monoclonal antibod-

ies and then rested for 8 weeks respond quite well to an immunization with Qa-1 plus helper determinants (Fig. 3c). In contrast, mice immunized with Qa-1 during the period of T helper cell depletion did not recover the ability to respond to Qa-1 (Fig. 3d), and mice immunized with both Qa-1 and H-Y during the depleted period became unresponsive to both antigens (Fig. 3e).

We thus show that whenever Signal 2 is not available, whether due to the lack of T helper cells or to the absence of a T helper determinant, CTL precursors are rendered unresponsive by the recognition of Signal 1.

Tolerance of Memory Cells

Any important mechanism for the maintenance of self-tolerance should not be limited to unprimed, naive CTL precursors but should also govern previously activated "memory" cells. To test this, we ran essentially the same protocol of T helper cell depletion as before, but this time using long-term primed memory mice as responders. The mice were primed with an immunogenic dose of Qa-1[b] + H-Y and rested for 4 weeks. They were then treated, or not, with αCD4 monoclonal antibodies and injected with cells bearing Qa-1[b] alone or Qa-1[b] + H-Y. Eight weeks later, they were immunized with Qa-1[b] plus various helper determinants. Figure 4 shows that once the mice have been primed appropriately, they are not affected by an injection of cells bearing Qa-1 alone (Fig. 4a); however, if they have been depleted of T helper cells, an injection of

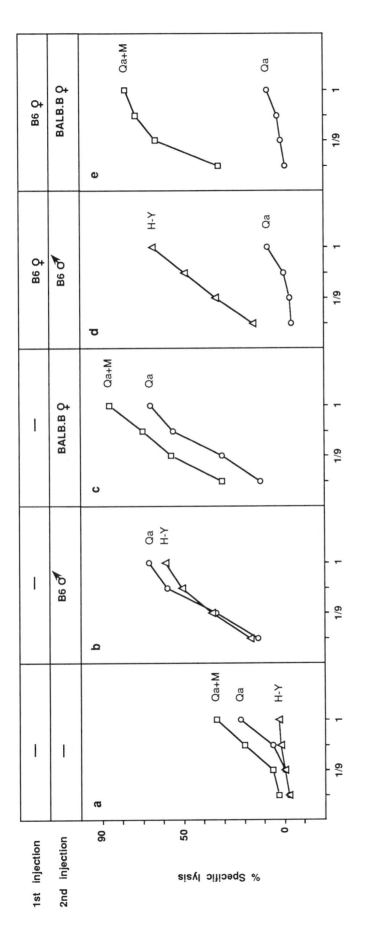

Responder dilution

Figure 2. Recognition of Qa-1 in the absence of a helper determinant is tolerogenic for CTL. B6.A female mice were primed (first injection) and were then boosted (second injection) 2 weeks later with 10^7 spleen cells, as indicated (above each panel). Two weeks after the second injection, the spleen cells were cultured as in Fig. 1 and tested 5 days later for killing activity. Only the activity against the stimulatory target is shown. Therefore, the activity against Qa-1 corresponds to lysis of B6 female targets after restimulation in vitro with B6 female spleen cells (○); the activity against Qa-1 plus minor histocompatibility antigens (Qa-1 + M) corresponds to lysis of BALB.B female targets after stimulation with BALB.B spleen cells (□), and the activity against H-Y corresponds to the lysis of B6.A male targets after stimulation with B6.A male spleen cells (△). In this and all following experiments, the highest dilution for the Qa and Qa + M activity corresponds to an E:T ratio of 100:1, whereas the highest dilution for the H-Y activity corresponds to an E:T ratio of 133:1.

802

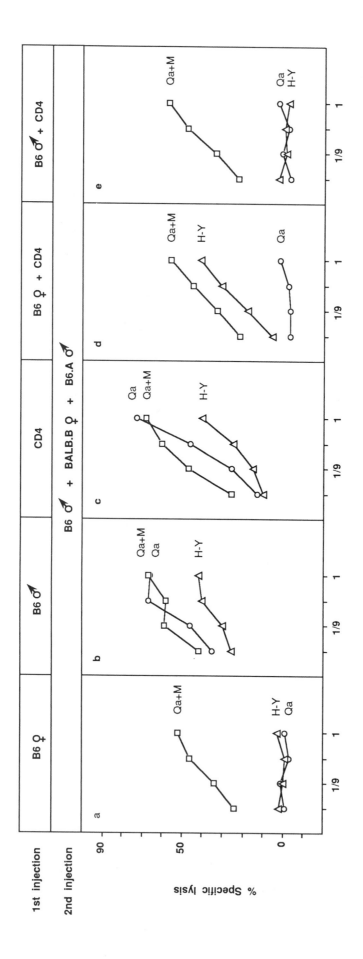

Figure 3. Tolerance induction after elimination of CD4[+] T helper cells. B6.A female mice were injected twice (c,d,e), 24 hr apart, with a mixture of the monoclonal antibodies GK1.5 (Dianalys et al. 1983) and YTA3.1.2 (Quin et al. 1989; a kind gift from H. Waldmann, Cambridge, England), which recognize different epitopes on the mouse CD4 molecule. Each injection corresponds to 1 mg of GK1.5 and 0.1 mg of YTA3.1.2 used as a 50% ammonium sulfate cut of ascites fluid. Six hours after the last injection of anti-CD4, the mice were injected with 10[7] spleen cells of B6 female mice (a,d) or were left uninjected. Nine weeks later, all of the mice were boosted with a mixture of 10[7] B6 male, 10[7] BALB.B female, and 10[7] B6.A male spleen cells. After 2 weeks, the spleen cells were set up in a mixed lymphocyte reaction and tested as described in Fig. 1.

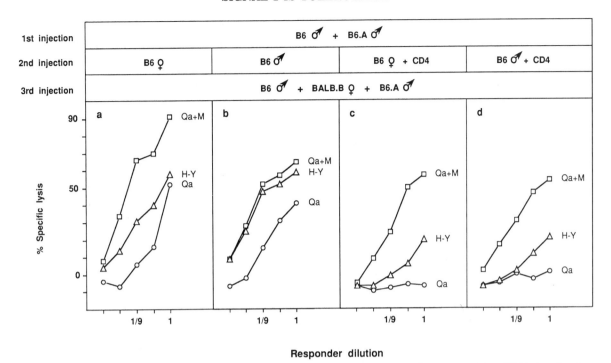

Figure 4. Tolerance induction of memory CTLs. B6.A female mice were primed with 10^7 B6 male and 6×10^6 B6.A male spleen cells. Four weeks later, some of the mice (*c,d*) were injected twice, 24 hr apart, with 1 mg GK1.5 and 0.1 mg YTA3.1.2. The mice were then injected with 10^7 B6 female spleen cells (*a,c*) or 10^7 B6 male spleen cells (*b,d*). The mice in *c* and *d* were injected on weeks 4 and 7 after antibody treatment with 10^7 B6 female spleen cells. Nine weeks after the anti-CD4 treatment, all of the mice were injected with 8×10^6 B6 male, 10^7 BALB.B female, and 8×10^6 B6.A male spleen cells. Two weeks later, the spleen cells of the mice were set up as described in Fig. 1 and tested 5 days later for killing activity.

cells bearing Qa-1 alone (Fig. 4c) or Qa-1 + H-Y (Fig. 4d) renders them unresponsive to further immunization. Thus, it appears that memory CTLs, like naive cells, are also dependent on Signal 2 and become unresponsive if they receive Signal 1 in its absence.

Strangely, in the case of primed mice, the helper antigens are no longer necessary for immunization as long as the T helper populations are left intact. Nevertheless, the primed CTLs become unresponsive when they encounter Qa-1 in the absence of T helper cells. Clearly, Signal 2 is necessary. Where does it come from in primed mice injected with Qa-1 alone? There are two possibilities:

1. Although unprimed mice obviously do not have a sufficient level of Qa-1-specific T helper cells to mount an immune response after immunization with Qa-1 alone, a low frequency of such cells might exist which, like the CTL precursors, can be expanded to functional numbers by immunization with Qa-1 plus helper determinants. Thus, a second injection would find an animal with sufficient numbers of Qa-1-specific T helper cells to mount a secondary response.
2. Perhaps a population of Qa-1-specific T helper cells exists which, for some reason, has only a weak functional capacity—not enough to aid in the activation of naive CTL precursors, but enough to help in a secondary response. This would imply that naive

and memory CTLs have different activation requirements (Byrne et al. 1988).

At the moment, we have no way of distinguishing between these two possibilities. In either case, the fact remains that CTLs do need help, whether in primary or secondary responses, and that an encounter with antigen in the absence of help renders them tolerant in both situations.

Fail-safe Mechanisms for Self-tolerance

Most, if not all, autoreactive T cells are deleted during thymic development (Kappler et al. 1987, 1988; MacDonald et al. 1988); however, there are at least two reasons why this step cannot by itself be sufficient to maintain self-tolerance: First, tolerance is maintained to antigens not found in the thymus. Second, T cells do not seem to mutate at the same rate as B cells (Chien et al. 1984; Ikuta et al. 1985), but, because they synthesize DNA, they can nevertheless mutate. If there were no fail-safe mechanisms in the periphery to ensure self-tolerance, an individual would certainly generate many dangerous autoreactive mutations in its lifetime.

As a backup system for self-tolerance, the model of Bretscher and Cohn is ingenious. Unlike networks (Pereira et al. 1989) or models involving T suppressors (Gershon and Kondo 1971; Dorsch and Roser 1977), it allows the specificity of the induction of tolerance to be the same as the specificity of activation. Tolerance is part and parcel of cellular activation; it occurs when Signal 2 does not follow the initial activation events induced by recognition of antigen. Hence, the specificity for cellular activation or tolerance is the same, manifest in one recognition event. Actually, there are two circumstances in which autoreactive cells may receive help and be activated. The first is the unlikely circumstance that a newly arisen, autoreactive T helper cell encounters an autoreactive CTL. This event should have a low but finite probability and must occur in some individuals. The likelihood of this event drops almost to impossibility in an immune system that requires a *three*-cell interaction to initiate a response. However, such a system would have a severely diminished capacity to mount normal immune responses. The two pressures—to prevent autoreactivity while allowing responses to foreign antigens—are best balanced by an immune system in which the minimal interactive unit comprises two antigen-specific cells.

A second potentially dangerous situation would be a "bystander effect," aptly illustrated by the anti-Qa-1 response and the response to Thy-1 (Lake and Mitchison 1976), where the T helper cell does not recognize the same antigen as the effector cell. If an autoreactive CTL precursor were to bind to an antigen-presenting cell (APC) that was also presenting a foreign antigen to a T helper (e.g., during a virus infection), the CTL could become activated. This would lead to temporary autoimmunity during the course of that virus infection. However, as soon as the infection was finished, the T helper cells would no longer be activated, and the CTLs would begin to recognize their autoantigen in the absence of helper cells and be tolerized.

The fact that both primary and memory CTLs are tolerizable implies that CTLs must distinguish between APCs and target cells. APCs are stimulatory cells that can pull a resting CTL into an active state (Greineder and Rosenthal 1975; Chesnut et al. 1982; Inaba et al. 1987), a potentially dangerous step that requires the aid of a T helper cell. Target cells, however, are killed quickly and efficiently by activated CTLs in the complete absence of any help (Zagury et al. 1975; Martz 1976). How then do CTLs distinguish between the two recognition events so that one leads to tolerance in the absence of help and the other does not? The distinction between APC and target cell cannot be made simply on the basis of cell type, because APCs such as macrophages and dendritic cells can also serve as targets (Zinkernagel and Doherty 1974; Parish and Müllbacher 1983; Inaba et al. 1987). The distinction could potentially depend on the CTL's state of activation or its state of differentiation.

1. *Differentiation.* It is not known whether the activated CTL which kills target cells is also the progenitor cell which divides to continue the line and maintain memory. If, like a plasma cell, the activated killer is terminally differentiated—geared to

kill for a certain period before dying—tolerance induction might not be critical. All cells bearing the right antigen would be treated as targets. However, to the progenitor cell that maintains the lineage, there are no targets. It is not a killer and can be activated only by a professional APC bearing the right antigen in the presence of help.

2. *Activation.* Most likely, killer cells are not terminally differentiated. They survive their lytic encounters (Zagury et al. 1975; Martz 1977) and are periodically able to revert to a resting state from which they can later be reactivated. Let us call the events that lead to the activation of a resting CTL the "activation" stimulus, and the events that induce an activated CTL to lyse its target the "triggering" stimulus. Because APCs can be targets, the difference between the two stimuli must be a difference perceived by the CTL rather than expressed by the cell being recognized. The simplest scenario would be that the early events of the two stimuli, involving calcium mobilization and perhaps phosphorylation (Tsien et al. 1982; Samelson et al. 1985), are the same. At this stage, differences must appear. Binding of activated CTLs to their targets should trigger the release of cytotoxic granules that lyse the target (Young and Liu 1988), whereas resting CTLs must be activated to initiate transcriptional and translational processes leading to cell division, granule formation, etc. Thus, activation and triggering, having different end points, result from different internal consequences of the same external event: the recognition of antigen. It thus becomes very easy to suggest that the resting CTL requires a second signal before it becomes activated, whereas the triggered activated killer simply releases its toxic substances immediately, requires nothing else, and is consequently not affected by the absence of help.

In either case, whether the discrimination between target cells and APCs is done by different cells or the same cell in different states of activation, the phase of a killer's life in which it can actively lyse targets must be rather short. Every killer must either die or revert to an activatable/tolerizable state before its capacity for running amuk can destroy a vital organ. Thus, the periodic need for activation or reactivation leaves the system with a constant opportunity to survey its killers and tolerize them if necessary.

But what about T helper cells? Who controls the controllers? If it is the presence of help that determines whether CTLs and B cells are activated or inactivated when they encounter antigen, what governs the activation of the helpers? More helpers? Cohn suggests that T helper cells, like CTLs, cycle between active and resting states and that they too need help to be activated by antigen (Cohn 1989). This deals with tolerance, but it leaves a major problem with the initiation of normal immune responses. If every helper needs help, what activates the first helper? This is a major shortcoming of the Bretscher-Cohn model; at first glance, it seems to make the model unworkable. We see no way out of this dilemma. Yet, because the idea of two signals works so beautifully and because of the increasing amount of data supporting it, we believe it to be the best working model presently available.

ACKNOWLEDGMENTS

We thank Antonio Lanzavecchia, Charles (W.B.) Mackay, Ronald Palacios, Rich Scheuerman, and Charley Steinberg for reading and improving the manuscript with their cogent arguments and Janette Millar for typing several versions. The Basel Institute was founded and is supported by Hoffmann-La Roche and Co. Ltd. (Basel, Switzerland).

REFERENCES

Bailey, D.W. and L.E. Mobraaten. 1969. Estimates of the number of loci contributing to the histocompatibility between strains C57BL/6 and BALB/c. *Transplantation* 7: 394.

Bretscher, P. and M. Cohn. 1970. A theory of self-nonself discrimination. Paralysis and induction involve the recognition of one and two determinants on an antigen, respectively. *Science* 169: 1042.

Buller, R.M.L., K.L. Holmes, A. Hügin, T.N. Frederickson, and H.C. Morse III. 1987. Induction of cytotoxic T-cell responses in vivo in the absence of CD4 helper cells. *Nature* 328: 77.

Byrne, J.A., J.L. Butler, and M.D. Cooper. 1988. Differential requirements for virgin and memory T cells. *J. Immunol.* 141: 3249.

Chesnut, R.W., S.M. Colon, and H.M. Grey. 1982. Antigen presentation by normal B cells, B cell tumors, and macrophages: Functional and biochemical comparison. *J. Immunol.* 128: 1764.

Chien, Y., N.R.J. Gascoigne, J. Kavalerm, N.E. Lee, and M. Davis. 1984. Somatic recombination in a murine T-cell receptor gene. *Nature* 309: 322.

Cohn, M. 1989. The a priori principles which govern immune responsiveness. In *Cellular basis of immune modulation*, p. 11. A.R. Liss, New York.

Dianalys, P., D.B. Wild, P. Marrack, A. Pierres, K.A. Wall, W. Havran, G. Otten, M.R. Loken, M. Pierres, J. Kappler, and F.W. Fitch. 1983. Characterization of the murine antigenic determinant, designated L3T4a, recognized by monoclonal antibody GK1.5: Expression of L3T4a by functional T cell clones appears to correlate primarily with class II MHC antigen-reactivity. *Immunol. Rev.* 74: 29.

Dorsch, S. and B. Roser. 1977. Recirculating, suppressor T cells in transplantation tolerance. *J. Exp. Med.* 145: 1144.

Flaherty, L. and E. Rinchik. 1980. A new allele and antigen at the Tla locus. *Immunogenetics* 11: 205.

Gershon, R.K. and K. Kondo. 1971. Infectious immunological tolerance. *Immunology* 21: 903.

Greineder, D. and A.S. Rosenthal. 1975. Macrophage activation of allogeneic lymphocyte in the guinea pig mixed leukocyte culture. *J. Immunol.* 114: 1541.

Ikuta, K., T. Ogura, A. Shimizu, and T. Honjo. 1985. Low frequency of somatic mutation in β-chain variable regions of human T-cell receptors. *Proc. Natl. Acad. Sci.* 82: 7701.

Inaba, K.I., J.W. Young, and R.M. Steinman. 1987. Direct activation of CD8[+] cytotoxic T lymphocytes by dendritic cells. *J. Exp. Med.* 166: 182.

Jenkins, R.N., C.J. Aldrich, N.F. Landolfi, and R.R. Rich. 1983. Correlation of Qa-1 determinants defined by antisera and by cytotoxic T lymphocytes. *Immunogenetics* 21: 215.

Kappler, J.W., N. Roehm, and P. Marrack. 1987. T cell tolerance by clonal elimination in the thymus. *Cell* 49: 273.

Kappler, J., U. Staerz, J. White, and P. Marrack. 1988. Self-tolerance eliminates T cells specific for Mls-modified products of the major histocompatibility complex. *Nature* 332: 35.

Keene, J. and J. Forman. 1982. Helper activity is required for the in vivo generation of cytotoxic T lymphocytes. *J. Exp. Med.* 155: 768.

Lake, P. and N.A. Mitchison. 1976. Associative control of the immune response to cell surface antigens. *Immunol. Commun.* 5: 795.

MacDonald, H.R., R. Schneider, R.K. Lees, R.C. Howe, H. Acha-Orbea, H. Festenstein, R.M. Zinkernagel, and H. Hengartner. 1988. T-cell receptor V$_\beta$ use predicts reactivity and tolerance to Mls^a-encoded antigens. *Nature* 332: 40.

Martz, E. 1976. Multiple target cell killing by the cytolytic T lymphocyte and the mechanism of cytotoxicity. *Transplantation* 21: 5.

———. 1977. Mechanism of specific tumor-cell lysis by alloimmune T lymphocytes: Resolution and characterization of discrete steps in the cellular interaction. *Contemp. Top. Immunol.* 7: 301.

Parish, C.R. and A. Müllbacher. 1983. Automated colorimetric assay for T cell cytotoxicity. *J. Immunol. Methods* 58: 225.

Pereira, P., A. Bandeira, and A. Coutinho. 1989. V region connectivity in T cell repertoires. *Annu. Rev. Immunol.* 7: 209.

Pilarski, L.M. 1977. A requirement for antigen-specific helper T cells in the generation of cytotoxic T cells from thymocyte precursors. *J. Exp. Med.* 145: 707.

Quin, S., S. Cobbold, R. Benjamin, and H. Waldmann. 1989. Induction of classical transplantation tolerance in the adult. *J. Exp. Med.* 169: 779.

Raulet, D.H. and M.J. Bevan. 1982. Helper T cells for cytotoxic T lymphocytes need not be I region restricted. *J. Exp. Med.* 155: 1766.

Samelson, L.E., J.B. Harford, and R.D. Klausner. 1985. Identification of the components of the murine T cell antigen receptor complex. *Cell* 43: 223.

Tsien, R.Y., T. Pozzan, and T.J. Rink. 1982. T-cell mitogens cause early changes in cytoplasmic free Ca^{2+} and membrane potential in lymphocytes. *Nature* 295: 69.

von Boehmer, H., P. Kisielow, W. Leiserson, and W. Haas. 1984. Lyt-2 T cell-independent functions of Lyt-2[+] cells stimulated with antigen or concanavalin A. *J. Immunol.* 133: 59.

Young, J.D.E. and C.C. Liu. 1988. Multiple mechanisms of lymphocyte-mediated killing. *Immunol. Today* 9: 140.

Zinkernagel, R. and P. Doherty. 1974. Restriction of in vitro T cell-mediated cytotoxicity in lymphocytic choriomeningitis within a syngeneic or semiallogeneic system. *Nature* 248: 701.

Zagury, D., J. Bernard, N. Thierness, M. Feldman, and G. Berke. 1975. Isolation and characterization of individual functionally reactive cytotoxic T lymphocytes: Conjugation, killing and recycling at the single cell level. *Eur. J. Immunol.* 5: 818.

Extrathymic Acquisition of Tolerance by T Lymphocytes

J.F.A.P. MILLER, G. MORAHAN, AND J. ALLISON
Walter and Eliza Hall Institute of Medical Research, P.O. Royal Melbourne Hospital, Victoria 3050, Australia

There is now convincing evidence for the imposition of self-tolerance by means of the clonal deletion of self-reactive T cells operating within the thymus. Experiments with monoclonal antibodies directed to T-cell receptors (TCRs) that bind the class II major histocompatibility complex (MHC) molecule, I-E, or the products of the Mls^a allele of the minor lymphocyte-stimulating (Mls) locus, have demonstrated the existence of cells with anti-self TCR in I-E$^+$ or Mls^{a+} mice in the immature population of thymus lymphocytes but not in the mature intrathymic or peripheral T-cell pools (Kappler et al. 1987, 1988; MacDonald et al. 1988). Likewise, in transgenic mice expressing in many of their thymus cells a TCR specific for the male (H-Y) antigen in the context of the class I H-2D^b MHC molecule, H-Y autospecific T cells are deleted in male, although not in female, mice (Kisielow et al. 1988). The most widely accepted model of deletion of self-reactive T cells attributes a censorship function to cells of the dendritic/macrophage lineages, which are rich in class I and II molecules and situated predominantly at the corticomedullary junction (Sprent and Webb 1987). A simpler way in which deletion might occur, at least for class I reactive lymphocytes, would be via the postulated "intracellular censorship" (Miller and Watson 1988): As the TCR is assembled in a self-reactive cell, it should complex with its ligand (either self-class I or self-class I associated with self-peptide) and the accumulation of complexes in the endoplasmic reticulum would be incompatible with cell survival.

If the induction of self-tolerance is limited to antigens synthesized by thymic stromal cells during T-cell maturation, a major dilemma must be faced. Must the entire array of self-antigens in the body be exhibited in the thymus? Otherwise, how could T cells capable of recognizing self-components not encountered in the thymus but unique to other tissues be negatively selected? Can T cells ever become tolerant to unique extrathymic antigens? Some autoantigens could be shed in the circulation and reach thymic macrophages or dendritic cells, which would then impart tolerance (Lorenz and Allen 1988; Nieuwenhuis et al. 1988; Boguniewicz et al. 1989). If, however, as has been documented (Braciale et al. 1987), exogenous antigen taken up by antigen-presenting cells becomes associated with class II MHC components, not with class I, how could differentiating class-I-restricted thymus cells be negatively selected by circulating antigen shed from extrathymic tissues? On the other hand, because antigen synthesized within cells generally becomes associated with class I molecules, how would fully mature class-I-restricted T cells become tolerant to self-components produced exclusively by some extrathymic tissue?

In some cases, T-cell tolerance may not have to be imposed. Thus, some autoantigens may be anatomically secluded from immunocompetent cells; others may occur on cells that do not normally express MHC class I or II molecules and hence are not able to stimulate T cells; others still may be exposed on cells that do express these MHC molecules but lack costimulator properties required for activation of T cells (Lafferty et al. 1980). Whatever the case may be, the fate of T cells potentially reactive to self-antigens synthesized outside the thymus should be examined critically. For this purpose, we used the transgenic approach, as it enables specific genes to be introduced into inbred strains and to be expressed and treated as self-molecules. By linking the gene to a specific promoter, its expression can be directed to particular cell types. This therefore allows an investigation of the in vivo effect on the immune system of an antigen synthesized in an extrathymic tissue, in the absence of any trauma or inflammation that is usually associated with tissue transplantation.

EXPERIMENTAL PROCEDURES

Mice. Mice of the inbred strains C57BL/6, C57BL/10 (both H-2^b), B10^{bm1} (H-2^{bm1}), B10.BR (H-2^k), B10.A(5R) (K^{b}D^d), and SJL (H-2^s) and various F$_1$ and F$_2$ hybrids between these strains were obtained from the specific pathogen-free colonies of the Walter and Eliza Hall Institute or from the Animal Resources Centre, Perth, Western Australia. Irradiation (750 rads) was administered from a ^{60}Co source in some experiments.

Production of transgenic mice. The rat insulin promoter (RIP), obtained from Hanahan (1985), was linked to the coding sequences of H-2K^b class I MHC protein, as described elsewhere (Allison et al. 1988). The sheep metallothionein promoter (sMTp) was provided by M.G. Peterson and K.H. Choo (Peterson and Mercer 1986; Choo et al. 1987) and linked to the H-2K^b gene, as described previously (Morahan et al. 1989b). The purified constructs were microinjected into fertilized eggs, and progeny were screened at weaning by hybridizing tail-blot DNA to appropriate ^{32}P-labeled probes. Transgene expression was detected by Northern blotting and immunoperoxidase staining.

Histology. Organs were fixed in buffered formalin and embedded in paraffin. Sections were stained with hematoxylin and eosin. Immunoperoxidase staining for H-2K[b] was performed with the monoclonal antibody B8-24-3, as described previously (Allison et al. 1988).

Cytolytic T-lymphocyte (CTL) assays. Spleen cells from transgenic H-2[s] mice or their nontransgenic littermates were cocultured with irradiated (2000 rads) B10.A(5R) spleen cells for 4 days and then with the target cells EL4 (H-2K[b]) or P815 (H-2K[d]) labeled with [51]Cr. The percentage of specific lysis was calculated from the formula ([test release–background release]/ [maximum release–background release]) × 100. The data show the mean of triplicate samples tested at various effector/target ratios; standard errors are shown by bars. In some assays, the cells were supplemented with supernatants from concanavalin-A-stimulated spleen cells (CAS) or recombinant interleukin-1 and -2 (rIL-1, rIL-2), kindly provided by Cetus Corporation and Hoffmann-La Roche.

Skin grafts. Transgenic mice of the 43-5 or 50-1 lines were mated with B10.H-2[bm1] mice, which differ from the congenic C57BL/10 mice only at the H-2K locus. Progeny were screened for the transgene and grafted with H-2K[b]-bearing C57BL/10 skin by the technique of Billingham and Medawar (1951).

Polymerase chain reaction. Total RNA from 30-day transgenic thymus and pancreas was converted to cDNA using reverse transcriptase and analyzed for expression of H-2K[b] transgene mRNA using the polymerase chain reaction (PCR). Two sets of oligonucleotides were used. One set specific for the transgene hybridized to a polylinker sequence present only in transgenic RNA and to a sequence in exon 4 of H-2K[b], giving a reaction product of 680 bp. The other set was general for H-2 and hybridized to the same sequence in exon 4 and to a sequence in exon 2 of H-2K[b]; it should detect several of the class I genes, giving a reaction product of 480 bp. The PCR was performed for 25 cycles at 94°C (90 sec), 60°C (2 min), and 72°C (3 min). The reaction product was processed by Southern analysis and detected with an H-2K[b] cDNA probe.

RESULTS

Transgenic Mice Expressing Class I Molecules in Pancreatic Islet β Cells

Transgenic offspring of eggs inoculated with the RIP-H-2K[b] construct showed abundant expression of H-2K[b] heavy-chain protein in the islet β cells. These normally express only very low levels of class I molecules (Baekkeskov et al. 1981). Expression could not be detected in the thymus by a variety of techniques, including

Northern blots, nuclease S1 mapping, and immuno-peroxidase histochemistry; however, it could be detected by using the PCR. As shown in Figure 1, thymus and pancreas from transgenic or control mice were analyzed for expression of transgenic H-2K[b] mRNA under semiquantitative reaction conditions (see Experimental Procedures). The pancreas contained only 1% of its mass as β cells; in a 30-day diabetic mouse, more than 75% of these cells were destroyed. The lower-molecular-weight band created with the H-2 general oligonucleotides is a nonspecific reaction product. Although the PCR detected a band in thymus tissue, it is not clear whether the transgene is expressed at the protein level or in cells specialized to impart tolerance. T cells differentiating in the thymus may not therefore have encountered the transgene product on cells able to impose tolerance; hence, the clones of T cells reactive to H-2K[b] might not have been eliminated. Because immunoperoxidase staining techniques did not reveal H-2K[b] protein in the thymus (Morahan et al. 1989a), we expected a T-cell response against the β cells and hence insulin-dependent diabetes mellitus (IDDM), but only in mice in which the transgene product was allogeneic. We were therefore surprised to find that the IDDM occurred at a very early age, regardless of whether the mice were syngeneic or allogeneic with respect to the transgene product and in the absence of T-cell involvement (Allison et al. 1988). Histology of the pancreas from diabetic mice revealed markedly abnormal islets, depleted of β cells, but containing normal numbers of glucagon-producing α cells and somatostatin-producing δ cells. The α and δ cells persisted as the disease progressed, but most of the β cells were lost by ~50 days after the onset of IDDM. The H-2K[b] protein, detected by immunocytochemistry with specific monoclonal antibodies, was expressed at least as early as day 16 in the transgenic embryo. However, the staining pattern was predominantly cytoplasmic, as expected, because the heavy chain requires β_2-microglobulin (β_2m) for transport to the cell surface. There was a low level of surface expression, as demonstrated by flow cytometric analysis (Allison et al. 1988).

No lymphocytic infiltration was observed at any stage. Moreover, transgenic mice depleted of T lymphocytes by neonatal thymectomy also developed IDDM, as did nude mice transgenic for the H-2K[b]

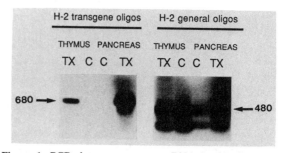

Figure 1. PCR detects transgene mRNA in the thymus of RIP-K[b] mice. (TX) Transgenic mice; (C) control mice.

gene. The absence of lymphocyte infiltration in transgenic mice expressing allogeneic MHC molecules on the β-cell membrane suggested that the mice were immunologically tolerant of the transgene product. Deliberate immunization with H-2K^b-bearing cells failed to provoke any lymphocytic infiltration in the islets (Morahan et al. 1989a). Likewise, no infiltration was observed in transgenic recipients of normal spleen cells from syngeneic nontransgenic donors. Spleen cells from 12-day-old RIP-K^b mice of the 31-2 line (of SJL background and developing severe IDDM early in life) were tested for specific tolerance to the transgene product using a cytotoxic assay (Table 1). Spleens from RIP-K^b mice and their nontransgenic littermates were cultured at 2×10^6/ml with an equal number of irradiated B10.A(5R) (K^{b}D^d) stimulator cells. After 4 days, the cultures were harvested, and the cells were tested in triplicate for their ability to lyse ^{51}Cr-labeled EL4 (H-2^b) and P815 (H-2^d) targets at an effector/target ratio of 50:1. Standard errors of the mean of triplicate samples are shown. The cells killed third-party H-2^d targets but not targets bearing H-2K^b. Responsiveness to these targets was observed when spleen cells were tested 1–2 weeks later (Morahan et al. 1989a). At this stage, severe IDDM had developed and islet β cells were markedly depleted. Tolerance was therefore dependent on the continued presence of critical amounts of the H-2K^b antigen and occurred in spite of the fact that transgene expression was not detectable in the thymus by immunoperoxidase staining.

Thymocytes were collected from 16-day-old mice and cultured at 5×10^6/ml. Cells obtained from individual nontransgenic, transgenic, or pooled transgenic thymocyte cultures were analyzed for their ability to lyse ^{51}Cr-labeled P815 or EL4 targets (Fig. 2). The thymocytes could kill both H-2K^b and H-2K^d targets, implying that developing anti-H-2K^b thymus cells were not clonally eliminated within the thymus.

CTLs were generated from spleen cells of transgenic mice and assayed for their ability to lyse EL4 and P815, as described above, except that some cultures were supplemented with CAS (2% v/v), rIL-1 (10 μg/ml), or rIL-2 (10 μg/ml) (Fig. 3). Lymphokines provided by Hoffmann-La Roche and Cetus gave similar results. Addition of CAS or rIL-2, but not rIL-1, to cultures of spleen cells from 12-day-old mice enabled the killing of

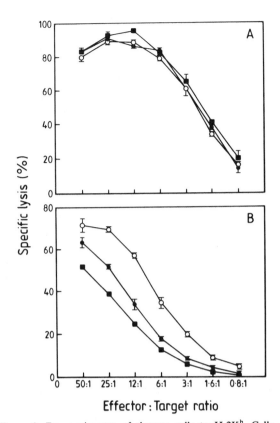

Figure 2. Responsiveness of thymus cells to H-2K^b. Cells obtained from individual nontransgenic (○), transgenic (●), or pooled transgenic (■) thymocyte cultures were analyzed for their ability to lyse ^{51}Cr-labeled P815 (*A*) or EL4 (*B*) targets.

both targets, thus effectively reversing the state of specific immunological tolerance and establishing the existence of anti-H-2K^b reactive T cells.

In vivo tests of tolerance were performed by skin grafting. After ∼3–5 weeks, mice of the 50-1 line of

Table 1. Responsiveness of Spleen Cells to H-2K^b: Effect of Age and Transgene Expression

Age of spleen donor	Transgene status	Specific lysis (%)	
		EL4	P815
12 days	transgenic	5 ± 2	35 ± 1
	nontransgenic	34 ± 2	40 ± 6
17 weeks	transgenic	95 ± 6	71 ± 3
	nontransgenic	85 ± 6	88 ± 4

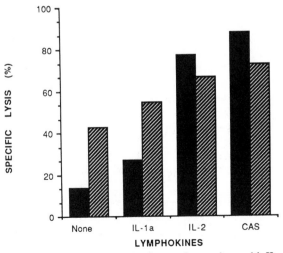

Figure 3. Reversal of unresponsiveness by coculture with IL-2. (*Solid bars*) EL4; (*hatched bars*) P815.

Table 2. Survival of C57BL/10 Skin Grafts on Transgenic RIP-K^b Mice

Mice	Number	Graft survival (days)			
		<20	20–30	31–50	>60
Transgenic (6 weeks old)	3	0	0	0	3
Transgenic (10–12 weeks old)	6	3	2	1	0
Nontransgenic (6–12 weeks old)	10	10	0	0	0

Transgenic RIP-K^b mice from the 50-1 line were crossed to bm1, and the progeny were grafted with C57BL/10 skin. Hair growth was noted on surviving grafts.

endogenous H-2^k haplotype and CBA background develop a less severe form of IDDM that does not initially require insulin treatment. These mice were crossed to C57BL/10^{bm1}, and the progeny grafted with C57BL/10 skin. As shown in Table 2, 6-week-old transgenic mice did not reject skin grafts, whereas 10-week-old mice did, again suggesting waning of tolerance with time and with increasing severity of IDDM. Grafting skin onto mice of the 31-2 line was attempted; however, few mice survived the operation because of the severity of IDDM in this line.

Transgenic Mice Expressing Class I Molecules in Hepatocytes

To investigate the effects of increased expression of class I MHC molecules in cells other than pancreatic β cells, sMTp was used to direct expression of the H-2K^b gene to various tissues (Morahan et al. 1989b). Zinc administration enhanced transgene expression, being greatest in liver, kidney, and exocrine pancreas. As was the case with mice expressing allogeneic class I in β cells, no lymphocyte infiltration was detected in transgene-producing tissues of sMTp transgenic mice allogeneic to H-2K^b. In contrast to the situation with the RIP class I transgenic mice, however, the sMTp transgenic mice had no dysfunction in organs expressing the transgene. This strengthens the notion that pancreatic β cells are unusually sensitive to the effects of overexpression of MHC molecules.

In vivo tests of tolerance were conducted by grafting C57BL/10 skin onto the progeny of sMTp-K^b mice crossed to B10.H-2^{bm1} mice. Although the nontransgenic progeny showed a first-set rejection of their grafts, none of the transgenic mice showed signs of rejection of the H-2K^b-bearing skin grafts over a period in excess of 60 days (Table 3). Despite this and the lack of lymphocytic infiltration in the tissues of sMTp transgenic mice, T cells could be stimulated in vitro to lyse H-2K^b-bearing target cells (Morahan et al. 1989b).

Table 3. Survival of C57BL/10 Skin Grafts on Transgenic sMTp-K^b Mice

Mice	Number	Graft survival (days)		
		<13	15–20	>60
Transgenic	9	0	0	9
Nontransgenic	4	3	1	0

Transgenic sMTp-K^b mice were crossed to bm1, and the progeny were grafted with C57BL/10 skin. Hair growth was noted on surviving grafts.

Tolerance was thus evident in vivo, although not in vitro.

To investigate the basis for the in vivo specific tolerance, transgenic mice were injected with spleen cells from normal mice syngeneic except for the transgene. No lymphocyte infiltration resulted. Transgenic mice were then irradiated (750 rads) and reconstituted with T-cell-depleted bone marrow or spleen cells from nontransgenic syngeneic donors (Morahan et al. 1989b). Whether zinc-induced or not, there was no evidence of graft-versus-host reactions (GVHR) in recipients of bone marrow. Differentiation of T cells within the transgenic recipients must have thus resulted in their inability to respond to the transgene product. In contrast, transgenic recipients of mature T cells developed GVHR in those tissues expressing the transgene product (liver, kidney, and pancreas), whereas other organs including the thymus and spleen were histologically normal after complete reconstitution. Signs of acute hepatitis were observed: apoptotic hepatocytes, intralobular infiltrating lymphocytes, focal necrosis, and mitotic activity, suggestive of some degree of liver regeneration. Dense collections of activated lymphocytes occurred in the portal tracts and mediated piecemeal necrosis of periportal hepatocytes (Morahan et al. 1989b), giving a picture similar to that seen in human chronic active hepatitis (Mackay 1985). After an additional 3 weeks, the lobular infiltrates had decreased and there was less hepatocellular death and piecemeal necrosis. The pathology diminished progressively, and by 12 weeks after reconstitution, many of the portal tracts were free of infiltration, whereas others showed no accompanying necrosis. The picture at this stage was reminiscent of that seen in chronic persistent hepatitis (Mackay 1985). These results strongly suggest that peripheral mechanisms, not involving clonal deletion or permanent clonal anergy, prevent immune responses to self-molecules, including MHC antigens.

DISCUSSION

We have documented evidence for the occurrence of specific tolerance of H-2K^b in both RIP-K^b and sMTp-K^b transgenic mice. This is evident in vivo by the absence of lymphocyte infiltration in transgene-producing tissues and by the failure to reject appropriate skin grafts. In the RIP-K^b model, tolerance waned as the islet β cells became depleted and the severity of IDDM increased. Among the possible mechanisms that induce tolerance in these models, the following are considered.

Is Tolerance Induced by the Intrathymic Clonal Elimination of Potentially Reactive Anti-H2-K^b T Cells?

As mentioned above, transgene expression was not detectable in the thymus of the RIP-K^b mice by a variety of techniques. It was detected at the RNA level in sMTp-K^b mice (Morahan et al. 1989b) and became detectable in the thymus of RIP-K^b mice only when the highly sensitive PCR was used (Fig. 1). However, we have not been able to demonstrate whether the transgene is expressed at the protein level in the thymus. In the RIP-K^b model, the fact that tolerance waned with age militates against the possibility that transgene expression in the thymus, although so low as to be undetectable by immunoperoxidase staining, nevertheless was able to impose tolerance. However, it may be suggested that H-2K^b molecules were shed from the β cells into the circulation and presented in the thymus by cells of the dendritic or macrophage lineages, which then induced tolerance in developing T cells. This is unlikely to be the case for three reasons: (1) Thymus cells of young and old transgenic mice were able to kill both H-2^d and H-2^b targets. (2) Transgenic mice secreting class I MHC molecules lacking the transmembrane domain have, in other experiments, produced neither T- nor B-cell tolerance to the membrane-bound form of that molecule (Arnold et al. 1988). (3) Tolerance of T cells in our young transgenic mice could be abolished in vitro by rIL-2.

Unlike the situation in the RIP-K^b model, spleen cells from sMTp transgenic mice were fully capable of killing targets bearing H-2K^b in vitro. Tolerance in both models is thus unlikely to be imposed by intrathymic clonal elimination of anti-H-2K^b T cells. Is it imposed extrathymically?

How is Peripheral Tolerance Imposed?

Of the many possible mechanisms that could induce tolerance to peripheral antigens, some can be eliminated as explanations for the sMTp-K^b model. For example, the "veto effect" (Fink et al. 1988) is unlikely to be operative because the transgene was not expressed in lymphoid organs. Furthermore, irradiated transgenic mice reconstituted with nontransgenic bone marrow cells displayed no signs of GVHR. Another possible mechanism involves the requirement for a second signal to activate T cells (Lafferty et al. 1980). Lack of such a signal cannot explain the tolerance in either transgenic model, because immunization with C57BL/6 spleen cells failed to induce lymphoid infiltration into transgene-expressing tissues.

Peripheral acquisition of tolerance may result from inappropriate antigen presentation by pancreatic β cells. Evidence for this comes from recent work (Markmann et al. 1988) in which isolated Ins-I-E β cells were able to tolerize T-cell lines in vitro.

Another possible peripheral T-cell tolerance-inducing mechanism may involve the activation of some type of suppressor cell. To date, however, we have been unable to demonstrate suppression in either transgenic model.

Is Tolerance Achieved by the Intrathymic Clonal Elimination of Potentially Reactive CD4$^+$ Helper T Cells?

Peripheral, not thymic, lymphocytes from young RIP-K^b mice were specifically tolerant of the H-2K^b transgene product (Morahan et al. 1989a). These results differ from those of Lo et al. (1988), who showed nonresponsiveness in thymocytes to class II molecules expressed by pancreatic β cells. T cells from their transgenic mice were suggested to have been inactivated by aberrant antigen presentation by β cells (Markham et al. 1988); if so, it is unclear how tolerance could have been achieved among thymocytes in these mice. Comparison of these observations with ours suggests the existence of distinct mechanisms imposing tolerance to class-I- and class-II-restricted T cells reactive to antigens expressed extrathymically. The difference may result from the separate processing pathways operating for the two classes of MHC molecules (Braciale et al. 1987). Thus, extrathymic antigens may be shed, processed, and presented in association with class II molecules by cells that impose negative selection in the thymus. In contrast, antigens presented in association with class I molecules are usually synthesized intracellularly. This would account for the inability of soluble (Arnold et al. 1988) or extrathymic class I molecules to impose tolerance by clonal elimination. In both our transgenic models therefore, class-II-restricted CD4 helper T cells that encounter shed extrathymic antigens presented intrathymically may be clonally eliminated. In contrast, class-I-restricted CTLs reactive to extrathymic antigens are neither eliminated in the thymus nor permanently silenced. Indeed, there may be no need to impose tolerance on these cells per se: withholding help would ensure an effective state of tolerance in vivo, as observed here. Elimination of the helper cells would be sufficient to maintain tolerance. The potentially reactive CTLs would persist and be activated only when the concentration of tolerogen falls below some threshold (e.g., in the older RIP-K^b mice) or on delivery of both antigen and help (e.g., in the IL-2-supplemented CTL assays). If this is the case, however, one must explain why thymocytes do not behave as tolerant cells in the RIP-K^b system and why spleen cells from sMTp-K^b transgenic mice are not tolerant in vitro. In the RIP-K^b model, the inactivation of anti-K^b CTLs may be a dynamic process dependent on critical levels of tolerogen. Lack of tolerance among thymocytes could be explained as follows. A decrease in tolerogen levels might incompletely inactivate the appropriate cell type in the thymus. This could have preceded the lack of tolerance in the periphery by ~1 week. In the sMTp-K^b model in which spleen cells are not tolerant in vitro, some other mechanism must be invoked to explain the observed in vivo tolerance.

Is Tolerance Achieved by the Inactivation or Elimination of Some Other Subset of Potentially Reactive T Cells?

The sensitivity of some T-cell subsets to a negative signal may continue for a short period after leaving the thymus; thus, encounter with antigen during this critical period would lead to their inactivation. Evidence in favor of this explanation comes from Matzinger and Guerder (1989), who showed that the same signal could tolerize thymocytes but activate splenic T cells. Evidence against this is that there has been no difference demonstrated between recent thymic emigrants and mature T cells as yet (R. Scollay, pers. comm.).

The target cell for tolerance could be the $CD8^+$ T-cell subset shown by Singer et al. (1987) to be unique in helping class I alloresponses. Tolerance would not be imposed on these cells within the thymus because class I molecules do not present exogenous antigens and $CD8^+$ cells will not "see" shed antigens. Hence, these cells could help the alloresponse of thymus lymphocytes. In contrast, tolerance would be imposed on these cells in the periphery so that the specific delivery of IL-2 would be limited in the spleen but not in the thymus.

In both transgenic models discussed above, tolerance might be imposed only on those T cells having receptors with the highest affinity for $H-2K^b$, with lower affinity T cells being spared. In the RIP-K^b model, the low-affinity cells would be able to function in vitro provided they received exogenous help (IL-2). Such help in vitro would allow them to lyse $H-2K^b$ targets. In vivo, however, exogenous help may not be sufficient to allow the cells to reject skin grafts. A precedent for this has been documented in the response of B6 mice to $B10^{bm6}$ (Singer et al. 1987). A B6 anti-bm6 CTL response may be obtained in vitro only if IL-2 is added or CD4 cells are present. In contrast, other in vitro responses, such as the B6 anti-bm1 response, do not require exogenous help. In vivo, B6 mice show great difficulties in rejecting bm6 skin grafts despite the presence of $CD4^+$ cells. Conceivably, therefore, the B6 anti-bm6 response involves only low-affinity cells that are poorly equipped to work in vivo but can respond in vitro when provided with exogenous help.

In the sMTp-K^b model, responsiveness is observed in vitro, possibly because only cells with the highest affinity for $H-2K^b$ have been inactivated, leaving cells with sufficient affinity to respond in vitro in the absence of exogenous help but still insufficiently well equipped to reject skin grafts in vivo.

ACKNOWLEDGMENTS

We are grateful to Dr. Marc Feldmann and Hoffmann-La Roche, to the Cetus Corporation for their generous gifts of rIL-2 and r-IL-1, and to Dr. Nick Gough for invaluable help with the PCR analysis. We thank Marisa Brugliera and Leonie Malcolm for excellent technical assistance. The investigations were supported by grants from the National Health and Medical Research Council of Australia, the Utah Foundation, the Buckland Foundation, the Apex-Australian Diabetes Foundation Research and Education Grant, the Jack Brockhoff Foundation, the Sunshine and H.B. McKay Charitable Trust, and the Multiple Sclerosis Foundation of Australia.

REFERENCES

Allison, J., I.L. Campbell, G. Morahan, T.E. Mandel, L. Harrison, and J.F.A.P. Miller. 1988. Diabetes in transgenic mice resulting from overexpression of class I histocompatibility molecules in pancreatic β cells. *Nature* **333:** 529.

Arnold, B., O. Dill, G. Kublbeck, L. Jatsch, M.M. Simon, J. Tucker, and G.J. Hammerling. 1988. Alloreactive immune responses of transgenic mice expressing a foreign transplantation antigen in a soluble form. *Proc. Natl. Acad. Sci.* **85:** 2269.

Baekkeskov, S., T. Kanatsuna, L. Klareskog, D. Nielsen, P. Peterson, A.A.H. Rubensten, D.F. Steiner, and A. Lernmark. 1981. Expression of major histocompatibility antigens on pancreatic islet cells. *Proc. Natl. Acad. Sci.* **78:** 6456.

Billingham, R.E. and P.B. Medawar. 1951. The technique of free skin grafting in mammals. *J. Exp. Biol.* **28:** 385.

Boguniewicz, M., G.H. Sunshine, and Y. Borel. 1989. Role of the thymus in natural tolerance to an autologous protein antigen. *J. Exp. Med.* **169:** 285.

Braciale, T.J., L.A. Morrison, M.T. Sweetser, J. Sambrook, M.-J. Gething, and V.L. Braciale. 1987. Antigen presentation pathways to class I and class II MHC-restricted T lymphocytes. *Immunol. Rev.* **98:** 95.

Choo, K.H., K. Raphael, W. McAdam, and M.G. Peterson. 1987. Expression of active human blood clotting factor IX in transgenic mice: Use of a cDNA with complete mRNA sequence. *Nucleic Acids Res.* **15:** 871.

Fink, P.J., R.P. Shimonkevitz, and M.J. Bevan. 1988. Veto cells. *Annu. Rev. Immunol.* **6:** 115.

Hanahan, D. 1985. Heritable formation of pancreatic β-cell tumours in transgenic mice expressing recombinant insulin/simian virus 40 oncogenes. *Nature* **315:** 115.

Kappler, J.W., N. Roehm, and P. Marrack. 1987. T cell tolerance by clonal elimination in the thymus. *Cell* **49:** 273.

Kappler, J.W., U. Staerz, J. White, and P. Marrack. 1988. Self tolerance eliminates T cells specific for the Mls modified products of the major histocompatibility complex. *Nature* **332:** 35.

Kisielow, P., H. Bluthmann, U.D. Staerz, M. Steinmetz, and H. von Boehmer. 1988. Tolerance in T-cell-receptor transgenic mice involves deletion of nonmature $CD4^+8^+$ thymocytes. *Nature* **333:** 742.

Lafferty, K.J., L. Andrus, and S.J. Prowse. 1980. Role of lymphokine and antigen in the control of specific T cell responses. *Immunol. Rev.* **51:** 279.

Lo, D., L.C. Burkly, G. Widera, C. Cowing, R.A. Flavell, R.D. Palmiter, and R.L. Brinster. 1988. Diabetes and tolerance in transgenic mice expressing class II MHC molecules in pancreatic beta cells. *Cell* **53:** 159.

Lorenz, R.G. and P.M. Allen. 1988. Direct evidence for functional self-protein/Ia-molecule complexes in vivo. *Proc. Natl. Acad. Sci.* **85:** 5220.

MacDonald, H.R., R. Sneider, R.K. Lees, R.C. Howe, H. Acha-Orbea, H. Festenstein, R.M. Zinkernagel, and H. Hengartner. 1988. T cell receptor V_β use predicts reactivity and tolerance to Mls^a-encoded antigens. *Nature* **332:** 40.

Mackay, I.R. 1985. Autoimmune diseases of the liver: Chronic active hepatitis and primary biliary cirrhosis. In *The autoimmune diseases* (ed. N.R. Rose and I.R. Mackay), p. 291. Academic Press, London.

Markmann, J., D. Lo, A. Naji, R.D. Palmiter, R.L. Brinster, and E. Heber-Katz. 1988. Antigen presenting function of class II MHC expressing pancreatic beta cells. *Nature* **336:** 476.

Matzinger, P. and S. Guerder. 1989. Does T-cell tolerance require a dedicated antigen-presenting cell? *Nature* **338:** 74.

Miller, J.F.A.P. and J.D. Watson. 1988. Intracellular recognition events eliminate self-reactive T cells. *Scand. J. Immunol.* **28:** 389.

Morahan, G., J. Allison, and J.F.A.P. Miller. 1989a. Tolerance of class I histocompatibility antigens expressed extrathymically. *Nature* **339:** 622.

Morahan, G., F. Brennan, P.S. Bhathal, J. Allison, K.O. Cox, and J.F.A.P. Miller. 1989b. Expression in transgenic mice of class I histocompatibility antigens controlled by the metallothionein promoter. *Proc. Natl. Acad. Sci.* **86:** 3782.

Nieuwenhuis, P., R.J.M. Stet, J.P.A. Wagenaar, A.S. Wubbena, J. Kampinga, and A. Karrenbeld. 1988. The transcapsular route: A new way for (self-) antigens to by-pass the blood-thymus barrier? *Immunol. Today* **9:** 372.

Peterson, M.G. and J.F.B. Mercer. 1986. Structure and regulation of the sheep metallothionein-Ia gene. *Eur. J. Biochem.* **160:** 579.

Singer, A., T.I. Munitz, H. Golding, A.S. Rosenberg, and I. Mizuochi. 1987. Recognition requirement for the activation, differentiation and function of T-helper cells specific for class I MHC alloantigens. *Immunol. Rev.* **98:** 143.

Sprent, J. and S.R. Webb. 1987. Function and specificity of T cell subsets in the mouse. *Adv. Immunology* **41:** 39.

Clonal Anergy of I-E-tolerant T Cells in Transgenic Mice with Pancreatic Expression of MHC Class II I-E

L.C. BURKLY,* D. LO,† O. KANAGAWA,‡ R.L. BRINSTER,† AND R.A. FLAVELL*§

*Biogen Inc., Cambridge, Massachusetts 02142; †Laboratory of Reproductive Physiology, School of Veterinary Medicine, University of Pennsylvania, Philadelphia, Pennsylvania 19104; ‡Lilly Research Laboratory, La Jolla, California 92037; §Howard Hughes Medical Institute, Section of Immunobiology, Yale University School of Medicine, New Haven, Connecticut 06510

Experimental conditions whereby T-cell tolerance can be established and maintained have been investigated and defined in many systems. However, the mechanisms of tolerance in these systems and their relevance to tolerance induction during normal T-cell development in vivo is still not fully understood. In vivo evidence for clonal deletion has been documented recently, made possible by the development of monoclonal antibodies (MAbs) to T-cell receptor (TCR) V_β chains and by the observation that certain (variable) V_β chains are associated with reactivity to I-E (Kappler et al. 1987b) and minor lymphocyte-stimulating antigens (Mls) (Kappler et al. 1988; MacDonald et al. 1988). For example, T cells utilizing the $V_\beta 17a$ TCR gene identified by MAb KJ23 are generally reactive to I-E (Kappler et al. 1987b) and are present in I-E$^-$ mice but deleted in the thymus of I-E-expressing mouse strains (Kappler et al. 1987a; Marrack et al. 1988). The ability to monitor the presence or absence of antigen-reactive T cells offers a valuable alternative to functional measurements and provides a means to determine whether mechanisms of T-cell tolerance other than clonal deletion occur. There is now ample evidence for clonal paralysis of T cells in vitro. T-cell clones are reportedly inactivated upon exposure to antigen in the presence of human T-cell clones (Lamb et al. 1983), chemically modified spleen cells (Jenkins and Schwartz 1987), purified major histocompatibility complex (MHC) class II on planar membranes (Quill and Schwartz 1987), class II$^+$ keratinocytes (Gaspari et al. 1988), and I-E$^+$ islet cells (Markmann et al. 1988). It is hypothesized that antigen presentation to T cells in the absence of appropriate costimulatory signals results in T-cell paralysis rather than activation. An in vivo situation in which MHC class II molecules are borne on nonlymphoid cell types would allow one to determine the consequences of this presentation for normal T-cell function.

We have reported previously about Ins-I-E transgenic mice (Lo et al. 1988) that express MHC class II I-E on pancreatic islet β cells and kidney tubule epithelium but not in the thymus or cells of peripheral lymphoid organs. These mice bear no evidence of au-

toreactive T-cell infiltrates, even after in vivo priming with I-E$^+$ spleen cells (D. Lo, unpubl.). The transgenic T cells were found to be specifically tolerant to the I-E molecule since they fail to mount a primary mixed lymphocyte reaction when cultured with conventional I-E$^+$ splenic antigen-presenting cells (APC). In this paper, we present the basis for tolerance to the I-E molecule in Ins-I-E mice by using two independent anti-TCR MAbs that detect I-E-reactive T cells.

EXPERIMENTAL PROCEDURES

Mice. SJL/J and C57BL/6 mice were obtained from the Jackson Laboratory (Maine). Transgenic animals described previously, Ins-I-E mice (Lo et al. 1988), EL-I-E (Lo et al. 1989), −1.4-kb E_α^d (v$^+$) (Widera et al. 1987; Burkly et al. 1989), and 107-1 (Widera et al. 1987), were bred at the University of Pennsylvania. Transgenic mice were backcrossed several times to the SJL/J strain to obtain mice homozygous for the $V_\beta 17a$ gene (Kappler et al. 1987b) for analysis of T cells bearing $V_\beta 17a^+$ TCR. These mice were identified by DNA dot hybridization by the absence of $V_\beta 8$ TCR genes because $V_\beta 8$ genes are lacking in the SJL/J genome. For analysis of $V_\beta 5^+$ T cells, each transgenic line was backcrossed several times to the C57BL/6 strain so that they were $V_\beta 5$-gene-positive and $V_\beta 17a$ gene negative. All progeny were also analyzed as described previously (Widera et al. 1987) for the presence of the transgenes by DNA dot hybridization, and only transgene$^+$ individuals were used.

Cytofluorographic analyses. $V_\beta 17a$-bearing T cells were detected by immunofluorescent staining of lymph node T cells prepared by treatment with the B-cell-specific MAb J11d (Bruce et al. 1981) followed by rabbit complement (Pel Freez, Wisconsin). The frequency of positive cells is calculated as the percentage of cells staining with cell-culture supernatant containing the KJ23 MAb followed by fluorescein isothyocyanate (FITC) goat anti-mouse immunoglobulin (Ig) minus the percentage staining with second step alone. $V_\beta 5$-bearing T cells were measured by staining total lymph node cells with the MR9-4 MAb (J. Bill et al., in prep.) followed by FITC goat anti-mouse IgG Fc-specific antibody (Jackson Immunoresearch, Pennsylvania). The frequency of B cells detected with this secondary reagent is < 3%. Stained cells were analyzed by flow cytofluorimetry on a Becton Dickinson FACStar, and contour plots shown have logarithmic scales.

T-cell proliferation. Stimulation of T cells with anti-$V_\beta 17a$ KJ23 MAb was performed with B-cell-depleted T cells or L3T4$^+$ T-cell populations prepared by treatment with J11d and anti-Lyt-2 (53-6.7, rat IgG2a) MAb + complement. T cells were coated with KJ23-containing ascites fluid (1/10) for 30 minutes at 4°C. After washing to remove unbound antibody, the cells were then plated at 2×10^6 responder cells per well in Costar 24-well plates (3524). Syngeneic mitomycin-c-treated splenic stimulators (2.5×10^6) T-cell-depleted by anti-Thy-1.2 (mouse IgM, New England Nuclear, Massachusetts) + complement were added per well. After 4 days, cells were transferred to Falcon 96-well plates (3072) at 2×10^5 cells/well, and triplicate wells were pulsed with [^{3}H]thymidine deoxyribose (TdR) on days 4, 5, or 6 for the final 6 hours of culture. Wells were harvested, and data reported are shown for day 5. T-cell proliferation induced by anti-$V_\beta 5$ MR9-4 MAb was performed with total spleen cells as follows. Falcon 96-well plates were coated with goat anti-mouse IgG at 20 μg/ml in phosphate-buffered saline for 4 hours at room temperature. After washing, TCR-specific MAbs were added (50 μl of undiluted cell culture supernatant or ascites fluid at 1/100) for 2 hours at room temperature, wells were washed again, and 2×10^5 spleen cells were added per well. Cells were cultured for 5 days with [^{3}H]TdR added during the final 6 hours. Cultures were performed in RPMI 1640 medium containing 2×10^{-5} 2-mercaptoethanol, L-glutamine, penicillin, and streptomycin, and 10% (v/v) fetal calf serum (Hyclone Laboratories, Utah) or 1% (v/v) fresh normal mouse sera where indicated. Stimulation with anti-T3 MAb 145-2C11 (Leo et al. 1987) was performed either with 1×10^5 responder cells and 2×10^5 T-depleted mitomycin-c-treated stimulator cells ($V_\beta 17a$ experi-

ments) or 2×10^5 whole spleen cells ($V_\beta 5$ experiments) added to wells of a 96-well plate. Cells were cultured for 3 days in the presence of 145-2C11 MAb containing cell culture supernatant and were pulsed with [^{3}H]TdR during the final 18 hours.

RESULTS

To determine whether the tolerance in our Ins-I-E mice resulted by deletion of I-E reactive T cells, we used the $V_\beta 17a$-specific MAb KJ23 and the MR9-4 MAb, which recognizes T cells expressing $V_\beta 5.1^+$ and $V_\beta 5.2^+$ TCR (Bill et al. 1988), to measure the frequency of these I-E reactive populations among Ins-I-E peripheral T cells. Immunofluorescent staining of lymph node T cells (Table 1) reveals no significant reduction in the frequency of $V_\beta 17a$ T cells in these animals when compared with the SJL/J$^+$ control strain. Furthermore, Ins-I-E and SJL/J $V_\beta 17a^+$ T-cell populations appear indistinguishable (Fig. 1) in that the intensity of $V_\beta 17$ staining is comparable, indicating that the density of TCR molecules per cell is similar. Also (Fig. 1), the proportion of $V_\beta 17a^+$ T cells that is CD4$^+$ (65–70%) versus CD8$^+$ (30–35%) is comparable in the two strains. Transgenic 107-1 mice expressing I-E in a normal fashion on thymus epithelium, mϕ, DC, and B cells have a low frequency of $V_\beta 17a^+$ T cells (Table 1), reflecting clonal elimination of these T cells in the thymus (Marrack et al. 1988). Analysis of $V_\beta 5^+$ lymph node cells shows that a considerable frequency of $V_\beta 5^+$ T cells are present in Ins-I-E mice as compared with B6 controls (Table 1), whereas 107-1 mice on the C57BL/6 background exhibit elimination of the $V_\beta 5^+$ T-cell population. Since 107-1 transgenic mice differ from C57BL/6 mice only by expression of the I-E transgene, this result formally demonstrates the deletion of $V_\beta 5$-bearing T cells because of expression of the I-E molecule. Thus, in vivo tolerance in Ins-I-E mice is not due to clonal deletion of these I-E-reactive T-cell populations.

To determine if T cells from the Ins-I-E mice were clonally paralyzed, we attempted to activate these I-E-

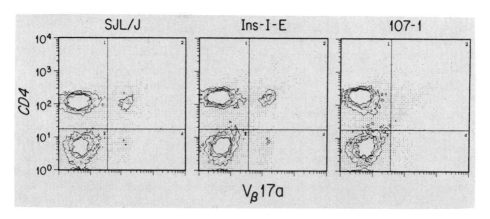

Figure 1. Log fluorescence intensity of CD4 versus $V_\beta 17a$ on lymph node T cells.

Table 1. T Cells Bearing I-E-specific Receptors Are Not Deleted in Ins-I-E Transgenic Mice

I-E expression	Mouse	$V_\beta 17a^+$ (%)	Mouse	$V_\beta 5^+$ (%)
None	SJL/J	9.7 +/− 1.0 (5)	C57BL/6	5.7 +/− 0.9 (4)
Pancreatic β cells, kidney	Ins-I-E	8.3 +/− 0.5 (6)	Ins-I-E	4.2 +/− 0.6 (4)
Wild type	107-1	2.2 +/− 0.5 (5)	107-1	0.1 +/− 0.1 (2)

Percentage represents the average +/− S.E.M. of n independent determination (n value is given in parentheses).

specific T cells. Normally, T cells can be activated by receptor cross-linking with MAbs recognizing their TCR in the presence of Fc receptor$^+$ accessory cells or by insolubilized anti-TCR antibodies in the presence of accessory cells or soluble costimulatory signals (Kaye et al. 1983; Frelinger et al. 1984; Crispe et al. 1985; Manger et al. 1985). If Ins-I-E T cells were rendered anergic by inappropriate exposure to I-E in vivo, they should not proliferate on reexposure to antigen (Jenkins and Schwartz 1987; Quill and Schwartz 1987) or through receptor cross-linking with anti-TCR antibodies. Tables 2 and 3 show representative data generated with the $V_\beta 17a$- and $V_\beta 5$-specific monoclonal antibodies, and Figure 2 summarizes the results of many experiments. Stimulation of T cells with MAb 145-2C11 (Leo et al. 1987) specific for the T3 molecule of the T3/antigen receptor complex was used as a positive control to demonstrate the general responsiveness of all T-cell populations.

Whereas anti-$V_\beta 17a$ monoclonal antibody could induce proliferation in SJL/J control T cells, Ins-I-E transgenic T cells showed little if any proliferation under the conditions described at various time points tested (Table 2). Only one responsive individual was found (Fig. 2). The 107-1 mice that have deleted most $V_\beta 17a^+$ T cells serve as a negative control.

Stimulation of spleen cells with anti-$V_\beta 5$ MAb MR9-4 insolubilized on anti-Ig-coated wells (Table 3, Fig. 2) revealed a positive response from C57BL/6 strain spleen cells. In this case, insolubilized $V_\beta 17a$ served as a negative control antibody. In contrast with B6 cells, proliferation of Ins-I-E T cells was absent or greatly diminished. Only one of six individuals gave a considerable response (Table 3, Exp. 2).

We have also analyzed El-I-E transgenic mice that only express I-E extrathymically on pancreatic acinar cells, are tolerant to I-E (Lo et al. 1989), and have normal percentages of $V_\beta 17a^+$ (8.6 ± 0.9) and $V_\beta 5^+$ (6.1 ± 0.1) T cells. In contrast with Ins-I-E mice, El-I-E T cells proliferate in response to anti-$V_\beta 17a$ at levels comparable with SJL/J T cells (Fig. 2). Although El-I-E mice respond to anti-$V_\beta 17a$ at control levels, anti-$V_\beta 5$ induced low levels of proliferation as compared with B6 controls. Thus, $V_\beta 5^+$ and $V_\beta 17a^+$ T cells differ in their ability to be tolerized by the I-E presented in El-I-E mice.

DISCUSSION

We have used anti-TCR monoclonal antibodies that detect I-E-reactive T-cell populations in order to examine I-E-tolerant Ins-I-E mice. Our data indicate that $V_\beta 17a^+$ and $V_\beta 5^+$ T cells are not clonally deleted in Ins-I-E mice. However, these T cells respond poorly, if at all, to receptor cross-linking. Exposure to I-E on nonlymphoid cells in vivo apparently rendered the T-cells anergic. Our results parallel those described for the induction of T-cell unresponsiveness in vitro. In particular, Markmann et al. (1988) demonstrated that T-cell clones exposed to I-E$^+$ Ins-I-E transgenic islet cells were clonally paralyzed. Previous indications that clonal paralysis can occur in vivo include tolerance established by injection of chemically fixed APC (Jenkins and Schwartz 1987) and MHC class II L-cell transfectants (Madsen et al. 1988) and induction of in vivo tolerance to Mls (Rammensee et al. 1989). However, our experiments provide the first evidence that

Table 2. Ins-I-E Transgenic T Cells Are Not Activated by Anti-$V_\beta 17a$ Monoclonal Antibody

		[^{3}H]TdR-incorporation induced by TCR-specific MAbs					
		$V_\beta 17a$-specific MAb				T3-specific MAb	
		(−)	(+)				
Exp.	Responder	cpm × 10^{-3}		Δcpm	(SI)	Δcpm	(SI)
1	SJL/J	3.3	24.9	21.6	(7.5)		
	Ins-I-E	0.9	1.1	0.2	(1.2)		
	107-1	0.4	0.3	−0.1	(0.8)		
2	SJL/J	13.0	55.1	42.1	(4.2)	69.2	(139.4)
	Ins-I-E	6.5	10.1	3.6	(1.6)	186.4	(144.4)
3	SJL/J	11.5	67.9	56.4	(5.9)	288.2	(388.4)
	Ins-I-E	14.7	21.0	6.3	(1.4)	268.5	(355.3)
	107-1	3.3	3.1	−0.2	(0.9)	266.0	(205.6)

Responder cells are B-cell-depleted lymph node T cells (Exp. 1) and L3T4$^+$ lymph node T cells (Exp. 2 and 3).

Table 3. Ins-I-E Transgenic T Cells Are Not Activated by Anti-$V_\beta 5$ Monoclonal Antibody

		[³H]TdR-incorporation induced by MAb specific for					
		$V_\beta 17a$	$V_\beta 5$			T3	
Exp.	Responder	total cpm × 10⁻³		Δcpm	(SI)	Δcpm	(SI)
1	C57BL/6	0.2	19.5	19.3	(97.5)	144.9	(52.8)
	C57BL/6	0.3	39.2	38.9	(130.7)	265.4	(62.7)
	Ins-I-E	3.5	3.9	0.4	(1.1)	115.2	(58.6)
	Ins-I-E	3.5	3.2	−0.3	(0.9)	98.1	(110.0)
	107-1	1.0	4.3	3.3	(4.3)	111.5	(30.3)
2	C57BL/6	0.5	11.6	11.1	(23.2)	133.4	(223.3)
	Ins-I-E	1.8	4.6	2.8	(2.6)	200.6	(223.9)
	Ins-I-E	2.3	18.8	16.5	(8.2)	128.9	(118.2)
	107-1	1.0	1.2	0.2	(1.2)	267.0	(268.0)

In Exp. 1, cultures were supplemented with 1% (v/v) fresh normal mouse serum.

paralysis of T cells does occur during normal T-cell development in a transgenic mouse system.

Low levels of proliferation were sometimes observed from Ins-I-E mice on TCR cross-linking with anti-$V_\beta 17a$ (Fig. 2). This might be expected since individual $V_\beta 17a^+$ T cells differ in their reactivity to allogeneic forms of the I-E molecule (Kappler et al. 1987b; Marrack et al. 1988). It is possible that not all $V_\beta 17a^+$ T cells recognize the I-E expressed in Ins-I-E mice ($E_\alpha{}^d E_\beta{}^b$) equally well, and thus not all $V_\beta 17a^+$ T cells will be tolerized. Whether or not the same is true of $V_\beta 5^+$ T cells has not been determined. Although $V_\beta 5^+$ T cells are clonally eliminated in I-E-expressing strains, $V_\beta 5^+$ T-cell hybrids are not demonstrably reactive to I-E⁺ spleen stimulator cells (Bill et al. 1988). This observation offers a second explanation for the proliferation sometimes evident in Ins-I-E mice (Fig. 2). The concept has been put forth that allogeneic I-E molecules are I-E/peptide complexes (Matzinger and Bevan 1977) with the I-E-associated peptides dependent on the I-E⁺ cell type (Marrack and Kappler 1988) and thus possibly on the non-MHC background genes (Bill et al. 1989). I-E/peptide complexes may vary between

individual Ins-I-E mice because of the fact that this transgenic line is not inbred. Animals analyzed were backcrossed four to six times onto SJL/J or C57BL/6, respectively. Thus, in some mice, particular $V_\beta 17a^+$ or $V_\beta 5^+$ I-E-reactive T cells may not be exposed to their appropriate ligand and thereby escape tolerance.

Our experiments with $V_\beta 17a$ demonstrate clonal anergy of peripheral CD4⁺ Ins-I-E T cells. Curiously, 30–35% of $V_\beta 17a^+$ T cells and the vast majority of $V_\beta 5^+$ T cells are CD4⁻ CD8⁺ in both normal and transgenic mice. Unlike normal CD8⁺ T cells, which respond to receptor cross-linking (Crispe et al. 1985; O. Kanagawa, unpubl.), our experiments indicate that the CD8⁺ transgenic T cells are apparently unresponsive as well. Although CD8⁺ T cells are commonly restricted to class I, their use of particular Vβ genes may confer sufficient reactivity to I-E to be paralyzed. Paralysis could result from contact with I-E⁺ islet cells, which lack APC function (Markmann et al. 1988), or from exposure to I-E in the absence of T-cell help.

We have suggested the possibility that clonal anergy of I-E-tolerant Ins-I-E T cells occurs by exposure to I-E⁺ islet cells in vivo. However, we have reported

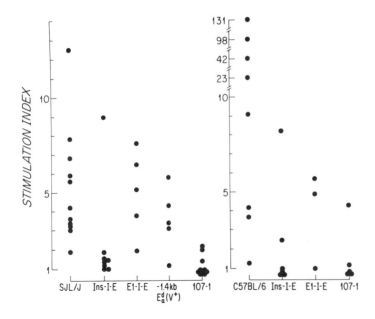

Figure 2. Summary of TCR-cross-linking experiments with anti-$V_\beta 17a$ (*left*) and anti-$V_\beta 5$ (*right*). Each dot represents the stimulation index (SI) for an individual mouse where SI is the cpm incorporated with KJ23 MAb over incorporation without MAb (*left*) and incorporation with MR9-4 MAb over incorporation with KJ23 as negative control antibody (*right*).

previously (Lo et al. 1988) that both peripheral T cells and thymocytes of Ins-I-E mice are specifically tolerant to I-E. In contrast, studies reported by Morahan et al. (1989) describe tolerance to the H-2 K^b molecule among peripheral T cells but not thymocytes in transgenic mice expressing K^b only on islet cells. Given the tolerant Ins-I-E thymocytes, we must consider the possibility that I-E was transported from the pancreas or kidney and presented in processed form in the thymus to induce tolerance there. The possibility that an I-E-derived peptide is presented by I-A molecules has been reported recently (Murphy et al. 1989). Nonetheless, our conclusion that tolerance in Ins-I-E mice is not due to clonal deletion is still valid. It is possible that tolerance may occur in the thymus by deletion versus paralysis depending on the quantity or site of presented antigen.

Ins-I-E mice contain significant numbers of potentially I-E-reactive T cells. Yet, it is possible that a very small percentage of I-E-reactive T cells was deleted that is required for function of the remaining I-E-specific population. We consider this possibility unlikely given results obtained with transgenic -1.4-kb E_α^d (v^+) mice, which have a readily detectable, partial reduction of $V_\beta 17a^+$ T cells ($5.9 \pm 0.3\%$, value obtained from Marrack et al. 1988). These mice express I-E on thymic epithelial cells (Widera et al. 1987; Burkly et al. 1989) but not on marrow-derived cells in the thymus or on peripheral cell types. Despite a significant reduction of $V_\beta 17a^+$ cells, T cells of these mice still proliferate in the presence of KJ23 MAb (Fig. 2).

We have also analyzed El-I-E mice for $V_\beta 17a^+$ and $V_\beta 5^+$ T cells and conclude that tolerance to I-E in these mice occurs by a nondeletional mechanism. However, El-I-E $V_\beta 17a^+$ T cells do proliferate on receptor cross-linking. The difference between Ins-I-E and El-I-E $V_\beta 17a^+$ T cells (both lines backcrossed four to six times to SJL/J) indicates that I-E expression in these two transgenic strains is not equivalent. Since both lines express I-E at high levels (Lo et al. 1988, 1989), our data argue in favor of a qualitative difference in I-E. We suggest that $V_\beta 17a^+$ T cells do not recognize the particular I-E/peptide complexes presented in El-I-E mice. In contrast, the $V_\beta 5^+$ population appears to be functionally impaired in El-I-E mice.

In summary, we have analyzed two transgenic lines with nonlymphoid expression of MHC class II I-E. We demonstrate tolerance to I-E occurs in these mice by a mechanism other than clonal deletion and provide functional evidence for clonal paralysis of normal I-E-specific T cells in vivo.

ACKNOWLEDGMENTS

We thank K. Hughes for technical assistance and M. Pomeroy for operating the flow cytofluorimeter.

REFERENCES

Bill, J., V.B. Appel, and E. Palmer. 1988. An analysis of T-cell receptor variable region gene expression in major histocompatibility complex disparate mice. *Proc. Natl. Acad. Sci* **85**: 9184.

Bill, J., O. Kanagawa, D.L. Woodland, and E. Palmer. 1989. The MHC molecule I-E is necessary but not sufficient for the clonal deletion of $V_\beta 11$-bearing T cells. *J. Exp. Med.* **169**: 1405.

Bruce, J., F.W. Symington, T.J. McKearn, and J.J. Sprent. 1981. A monoclonal antibody discriminating between subsets of T and B cells. *J. Immunol.* **127**: 2496.

Burkly, L.C., D. Lo, R.L. Brinster, and R.A. Flavell. 1989. I-E transgenic mice: A model system to dissect the regulation and function of MHC class II genes in vivo. *Immunol. Res.* (in press).

Crispe, I.N., M.J. Bevan, and U. Staerz. 1985. Selective activation of Lyt 2^+ precursor T cells by ligation of the antigen receptor. *Nature* **317**: 627.

Frelinger, J., A. Sing, A. Infante, and C.G. Fathman. 1984. Clonotypic antibodies which stimulate T cell clone proliferation. *Immunol. Rev.* **81**: 21.

Gaspari, A.A., M.K. Jenkins, and S.I. Katz. 1988. Class II MHC-bearing keratinocytes induce antigen-specific unresponsiveness in hapten-specific TH1 clones. *J. Immunol.* **141**: 2216.

Jenkins, M.K. and R.H. Schwartz. 1987. Antigen presentation by chemically modified splenocytes induced antigen-specific T cell unresponsiveness in vitro and in vivo. *J. Exp. Med.* **165**: 302.

Kappler, J.W., N. Roehm, and P. Marrack. 1987a. T cell tolerance by clonal elimination in the thymus. *Cell* **49**: 273.

Kappler, J.W., U. Staerz, J. White, and P. Marrack. 1988. Self-tolerance eliminates T cells specific for Mls-modified products of the major histocompatibility complex. *Nature* **332**: 35.

Kappler, J.W., T. Wade, J. White, E. Kushnir, M. Blackman, J. Bill, N. Roehm, and P. Marrack. 1987b. A T cell receptor V_β segment that imparts reactivity to a class II major histocompatibility complex product. *Cell* **49**: 263.

Kaye, J.A., S. Porcelli, J. Tite, B. Jones, and C.A. Janeway, Jr. 1983. Both a monoclonal antibody and antisera specific for determinants unique to individual cloned helper T cell lines can substitute for antigen and antigen-presenting cells in the activation of T cells. *J. Exp. Med.* **158**: 836.

Lamb, J.R., B.J. Skidmore, N. Green, J.M. Chiller, and M.J. Feldmann. 1983. Induction of tolerance in influenza virus-immune T lymphocyte clones with synthetic peptides of influenza hemagglutinin. *J. Exp. Med.* **157**: 1434.

Leo, O., M. Foo, D.H. Sachs, L.E. Samelson, and J.A. Bluestone. 1987. Identification of a monoclonal antibody specific for a murine T3 polypeptide. *Proc. Natl. Acad. Sci.* **84**: 1374.

Lo, D., L.C. Burkly, R.A. Flavell, R.D. Palmiter, and R.L. Brinster. 1989. Tolerance in transgenic mice expressing class II MHC on pancreatic acinar cells. *J. Exp. Med.* **170**: 87.

Lo, D., L.C. Burkly, G. Widera, C. Cowing, R.A. Flavell, R.D. Palmiter, and R.L. Brinster. 1988. Diabetes and tolerance in transgenic mice expressing class II MHC molecules in pancreatic beta cells. *Cell* **53**: 159.

MacDonald, H.R., R. Schneider, R.K. Lees, R.C. Howe, H. Acha-Orbea, H. Festenstein, R.M. Zinkernagel, and H. Hengartner. 1988. T cell receptor use predicts reactivity and tolerance to Mls^a-encoded antigens. *Nature* **332**: 40.

Madsen, J.C., R.A. Superina, K.J. Wood, and P.J. Morris. 1988. Immunological unresponsiveness induced by recipient cells transfected with donor MHC genes. *Nature* **332**: 161.

Manger, B., A. Weiss, C. Weyand, J. Goronzy, and J.D. Stobo. 1985. T cell activation: Differences in the signals required for IL-2 production by nonactivated and activated T cells. *J. Immunol.* **135**: 3669.

Markmann, J., D. Lo, A. Naji, R.D. Palmiter, R.L. Brinster, and E. Heber-Katz. 1988. Antigen presenting function of class II MHC expressing pancreatic beta cells. *Nature* **336**: 476.

Marrack, P. and J. Kappler. 1988. T cells can distinguish between allogeneic major histocompatibility complex products on different cell types. *Nature* **332:** 840.

Marrack, P., D. Lo, R. Brinster, R. Palmiter, L. Burkly, R.A. Flavell, and J.W. Kappler. 1988. The effect of thymus environment on T cell development and tolerance. *Cell* **53:** 627.

Matzinger, P. and M.J. Bevan. 1977. Hypothesis: Why do so many lymphocytes respond to major histocompatibility antigens? *Cell. Immunol.* **29:** 1.

Morahan, G., J. Allison, and J.F.A.P. Miller. 1989. Tolerance of class I histocompatibility antigens expressed extrathymically. *Nature* **339:** 622.

Murphy, D.B., D. Lo, S. Rath, R.L. Brinster, R.A. Flavell, A. Slanetz, and C.A. Janeway, Jr. 1989. A novel MHC class II epitope expressed in thymic medulla but not cortex. *Nature* **338:** 765.

Quill, H. and R.H. Schwartz. 1987. Stimulation of normal inducer T cell clones with antigen presented by purified Ia molecules in planar lipid membranes: Specific induction of a long-lived state of proliferative nonresponsiveness. *J. Immunol.* **138:** 3704.

Rammensee, H.-G., R. Kroschewski, and B. Frangoulis. 1989. Clonal anergy induced in mature $V_\beta 6^+$ T lymphocytes on immunizing Mls-1^b mice with Mls-1^a expressing cells. *Nature* **339:** 541.

Widera, G., L.C. Burkly, C.A. Pinkert, E. Boettger, C. Cowing, R.D. Palmiter, R.L. Brinster, and R.A. Flavell. 1987. Transgenic mice selectively lacking MHC class II (I-E) antigen expression on B cells: An in vivo approach to investigate Ia gene function. *Cell* **51:** 175.

Alternative Self or Nonself Recognition of an Antigen Expressed in a Rare Cell Type in Transgenic Mice: Implications for Self-tolerance and Autoimmunity

D. Hanahan,*† C. Jolicoeur,*† S. Alpert,†‡ and J. Skowronski†
*Department of Biochemistry and Biophysics and Hormone Research Institute, University of California,
San Francisco, California 94143-0534; †Cold Spring Harbor Laboratory, Cold Spring Harbor, New York 11724

During its development, the immune system acquires the ability to recognize and respond to a wide variety of cells and other entities from the outside environment (Hood et al. 1984; Roitt et al. 1985). A necessary feature of this capacity is the ability to discriminate between what is a normal component of the body (self) and what is not (foreign or nonself). The existence of immunological tolerance toward self has been well-established for many years, and mechanisms that could serve to achieve it have been postulated and increasingly refined as our knowledge of the development, organization, and function of the immune system has progressed (Burnet 1959; Dresser and Mitchison 1968; Bretscher and Cohn 1970; Weigle 1973; Howard and Mitchison 1975; Nossal 1983; Schwartz 1989). The importance of self-tolerance can be seen in the damages wrought by autoimmune diseases, such as insulin-dependent diabetes, in which the immune system becomes self-reactive against specific cells and seeks to destroy them. In the case of diabetes, the autoimmune response succeeds in destroying the pancreatic β cells, resulting in a condition of insulin insufficiency and consequent deleterious effects throughout the body (Rossini et al. 1985). Regarding the principles of self, the possibility is evident that failures to establish or maintain a condition of nonresponsiveness toward self-antigens could be a factor in the induction of autoimmune responses. Thus, one may in principle be able to relate the conditions of tolerance and autoimmunity through the mechanisms of self/nonself recognition.

Several new approaches have contributed to our current understanding of the cellular mechanisms of self-tolerance. One of these applies the knowledge of T-cell receptor (TCR) gene structure and germ-line diversity to the analysis of the consequences of exposure to certain "super antigens" that have been found to have widespread effects on the immune response (Kappler et al. 1988, 1989; MacDonald et al. 1988; Pullen et al. 1988; Robertson 1988; Janeway et al. 1989; Mollick et al. 1989). The combination of reagents specific for particular TCR chains and an antigen that can be selec-

tively presented has allowed the response of developing T cells to that antigen to be visualized. This experimental approach has revealed that both cell death (clonal deletion) and functional inactivation (clonal anergy or paralysis) are mechanisms for achieving selective nonresponsiveness in the T-cell compartment (Kappler et al. 1987, 1988; MacDonald et al. 1988; Rammensee et al. 1989).

A second new method for studying self-tolerance has used the stable introduction of genes into lines of transgenic mice to address different aspects of the development and maintenance of selective recognition and nonresponsiveness toward components of self. Two different and complementary strategies have proved informative about the properties of self-recognition. One involves the introduction of rearranged immunoglobulin (Ig) or TCR genes to produce transgenic mice that express the antigen receptor encoded by the transgene on a large fraction of B or T cells. This approach provides a means to visualize the response of developing lymphocytes toward self-antigens recognized by these antigen receptors and has been used to demonstrate unambiguously that both clonal deletion and clonal anergy (or paralysis) of self-reactive lymphocytes are mechanisms for achieving nonresponsiveness by B cells and T cells (Goodnow et al. 1988 and this volume; Kisielow et al. 1988a,b; Sha et al. 1988a,b; Teh et al. 1988; Nemazee and Burki 1989).

Another transgenic strategy centers on the introduction of genes that encode new self-antigens into lines of transgenic mice to evaluate the responses of the immune system to a protein that was heretofore not a normal component of a mouse but now has become a stable part of the genome and the milieu of antigens it elaborates. One of the first examples of this approach involved targeted expression to pancreatic β cells in transgenic mice of a protein called large T antigen (Tag), which is encoded within the early region of SV40 (Adams et al. 1987). Mice in one lineage were found to be selectively nonresponsive to this new self-antigen, demonstrating that tolerance to an antigen expressed on a rare cell type could be established. However, tolerance was not obligatory since mice in several other lineages were consistently not tolerant to T antigen. Moreover, mice in the nontolerant lines

---

‡Present address: Department of Microbiology and Immunology, University of California, San Francisco, California 94143.

developed spontaneous autoimmunity against the transgenic self-antigen and the cells that expressed it. These two alternative responses were genetically stable within independent transgenic lines. The reproducibility of the tolerant and nontolerant phenotypes has provided a format to study the principles underlying the development of an ability to recognize and become nonresponsive toward rare self-antigens. Furthermore, it has allowed investigators to address the mechanisms by which an autoimmune response can be generated when recognition of a self-protein occurs but nonresponsiveness toward it does not. In this paper, we intend to review the characteristics of the transgenic lines that differentially express the same protein in their pancreatic β cells and then to consider the alternative immune responses to these distinct patterns of self-antigen expression.

MATERIALS AND METHODS

Hybrid genes and transgenic lineages. The transgenic lines used in this paper have been generated and propagated using standard techniques, which have been described previously (Hogan et al. 1986). The construction of the rat insulin promoter (RIP1)-Tag and rat insulin reverse (RIR)-Tag hybrid genes as well as the generation and initial characterization of the RIP1-Tag2, -Tag3, and -Tag4 lineages were presented previously (Hanahan 1985). The RIR-Tag2 line was characterized by Efrat and Hanahan (1987). The RIR3-Tag gene represents a deletion of part of the RIR-Tag regulatory region so that sequences from + 180 to −278 of the insulin gene are retained, whereas those from −278 to −540 are removed. This construct and the characterization of the transgenic lineage carrying it will be described in depth elsewhere (S. Efrat and D. Hanahan, unpubl.). Unless otherwise noted, transgenic males were bred to C57BL/6J females, and transgenic progeny were identified by DNA analysis of tail biopsies.

Expression of T antigen. The immunochemical identification of T antigen expression in the various lineages was performed on tissue sections, as has been described previously (Hanahan 1985; Efrat et al. 1987; Efrat and Hanahan 1987; Alpert et al. 1988; Teitelman et al. 1988). Confirmation of T-antigen immunoreactivity as a reflection of synthesis of the bona fide protein involved immunostaining for the cellular protein p53, which can only be detected in β cells if it is stabilized by large T protein (Efrat et al. 1987). Solid tumor formation under the influence of the hybrid insulin/T antigen genes occurs in every individual, except for the RIR3-Tag2 line in which the mice only develop sporadic islet hyperplasia at old ages. The solid tumors derive from the pancreatic β cells, and all of the tumor cells express T antigen, p53, and insulin (Hanahan 1985; Efrat et al. 1987; Efrat and Hanahan 1987). The population of islets expressing the large T oncoprotein undergo various changes prior to the formation of a few solid

tumors, as has been described previously (Teitelman et al. 1988; Folkman et al. 1989). The characteristics of these and other transgenic tumorigenesis models have been reviewed and discussed previously (Hanahan 1988).

Characterization of cellular and humoral responses. Cellular infiltration of the islets was analyzed first by staining of pancreatic sections with hematoxylin and eosin (H&E) and subsequently by immunostaining with antibodies for cell-surface markers that identify specific leukocyte subsets. The monoclonal antibodies used for this characterization recognize the Lyt-2, L3T4, B220, and Mac-1 cell-surface determinants on $CD8^+$ T cells, $CD4^+$ T cells, B cells, and macrophages, respectively. Their specificities and utilization have been described previously (Ledbetter and Herzenberg 1979; Springer et al. 1979; Springer 1981; Morse et al. 1982; Dialynas et al. 1983; Sanchez-Madrid et al. 1983).

Large T protein was purified from HeLa cells infected with an adeno/SV40 hybrid virus using an immuno-affinity column (Simanis and Lane 1985) prepared with the anti-T-antigen monoclonal antibody PAb419 (Harlow et al. 1981). The purified T antigen was used in the immunization experiments to assess tolerance and to serve as the solid-phase substrate in the radioimmunoassay (RIA). For immunizations, 5–10 μg of purified T protein was injected intraperitoneally into each mouse in a mixture with either complete Freund's adjuvant (CFA) (primary immunization) or incomplete Freund's adjuvant (IFA) (secondary boost).

The solid-phase RIA used for quantification of both the induced and spontaneous antibody response against T antigen is described in depth elsewhere (J. Skowronski et al., in prep.). The initial assays for both induced and autoimmune responsiveness toward T antigen, which also represent one confirmation of the specificity of the RIA, involved immunoprecipitation from extracts of radiolabeled COS cells (Gluzman 1981) that express large T antigen, using serum collected from primary or secondary immunizations of control or transgenic mice (Adams et al. 1987). For the RIA, the *Escherichia coli* protein, β-galactosidase (β-Gal), was used as an internal standard in the immunizations. A monoclonal antibody specific for T-antigen and normal mouse serum antibodies obtained by immunization with β-Gal protein were used as positive controls in the assay, and neither these control antibodies nor antisera induced in the transgenic mice against either β-Gal or T antigen cross-reacted with the other protein (J. Skowronski et al., in prep.).

RESULTS

Two Expression Patterns of Hybrid Insulin/T Antigen Genes

The basic strategy of our experimental approach has been to construct hybrid genes to direct the synthesis of selected proteins to the pancreatic β cells in transgenic mice and then to examine both the patterns of expression and the consequences of that expression. The prototype chosen was the SV40 large T antigen. This 96-kD protein has a number of interesting properties among which are its antigenicity and oncogenic activities (Tooze 1981). Immunization with purified large T protein produces both humoral and cytotoxic T-cell responses (Chang et al. 1979; Tevethia et al. 1980). Large T is predominantly localized to the nucleus by virtue of a nuclear localization signal sequence contained within it (Kalderon et al. 1984; Lanford and Butel 1984). However, it is well established that large T can be recognized on the cell surface of many cultured cells expressing the SV40 early region. The most consistent means of identifying the cell-surface component of T antigen has been with cytotoxic T-cell lines induced in mice by SV40 viral infection or after transplantation of SV40-transformed cell lines (Trinchieri et al. 1976; Gooding 1979; Knowles et al. 1979; Gooding and O'Connell 1983; Pan and Knowles 1983; Gooding et al. 1984; Tevethia and Tevethia 1984; Pan et al. 1987; Rawle et al. 1988). These T-cell clones are class I major-histocompatibility-complex (MHC)-restricted, and given the (self)-antigen-presenting properties of class I molecules it would seem reasonable to conclude that the cell-surface component of large T is in fact processed peptides of the protein that are effectively presented in the context of class I MHC molecules. However, in certain cell lines a cell-surface component of large T antigen has also been identified by immunostaining (Deppert et al. 1980; Soule et al. 1980; Ismail et al. 1981; Deppert and Walter 1982), most recently with monoclonal antibodies specific for either amino- or carboxy-terminal epitopes of T antigen (Ball et al. 1984; Gooding et al. 1984). This raises the possibility that larger fragments of the protein are presented on the cell surface by other means. In fact, one study reported that the membrane fraction of an SV40-transformed cell line contained a 96-kD protein indistinguishable from the one present in the nuclear fraction as assessed by immunoprecipitation (Soule and Butel 1979). However, the localization of intact large T protein to the membrane has not been reported for other cell types. Nevertheless, what is clear from all of these studies is that expression of large T in a variety of cell types can be detected in living cells by components of the immune system, which indicates that the protein is effectively presented for immunological recognition on the cell surface. This quality renders the large T protein an attractive molecule for studying interactions of a new self-antigen with the immune system in transgenic mice, given that normal mice do not normally experience it.

Several different configurations of the rat insulin II gene regulatory region have been used to direct the expression of large T antigen to the insulin-producing β cells of transgenic mice. One construct aligned the insulin promoter to transcribe the SV40 early region much as it would the insulin gene (Hanahan 1985). This hybrid gene, called RIP1-Tag, has 695 bp of 5'-flanking DNA to the insulin gene, including the transcriptional enhancer, which is known to be cell-type-specific in vitro (Walker et al. 1983). In the second construct, the insulin promoter was inverted so that sequences upstream of the enhancer abutted the T-antigen-coding region, and the insulin promoter was at the distal (5') end of the construct aligned to transcribe in the opposite direction to the T-antigen-coding region (Hanahan 1985). Surprisingly, this construct, called RIR-Tag, is expressed in a manner comparable with the RIP1-Tag hybrid gene, which utilizes the insulin promoter element. The RIR-Tag construct appears to function by virtue of a cryptic promoter element residing at the 5' boundary of the enhancer on the opposite strand and with opposite orientation to that of the bona fide insulin promoter (Efrat and Hanahan 1987).

Both the RIP1-Tag and the RIR-Tag hybrid genes were established in several independent lines of transgenic mice. In every case, large T antigen was synthesized in the pancreatic β cells of adult mice. Given that the β cells are localized into approximately 400 focal clusters called the islets of Langerhans, which comprise only 1% of the pancreas, immunohistochemical techniques have been the primary means of identifying the cells synthesizing large T antigen. Several criteria have been used to establish the presence of large T. The most direct criterion involved the visualization of large T protein in situ with either rabbit polyclonal antisera raised against the purified protein or with one of a series of monoclonal antibodies specific for different epitopes of the protein (Harlow et al. 1981).

The presence of authentic large T protein has been confirmed by two of its properties. One is that large T binds to and stabilizes the steady-state levels of a cellular protein known as p53, so that it can be visualized by immunostaining, which is normally not possible. Thus, the presence of p53 in cells supports the conclusion that large T itself is present in an intact conformation. The second property of large T that can be used to assess transgene expression is its ability to transform cells. In most lineages, every mouse inheriting a hybrid insulin/T antigen gene inevitably developed a few pancreatic β-cell tumors and succumbed as a consequence. Biochemical analysis demonstrated that the tumors express both large T protein and p53 (Efrat et al. 1987). This supports the assumptions of the immunohistochemical analyses discussed above. An exception to the β-cell specificity has been observed in one line, RIP1-Tag2, in which about 5–10% of the mice also develop neuroendocrine tumors of the intestine capable of transcribing (S. Grant et al., in prep.). In every other case, the immunohistochemical and phenotypic evidence supports the conclusion that the insulin gene regulatory region targets expression of large T antigen to the insulin-producing β cells in adult transgenic mice.

Although mice in every line of insulin/T antigen transgenics express large T in their β cells and most develop β-cell tumors later in life, there are significant differences in the temporal patterns of expression among the independent lines. Two general classes are evident as illustrated in Figure 1. In the first class, the transgenic mice begin to express T antigen during embryogenesis and express T antigen uniformly in their β cells as adults. Two lineages showing this pattern of developmental expression of the insulin/T antigen hybrid gene have been extensively characterized: RIP1-Tag2 and RIR-Tag2. Mice in each line first express detectable levels of T antigen beginning at embryonic day 10, both in the pancreatic diverticulum off the gut and transiently in neuroblasts in the neural tube and neural crest (Alpert et al. 1988). When insulin immunoreactivity is first evident 2 days later in the nascent pancreas, all the insulin-producing cells also coexpress large T. The transgene has a selectively wider pattern of developmental expression than the endogenous insulin genes in that it is also transiently detected in cells that express the other three islet cell hormones, as well as in neuroblasts. T-antigen expression becomes restricted to the β cells of adult mice in these two lineages, initially without consequence. However, beginning at about 6 weeks of age, abnormal cell proliferation and islet hyperplasia become evident. A period of islet hyperplasia is followed by the emergence of a few β-cell tumors that kill the mice by overproducing insulin and thereby inducing acute hypoglycemia. The characteristics of these two lineages are summarized in

Table 1, and an analysis of T-antigen expression in the embryonic pancreas is presented in Figure 2.

A second and clearly distinct class of transgenic mice was also produced. Mice in these lines did not express the insulin/T antigen genes during embryogenesis nor as neonates. Rather, there was a delayed onset of transgene expression to adulthood, as is documented in Figure 1 by immunostaining for both T antigen and p53. Beginning at about 10–12 weeks, scattered β cells expressing T antigen could be detected in the islets (Adams et al. 1987; Efrat et al. 1987). Over time, the number of T-antigen-positive β cells increases until a majority (but not all) evidence transgene expression. The β cells were the only site of synthesis that could be detected, and again expression of the large T oncoprotein eventually elicited β-cell proliferation, islet hyperplasia, and the formation of solid tumors in the pancreas. The characteristics of two delayed onset lines are summarized in Table 1 for the purposes of this discussion.

The delayed onset phenotype has been observed in about one-half of the lines of insulin/T antigen transgenic mice and is stable upon continuous backcrossing to inbred mice. We attribute this pattern of expression to the chromosomal position into which the insulin gene regulatory region has become integrated. Regardless of the molecular mechanism underlying this

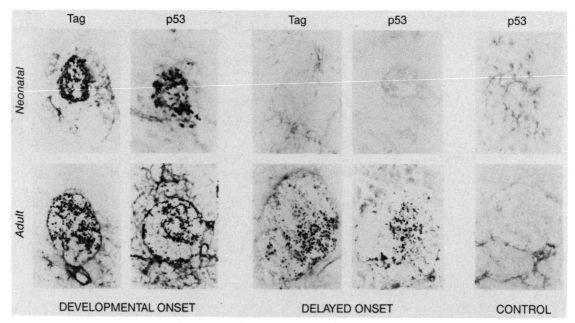

Figure 1. Two heritable patterns of transgene expression. Neonatal and young adult mice from two transgenic lineages, RIP1-Tag2 and RIP1-Tag4, were analyzed for expression of the product of the hybrid insulin/T antigen gene. T-antigen protein was detected by immunostaining pancreatic tissue sections with rabbit polyclonal antisera raised against immunoaffinity-purified SV40 large T protein, and the association was visualized by a horseradish-peroxidase (HRP)-conjugated secondary antibody specific for rabbit IgG following its reaction with diaminobenzidine (DAB), nickel sulfate, and hydrogen peroxide. Expression of authentic large T protein was confirmed by immunostaining for the mouse p53 protein, which cannot be detected in neonatal or adult controls islets (*right*). The binding of large T stabilizes p53 and renders it visible by immunostaining as is shown in neonatal islets of the RIP1-Tag2 mice and in adult islets (shown) and tumors (not shown) of both RIP1-Tag2 and RIP1-Tag4 mice. Similar patterns characterize RIR-Tag2 mice and RIP1-Tag3 mice (not shown) that thereby divide the lineages into those showing either developmental onset (*left*) or delayed onset (*middle*) (into adulthood) of expression of the insulin/T-antigen transgenes. (Data from Efrat et al. 1987.)

Table 1. Stable Tolerant and Nontolerant Phenotypes among RIP-Tag Transgenic Lineages

Lineage	Pattern of self-antigen expression	Humoral response to purified T antigen	Response to T antigen in β cells
RIP1-Tag2	developmental onset	nonresponsive	none
RIR-Tag2	developmental onset	nonresponsive	none
RIP1-Tag3	delayed onset	fully responsive	autoimmunity
RIP1-Tag4	delayed onset	fully responsive	autoimmunity

phenotype, the stability of the delayed onset phenotype has allowed us to examine the immunological consequences of this unusual temporal synthesis of a new self-antigen in the β cells and to compare them with those of transgenic mice that express the same protein during late embryogenesis and throughout postnatal life.

Stable Tolerance or Nontolerance among the RIP-Tag Lineages

One measure of tolerance toward a protein is the humoral response after immunization with that protein in a mixture with an adjuvant that stimulates the immune system. In this case, nonresponsiveness compared with controls is taken to be a condition of tolerance (Dresser and Mitchison 1968; Weigle 1973; Howard and Mitchison 1975). Self-tolerance to T antigen in the transgenic lineages was initially assessed by taking immunopurified large T protein and presenting it to both control and transgenic mice in a standard immunization regimen (Adams et al. 1987). The development of antibodies specific for large T was assessed by immunoprecipitation with extracts of radiolabeled COS cells, which is a monkey cell line expressing high levels of T antigen (Gluzman 1981). The immunoprecipitates

were analyzed on SDS-protein gels. The induction of immunoprecipitating antibodies for T antigen confirmed that the protein was a potent immunogen in normal control mice. Both a primary response and an amplified secondary response could be visualized by the extent of protein immunoprecipitated, which in the secondary response was comparable with that brought down by a monoclonal antibody specific for large T. An example of this analysis is presented in Figure 3. Among transgenic mice analyzed from the different lineages, a clear pattern emerged. Mice from several lines showed a response to immunization with T antigen that was indistinguishable from the control mice, which do not carry the genetic information for the T protein. By this criterion, they were nontolerant to T antigen. In contrast, mice from another lineage (RIP1-Tag2) showed a dramatically reduced responsiveness to T antigen in that little or no large T protein was immunoprecipitated by the immunoglobulins in either primary or secondary bleeds (Fig. 3). Therefore, these mice were judged to be nonresponsive to large T and thus potentially self-tolerant to the protein whose genetic information they carry.

The alternative responsive and nonresponsive phenotypes have consistently segregated with the integrated transgenes upon their transmission to progeny as

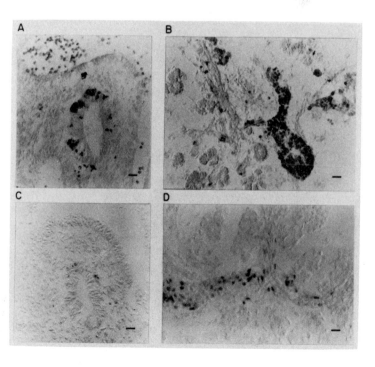

Figure 2. Differences in the levels of transgene expression during pancreatic development. Embryos from the two developmental onset lineages were analyzed for expression of T antigen. The panels illustrate consistent differences in the amount of T antigen as visualized by simultaneous immunostaining, again using an HRP/DAB histochemical reaction as described in Figure 1. (*Top*) Pancreatic sections of RIP1-Tag2 embryos at embryonic day e10 (*A*) and day e17 (*B*). (*Bottom*) RIR-Tag2 embryos at e10 (*C*) and e17 (*D*). In each case, the e10 sections are taken through the pancreatic diverticulum off the gut, and the e17 sections illustrate an islet budding away from a duct. (Reprinted, with permission, from Alpert et al. 1988.)

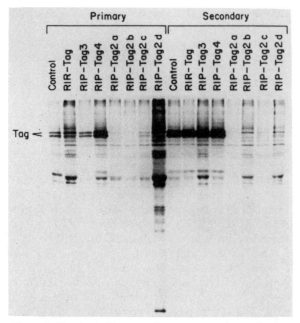

Figure 3. Two heritable types of response upon immunization with T antigen. Immunopurified large T protein was used to immunize four control mice and four mice each from several of the insulin/T antigen transgenic lineages in a standard adjuvant regimen. Both primary and secondary responses were analyzed by using serum samples to immunoprecipitate the SV40 large T antigen being synthesized in radiolabeled COS cells that express the SV40 viral genome. The immunoprecipitates were analyzed on SDS protein gels. An example is shown for one each of the control and the three delayed onset lineages, RIP-Tag3, -Tag4, and RIR-Tag1. All show a primary and an increased secondary response against large T that migrates as a dimer following immunoprecipitation from COS cells. The responses of all four mice from the developmental onset lineage RIP1-Tag2 are shown to document their nonresponsiveness relative to controls and the delayed onset transgenics. (Reprinted, with permission, from Adams et al. 1987.)

mice from a given line have all been either reproducibly tolerant or reproducibly nontolerant to T antigen using this immunization/immunoprecipitation assay. Remarkably, these two distinctive immunological characteristics correlate with the two classes of transgene expression. Mice from the RIP1-Tag2 line that expressed T antigen during embryogenesis were immunologically nonresponsive as adults, whereas mice from the RIP1-Tag3 and RIP1-Tag4 lines showing delayed onset of β-cell-specific expression of T antigen were fully responsive to the purified protein (Table 1). Thus, among a series of independent lines of transgenic mice, two genetically stable immunological phenotypes were produced toward a self-protein that was known, well-characterized, and available in purified form as were the specific immunological reagents to detect it. These characteristics, in conjunction with the knowledge of the temporal and spatial expression patterns of T-antigen expression, present an opportunity for detailed studies on the requirements for the establishment of tolerance and the qualities and the consequences of nontolerance to a self-antigen. Both issues have proved amenable to study, and the current

status of our investigations into each is presented below.

Consequences of Nonself Recognition

Transgenic mice in the delayed onset class are fully responsive upon presentation of exogenous large T protein. This raises the question of whether they are responding to the same protein being synthesized in their pancreatic β cells. A screen of random serum samples revealed that a subset of the delayed onset mice had circulating autoantibodies that were capable of selectively immunoprecipitating large T antigen (Adams et al. 1987). Autoantibodies were never seen in the tolerant lines. Thus, nontolerance and delayed onset of T-antigen expression resulted in sporadic humoral autoimmunity. More extensive sampling allowed statistical analysis of the appearance of T antigen autoantibodies. Every nontolerant line had an appreciable incidence of autoantibodies, which was 65% in randomly bred and sampled RIP1-Tag3 mice and 35% among RIP1-Tag4 mice. The fact that nontolerant did not obligate autoantibodies suggested that additional factors to the delayed onset of T-antigen expression might be involved in the induction of the autoimmune reaction.

To dissect further the development of the humoral autoimmune response against T antigen, a temporal study was conducted over the lifetimes of a number of members of the RIP1-Tag3 lineage. We exploited the ability to collect serum samples and thereby noninvasively monitor the development of circulating autoantibodies against the large T protein. The study was broadened to encompass another possible factor in the variable incidences of autoimmunity, namely, genetic differences in general and specific differences in the MHC haplotype in particular. Many diseases of apparent autoimmune nature are associated with and presumably influenced by specific haplotypes of the MHC complex (Todd et al. 1987; Wraith et al. 1989). Correlations of this type could be presumed to reflect a differential ability of allelic MHC molecules to present peptides of the autoantigens that are inducing the immune response. In this regard, it is significant that the original founders for the insulin/T antigen lineages developed from F_2 embryos derived from C57BL/6J and DBA/2J inbred mice, which carry the $H-2^b$ and $H-2^d$ MHC complexes, respectively. Thus, each founder was a mixture of these two genotypes. The transgenic lines were initially established by backcrossing to C57BL/6J and also by intercrossing to produce homozygotes for the transgene. Each line therefore contained a mixture of two genotypes and potentially of the two MHC haplotypes, at least in the early generations, which motivated an evaluation of possible genetic influences on the incidence of autoimmunity.

A time course of autoantibody production was conducted on RIP1-Tag3 mice that were derived from a transgenic male parent that had been haplotyped as homozygous for the $H-2^b$ MHC and then mated with inbred females. A preliminary screen of four different backcrosses to C57BL/6, DBA/2, C3HeB, and B10.BR showed variable incidences and titers of anti-large T antibodies at 5–5.5 months of age, with the two parental backgrounds C57BL/6 and DBA/2 being the most diverse in both parameters (not shown). Therefore, backcross progeny of RIP1-Tag3 (H-2^b/H-2^b) to either C57BL/6 (H-2^b) or DBA/2 (H-2^d) were routinely examined for serum autoantibodies beginning at 3 months and continuing throughout their lives (Fig. 4). It is evident that there are genetic differences in the responses seen in the two cases. Mice homozygous for the H-2^b MHC show a low incidence and a low titer of autoantibodies. In marked contrast, mice carrying both H-2^d and H-2^b showed a 100% incidence of autoantibodies. The serum titers were substantially higher, reaching levels comparable with those induced by immunization of mice with purified large T protein. In both cases, spontaneous autoantibodies were first apparent beginning at 4 months of age, which is 4–6 weeks after the synthesis of T antigen in the β cells ensues. From this, we infer that the appearance of T antigen can result in the induction of autoantibodies

and that there is a genetic component to the character of that response.

The implication from the time course of a genetic control of autoimmunity raised the prospect that the distinctive MHC alleles were a major factor, given their association with various autoimmune diseases and the demonstrated ability of both class I and II molecules to present antigens to the immune system. This possibility has begun to be addressed from several perspectives. To assess the specific contribution of MHC alleles, RIP1-Tag3 males were backcrossed to C57BL/10 mice and to B10.D2 mice. C57BL/6 and C57BL/10 are closely related, and B10.D2 is congenic with C57BL/10 except for the presence of the H-2^d MHC complex. In preliminary results from this analysis, RIP1-Tag3 backcrosses to C57BL/10 were found to be indistinguishable from C57BL/6 with regard to incidence and titer, whereas those to B10.D2 were similar to DBA/2. A second experiment outcrossed the H-2^b/H-2^b transgenics to B6D2 mice, which are F$_1$ hybrids of C57BL/6 and DBA/2. These progeny were analyzed both for autoantibodies and MHC haplotype, and again the incidence of autoimmunity was substantially higher in the

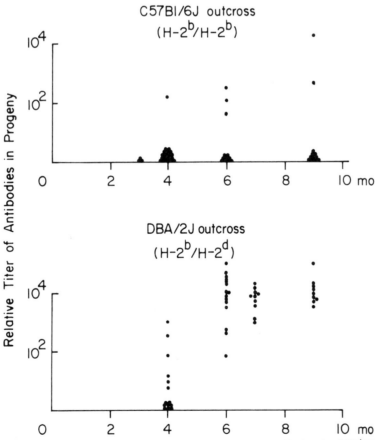

Figure 4. Time course of T-antigen autoantibodies in two MHC backgrounds. RIP1-Tag3 males (H-2^b/H-2^b) were mated with C57BL/6J (H-2^b) or DBA/2J (H-2^d) females, and their transgenic progeny followed over the course of their lives for the development of serum autoantibodies against T antigen. Each dot represents the analysis of serum taken from one individual at the timepoint indicated on the ordinate. The titer of anti-T-antigen antibodies is given on the axis as determined using a quantitative solid-phase RIA (J. Skowronski et al., in prep.). Some individuals did not live to reach the later timepoints.

mice carrying an H-2^d allele (Fig. 5). These analyses are consistent with the interpretation that the H-2^d allele confers a strong predisposition for development of humoral autoimmunity, whereas H-2^b alone is considerably less effective in inducing the response. Further support for the conclusion that allelic differences in the MHC influence the autoimmunity comes from crosses to mice carrying H-2^k, in which transgenic progeny show an intermediate incidence and intensity of the humoral response to T antigen. It should be mentioned that the transgenic mice of every H-2 type evidence similar patterns of expression of T antigen in that onset occurs beginning at 10–12 weeks, and by 20 weeks virtually every one of the pancreatic islets contains β cells synthesizing T antigen.

The cellular response toward the β cells expressing T antigen has initially been addressed by histological analyses of tissue sections. Evaluation of pancreases from mice in the RIP1-Tag3 lineage revealed lymphocyte infiltration of the pancreatic islets in virtually every mouse, as indicated by staining with H&E. A series of

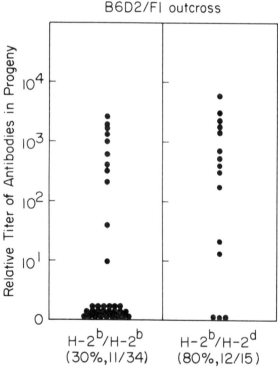

Figure 5. Relation of autoantibody response to segregating MHC haplotypes. RIP1-Tag3 males were outcrossed to B6D2F$_1$ females, and their progeny were analyzed for autoantibodies at 6 months and subsequently typed for MHC haplotype using restriction-fragment-length polymorphism analysis for the Aβ chain of the class II I-A gene as described elsewhere (J. Skowronski et al., in prep.). Note that, whereas H-2^d MHC confers the high-frequency incidence, other alleles in the DBA background appear to influence the titer of antibodies that develop in the H-2^b/H-2^b MHC background. (Compare this 6-month timepoint of H-2^b/H-2^b mice with that in Fig. 4).

monoclonal antibodies that recognize specific lymphocyte subsets was used to identify the cells infiltrating the islets as either CD8$^+$ cytotoxic T cells, CD4$^+$ T helper cells, B cells, or macrophages, by virtue of their expression of the Lyt-2, L3T4, B220, and Mac-1 determinants, respectively. Immunostaining of pancreatic sections showed that all four classes of leukocytes could be detected in the infiltrated islets. In contrast, nontransgenic control mice showed only rare macrophages associated with the periphery of the islets. The extent of infiltration varied among the islets of an affected individual, with some islets being highly infiltrated whereas others were unaffected. This heterogeneity of infiltration is similar to that observed in a number of cases of natural autoimmunity against the pancreatic β cells such as in human type-1 diabetes (Gepts and Lecompte 1988) and in the diabetes seen in the BB rat and the nonobese diabetic (NOD) mouse (Fujita et al. 1982; Kanazawa et al. 1984; Logothetopoulos et al. 1984; Dean et al. 1985). When examined at 5 months of age, every RIP1-Tag3 mouse evidenced cellular infiltration. An example of this analysis is presented in Figure 6. What is clear is that within 2 months of the delayed onset of T-antigen expression in the pancreatic β cells of RIP1-Tag3 mice, every mouse had developed leukocyte infiltration of the pancreatic islets consisting of B and T cells and macrophages. This infiltration is not evident in mice from the same line at 3 months of age when expression of T antigen is just ensuing.

Regarding the cellular response to T antigen, it is remarkable that, whereas every islet expresses T antigen by 4–5 months, in an H-2^b/H-2^b background only 30% of the mice develop autoantibodies during their lifetimes despite the fact that all eventually succumb to pancreatic β-cell tumors. This dichotomy has motivated further comparison of RIP1-Tag3 mice derived from backcrosses to low-responder (C57BL/10) and high-responder (B10.D2) MHC backgrounds. The transgenic progeny derived from these crosses were analyzed for lymphocyte infiltration initially at 5 months as part of a time course of the cellular response. In all four cases, leukocyte infiltration of the islets could be detected. There was variation among the islets of an individual regarding the extent of infiltration as was discussed above. However, there was no obvious difference between the four cases regarding the number of infiltrated islets nor the types of leukocytes that were infiltrating. The only variation was that in the autoantibody-positive, high-responder H-2^d background there appeared to be substantially more B cells within the islets. The numbers of CD4$^+$ and CD8$^+$ T cells and macrophages were similar in antibody-positive and -negative mice of either low- or high-responder MHC haplotype (not shown). These results are provocative because they imply that the immune system in all cases recognizes and is attracted to the location of T-antigen synthesis but that attraction does not necessarily lead to activation of the immune response, as measured by the appearance of circulating autoantibodies to T antigen.

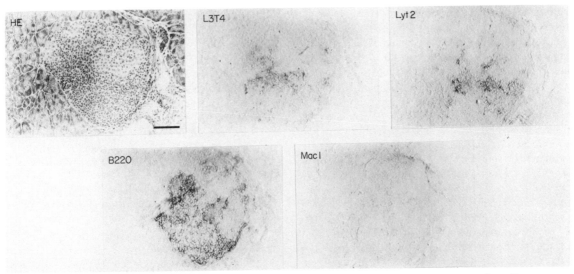

Figure 6. Leukocyte infiltration of islets in transgenic mice nontolerant for T antigen. RIP1-Tag3 (H-2^b/H-2^b) males were outcrossed to B10.D2 (H-2^d/H-2^d) females, and their transgenic progeny were analyzed for leukocyte infiltration at various timepoints. The representative example shown here is of an autoantibody-positive transgenic mouse at 5 months of age. The panels show histochemical staining with H&E and immunostaining with antibodies that recognize the following determinants: L3T4 on CD4$^+$ T-helper cells; Lyt-2 on CD8$^+$ cytotoxic T cells, B220 on B cells, and Mac-1 on macrophages. The bar represents 100 μm.

Characteristics of the Tolerance Induced by Developmental Expression

Developmental onset of expression and its continuation throughout life in the pancreatic β cells of RIP-Tag2 mice leads to a nonresponsive condition. This conclusion was initially based on assays in which the mice were immunized with purified large T in adjuvant and the response assessed by immunoprecipitation of extracts from radiolabeled COS cells with serum collected before and after primary and secondary immunizations, as was described above. These assays did not provide information about the general responsiveness of mice in the various lineages nor regarding possible differences in the extent of their nonresponsiveness. To address both of these issues, a semiquantitative solid-phase RIA was established. Equal quantities of large T protein and the *E. coli* protein β-Gal were used to immunize both control and transgenic mice in a standard regimen of CFA followed by IFA. Serum from prebleeds and bleeds taken after the primary and secondary immunizations were serially diluted and assayed for binding to either large T or β-Gal proteins immobilized on a solid phase. The binding reaction was visualized with an iodinated secondary antibody reactive with IgG and quantitated in a gamma counter. The use in parallel of antibodies specific for large T and for β-Gal allowed relative titers to be established from the half-maximum of the dilution curves. There was no cross-reactivity between T-antigen and β-Gal as assessed by their separate immunization and evaluation with the two control antibodies (J. Skowronski et al., in prep.).

Table 2. Characteristic Nonresponsiveness to Large T Antigen

| Mouse lineage | T-antigen expression | | | | Immunological responsiveness to T antigen | |
	onset	relative levels[a]	stabilization of p53[a]	β-cell tumors	by immunization with Tag[b]	by lymphocyte infiltration of islets[c]
C57BL/6J	—	—	—	—	1	none
RIP1-Tag3	10–12 weeks	(−)→ + +	(−)→ + +	30–60 weeks	1	extensive
RIP1-Tag2	e10	+ + +	+ + +	10–14 weeks	<10^{-3}	none
RIR-Tag2	e10	+ +	+ +	16–24 weeks	10^{-1}–10^{-2}	none
RIR3-Tag2	n.d.	+	+	none (hyperplasia)	1/2	none

[a] Relative levels of T antigen were determined by immunostaining adjacent sections with antibodies to SV40 large T and mouse p53 that were visualized with HRP-conjugated secondary antibodies upon reaction with DAB. Comparisons between the lines were established following DAB reactions performed in parallel on several occasions. n.d. indicates not determined.

[b] Sera collected after immunization with purified large T protein in CFA/IFA were titered for antibodies to large T by a solid-phase RIA. The titers are given relative to C57BL/6J control mice, which develop an antibody titer of ~5 × 10^4/ml. All mice responded with similar titers of anti-β-Gal antibodies when coimmunized with purified *E. coli* β-Gal as part of the same regimen.

[c] Leukocyte infiltration assessed by H&E staining of pancreatic tissue sections fixed with paraformaldehyde.

Groups of four individuals from control mice (B6D2) and from the transgenic lineages were analyzed for their responsiveness to T antigen and β-Gal. The results are summarized in Table 2. All of the mice responded similarly to β-Gal, which indicates that the transgenic mice are not generally immunodeficient. Comparison of the responses to T antigen confirmed the previous observation that RIP1-Tag2 mice are nonresponsive. The control nontransgenic mice mounted a discernible primary and a strong secondary response to T antigen. In contrast, RIP1-Tag2 mice did not evidence a primary response, and the second response was either undetectable or barely detectable in this assay, giving a relative titer of $< 10^{-3}$ when compared with those of the controls. The analysis of mice in the RIR-Tag2 lineage also demonstrated nonresponsiveness but to a lesser extent. In these mice, a primary response was again not evident, and the secondary response was reduced to 10^{-1} to 10^{-2} of that of the control mice. The nonresponsiveness upon immunization was reproducible and judged to be significant since mice in this line are tolerant by the criteria that they do not spontaneously develop either autoantibodies against T-antigen or leukocyte infiltration of the pancreatic islets.

There is a clear correlation between onset of T-antigen expression during embryogenesis and the subsequent nonresponsiveness of the mice as adults. Thus, neither RIP1-Tag3 mice nor RIP1-Tag4 mice express T antigen during development, and each are nontolerant and fully responsive. Both RIP1-Tag2 and RIR-Tag2 mice express T antigen beginning at embryonic day 10 (Fig. 2) and continue to do so throughout their lives. The expression of large T during the primary development of the immune system therefore appears to be a necessary condition for the establishment of self-tolerance to this protein when it is expressed as an antigen in the pancreatic β cells.

A second characteristic of the establishment of self-tolerance indicated in these transgenic experiments is a relationship between the levels of expression of the self-antigen and the subsequent degree of immunological nonresponsiveness toward that antigen. Although both RIP1-Tag2 and RIR-Tag2 mice begin to express T antigen in the pancreas and the nervous system at embryonic day 10, there are consistent differences in the levels of T antigen throughout embryogenesis and subsequent postnatal life. Three criteria support the conclusion of quantitative differences in T-antigen expression: (1) Immunostaining for large T itself with both rabbit polyclonal and mouse monoclonal antibodies shows reproducible differences in the intensity of immunoreactivity; (2) immunostaining for the cellular protein p53, which can only be seen as a stable complex with large T, shows similar differences in immunoreactivity between the two lines; and (3) mice in the RIP1-Tag2 line develop tumors and die between 12 and 16 weeks of age, whereas in RIR-Tag2 mice this occurs between 16 and 24 weeks of age. Thus, we conclude that there are significant differences in the amounts of T antigen produced in the two lineages. Moreover, these differences influence the degree of nonresponsiveness that is established, giving a relative responsiveness of $< 10^{-3}$ in RIP1-Tag2 mice and 10^{-1} to 10^{-2} in RIR-Tag2 (Table 2).

The evidence for quantitative effects on nonresponsiveness toward self-antigens is further supported by analysis of a third line RIR3-Tag2. Mice in this line express even lower levels of both T antigen and p53 as assessed by immunostaining of young adults (S. Efrat and D. Hanahan, unpubl.). Significantly, these mice do not develop solid tumors although β-cell hyperplasia can arise in older mice. All three criteria indicate that T antigen is expressed but at very low levels. When mice in this line were analyzed after immunization with T antigen and β-Gal, they were found to be no more than two-times less responsive than controls. Yet, these mice do not develop spontaneous lymphocyte infiltration of the islets. Thus, we suspect that the reduced humoral response upon immunization is significant. However, it is also possible that the levels of T antigen are simply too low to be effectively presented for induction of either self-tolerance or autoimmune responses to it. These observations clearly motivate us to extend the tolerance assays into the T-cell compartment.

A final aspect of self-tolerance that has been explored is the possibility that specific haplotypes of the MHC influence the self-learning process. This possibility was suggested by the effects that MHC haplotypes have on the incidence and intensity of the autoimmunity that develops in the delayed onset class of transgenic mice. One might suppose that whichever MHC molecule was presenting T-antigen peptides during the induction of autoimmunity would also be similarly effective in the establishment of self-tolerance in those circumstances where T antigen was present during immunological development. This possibility was addressed in mice from the RIR-Tag2 lineage. These mice show a reduced but measurable response, and therefore we

Table 3. Assessing MHC Influences on Tolerance in RIR-Tag2 Mice

Genetic background (F × M)	MHC haplotype of progeny	Responsiveness to T antigen[a]	Responsiveness to β-Gal[a]
C57BL/10J × C57BL/10J	H-2^b/H-2^b	1	1
C57BL/10J × RIR-Tag2	H-2^b/H-2^b	10^{-2}–10^{-3}	1
B10.D2 × RIR-Tag2	H-2^b/H-2^d	10^{-2}–10^{-3}	1
B10.Br × RIR-Tag2	H-2^b/H-2^k	10^{-2}–10^{-3}	1

[a] Responsiveness is given relative to nontransgenic control mice (C57BL/10J). In each case, 10 μg of T antigen plus 10 μg of β-Gal were used to immunize mice in a standard Freund's regimen. The titers of antibodies in the secondary response of the controls was about 5×10^4 for Tag and 1×10^5 for β-Gal.

reasoned that any changes in the degree of nonresponsiveness conferred by different MHC alleles could be detected. RIR-Tag2 mice in an H-2^b/H-2^b background were crossed to C57BL/10, B10.D2, and B10.BR mice, which carry the b, d, and k haplotypes, respectively. The transgenic progeny of these matings were immunized and analyzed for their responsiveness to T antigen. No significant differences in the extent of nonresponsiveness were detected in the three MHC backgrounds (Table 3) from which we conclude that there is no obvious effect of these alleles on the tolerance process.

DISCUSSION

The lines of transgenic mice carrying hybrid insulin/T-antigen genes constitute an attractive model with which to explore interactions of the antigens expressed in rare cell types with the immune system. The two genetically stable patterns of transgene expression have revealed a fortuitous if somewhat mysterious phenomenon. Of particular interest is the delayed onset of β-cell-specific expression into adulthood, a condition that has been observed in about one-half of the independent lines of transgenic mice carrying hybrid insulin genes. The stability of the phenotype after continuous backcrossing to various strains of inbred mice suggests that the delayed onset is dictated by chromosomal position. The question then arises as to whether this is a special feature of the insulin gene regulatory region, the pancreatic β cell, or both. In this regard, it is of note that all four of the transgenic lines produced with a glucagon promoter/T-antigen gene express T antigen during embryogenesis (Efrat et al. 1989). This result suggests that neither the T-antigen gene nor bacterial plasmid sequences are responsible for the delayed onset since both of these sequences are in common with the hybrid insulin genes. Yet, of the 11 insulin/T-antigen lines generated, 6 evidenced the delayed onset phenotype. Moreover, several other hybrid insulin genes appear to be showing either delayed onset or heterogeneous expression phenotypes (Edwards et al. 1989; and our unpublished observations). Thus, one might suspect that either the β cell and/or insulin gene regulatory elements are particularly sensitive to the chromosomal location into which a β-cell-specific gene has been integrated. We have recently studied the transgene integration sites in four of these lineages using plasmid rescue into *E. coli* strains that carry mutations in methylated cytosine-dependent restriction activities. The results clearly indicate that the delayed onset integrations are much more highly modified (methylated) than those showing developmental onset, in a manner that could be presumed to influence their accessibility to transcription (S. Grant et al., in prep.). One could speculate that normal cellular genes might also be integrated into chromosomal locations that are subject to this type of epigenetic control that might render their expression irregular in cell types such as the β cell. The delayed onset or heterogeneous expression of these genes may be functionally or immunologically significant in disease states of the β cell such as in diabetes.

Whatever the explanation for the epigenetic control of transgene expression, the different patterns of expression have proven to be extremely valuable in that we have had the opportunity to compare the immunological consequences of expressing the same antigen either during embryogenesis and subsequent life or beginning only during adulthood. Moreover, the antigen, the large T protein of SV40, is well-characterized, available in purified form, and readily detectable using either polyclonal or monoclonal antibodies. The two temporal patterns of expression produce two consistent immunological responses. Onset during embryogenesis confers nonresponsiveness toward large T protein, as assessed both by immunization with purified protein and by the lack of autoimmune phenomena. In contrast, delayed onset results in nonself recognition of T antigen as demonstrated by strong responsiveness toward exogenous protein and the frequent induction of an autoimmune response against what is a "self-protein" and the cells that synthesize it. These transgenic mice are thereby allowing investigations into the mechanisms of alternative self-tolerance and autoimmunity for a β-cell antigen.

Principles of Self Recognition

A comparison of the developmental onset and delayed onset lines of transgenic mice has revealed that the presence of the self-antigen during the primary development of the immune system is necessary to establish a condition of nonresponsiveness or self-tolerance toward T antigen expressed in the pancreatic β cells. This result supports the classical concept of a temporal window of self-education during which a developing immune system comes to recognize and become nonresponsive toward components of its host organism (Burnet 1959). Among the transgenic lines with developmental onset, different levels of T antigen are apparent by several criteria. These levels seem to correlate with the subsequent degree of nonresponsiveness as assessed by the humoral response upon immunization with purified large T protein. Yet, all the developmental onset mice are similarly tolerant by the criterion that none evidence spontaneous autoimmune responses against the endogenous protein or the β cells that synthesize it. It is clear that the T-cell response to exogenous T antigen should now be examined to ascertain the characteristics of both helper and cytotoxic T cells when presented with the protein.

The set of developmental onset lines, with their distinctive levels of expression, should prove valuable in future investigations into the cellular mechanisms underlying the nonresponsive condition. Other studies in transgenic mice and in mice with polymorphic self-antigens have revealed that both clonal deletion and functional inactivation of self-reactive lymphocytes are mechanisms by which selective nonresponsiveness is achieved (Kappler et al. 1987, 1988; Goodnow et al.

1988; Kisielow et al. 1988a,b; Sha et al. 1988a,b; Teh et al. 1988; Blackman et al. 1989; Matzinger and Guerder 1989; Nemazee and Burki 1989; Scott et al. 1989). Most of these studies have used antigens that are widely dispersed and presumably accessible to the thymus and fetal liver/bone marrow in which the primary development of the immune system takes place. However, it is important to ask what happens in the case of antigens expressed in rare cell types? It is not clear how the information about the components of rare cells is communicated to the developing immune system. One possibility is that there is a mechanism for transporting information back to the major lymphoid organs, perhaps by macrophages or T cells that are specially instructed during the self-learning period. Alternatively, there may be mechanisms for establishing and maintaining self-tolerance in the periphery. The recent experiments of Miller and his colleagues using a polymorphic H-2 antigen expressed in the β cells of transgenic mice have provided evidence for a peripheral tolerance mechanism (Morahan et al. 1989; Miller et al., this volume). It will be of interest to compare their results with MHC antigens with those obtained with non-MHC antigens such as T antigen, especially considering the likelihood that antigen presentation by the MHC is involved in the establishment of self-tolerance. In this regard, it is notable that our results to date have not revealed variations among distinct MHC alleles in the degree of nonresponsiveness that is established by developmental expression in contrast with the apparent MHC influences on the incidence and intensity of humoral autoimmunity.

One could propose that the MHC molecules involved in antigen presentation during self-learning are different from those that act in the induction of an autoimmune response. Thus, one type of MHC molecule could be involved in the establishment of self-tolerance to T antigen in the developmental onset mice, whereas a different MHC gene mediates the induction of autoimmunity in the delayed onset RIP-Tag mice. Perhaps the *attraction* of lymphocytes to the islets in the nontolerant mice involves the same MHC gene that acts in the establishment of tolerance (e.g., a class I gene), whereas the *activation* of the autoimmune response involves a distinct gene (e.g., a class II gene) that shows differential ability to present T antigen among its alleles.

A Model of Autoimmunity

The failure to express T antigen during embryogenesis has two important and interrelated consequences. The first is that the mice do not come to recognize this self-antigen as such, despite the fact that its gene is a stable component of the germ line and hence is genetically self. This result supports the proposition that self-antigen expression during immunological development is important for subsequent self-tolerance and would seem to argue against the notion that every protein coding region is somehow transiently expressed in the developing thymus so as to effect tolerance. The second consequence of delayed onset of β-cell-specific expression is autoimmunity, which is manifested at both the cellular and humoral levels. The characteristics of the autoimmune process are intriguing and have the prospect of being a model for other cases of autoimmunity in which the autoantigens are presently unknown or inaccessible.

Humoral autoimmunity is detected beginning at least 4–6 weeks after the synthesis of large T is initiated in the β cells. Both the incidence and the titer of circulating autoantibodies appear to be influenced by the MHC haplotype. Significant correlations of MHC haplotype with several autoimmune diseases have been noted previously (Todd et al. 1987; Wraith et al. 1989; McDevitt et al., this volume), and this model appears to share that property, which supports its significance and generality. It is now well-accepted that differential autoantigen presentation by MHC molecules is likely to underlie the observed correlations between autoimmunity and MHC haplotype. SV40 T antigen elicits distinguishable cytotoxic T-cell responses among mice of different MHC haplotypes that were either immunized with cells expressing large T antigen or infected with SV40 virus. However, the MHC correlation in the cytotoxic assays is opposite to that observed for the humoral response in this model. Here, we see H-2^d conferring a 100% incidence of humoral autoimmunity and a titer of autoantibodies approaching that achieved by immunization of control mice with purified large T antigen. In contrast, H-2^b confers an incomplete incidence (30%) and lower titers of autoantibodies. These associations are opposite of those observed in cytotoxic T-cell assays performed either in vitro or via tumor transplantation, where H-2^b is a high-responder and H-2^d is a low-responder haplotype (Gooding 1979; Knowles et al. 1979; Pan et al. 1987).

The dichotomy between the autoimmune response and the tumor transplantation response to T antigen suggests that the MHC genes involved in the autoimmune reaction against the β cells are different from those that participate in the response against large T as a tumor transplantation antigen. In this regard, it is of note that the autoimmunity in these mice does not confer tumor immunity. The mice eventually succumb to the effects of β-cell tumors and not insulin-dependent diabetes. The solid tumors in general appear relatively devoid of lymphocyte infiltration, in contrast with the islets that not only show significant leukocyte infiltration but also evidence of varying degrees of β cell destruction (Adams et al. 1987; C. Jolicoeur, unpubl.). Thus, it appears that the β-cell tumors manage to avoid the attentions of the immune system, perhaps by attenuating class I MHC expression or by modulating its presentation of the large T autoantigen. It has been shown previously that normal β cells express class I MHC (Baekkeskov et al. 1981; Allison et al. 1988) and the β-cell tumors continue to express class I molecules as assessed by immunoprecipitation (S. Baekkeskov, pers. comm.). Therefore, one might suggest that differences in antigen presentation are responsible for the relative invisibility of the tumors.

The mechanism of immunological recognition and response to T antigen following its delayed appearance in the β cells of an adult mouse is proving to have unexpected complexity. Contrary to our simplest expectations, lymphocyte infiltration was observed in all cases beginning 4–6 weeks after synthesis of T antigen ensued. Thus, regardless of the MHC haplotype of the RIP1-Tag3 transgenic mice, lymphocytes quickly recognized the presence of something unusual in the pancreatic islets and therefore began to infiltrate them. Four classes of leukocytes were evident in both high-responder ($H-2^d/H-2^b$) and low-responder ($H-2^b/H-2^b$) backgrounds: $CD4^+$, $CD8^+$, $B220^+$, and $Mac-1^+$ cells, representing helper and cytotoxic T cells, B cells, and macrophages, respectively. Yet, despite the fact that immunological recognition of T-antigen synthesis in the β cells occurs in every mouse, activation of the humoral immune response is not an obligatory consequence of infiltration. Moreover, the MHC haplotype appears to influence activation of the humoral autoimmunity, rather than recognition of the nonself-antigen per se. It is particularly notable that in low-responder $H-2^b$ mice, lymphocytes can infiltrate and persist in the islets throughout the lives of these individuals and yet not become activated to produce antibodies. This is especially remarkable when one again recalls that these mice develop β-cell tumors as a consequence of T antigen synthesis, and even tumorigenesis does not activate humoral autoimmunity against T antigen.

It will now be of interest to compare the infiltrating leukocytes in both low- and high-responder MHC backgrounds using reagents that identify functionally activated cells to determine whether the infiltrating T cells and macrophages only become activated in certain cases, as are the B cells, and to ascertain whether that activation is influenced by particular MHC haplotypes. This model for the recognition of a nontolerant self-antigen by the immune system appears to have revealed a significant property, namely that the *attraction* of the immune system is functionally separable from its *activation*. In this regard, it will be important to subdivide the MHC complex using recombinants between $H-2^d$ and $H-2^b$ in order to identify the MHC gene responsible for activation of the immune response. Separation of attraction and activation has also been inferred from genetic studies of the NOD mouse. Certain genetic outcrosses evidenced lymphocyte accumulation around the islets (attraction) but not destructive autoimmunity, whereas in other backcrosses and in the homozygous NOD animals the immune response actively destroyed the β cells and thereby effected a diabetic condition (Prochazka et al. 1987). In this case, however, the autoantigen and its pattern of expression is unknown.

There are also indications that other variables may contribute to the induction of autoimmunity in the RIP-Tag transgenic mice. The case for factors in addition to MHC comes from the observation that every islet expresses the autoantigen and yet only a subset becomes infiltrated, and even then activation is neither immediate nor obligatory. Thus, one could infer that local differences among the 400 pancreatic islets may dictate their visibility to the immune system in both low and high responders. Among the possibilies are anatomical location within the pancreas and differences in the character of the islets, which do, for example, evidence both β-cell senescence and hyperplasia in a nonuniform manner in these mice (Teitelman et al. 1988). A second factor is implicated by the remarkably persistent failure to develop humoral autoimmunity in a majority of mice from the low responder ($H-2^b$) MHC background, which may belie significant differences in their immunological repertoire. For example, it is possible that a super antigen is inducing the clonal deletion of major classes of T-cell receptors during T-cell development. The absence of T cells bearing these receptors might be retarding effective activation of the autoimmune response when $H-2^b$ molecules present T antigen. In this regard, it is of note that a recent study has revealed that $H-2^b$ mice have very low levels of $CD4^+ V_\beta 17a^+$ cells when compared with other haplotypes (Blackman et al. 1989). This observation is consistent with the notion that differences in deletion or positive selection could be manifesting the infrequent autoimmunity toward T antigen in the $H-2^b$ background.

In summary, the interactions of T antigen with the immune system of transgenic mice present a model that is contributing to our understanding of the mechanisms by which immunological recognition of antigens expressed in rare cell types is achieved. The benefits of this system come from the existence of characteristic patterns of either developmental or delayed onset of expression among stable lineages of transgenic mice, the knowledge and accessibility of the self-antigen, and the implications that distinctive cellular interactions operate in the alternative induction of self-tolerance or autoimmunity.

ACKNOWLEDGMENTS

This research was funded by grants from the National Cancer Institute and the Juvenile Diabetes Foundation (D.H.) and by a grant from Monsanto Company to Cold Spring Harbor Laboratory. We thank Shimon Efrat for the RIR3-Tag2 transgenic mice and Leslie Spector for excellent preparation of the manuscript.

REFERENCES

Adams, T.E., S. Alpert, and D. Hanahan. 1987. Non-tolerance and autoantibodies to a transgenic self antigen expressed in pancreatic β cells. *Nature* **325:** 223.

Allison, J., I.L. Campbell, G. Morahan, T.E. Mandel, L.C. Harrison, and J.F.A.P. Miller. 1988. Diabetes in transgenic mice resulting from over-expression of class I histocompatibility molecules in pancreatic β cells. *Nature* **333:** 529.

Alpert, S., D. Hanahan, and G. Teitelman. 1988. Hybrid

insulin genes reveal a developmental lineage for pancreatic endocrine cells and imply a relationship with neurons. *Cell* **53:** 295.

Baekkeskov, S., T. Kanatsuna, L. Kareskog, D.A. Nielsen, P.A. Peterson, A.H. Rubenstein, D.F. Steiner, and A. Lernmark. 1981. Expression of major histocompatibility antigens on pancreatic islet cells. *Proc. Natl. Acad. Sci.* **78:** 6456.

Ball, R.K., J.L. Siegel, S. Quelhorst, G. Brandner, and D.G. Braun. 1984. Monoclonal antibodies against simian virus 40 nuclear large T tumor antigen: Epitope mapping, papovavirus cross-reactions and cell surface staining. *EMBO J.* **3:** 1485.

Blackman, M., P. Marrack, and J. Kappler. 1989. Influence of the major histocompatibility complex on positive thymic selection of $V_\beta 17a^+$ T cells. *Science* **244:** 214.

Bretscher, P. and M. Cohn. 1970. A theory of self-nonself discrimination. *Science* **159:** 1042.

Burnet, F.M. 1959. *The clonal selection theory of acquired immunity.* Cambridge University Press, England.

Chang, C., R.G. Martin, D.M. Livingston, S.W. Luborsky, C.P. Hu, and P.T. Mora. 1979. Relationship between T-antigen and tumor-specific transplantation antigen in simian virus 40 transformed cells. *J. Virol.* **29:** 69.

Dean, B.M., R. Walker, A.J. Bone, J.D. Baird, and A. Cooke. 1985. Pre-diabetes in the spontaneously diabetic BB/E rat: Lympholytic subpopulations in the pancreatic infiltrate and expression of rat MHC class II molecules in endocrine cells. *Diabetologia* **28:** 464.

Deppert, W. and G. Walter. 1982. Domains of simian virus 40 large T-antigen exposed on the cell surface. *Virology* **122:** 56.

Deppert, W., K. Hanke, and R. Henning. 1980. Simian virus 40 T-antigen related cell surface antigen: Serological demonstration on simian virus 40 transformed monolayer cells in situ. *J. Virol.* **35:** 505.

Dialynas, D.P., Z.S. Quan, K.A. Wall, A. Pierres, I. Quintans, M.R. Loken, and F.W. Fitch. 1983. Characterization of the murine T cell surface molecules, designated L3T4, identified by monoclonal antibody GK1.5: Similarity of L3T4 to the human Leu3/T4 molecule. *J. Immunol.* **131:** 2445.

Dresser, D.W. and N.A. Mitchison. 1968. The mechanism of immunological paralysis. *Adv. Immunol.* **8:** 129.

Edwards, R.H., W.J. Rutter, and D. Hanahan. 1989. Directed expression of NGF to pancreatic β cells in transgenic mice leads to selective hyperinnervation of the islets. *Cell* **58:** 161.

Efrat, S. and D. Hanahan. 1987. Bidirectional activity of the rat insulin promoter/enhancer region in transgenic mice. *Mol. Cell. Biol.* **7:** 192.

Efrat, S., S. Baekkeskov, D. Lane, and D. Hanahan. 1987. Coordinate expression of the endogenous p53 gene in β-cells of transgenic mice expressing hybrid insulin-SV40 T-antigen genes. *EMBO J.* **6:** 2699.

Efrat, S., G. Teitelman, D. Ruggiero, and D. Hanahan. 1989. Glucagon gene regulatory region directs oncoprotein expression to neurons and pancreatic a cells. *Neuron* **1:** 605.

Folkman, J., K. Watson, D. Ingber, and D. Hanahan. 1989. Induction of angiogenesis during the transition from hyperplasia to neoplasia. *Nature* **339:** 58.

Fujita, T., R. Yui, Y. Kusumoto, Y. Serizawa, S. Makino, and Y. Tochino. 1982. Lymphocyte insulitis in a "non-obese diabetic (NOD)" strain of mice: An immunohistochemical and electron microscope investigation. *Biochem. Res.* **3:** 429.

Gepts, W. and P. Lecompte. 1988. The pathology of type I (juvenile) diabetes. In *The diabetic pancreas* (ed. B.W. Volk and E.R. Anguilla), p. 337. Plenum Press, New York.

Gluzman, Y. 1981. SV40-transformed simian cells support the replication of early SV40 mutants. *Cell* **23:** 175.

Gooding, L.R. 1979. Specificities of killing by T lymphocytes

generated against syngeneic SV40 transformants: Studies employing recombinants within the H-2 complex. *J. Immunol.* **122:** 1002.

Gooding, L.R. and K.A. O'Connell. 1983. Recognition by cytotoxic T lymphocytes of cells expressing fragments of the SV40 tumor antigen. *J. Immunol.* **131:** 2580.

Gooding, L.R., R.W. Geib, K.A. O'Connell, and E. Harlow. 1984. Antibody and cellular detection of SV40 T-antigenic determinants on the surfaces of transformed cells. *Cancer Cells* **1:** 263.

Goodnow, C.C., J. Crosbie, S. Adelstein, T.B. Lavoie, S.J. Smith-Gill, R.A. Brink, H. Pritchard-Briscoe, J.S. Wotherspoon, R.H. Loblay, K. Raphael, R.J. Trent, and A. Basten. 1988. Altered immunoglobulin expression and functional silencing of self-reactive B lymphocytes in transgenic mice. *Nature* **334:** 676.

Hanahan, D. 1985. Heritable formation of pancreatic β-cell tumors in transgenic mice expressing recombinant insulin/ simian virus 40 oncogenes. *Nature* **315:** 115.

———. 1988. Dissecting multistep tumorigenesis in transgenic mice. *Annu. Rev. Genet.* **22:** 479.

Harlow, E., L.V. Crawford, D.C. Pim, and N.M. Williams. 1981. Monoclonal antibodies specific for simian virus 40 tumor antigens. *J. Virol.* **39:** 861.

Hogan, B.L.M., F. Costantini, and E. Lacy. 1986. *Manipulation of the mouse embryo: A laboratory manual.* Cold Spring Harbor Laboratory, Cold Spring Harbor, New York.

Hood, L.E., I.L. Weissman, W.B. Wood, and J.H. Wilson. 1984. *Immunology.* Benjamin-Cummings, Menlo Park, California.

Howard, J.G. and N.A. Mitchison. 1975. Immunological tolerance. *Prog. Allergy* **18:** 43.

Ismail, A., E.A. Baumann, and R. Hand. 1981. Cell surface T-antigen in cells infected with simian virus 40 or an adenovirus/simian virus 40 hybrid $Ad2^+D2$. *J. Virol.* **40:** 615.

Janeway, C.A., Jr., J. Yagi, P.J. Conrad, M.E. Katz, B. Jones, S. Vroegop, and S. Buxser. 1989. T-cell responses to Mls and to bacterial proteins that mimic its behavior. *Immunol. Rev.* **107:** 61.

Kalderon, D., B.L. Roberts, W.D. Richardson, and A.E. Smith. 1984. A short amino acid sequence able to specify nuclear location. *Cell* **39:** 499.

Kanazawa, Y., K. Komeda, S. Sato, S. Mori, K. Akanuma, and F. Takaku. 1984. Non-obese diabetic mice: Immune mechanisms of pancreatic β cell destruction. *Diabetologia* **27:** 113.

Kappler, J.W., N. Roehm, and P. Marrack. 1987. T cell tolerance by clonal elimination in the thymus. *Cell* **49:** 273.

Kappler, J.W., U.D. Staerz, J. White, and P.C. Marrack. 1988. Self-tolerance eliminates T cells specific for Mls-modified products of the major histocompatibility complex. *Nature* **332:** 35.

Kappler, J., B. Kotzin, L. Herron, E.W. Gelfand, R.D. Bigler, A. Boylston, S. Carrel, D.N. Posnett, Y. Choi, and P. Marrack. 1989. V_β specific stimulation of human T cells by Staphylococcus toxins. *Science* **244:** 811.

Kisielow, P., H.S. Teh, H. Blüthmann, and H. von Boehmer. 1988a. Positive selection of antigen-specific T cells in thymus by restricting MHC molecules. *Nature* **335:** 730.

Kisielow, P., H. Blüthmann, U.D. Staerz, M. Steinmetz, and H. von Boehmer. 1988b. Tolerance in T-cell-receptor transgenic mice involves deletion of nonmature $CD4^+8^+$ thymocytes. *Nature* **333:** 742.

Knowles, B.B., M. Koncar, K. Pfizenmaier, D. Solter, D.P. Aden, and G. Trinchieri. 1979. Genetic control of the cytotoxic T cell response to SV40 tumor associated specific antigen. *J. Immunol.* **122:** 1798.

Lanford, R.E. and J.S. Butel. 1984. Construction and characterization of an SV40 mutant defective in nuclear transport of T-antigens. *Cell* **37:** 801.

Ledbetter, I.A. and L.A. Herzenberg. 1979. Xenogeneic

monoclonal antibodies to mouse lymphoid differentiation antigens. *Immunol. Rev.* **47**: 63.

Logothetopoulos, J., N. Valiquette, E. Madura, and D. Cvet. 1984. The onset and progression of pancreatic insulitis in the overt, spontaneously diabetic young adult BB rat studied by pancreatic biopsy. *Diabetes* **33**: 33.

MacDonald, H.R., R. Schneider, R.K. Lees, R.C. Howe, H. Acha-Orbea, H. Festenstein, R.K. Zinkernagel, and H. Hengartner. 1988. T-cell receptor V_β use predicts reactivity and tolerance to Mls[a]-encoded antigens. *Nature* **332**: 40.

Matzinger, P. and S. Guerder. 1989. Does T cell tolerance require a dedicated antigen presenting cell? *Nature* **338**: 74.

Mollick, J.A., R.G. Cook, and R.R. Rich. 1989. Class II MHC molecules are specific receptors for Staphylococcus enterotoxin A. *Science* **244**: 817.

Morahan, G., J. Allison, and J.F.A.P. Mitter. 1989. Tolerance of class I histocompatibility antigens expresed extrathymically. *Nature* **339**: 622.

Morse, H.C.I., W.F. Davidson, R.A. Yetter, and R.L. Coffman. 1982. A cell surface antigen shared by B cells and Ly2[+] peripheral T cells. *Cell. Immunol.* **70**: 311.

Nemazee, D.A. and K. Burki. 1989. Clonal deletion of B lymphocytes in a transgenic mouse bearing anti-MHC class I antibody genes. *Nature* **337**: 562.

Nossal, G.J.V. 1983. Cellular mechanisms of immunologic tolerance. *Annu. Rev. Immunol.* **1**: 33.

Pan, S. and B.R. Knowles. 1983. Monoclonal antibody to SV40 T-antigen blocks lysis of cloned cytotoxic T cell line specific for SV40 TASA. *Virology* **125**: 1.

Pan, S., J. Abramczuk, and B.B. Knowles. 1987. Immune control of SV40 induced tumors in mice. *Int. J. Cancer* **39**: 722.

Prochazka, M., E.H. Leiter, D.V. Serreze, and D.L. Coleman. 1987. Three recessive loci required for insulin-dependent diabetes in nonobese diabetic mice. *Science* **237**: 286.

Pullen, A.M., P. Marrack, and J.W. Kappler. 1988. The T cell repertoire is heavily influenced by tolerance to polymorphic self-antigens. *Nature* **335**: 796.

Rammensee, H.G., R. Kroschewski, and B. Frangoulis. 1989. Clonal anergy induced in mature $V_\beta 6^+$ T lymphocytes on immunizing Mls-1[b] mice with Mls-1[a] expressing cells. *Nature* **339**: 541.

Rawle, F.C., K.A. O'Connell, R.W. Geib, B. Roberts, and L.R. Gooding. 1988. Fine mapping of an H-2K[k] restricted cytotoxic T lymphocyte epitope in SV40 T-antigen by using in-frame deletion mutants and a synthetic peptide. *J. Immunol.* **141**: 2734.

Robertson, M. 1988. Tolerance, restriction and the Mls enigma. *Nature* **332**: 18.

Roitt, I.M., J. Brostoff, and D.K. Morle. 1985. *Immunology.* Gower, London.

Rossini, A.A., J.P. Mordes, and A.A. Like. 1985. Immunology of insulin-dependent diabetes mellitus. *Annu. Rev. Immunol.* **3**: 289.

Sanchez-Madrid, F., P. Simon, S. Thompson, and T.A. Springer. 1983. Mapping of antigenic and functional epitopes on the α and β subunits of two related mouse glycoproteins involved in cell interactions, LFA-1 and Mac-1. *J. Exp. Med.* **158**: 586.

Schwartz, R.H. 1989. Acquisition of immunologic self-tolerance. *Cell* **57**: 1073.

Scott, B., H. Blüthmann, H.S. Teh, and V. von Boehmer. 1989. The generation of mature T cells requires interaction of the $\alpha\beta$ T cell receptor with major histocompatibility antigens. *Nature* **338**: 591.

Sha, W.C., C.A. Nelson, R.D. Newberry, D.M. Kranz, J.H. Russell, and D.Y. Loh. 1988a. Selective expression of an antigen receptor on CD8-bearing T lymphocytes in transgenic mice. *Nature* **335**: 271.

———. 1988b. Positive and negative selection of an antigen receptor on T cells in transgenic mice. *Nature* **336**: 73.

Simanis, V. and D.P. Lane. 1985. An immunoaffinity purification for SV40 large T-antigen. *Virology* **144**: 88.

Soule, H.R. and J.S. Butel. 1979. Subcellular localization of simian virus 40 large T-antigen. *J. Virol.* **30**: 523.

Soule, H.R., R.E. Lanford, and J.S. Butel. 1980. Antigenic and immunogenic characteristics of nuclear and membrane-associated simian virus 40 tumor antigen. *J. Virol.* **33**: 887.

Springer, T.A. 1981. Monoclonal antibody analysis of complex biological systems. *J. Biol. Chem.* **256**: 3833.

Springer, T., G. Galfre, D.S. Secher, and C. Milstein. 1979. Mac-1: A macrophage differentiation antigen identified by monoclonal antibody. *Eur. J. Immunol.* **9**: 301.

Teh, H.S., P. Kisielow, B. Scott, H. Kishi, Y. Uematsu, H. Blüthmann, and H. von Boehmer. 1988. Thymic major histocompatibility complex antigens and the $\alpha\beta$ T cell receptor determine the CD4/CD8 phenotype of T cells. *Nature* **335**: 229.

Teitelman, G., S. Alpert, and D. Hanahan. 1988. Proliferation, senescence and neoplastic progression of β cells in hyperplasic pancreatic islets. *Cell* **52**: 97.

Tevethia, S.S. and M.J. Tevethia. 1984. Localization of antigenic sites reactive with cytotoxic lymphocytes on the proximal half of SV40 T-antigen. *Cancer Cells* **1**: 271.

Tevethia, S.S., D.C. Flyer, and R. Tjian. 1980. Biology of simian virus 40 (SV40) transplantation antigen. VI. Mechanism of induction of SV40 transplantation immunity in mice by purified SV40 T-antigen (D2 protein). *Virology* **107**: 13.

Todd, J.A., J.I. Bell, and H.O. McDevitt. 1987. HLA-DQβ gene contributes to susceptibility and resistance to insulin dependent diabetes mellitus. *Nature* **329**: 559.

Tooze, J., ed. 1981. *Molecular biology of tumor viruses,* 2nd edition, revised: *DNA tumor viruses.* Cold Spring Harbor Laboratory, Cold Spring Harbor, New York.

Trinchieri, G., D.P. Aden, and B.B. Knowles. 1976. Cell-mediated cytotoxicity to SV40-specific tumor-associated antigens. *Nature* **261**: 312.

Walker, M.D., T. Edlund, A.M. Boulet, and W.J. Rutter. 1983. Cell-specific expression controlled by the 5′-flanking region of insulin and chymotrypsin genes. *Nature* **306**: 557.

Weigle, W.O. 1973. Immunological unresponsiveness. *Adv. Immunol.* **16**: 61.

Wraith D.C., H.O. McDevitt, L. Steinman, and H. Acha-Orbea. 1989. T cell recognition as the target for immune intervention in autoimmune disease. *Cell* **57**: 709.

Inflammatory Destruction of Pancreatic β Cells in γ-Interferon Transgenic Mice

N. Sarvetnick,* J. Shizuru,† D. Liggitt,* and T. Stewart*

*Department of Developmental Biology, Genentech, Inc., South San Francisco, California 94080;
†Department of Medicine, Division of Immunology and Rheumatology, Stanford University
Medical Center, Stanford, California 94305

The lesion "insulitis" was originally described by Gepts (1965) as a discrete accumulation of lymphocytes within and surrounding the islets of newly diagnosed, insulin-dependent diabetic patients. This was perhaps the first indication that human diabetes can be mediated by the cellular immune system, resulting in the loss of insulin-producing β cells from pancreatic islets. A similar inflammatory lesion has also been observed in nonobese diabetic (NOD) mice (Like and Weringer 1988) and BB rats (Tarui et al. 1986), two animal models of insulin-dependent diabetes mellitus (IDDM). The presence of antibodies directed against islet cell components has also been demonstrated in both humans and animal models (Sai et al. 1984), and these antibody data suggest that the immune sensitization to specific islet cellular components might be involved in the onset of the disease. Additionally, there is a strong genetic correlation with susceptibility to the disease (Arnheim et al. 1985; Sheehy et al. 1985; Nepom et al. 1986; Todd et al. 1987,1989) since the frequency of individuals that express the human leukemic A antigen (HLA) DR3 or DR4 haplotype are disproportionately increased in the IDDM population as compared with the frequency of this haplotype in the general population (Nerup 1978). This correlation suggests further that one or more host islet antigens can be presented to the host immune system in a major-histocompatibility-complex (MHC) -restricted manner. Most strikingly, pancreatic grafts between human identical twins discordant for the disease showed that selective destruction of the β cells ensued despite the fact that the transplanted tissue was MHC-matched (Sibley et al. 1985). This "experiment" directly demonstrated that long-term immunological sensitization of the diabetic immune system to islets may develop.

Taken together, the MHC-linked genetic susceptibility of IDDM and the documented humoral response expressed in prediabetic patients imply that a specific antigen or antigens within islets might be recognized by the immune system of the host. In other words, tolerance to self-constituents is broken down or was never properly established. How might this occur? Under nonpathogenic circumstances the host is tolerant or nonresponsive toward self-constituents. Three mechanisms for the generation and maintenance of self-tolerance have been described over recent years. These include the selective programmed demise of T cells reactive with self-components during their maturation in the thymus (Kappler et al. 1987; Kisielow et al. 1988; Sha et al. 1988; Roser 1989). This mechanism has been shown recently to be in effect for self-antigens that are present within the thymus. Tolerance to antigens confined to the periphery most likely occurs via a different mechanism. Experimental results from several systems demonstrate that autoreactive T lymphocytes are present but in a nonresponsive or paralyzed state in the periphery (Hooper et al. 1987; Hooper and Taylor 1987; Flavell 1988). A final mechanism is active "suppression" of autoreactive T cells by suppressor cells in the periphery. In individuals with IDDM, one or more of these mechanisms of self-tolerance have been impaired.

The work described here addresses possible pathways leading to the breakdown of self-tolerance in IDDM. One intriguing concept is that previously unencountered (peripheral) islet cell antigens emerge after self-tolerance has been established and are presented to the host immune system provoking a primary immune response (Bottazzo et al. 1983). Such an event might be triggered by a viral or bacterial infection of the pancreas. Viral infections are known to induce the host production of protective cytokines such as γ-interferon (IFN-γ). IFN-γ has been shown to induce the overexpression of MHC class I and II on a wide variety of cell types and thus may enhance antigen presentation by the host (Wong et al. 1984; Todd et al. 1985). Increased expression of MHC class I and II antigens has been reported on islet cells of diabetic patients (Bottazzo et al. 1985). Thus, it is possible that the pancreatic β cells placed in the IFN-γ rich microenvironment could act as antigen-presenting cells (APC) and directly present autoantigens to the immune system. Alternatively, during an infection, host antigens could be released from damaged cells and presented to the host by APCs near the site of the infection, thereby facilitating an autoreactive response. Damage to host cells could be mediated by other lymphokines produced in response to the infection. Of relevance here is the lymphokine interleukin-1 (IL-1), which has been demonstrated to have direct cytotoxic effects on β cells (Bendtzen et al. 1986).

To test whether the products of a microbial infection could lead to the breakdown of self-tolerance, we experimentally recapitulated the response to an infection in vivo (Sarvetnick et al. 1988). IFN-γ was constitutively expressed in the pancreatic islets in transgenic mice and consequences of this local expression of IFN-γ were examined. These transgenic mice became clinically diabetic and suffered an inflammatory rejection of the pancreatic islets.

EXPERIMENTAL PROCEDURES

Production of transgenic mice. To derive transgenic mice expressing IFN-γ in the pancreatic β cells, recombinant DNA plasmids were constructed that joined the controlling sequences of the human insulin gene to the mouse IFN-γ gene. DNA constructs were made by methods described previously (Sarvetnick et al. 1988), using the coding sequences from the genomic murine IFN-γ gene (Gray and Goeddel 1983) and hepatitis B 3' untranslated sequences 1.9 kb from the promoter of the human insulin B allele (Ullrich et al. 1980,1982).

Restriction fragments from these plasmids, free of plasmid sequences, were isolated from low-melting-temperature agarose gels by NaI glass bead extraction. BALB/c or CD-1 (outbred, closed stock) female mice (4 weeks old) were superovulated, and 1-cell-stage embryos were flushed from the oviducts of the mated female mice and microinjected with approximately 2 pl of DNA at a concentration of 1 ng/μl. The injected, fertilized eggs were then transferred to the ampullae of 1/2-day pseudopregnant recipient CD-1 female mice to complete their development. Tail DNA of mice from litters 4 weeks old or greater were analyzed by Southern blot analysis.

Determination of diabetes. Blood glucose measurements reaffirmed the diagnosis of spontaneous diabetes and were determined by analysis of either whole blood (Accucheck II, Boehringer Mannheim) or on serum or plasma by standard enzymatic methods. Mice were considered diabetic when the urine glucose was 2–5% and the nonfasting blood glucose was greater than 400 mg/dl for 3 consecutive days. Normal (nontransgenic) mice never showed glycosuria and had blood glucose concentrations of approximately 100–200 mg/dl.

Fetal pancreas and adult islet transplantation. Pancreases were harvested from BALB/c 18-day-old embryos. A single fetal pancreas was implanted into the kidney of IFN-γ^+ mice. Recipient mice were sacrificed 1 month posttransplant, and the kidney was excised, formalin-fixed, and paraffin-embedded.

Adult BALB/c islets were isolated by a modified form of collagenase digestion and density-gradient purification. Following cannulation of the common bile duct, a solution of 0.8 mg/ml type-IV collagenase dissolved in Hanks' balanced salt solution was infused into each pancreas. After a 25-minute incubation at 37°C, the pancreases were disrupted by pipeting of the tissue and were washed twice by centrifugation (200g for 1 min). The digested tissue was loaded onto a discontinuous Ficoll gradient. The banded islets were washed and then incubated in CMRL tissue culture media containing 10% fetal calf serum. Islets (800) were hand-picked under a dissecting microscope and infused into the liver by cannulation of the portal vein. These mice also received a simultaneous islet transplant of 200 islets per graft under the kidney capsule at the time of portal vein transplantation. Recipient diabetic mice were sacrificed for histological analysis of their livers at intermittent time points after transplantation.

Histological analysis. To analyze the expression of leukocyte surface antigens L3T4 (CD4) and Lyt-2 (CD8), 7 μm of unfixed cryostat sections were stained with monoclonal antibodies (Boehringer-Mannheim) and visualized by the indirect immunoperoxidase technique (Vector ABC) with diaminobenzidine/nickel sulfate as a chromogen. Sections were counterstained with methyl green.

RESULTS

Three independent lines of transgenic mice were established that harbored chimeric genes and expressed IFN-γ in pancreatic islets. Overt insulin-dependent diabetes mellitus developed in two of these three lines (Sarvetnick et al. 1988). The most well-characterized line, the 461-2 line, demonstrated hyperglycemia between 10–20 weeks of age. By 20 weeks of life, the blood glucose of all the transgenic progeny derived from this founder rose to >400 mg/dl. A second line of insulin promotor (Ins)-IFN-γ transgenics (462-4) became hyperglycemic starting at approximately 5 months of age. These mice demonstrated a more variable time of clinical onset ranging from 20 weeks to 40 weeks. The third line of mice, the 454-4 line, never exhibited the diabetic trait. In the case of the 461-2 and the 462-4 lines, the diabetes was accompanied by polyurea, polydipsea, and weight loss. When these animals were supplemented with exogenous insulin, they were able to breed.

If maintained without insulin for more than 1 month, the transgenic diabetic animals became ataxic and developed additional clinical signs of diabetes. Although these clinical signs were most likely the result of a lack of insulin, we wanted to eliminate the potential metabolic contributions that high levels of circulating IFN-γ might produce. We therefore attempted to measure circulating levels of IFN-γ in the serum of diabetic and prediabetic 461-2 mice. To accomplish this, serum from transgenic mice was tested in vitro for the ability to protect A549 cells from the cytomegalovirus cytopathic effect. Utilizing this biological assay, we were unable to detect IFN-γ in the serum of diabetic or prediabetic mice. Although presumably low levels of circulating IFN-γ were present in these mice, the levels were below the detection limits of this biological assay.

Histological analysis of pancreases from these animals revealed very dramatic differences from normal pancreas morphology. At the time of onset of the clinical disease, the microscopic structure of the pancreas was distorted and islets were not easily identifiable. The exocrine tissue was unevenly infiltrated by masses of mononuclear inflammatory cells. Furthermore, there was significant atrophy of exocrine tissue. Foci of exocrine tissue were present and were separated and isolated by fibrotic bands. Figure 1d shows a representative histological appearance of older animals (~16 weeks old). At this stage, the disease resembled a chronic/active pancreatitis with inflammatory cells accumulating within interstitial regions of the pancreas and fibrosis surrounding islet remnants and ducts.

To further characterize the progression of the disease, we studied the histological characteristics of prediabetic mice (transgenic line 461-2) at different stages of development. Histological examination of the younger pancreases revealed strikingly different morphologies (see Fig. 1b). The pancreas of a 1-month-old IFN-γ transgenic prediabetic mouse contained lymphocytes that surrounded the islets, whereas the exocrine pancreas appeared largely unaffected. This more discrete inflammation is reminiscent of the lesion described originally by Gepts (1965) as insulitis. Microscopic analysis also revealed the presence of venules lined with prominent endothelium in the vicinity of the inflammation. The size and complexity of the inflammatory lesions became generally larger as older pancreases were examined. At middle stages of the disease (7 weeks), some islets appeared hyperplastic, whereas others were densely atrophic. However, by 2 months of age (see Fig. 1c), the lymphocytic lesions had become quite large, and the islet structures were nearly obscured.

In older animals (see Fig. 1d), the pancreases had a very disorderly and sclerotic appearance. Islets were scant or more typically absent and sometimes difficult to recognize. Masses of mixed inflammatory cells could be seen throughout the interstitium, and there was a notable loss of exocrine tissue as well. A striking feature of these pancreases was the appearance of numerous duct cells forming primitive ducts found throughout the interstitium. These ducts, some of which were wide-

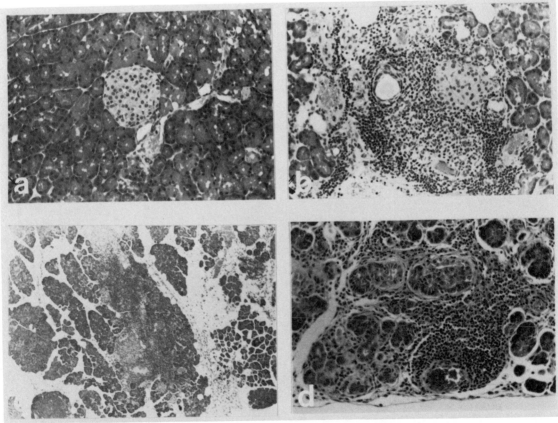

Figure 1. Islets of Langerhans from normal and diabetic Ins-IFN-γ transgenic mice stained with hematoxylin and eosin (H & E). (a) Normal BALB/c pancreas stained with H & E. The islet is the pale circular structure in the center. (b) Section of a pancreas from a 1-month-old Ins-IFN-γ prediabetic mouse. The islet is obscured by lymphocytes that stain darkly. The exocrine tissue adjacent to the islet is also affected. (c) Section of a 2-month-old pancreas stained with H & E. This lower magnification demonstrates the extensive lymphocytic inflammation at this stage in the prediabetic animal. Lymphocytes are accumulating in the interstitial region of the pancreas. (d) Section of a pancreas of a 16-week-old diabetic animal. This shows more chronic inflammation, acinar atrophy, and proliferation of duct cells.

ly dilated and incorporated within islet remnants, were surrounded by dense accumulations of collagen and fibroblasts.

To characterize the subsets of cells infiltrating the prediabetic animals, we used a series of monoclonal antibodies (MAbs) that react with antigens on leukocyte subsets. These were used to stain cryostat sections of 3-week-old transgenic pancreases. The antibody to leukocyte common antigen confirmed that the infiltrating cells were indeed leukocytes. The tissues were then analyzed with the MAb Mac-1, which recognizes a determinant on macrophages and natural killer cells. This experiment demonstrated that only a small proportion (5%) of the infiltrating cells were from this lineage. Studies with an anti-Thy-1 antibody and an anti-immunoglobulin G antibody revealed that the infiltrate was composed largely of T cells. Utilizing antibodies directed against helper (anti-L3T4) and cytotoxic T cells (anti-Lyt-2), it was established that the infiltrating cell population was largely helper T lymphocytes (70%) with some (25%) cytotoxic T cells (Fig. 2).

To address the question of whether or not diabetic transgenic mice were specifically sensitized to islet antigens, histocompatible islets were transplanted into diabetic and prediabetic recipients. Immunosensitized mice would be expected to "reject" an MHC-matched islet graft, whereas animals that became diabetic for nonimmune reasons would not be expected to demonstrate cell-mediated rejection. Thus, isolated adult BALB/c islets were infused into the portal vein of diabetic IFN-γ transgenic mice and, as a control, into diabetic Ins-I-A^d mice (nonimmune mediated, Sarvetnick et al. 1988). Introduction of sufficient numbers of histocompatible islets into the livers of diabetic recipients allows physiological normalization of blood glucose levels (normal glucose levels are 90–120 mg/dl).

Then, 800 islets were infused, an amount that has been shown previously to reconstitute glucose homeostasis permanently in mice made diabetic by the β-cell-specific toxin streptozotocin. Fetal and adult islets were also transplanted under the kidney capsule in prediabetic and diabetic transgenic mice as grafts for histological analysis only.

Within 24 hours posttransplant, the control diabetic Ins-I-A^d mice became normoglycemic and remained normoglycemic up until the time they were sacrificed, approximately 1 month later. In contrast, diabetic Ins-IFN-γ transgenic mice never achieved normoglycemia, each having stable blood glucose levels of > 400 mg/dl at all measured time points after surgery. These mice were sacrificed at intervals, and their livers were sectioned for histological evaluation of transplanted islets. Liver sections from reconstituted normoglycemic Ins-I-A^d transgenic mouse at 1 month posttransplant showed normal appearing islets. found scattered throughout the livers, nestled within and next to vessels and hepatic parenchyma. Immunohistochemical staining for islet hormones including insulin, glucagon, and somatostatin were found to be at normal intensity. No lymphocytic infiltrate was observed in either the liver sections or kidney capsule grafts from the Ins-I-A^d mice.

Histological examinations of the grafts from the Ins-IFN-γ transgenic mice were markedly different from those obtained from BALB/c control and Ins-I-A^d mice. As early as 4 days posttransplant, islets within the liver were surrounded by inflammatory cellular infiltrates. By 2.5 weeks posttransplantation, the few remaining islets were virtually obscured by dense collections of inflammatory cells. Adult islet and fetal pancreatic grafts in the kidney also demonstrated progressive mononuclear cell infiltrates as a tissue-specific re-

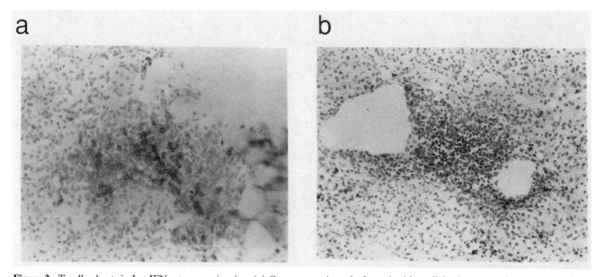

Figure 2. T-cell subsets in Ins-IFN-γ transgenic mice. (*a*) Cryostat section of a 3-week-old prediabetic transgenic pancreas stained with an anti-L3T4 monoclonal antibody that identifies helper T lymphocytes. The section is counterstained with methyl green. Approximately 70% of the infiltrating cells stain with this antibody. (*b*) Cryostat section of a 3-week-old transgenic pancreas stained with an anti-Lyt-2 monoclonal antibody that identifies cytotoxic T lymphocytes. The section is counterstained with methyl green. Approximately 25% of the infiltrating cells stain with this antibody.

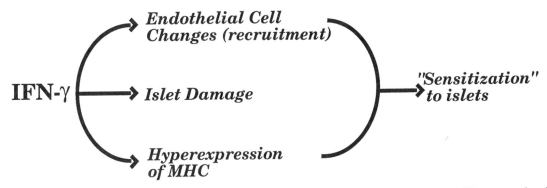

Figure 3. Diagrammatic representation of potential pathway leading to loss of islet tolerance in Ins-IFN-γ transgenic mice. Expression of IFN-γ by the β cells leads to endothelial changes, allowing recruitment of lymphoid cells into the pancreas. The presence of lymphocytes, in conjunction with islet permeability/damage and localized heightened MHC expression, all cooperate, resulting in eventual immunological sensitization to the islets.

sponse since BALB/c pituitary grafts in the contralateral kidney remained intact and without evidence of cell-mediated destruction.

DISCUSSION

The Ins-IFN-γ transgenic mice develop hyperglycemia concurrent with an aggressive inflammatory lesion directed against the islets, which ultimately leads to their destruction. This is undoubtedly a complex process that results in the specific sensitization immune system of the transgenic mice to islets. We do not know the mechanism by which it occurs.

One possibility is that β cell death is caused by direct toxicity from locally produced lymphokines. Toxicity to β cells by high levels of IFN-γ has been reported previously in in vitro studies (Campbell et al. 1988). Thus, overexpression of the IFN-γ itself could be toxic to β cells, leading to diabetes. Alternatively, combinations of lymphokines produced by the accumulating cellular infiltrate could cause the demise of the B cells. Tumor necrosis factor and IL-1 in combination have been shown to be particularly cytotoxic to β cells (Mandrup-Poulsen et al. 1987).

The localized production of IFN-γ may also have indirect effects on the recruitment of inflammatory cells into islet parenchyma. Specialized vessels, high-endothelial venules (HEVs), were observed upon microscopic examination of the pancreases. HEVs are composed of plump endothelial cells that allow the extravasation of leukocytes into surrounding tissue. Although HEVs are usually found in organized lymphoid tissue, they have also been reported to occur at sites of chronic inflammation. It has been demonstrated previously that IFN-γ can induce the expression of high-endothelial-cell surface antigens in vitro (Duijvestijn et al. 1986). Thus, in a similar manner the lymphokine could direct-

ly enhance vascular differentiation in the pancreas of the IFN-γ transgenic mice. Such vascular changes might then cause the efficient influx of inflammatory cells into the interstitium of the pancreas.

Damage, however mediated, certainly renders the β cells porous to release-sequestered antigens. β-Cell-specific antigens could potentially be presented by APCs within the inflammatory infiltrate or in the adjacent lymph nodes, thereby inducing a primary immune response. Another way in which an islet-specific response might be triggered is if β cells themselves function as APCs. IFN-γ has been shown to upregulate MHC classes I and II antigens on several cell types (Wong et al. 1984; Todd et al. 1985), and therefore the possibility that β cells may be directly presenting antigen themselves cannot be excluded. This latter mechanism appears less likely since it has been demonstrated recently that islet β cells expressing class II molecules induce tolerance in the form of immunological unresponsiveness when used as APCs to stimulate T-cell clones in vitro (Markmann et al. 1989). It is thought that antigen presentation resulting in T-cell activation requires secondary signals in addition to presentation of antigen plus MHC. Failure to produce the requisite second signal may result in T-cell anergy rather than activation. Thus, class-II-expressing β cells may lack the ability to produce the necessary stimulatory factors and are therefore inadequate as APCs. Finally, instead of inducing a primary response, the IFN-γ could be acting to effect a subset of T cells normally resident but quiescent within the periphery. Several systems have demonstrated the theoretical and physical presence of such autoreactive T cells, and it is likely that cells exist in normal animals that are potentially reactive with components on normal islets. As these quiescent cells traffic through the pancreas, they might be relieved of their quiescence through contact with IFN-γ and/or other factors, and the islet-specific compartment could proliferate thereby initiating and perpetuating a response.

It is likely that several of the above mechanisms could be interacting to produce the phenotype we have observed in the IFN-γ transgenic mice (see Fig. 3). The lesion combines the phenomena of chemotaxis, inflammation, fibrosis, and autoimmunity. The processes are similar to those observed in human disease although the similarly obscure etiology could be quite different. More extensive studies are required to unravel the complex physiological responses to overexpression of this lymphokine in vivo.

REFERENCES

Arnheim, N., C. Strange, and H. Erlich. 1985. Use of pooled DNA samples to detect linkage disequilibrium of polymorphic restriction fragments and human disease: Studies of the HLA class II loci. *Proc. Natl. Acad. Sci.* **82**: 6970.

Bendtzen, K., T. Mandrup-Poulsen, J. Nerup, J.H. Nielsen, C.A. Dinarello, and M. Svenson. 1986. Cytotoxicity of human p17 interleukin-1 for pancreatic islets of Langerhans. *Science* **232**: 1545.

Bottazzo, G.F., R. Pujol-Borrell, T. Hanafusa, and M. Feldmann. 1983. Role of aberrant HLA-DR expression and antigen presentation in induction of endocrine autoimmunity. *Lancet* **II**: 1115.

Bottazzo, G.F., B. Dean, J.M. McNally, E.H. MacKay, P.G.F. Swift, and D.R. Gamble. 1985. In situ characterization of autoimmune phenomena and expression of HLA molecules in the pancreas in diabetic insulitis. *N. Engl. J. Med.* **313**: 353.

Campbell, I.L., A. Iscaro, and L. Harrison. 1988. IFN-γ and tumor necrosis factor-α: Cytotoxicity to murine islets of Langerhans. *J. Immunol.* **141**: 2325.

Duijvestijn, A.M., A.B. Schreiber, and E.C. Butcher. 1986. Interferon-γ regulates an antigen specific for endothelial cells involved in lymphocyte traffic. *Proc. Natl. Acad. Sci.* **83**: 9114.

Flavell, R.A. 1988. *6th HLA/H2 Cloning Workshop*, Airlie, Virginia. Abstract 51.

Gepts, W. 1965. Pathologic anatomy of the pancreas in juvenile diabetes mellitus. *Diabetes* **14**: 619.

Grey, P.W. and D.V. Goeddel. 1983. Cloning and expression of murine immune interferon cDNA. *Proc. Natl. Acad. Sci.* **80**: 5842.

Hooper, D.C. and R.B. Taylor. 1987. Specific helper T cell reactivity against autologous erythrocytes implies that self tolerance need not depend on clonal deletion. *Eur. J. Immunol.* **17**: 797.

Hooper, D.C., J.L. Young, C.J. Elson, and R.B. Taylor. 1987. Murine T cells reactive against autologous erythrocytes: Evidence for in vitro and in vivo priming with mouse and rat red blood cells. *Cell. Immunol.* **106**: 53.

Kappler, J.W., N. Roehm, and P. Marrack. 1987. T cell tolerance by clonal elimination in the thymus. *Cell* **49**: 273.

Kisielow, P., H. Blüthmann, U.D. Staerz, M. Steinmetz, and H. von Boehmer. 1988. Tolerance in T-cell-receptor trans-genic mice involves deletion of nonmature CD4+8+ thymocytes. *Nature* **333**: 742.

Like, A.A. and E.J. Weringer, eds. 1988. *The pathology of the endocrine pancreas in diabetes*. Springer-Verlag, New York.

Mandrup-Poulsen, T., K. Bendtzen, C.A. Dinarello, and J. Nerup. 1987. Human tumor necrosis factor potentiates human interleukin 1-mediated rat pancreatic beta cell cytotoxicity. *J. Immunol.* **138**: 4077.

Markmann, J., D. Lo, A. Naji, R.D. Palmiter, R.L. Brinster, and E. Heber-Katz. 1989. Antigen presenting function of class II MHC expressing pancreatic beta cells. *Nature* **336**: 476.

Nepom, B.S., J. Palmer, S.J. Kim, J.A. Hansen, S.L. Holbeck, and G.T. Nepom. 1986. Specific genomic markers for the HLA-DQ subregion discriminate between DR4+ insulin-dependent diabetes mellitus and DR4+ seropositive juvenile rheumatoid arthritis. *J. Exp. Med.* **164**: 345.

Nerup, J. 1978. HLA studies in diabetes mellitus: A review. *Adv. Metab. Disord.* **9**: 263.

Roser, B.J. 1989. Cellular mechanisms in neonatal and adult tolerance. *Immunol. Rev.* **107**: 179.

Sai, P., M. Kremer, M.F. Nomballais, and G. Aillet. 1984. Antibodies spontaneously bound to islet cells in type-I diabetes. *Lancet* **II**: 233.

Sarvetnick, N., D. Liggitt, S.L. Pitts, S.E. Hansen, and T.A. Stewart. 1988. Insulin-dependent diabetes mellitus induced in transgenic mice by ectopic expression of class II MHC and interferon-gamma. *Cell* **52**: 773.

Sha, W.C., C.A. Nelson, R.D. Newberry, D.M. Kranz, J.H. Russell, and D. Loh. 1988. Positive and negative selection of an antigen receptor on T cells in transgenic mice. *Nature* **336**: 73.

Sheehy, M.J., J.R. Rowe, and M.J. Macdonald. 1985. A particular subset of HLA-DR4 accounts for all or most of the DR4 association in type I diabetes. *Diabetes* **34**: 942.

Sibley, R.K., D.E.R. Sutherland, F. Goetz, and A.F. Michael. 1985. Recurrent diabetes mellitus in the pancreas iso-and allograft. *Lab. Invest.* **53**: 132.

Tarui, S., Y. Tochino, and K. Nonaka. 1986. *Insulitis and type 1 diabetes—Lessons from the NOD mouse*. Academic Press, New York.

Todd, I., R. Pujol-Borrell, L.J. Hammond, G.F. Bottazzo, and M. Feldman. 1985. Interferon-gamma induces HLA-DR expression by the thyroid epithelium. *Clin. Exp. Immunol.* **61**: 261.

Todd, J.A., J.I. Bell, and H.O. McDevitt. 1987. HLA-DQβ gene contributes to susceptibility and resistance to insulin-dependent diabetes mellitus. *Nature* **329**: 599.

Todd, J.A., C. Mijovic, J. Fletcher, D. Jenkins, A.R. Bradwell, and A.H. Barnett. 1989. Identification of susceptibility loci for insulin-dependent diabetes mellitus by trans-racial gene mapping. *Nature* **338**: 587.

Ullrich, A., T.J. Dull, A. Gray, J. Brosius, and I. Sures. 1980. Genetic variation in the human insulin gene. *Science* **209**: 612.

Ullrich, A., T.J. Dull, A. Gray, J.A. Philips, and S. Peter. 1982. Variation in the sequence and modification state of the human insulin gene flanking regions. *Nucleic Acids Res.* **10**: 2225.

Wong, G.H.W., I. Clark-Lewis, A.W. Harris, and J.W. Schrader. 1984. Effect of cloned interferon-γ on expression of H-2 and Ia antigens on cell lines of hemopoietic, lymphoid, epithelial, fibroblastic and neuronal origin. *Eur. J. Immunol.* **14**: 52.

Reactivity and Tolerance of Virus-specific T Cells

R.M. Zinkernagel, H.P. Pircher, M. Schulz, T. Leist,
S. Oehen, and H. Hengartner
Laboratory of Experimental Pathology, Institute of Pathology, University of Zurich, Switzerland

Studies of immune responses to lymphocytic chorio-meningitis (LCM) virus (LCMV) have influenced immunological concepts repeatedly. Ideas about tolerance (Burnet and Fenner 1949) were in part based on transplacental or neonatal infection of mice with LCMV leading to a virus carrier state (Traub 1936; Hotchin 1962; Lehmann-Grube 1971); this tolerance was subsequently shown to be complete at the T-cell level but incomplete for B cells, leading to immune complex disease (Oldstone and Dixon 1967). The concept that antiviral cell-mediated immune responses may not always be beneficial but may sometimes induce immunopathology has been based essentially on observations in the LCMV system (Rowe 1954; Hirsch et al. 1967; Cole et al. 1972; Doherty and Zinkernagel 1974). The notion that cytotoxic T cells played a role in immunity against virus in general was first shown for LCMV (Oldstone and Dixon 1970; Marker and Volkert 1973). Subsequently, the role of classic transplantation antigens (class I) coded by the major histocompatibility gene complex (MHC) in cytotoxic T-cell recognition (Zinkernagel and Doherty 1974) and in positive selection of T cells in the thymus was discovered using LCMV (Zinkernagel et al. 1978). LCMV is used here to study T-cell specificity and tolerance.

LCMV is a member of the Arenaviruses and is a natural mouse pathogen (Hotchin 1962, 1971; Lehmann-Grube 1971). Its negative-stranded RNA genome consists of a small RNA coding in ambisense direction for the glycoprotein (GP) and the nucleoprotein (NP) (Bishop and Auperin 1987; Buchmeier and Parekh 1987; Southern and Bishop 1987; Whitton et al. 1988b); the larger viral RNA codes for a polymerase and probably for additional gene products.

Since LCMV is not cytopathic, it may readily induce a carrier state in vivo and in vitro (Hotchin 1962, 1971; Lehmann-Grube 1971). The immunological and more recent extensive virological analyses of LCMV have been reviewed comprehensively (Hotchin 1962, 1971; Lehmann-Grube 1971; Doherty and Zinkernagel 1974; Buchmeier et al. 1980; Bishop and Auperin 1987; Buchmeier and Parekh 1987; Southern and Bishop 1987).

During the past 6 years, several observations have influenced cell-mediated immunology profoundly: the description of the T-cell receptor structure (Hedrick et al. 1984; Toyonaga et al. 1984), the discovery of the three-dimensional structure of MHC class I products (Bjorkman et al. 1987), and the finding that T cells recognize antigen fragments bound by class II or class I MHC products (Yewdell et al. 1985; Townsend et al. 1986; Buus et al. 1987; Guillet et al. 1987).

In this paper, we review the following experiments done in close collaboration by the various authors and the laboratories indicated in the different sections. First, studies on LCMV-epitope mapping in vitro and in vivo revealed the excellent protective antiviral capacity of LCMV antigen fragments expressed in recombinant vaccinia virus; they also suggested that such vaccination may facilitate immunopathological disease under some conditions. Second, models of MHC-disease associations were analyzed by using LCMV. Third, mice carrying T-cell receptor (TCR) α and β chains specific for LCMV + D^b are described, and preliminary results on their T-cell reactivity and tolerance to LCMV are presented.

Target Antigens for LCMV-specific Cytotoxic T Cells In Vitro and In Vivo[1]

Recombinant vaccinia viruses expressing single antigens or antigen fragments of other viruses (Panicali et al. 1983; Chakrabati et al. 1985; Mackett et al. 1985; Yewdell et al. 1985; Townsend et al. 1986; Jonjic et al. 1988; Whitton et al. 1988a) have contributed greatly to our understanding of T-cell recognition. The crucial work of Townsend et al. (1986) on influenza viruses and similar studies on vesicular stomatitis virus (Yewdell et al. 1985), cytomegalovirus, and LCMV (Oldstone et al. 1988; Whitton et al. 1988a) have documented that virus-specific cytotoxic T cells recognize processed viral antigens in an H-2-dependent fashion. These analytical studies in vitro have been complemented by some studies in vivo that evaluated the protective capacity of such recombinant vaccinia viruses. These experiments have shown that protection against influenza virus (Andrew et al. 1987) or respiratory syncytial virus (King et al. 1987) is inducible with recombinant virus expressing hemagglutinin but not, or only marginally, by recombinants expressing NP. In the case of rabies virus (Rupprecht et al. 1986), Friend leukemia virus (Earl et al. 1986), and herpes simplex virus-I (Martin and Rouse 1987), recombinant vaccinia virus expressing viral GP have been shown to yield efficient protection against reinfection either via antibodies or via cellular immunity. However, clear evi-

---

[1]This section is based on the experimental work of M. Schulz and S. Oehen.

dence that viral antigens that are not recognized by neutralizing antibodies may provide efficient protection has been obtained for a nonstructural protein of murine cytomegalovirus (Jonjic et al. 1988).

It has been demonstrated by various methods that recovery from LCMV and protection against LCMV are virtually exclusively mediated by virus-specific cytotoxic T cells; neither antibodies nor helper T cells play a major role. Also, the LCMV-induced lethal choriomeningitis after intracerebral infections or the early phase (6–9 days) of the swelling reaction after local infection in the footpad are strictly cytotoxic T-lymphocyte-dependent (for review, see Hotchin 1971; Lehmann-Grube 1971; Doherty and Zinkernagel 1974; Buchmeier et al. 1980).

A vaccinia recombinant virus expressing the LCMV GP was originally obtained from M. Mackett, D.H.L. Bishop, and H. Overton, Institute of Virology, Oxford, United Kingdom (Mackett et al. 1985; Romanowski et al. 1985; Southern and Bishop 1987). Other vaccinia recombinant viruses were constructed by cloning truncated cDNA of the gene coding for LCMV NP into the vaccinia recombinant vector pSC11 of Moss et al. (Chakrabati et al. 1985). Details of the methods used are given by Hany et al. (1989) and M. Schulz et al. (in prep.). To evaluate the protective potential of vaccinia recombinant viruses in an acute virus infection, we have studied T-cell responses to LCMV and to vaccinia recombinant viruses expressing the LCMV GP or NP (Oldstone et al. 1988; Whitton et al. 1988a,b; Hany et al. 1989; Schulz et al. 1989) both in vitro and in vivo.

The viral antigen specificity of primary cytotoxic T-cell responses of $H-2^b$, $H-2^k$, $H-2^q$, $H-2^s$, $H-2^f$, and some H-2-recombinant mice against LCMV (WE isolate), as well as the specificity of some T-cell clones and T-cell lines, was defined on target cells infected with vaccinia-LCMV NP or vaccinia-LCMV GP. NP was recognized together with $H-2^q$ (D^q), $H-2^d$ (DL^d), $H-2^s$ and $H-2^b$ (D^b) (Table 1). GP specificity was restricted to $H-2^f$

and $H-2^b$ (K^b and D^b); $H-2^k$-restricted anti-LCMV responses were neither GP- nor NP-specific (Table 1).

The antiviral protective immunity induced by vaccinia-GP or vaccinia-NP recombinants was evaluated in mice. T-cell-mediated protection (Table 1) correlated well with the cytotoxic T-cell specificity defined in vitro. Some of the H-2 alleles plus NP, or H-2 plus GP combinations that were found to be nonresponder combinations in vitro were, however, protected to variable and low degrees by vaccinia recombinant viruses in vivo (Hany et al. 1989), indicating that antiviral protection is a more sensitive readout than cytotoxicity in vitro. After immunization with a vaccinia-NP recombinant, $H-2^d$ mice had, for example, 10^4 times lower LCMV titers in spleens than in vaccinia-primed controls. Although vaccinia-GP-immunized ($H-2^d$) mice revealed no cytotoxic T-cell activity in vitro, they nevertheless had 10^2 times lower LCMV titers in spleens than controls. Interestingly, antiviral protection, particularly in low-responder combinations, was usually short-lived and diminished after 3 weeks, whereas in a high-responder situation, protection was of a longer duration (> 8 weeks). Vaccination with vaccinia-NP or -GP recombinants protected mice against lethal T-cell-mediated LCM or prevented the local footpad swelling reaction; these in vivo effects were H-2-dependent and followed the identical roles established for cytotoxic T lymphocyte (CTL) recognition in vitro. These experiments document for LCMV NP that one viral protein may exhibit several protective antigenic determinants recognized by T cells in an H-2 K or D allele-specific manner.

From previous analyses (Whitton et al. 1988a,b; Hany et al. 1989), it was obvious that the NP is the main target in the $H-2^d$ haplotype, mapping the described T-cell epitope of nine amino acids (118–126) to L^d (Schulz et al. 1989). In addition, these analyses revealed that DL^d- and DL^q-restricted cytotoxic T cells recognize a common T-cell epitope in the amino-termi-

Table 1. Summary of Vaccinia-LCMV Recombinant Virus-specific CTL Activity In Vitro and Protection In Vivo against Virus Replication and/or against Lethal LCM

Mouse strain	H-2 K	H-2 D	Non-H-2 background	Vacc-GP	Vacc-NP	Vacc-WR	LCMV-WE control
B10.BR	k	k	B10	−(+/−)	−(+/−)	−	++
CBA/J	k	k	CBA	−(+/−)	−(+/−)	−	++
C57BL/6	b	b	B6	++	+	−	++
C57BL/10	b	b	B10	++	+	−	++
B10.D2	d	d	B10	−	++	−	++
BALB/c	d	d	BALB	−	++	−	++
B10.G	q	q	B10	−	++	−	++
DBA/1	q	q	DBA	−	++	−	++
B10.M	f	f	B10	++	−	−	++
B10.S	s	s	B10	−	++	−	++
B10.AKM	k	q	B10	−(+/−)	++	−	++
B10.A(5r)	b	d	B10	+	++	−	++

All strains listed were tested in vitro for CTL activity on infected syngeneic target cells 8 days after priming with LCMV-WE; other mice were tested 18–25 days after priming with respect to LCMV clearance or protection against lethal LCM; B10.M and B10.S mice were not tested for antiviral protection. (−) Indicates no protection; (+/−) indicates variably low degree of protection in the virus titer assay for antiviral protection but not protection against lethal LCM. (++) Means >3.4 $\log_{10}$ protection in the virus titer assay on day 6 after challenge and usually 100% protection against lethal LCM. These data were summarized from Hany et al. (1989).

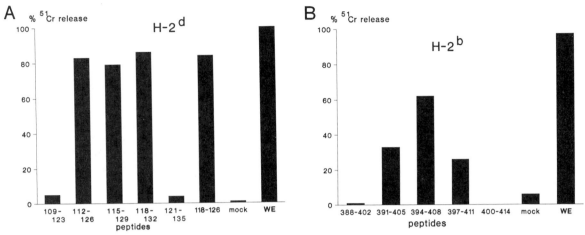

Figure 1. Epitope mapping with synthetic peptides. LCMV-WE NP peptides of 15 amino acids overlapping by 12 amino acids were made by solid-phase synthesis. The amino acid sequence of LCMV-WE from 109 to 130 is LKAKIMRTE*RPQAS-GVYM*GNLT; the nonapeptide forming an efficient fragment with H-2L^q is italicized. (*A*) Relevant peptides defining the T-cell epitopes of LCMV NP in H-2^d and H-2^q. Peptide 118-126 comprises the common sequence of the three shown positive peptides. (*B*) Relevant peptides defining the T-cell epitopes of LCMV NP for H-2^b; the common nonapeptide comprises amino acids 397-405 of NP (QPQNGQFIH) (Schulz et al. 1989).

nal region of the NP (The nonapeptide RPQAS-GVYM) (Schulz et al. 1989) (Fig. 1A).

These results also show that distinct single T-cell epitopes of an internal viral protein efficiently protected mice against various manifestations of viral disease. The location of these epitopes within amino- and carboxy-terminal regions of the nucleoprotein and their H-2 restriction fine specificity previously defined in vitro were confirmed in vivo (Tables 2 and 3). So far, the protective potential against mortality of a complete internal viral protein has been documented for cytomegalovirus immediate-early protein (Jonjic et al. 1988) and possibly NP of influenza A virus (Andrew et al. 1987). In respiratory syncytial virus a slight reduction in virus titer (0.7–0.8 log$_{10}$ pfu) was documented by vaccination with internal protein expressed in vaccinia virus (King et al. 1987).

The protective capacity of the LCMV-NP epitopes expressed in vaccinia virus is comparable to that of wild-type LCMV in mice. The implication of the data is that the defined fragments only protect mice possessing one or a very limited number of MHC alleles (Bennink and Yewdell 1988; Hany et al. 1989). To protect the entire mouse population against LCMV, it would be necessary to introduce all possible fragments into a potential recombinant vaccinia virus.

Role of MHC in Determining Susceptibility to Disease[2]

In infections involving noncytopathic viruses, the host cell is not destroyed by the virus directly, but rather by the immune response. Severity of disease in these latter infections, such as hepatitis B virus infec-

Table 2. Protection against Lethal LCM by Immunization with Recombinant Vaccinia Viruses Expressing Truncated LCMV-NP Genes

Mice immunized with	ICR (H-2^q)		C57BL/6 (H-2^b)	
	mortality	target	mortality	target
Uninfected	100%	−	100%	−
Vaccinia WR	100%	−	100%	−
NP6 (a.a. 1–558)	17%	+	0%	+
NP5 (a.a. 1–410)	n.t.	+	60%	+
NP4 (a.a. 1–375)	n.t.	+	100%	−
NP3 (a.a. 1–259)	n.t.	+	100%	−
NP2 (a.a. 1–202)	20%	+	100%	−
NP1 (a.a. 1–103)	100%	−	100%	−

Groups of five mice were vaccinated by i.v. injection of 3×10^6 pfu of the different recombinant vaccinia viruses and were challenged 18–25 days later i.c. with 150 pfu of LCMV-WE. Uninfected and wild-type vaccinia virus WR immunized mice were analyzed as controls. The coding capacity for nucleoprotein (complete 558 a.a.) of the different recombinant vaccinia viruses (NP1–NP6) is indicated. Lethal LCM occurred in all cases before day 9. Indicated for each recombinant vaccinia virus is its ability (+/−) to form target cells for LCMV immune spleen cells. Data are summarized from Schulz et al. (1989).

Table 3. Antiviral Protection by Vaccination of H-2^q Mice with Recombinant Vaccinia Viruses Expressing LCMV NP Epitopes

Mice immunized with	Prevention of footpad swelling reaction	Viral titers in spleens (log$_{10}$ pfu)
LCMV-WE vaccinia NP6	0–10%	<2
(a.a. 1–558) vaccinia NP2	0–10%	<2
(a.a. 1–202) vaccinia NP1	0–10%	<2
(a.a. 1–103) vaccinia WR	60–80%	5–6
vaccinia WR	60–80%	5

Vaccination and challenge infection: See legend to Table 2. Mice were challenged into the footpad or i.v. Data summarized from Schulz et al. (1989).

tion in man (Bianchi 1981; Mondelli and Eddleston 1984) or LCMV in mice (Hotchin 1962; Lehmann-Grube 1971; Doherty, and Zinkernagel 1974), is determined by the balance between the kinetics of virus spread and the kinetics of the T-cell immune response. Mice infected intracerebrally (i.c.) with low doses of the LCMV isolate WE (LCMV-WE) usually develop a fatal T-cell-mediated choriomeningitis (Hotchin 1962; Lehmann-Grube 1971; Cole et al. 1972; Doherty and Zinkernagel 1974). This disease is strictly dependent on induction of virus-specific cytotoxic T cells (Cole et al. 1972); it does not develop in T-cell-deficient mice and may be adoptively transferred by cloned cytotoxic T cells (Doherty and Zinkernagel 1974; Baenziger et al. 1986). There is no evidence for a crucial involvement of antibodies in LCM. Mice infected with high doses of LCMV-WE i.c. do not develop lethal T-cell-mediated disease and survive for reasons as yet poorly understood. This "high-virus-dose-immune-paralysis" (Hotchin 1962; Lehmann-Grube 1971) is in some ways comparable to induction of a hepatitis B virus carrier status in adult humans. This state may be attributed to an immune suppressive action of LCMV (Mims and Wainwright 1968; Leist et al. 1988), to differential re-

[2]These studies were performed by T. Leist and S. Oehen.

cruitment of effector cells to sites other than the meninges (Doherty and Zinkernagel 1974; Pfau et al. 1982), or to the rapid selection of virus variants (Pfau et al. 1982; Ahmed et al. 1984).

After infection of mice with low doses (10^2–10^3 plaque-forming units [pfu]) of the LCMV-DOCILE isolate (kindly provided by C. Pfau, Troy, New York) or high doses (10^5–10^6 pfu) of this virus, mice develop a more or less severe hepatitis that may be monitored histologically or by measuring enzyme levels in serum that are known to be increased in parallel with liver cell damage (Bianchi 1981; Mondelli and Eddleston 1984; Zinkernagel et al. 1986).

The influence of major transplantation antigens on susceptibility to T-cell-mediated hepatitis caused by infection with the noncytopathic LCMV was evaluated in B10 H-2-congenic mice (Table 4). Susceptibility to early T-cell-mediated liver cell destruction (day 7–9) and early mortality (i.e., before day 12) was H-2D^q-linked and correlated directly with early (day 6–8) and high cytotoxic T-cell activity. In contrast, susceptibility to become an LCMV carrier, inability to rapidly clear virus, or development of late hepatitis (day 14–17) was linked to D^k and correlated with absence of early cytotoxic T-cell activity. Thus, H-2D-regulated T-cell immune responses controlling both virus spread and immunopathology may directly determine the type and severity of disease. The results also illustrate that susceptibility to disease caused by one virus may be linked to distinct MHC alleles dependent on the disease parameter studied.

An interesting and novel aspect of MHC-disease association was discovered in mice vaccinated with vaccinia recombinant viruses expressing LCMV GP or NP (Whitton et al. 1988b; Hany et al. 1989). The susceptibility of these mice to LCM was studied after i.c. infection with LCMV. Effective vaccination usually protects a host against cytopathogenic viral infection by triggering an appropriate cellular or humoral immune response (Notkins 1975; Möller 1983). Evaluation of protective capacity of vaccinia recombinant viruses revealed, as expected from cytotoxic T-cell data and from other in vivo studies (Lehmann-Grube 1971; Hany et al. 1989), that preimmunization of various strains of mice with either a vaccinia recombinant virus express-

Table 4. MHC-disease Association Depends on the Symptom Studied in T-cell-mediated Hepatitis Triggered by LMCV-DOCILE

Host response anti-LCMV-CTL	High virus dose injected (10^5–10^6 pfu)[a]				Low virus dose injected (10^2–10^3 pfu)			
	T-cell-mediated hepatitis[b]		virus clearance[c]	virus presence	T-cell-mediated hepatitis		virus clearance	virus presence
	early	late			early	late		
High responder[d] D^q	severe	absent	early	<14 d	very mild absent	absent	early	<8 d
Low responder D^k	absent	mild	late	>14 d	absent	severe	late	>14 d

[a]Mice were injected i.v. with the indicated numbers of pfu.
[b]Hepatitis was assessed by measuring liver enzyme concentrations in the serum of mice at various time points (for details, see Zinkernagel et al. 1986) and by monitoring liver sections histologically.
[c]Virus titers were determined by in vivo titration of liver cell homogenates as detailed by T.P. Leist et al. (in prep.).
[d]H-2 congenic B10 mice were used; B10.AKM (K^k D^q), B10.BR (K^{k}D^k). (Data modified from T.P. Leist et al., in prep.)

ing LCMV GP, LCMV NP, or with LCMV-WE protected mice against low-dose i.c. challenge (Table 5) in an H-2-dependent manner; unprimed or vaccinia-virus-primed mice were susceptible to low i.c. challenge and died. In contrast, mice of some strains survived high doses of LCMV-WE injected i.c. because of high-dose-immune-paralysis (Fig. 2). In the same mouse strain, the following paradoxical effects of vaccination were observed. B10.BR(H-2^k) mice respond with cytotoxic T cells specific for LCMV fragments coded for by the large viral 9S RNA segment and not (or very little) to GP or NP (Oldstone et al. 1988; Whitton et al. 1988b; Hany et al. 1989). B10.BR mice were protected from low doses of LCMV-WE i.c. by priming with LCMV-WE but not by vacc-NP, whereas C57BL/6 (H-2^b) mice were protected by LCMV-WE, vacc-NP, and vacc-GP. In contrast to relevant B10.BR controls that survived a high dose challenge, mice prevaccinated with vacc-NP died of LCM (Fig. 2). Comparable results were found for H-2^d mice. H-2^d mice have been shown to generate cytotoxic T cells mainly against NP determinants; accordingly, they were protected partially or completely by vacc-NP but not vacc-GP against low-dose challenge with LCMV-WE i.c. After immunization with vacc-GP, and in contrast to control mice, H-2^d mice succumbed, however, to high LCMV-WE i.c. challenge doses.

The findings in both model diseases may be interpreted as follows: The balance between virus spread and immune response seems to be influenced according to the following rules: High immune responsiveness will rapidly limit virus spread and therefore only cause limited T-cell-mediated host-cell destruction of virus-infected cells. However, absence of an immune re-

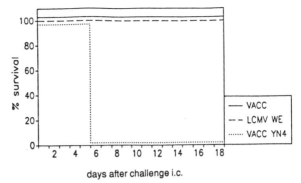

Figure 2. Susceptibility to immunopathological disease enhanced by vaccination. Six B10.BR mice were immunized i.v. with 2×10^6 pfu recombinant vaccinia virus expressing the LCMV NP (vacc-NP4), or with wild-type vaccinia virus (vacc), or with LCMV-WE (100 pfu). After 3 weeks, the mice were challenged i.c. with 10^4 pfu LCMV-WE. The time to death caused by LCMV was registered over a time period of 30 days.

sponse will result in a chronic virus infection or a virus carrier state of the host without overt disease because T-cell-mediated host-cell destruction cannot occur. In low responders, a protracted T-cell response will initially permit a wide spread of the virus and then cause destruction of many infected host cells. This may initiate inflammatory processes resulting in immunopathology progressing subacutely or chronically. These delicate host–parasite relationships are influenced by genetic factors of the host (including the MHC), by the virus (Zinkernagel et al. 1986), by the infectious dose, by the time after vaccination (i.e., the kinetics of immunological memory), by the immunocompetence of

Table 5. H-2 Dependence of Protection against Lethal Choriomeningitis Triggered by Intracerebral Injection of LCMV by Vaccination with Vaccinia Recombinant Virus Expressing the LCMV-GP or NP

Vaccination	Mouse strain (H-2K, D)	Major cytotoxic T-cell epitopes	Number of mice dead/injected	Mean time to death ±s.e.m.
Vaccinia	C57BL/6	GP+++	6/6	7.0 ± 0.2
Vacc-GP	(bb)	NP++	0/6	>20
Vacc-NP			0/6	>20
LCMV-WE			0/6	>20
None			6/6	7.0 ± 0.2
Vaccinia	B10.BR	epitope	6/6	7.3 ± 02
Vacc-GP	(kk)	coded by	6/6	6.0 ± 0.2
Vacc-NP		9s RNA	6/6	6.7 ± 0.2
LCMV-WE		GP −	1/6	19.0
None		NP −	6/6	7.0 ± 0.2
Vaccinia	DBA/2	NP+++	6/6	7.3 ± 0.2
Vacc-GP	(dd)	GP −	6/6	7.0 ± 0.3
Vacc-NP			0/5	>20
LCMV-WE			0/6	>20
None			6/6	7.0 ± 0.2

The number of mice indicated were vaccinated i.v. with 2×10^6 pfu recombinant vaccinia virus expressing either LCMV GP (vacc-GP, isolate vacc-G2), LCMV NP (vacc-NP, isolate vacc-NP6), vaccinia virus, or left unprimed. LCMV-immune mice were injected i.v. with 100 pfu LCMV-WE. After 24 days, mice were challenged i.c. with 200 pfu of a neurotropic LCMV (Amstrong). The time to death caused by LCM was registered over a time period of 20 days and the mean time to death ±s.e.m. of each group was calculated. The vaccinia recombinant viruses have been described in detail (Hany et al. 1989); vacc-G2 was a gift from D. Bishop, Oxford. The LCMV isolates were originally obtained from F. Lehmann-Grube, Hamburg (WE) (Lehmann-Grube 1971) and M. Buchmeier, La Jolla (Amstrong) (Buchmeier et al. 1980).

the host, and by many other factors. Vaccination may shift the balance from low- to high-responder status and thereby prevent immunopathologically mediated disease. However, vaccination may also enhance immunopathologically T-cell-mediated disease if a nonresponsive or very low responder host is vaccinated, because the balance is now shifted from an asymptomatic carrier status to a low or intermediate responder whose unfavorable balance between virus spread and immune response now favors development of immunopathological disease.

Analysis of Transgenic Mice Expressing a T-cell Receptor Specific for LCMV[3]

Transgenic mice were generated with T-cell receptor (TCR) $\alpha\beta$ genes originally isolated from a cytotoxic T-cell clone P14. This $CD8^+$ T cell clone recognizes LCMV GP in the context of H-$2D^b$. The α ($V_\alpha 2J_\alpha TA31$) and the β ($V_\beta 8,1D_\beta J_\beta 2.4$) TCR cDNA were cloned separately into an expression vector driven by a MHC class I promoter (Pircher et al. 1989). Both α and β constructs were coinjected into fertilized eggs of (C57BL/6 × DBA/2) F_2 mice. Transgenic offspring were mated with C57BL/6 (H-2^b) and BALB/c (H-2^d) mice. Heterozygote transgenics and transgene-negative offspring were analyzed in parallel. Because of the $V_\beta 8.1$ used, these transgenic mice express TCR specific not only for LCMV + D^b, but also for Mls^a (Kappler et al. 1988).

Thymocytes exhibited the following CD4/CD8 phenotypes (Table 6). Whereas control mice lacking the transgenes had 2% double-negative (DN) $CD4^-8^-$, 83% double-positive $CD4^+8^+$, 12% single $CD4^+$, and 3% single $CD8^+$ positive thymocytes, transgenic H-2^b mice possessed approximately 19% single $CD8^+$ versus 2% single $CD4^+$ positive T cells. The relative dominance of $CD8^+$ single-positive cells was also seen in lymph node cells (Table 7). Transgenic mice had 46% $CD8^+$ T cells (vs. 23% in controls), which expressed the transgenic $V_\beta 8$ chain to 94%. In contrast, transgenic mice possessed fewer $CD4^+$ T cells, i.e., 6% (of

which 70% were transgene $V_\beta 8$-positive). The skewing of T cells toward the $CD8^+$ subsets in TCR $\alpha\beta$ transgenic mice was only observed in H-2^b but not in H-2^d mice. The dominance of $CD8^+$ single-positive T cells reflects the origin of the transgenic T-cell receptor from a $CD8^+$- and H-2^b-restricted cytotoxic T-cell clone. These findings can be explained by mechanism of positive selection of T cells recognizing self-MHC molecules in the thymus. Similar results have been obtained with TCR $\alpha\beta$ transgenic mice by two other groups using H-Y-specific and alloreactive TCR (Sha et al. 1988b; Teh et al. 1988).

T-cell tolerance to LCMV was studied in P14 $\alpha\beta$ transgenic mice carrying the virus after neonatal infection. The following changes were seen in these LCMV-tolerant transgenic mice: Total thymocyte numbers were decreased to between 1% and 10% of control values (Tables 6 and 7). Transgenic LCMV carrier mice had fewer single $CD8^+$ and considerably more single $CD4^+$ thymocytes, whereas $CD4^+8^+$ double-positive cells were reduced by half. The $CD8^+$ peripheral T-cell subset was drastically reduced from 46% to 7% in transgenic carrier mice; of those, only 33% expressed $V_\beta 8$. $CD4^+$ peripheral T cells were present to about 5%, comparable to the 6% in control transgenes. Double staining with monoclonal antibodies specific for CD3, CD4, CD8, and TCR $V_\beta 8$ further revealed a larger number of double-negative $CD4^-8^-$ $CD3^+$ T cells (10–20%) that expressed the transgenic receptor. This result suggests that besides absence of transgenic receptor expressing $CD8^+$ T cells, failure to express CD8 may be an alternative pathway to achieve nonreactivity. This result complements data obtained in the H-Y and allo-MHC TCR transgenic models showing that T cells carrying a potentially autoreactive TCR are present but have down-modulated CD8 (Kisielow et al. 1988; Sha et al. 1988a). The double-negative ($CD4^-8^-$) T cells in the periphery are apparently different from those found in the thymus (Table 6). The 30–40% double-negative $CD4^-8^-$ thymocytes in the transgenic LCMV carrier mouse are high $CD3^+$ but are $V_\beta 8^-$ and TCR α,β^- and probably reflect the remaining number of δ^+ thymocytes that were not affected by tolerance induction. These results strongly suggest that immunological unresponsiveness to LCMV in the LCMV carrier mouse is due to clonal deletion of

---

[3]These studies were performed by H.P. Pircher and H. Hengartner with the generous help of the laboratories of Dr. Tak Mak, Ontario Cancer Institute, Toronto, and Dr. K. Bürki, Sandoz AG, Basel.

Table 6. Thymocyte Subsets in TCR $\alpha\beta$ Transgenic Mice

	Compartments				Number of thymocytes
	$CD4^-8^-$	$CD4^+8^+$	$CD4^+8^-$	$CD4^-8^+$	
Control	2%	82%	11%	3%	10×10^7
TCR $\alpha\beta$ transgenic	13%	66%	2%	18%	85×10^7
TCR $\alpha\beta$ transgenic Mls^a	12%	79%	4%	4%	20×10^7
TCR $\alpha\beta$ transgenic LCMV carrier	44%	31%	14%	9%	1×10^7

Single thymocyte suspensions of the indicated mice were stained with phycoerythrin-conjugated anti-CD4 (Becton Dickinson) and with fluorescein (FITC) conjugated anti-CD8 (Becton Dickinson) MAb. Two-color fluorescence analysis was performed on an EPICS Profile Analyzer and the percentages of single and double stained cells were calculated. The results of one representative set of experiments are shown.

Table 7. Lymph Node Cells in TCR $\alpha\beta$ Transgenic Mice

	CD4$^+$	CD8$^+$	CD3$^+$
Control	36%	23%	65%
% of the population expressing V$_\beta$8	12%	14%	13%
TCR $\alpha\beta$ transgenic	6%	46%	63%
% of the population expressing V$_\beta$8	69%	94%	94%
TCR $\alpha\beta$ transgenic LCMV carrier	5%	6%	33%
% of the population expressing V$_\beta$8	23%	33%	70%

Lymph node cells of the indicated mice were stained with anti-CD4, anti-CD8, anti-CD3, and anti-TCR V$_\beta$8 MAb and analyzed on an EPICS Profile Analyzer. The percentages of one representative set of experiments are shown.

LCMV-specific T cells in the thymus at the CD4$^+$8$^+$ stage. These findings in LCMV-tolerant transgenic mice are similar to those in the H-Y model (Kisielow et al. 1988) and contrast with those in Mls^a transgenic mice (Pircher et al. 1989); the latter exhibited about normal high levels of CD4^{++} and low levels of CD4$^-$8$^-$ thymocytes (Table 6). Thus, in the same transgenic mice expressing a TCR with the double specificity for LCMV + D^b and for Mls^a, tolerance induction to the two antigens differs drastically, probably reflecting different affinities of the TCR for the two antigens or distinct patterns of self-antigen expression in the thymus with respect to localization and possibly also with respect to kinetics of presentation during ontogeny.

The effector function of T cells from the transgenic mice has been analyzed in vitro and in vivo as summarized in Table 7. Upon stimulation in vitro with LCMV-infected macrophages, spleen cells or lymph node cells from transgenic mice but not from controls or trans-

Table 8. LCMV-specific Cytolytic Activity of Spleen Cells Derived from TCR $\alpha\beta$ Transgenic Mice

	Target cells	
Effectors	MC57G-LCMV	MC57G
Spleen cells activated in vitro for 3 days with LCMV-infected macrophages[a]		
control	–	–
TCR β transgenic mice	–	–
TCR $\alpha\beta$ transgenic mice	+++	–
Spleen cells from mice infected with LCMV on day -4[b]		
control	+	+
TCR $\alpha\beta$ transgenic mice	+++	–

Effector cells were tested in a ^{51}Cr-release assay for their cytolytic activity on LCMV-infected and noninfected MC57G (H-2^b) fibroblast target cells. Effector to target cell ratio was 10:1. Assay time 4–5 hr. Spontaneous release <25%. Specific lysis: – <10%, + <25%, +++ >60%.

[a] Spleen cells (5 × 10^6) from nonimmunized mice were cultured with 4 × 10^5 LCMV-infected macrophages for 3 days.

[b] Mice were primed with an i.v. injection of 10^6 pfu LCMV-WE 4 days before.

genic LCMV carrier mice generated cytotoxic T-cell activity within 2–3 days without previous priming in vivo. Similarly, transgenic mice but not normal controls generated high cytotoxic LCMV-specific T-cell activity within 4 days after infection in vivo. Preliminary studies revealed that the primary swelling reaction of footpads after local injection of LCMV was generated very rapidly in transgenic mice by day 3–4, peaking on day 4–5 and disappearing by day 7; control mice showed swelling first on day 6–7 that peaked on day 8–9 and disappeared by day 13–15. These observations fit the notion that virus replication locally in the foot recruits effector T cells rapidly in transgenic mice, similar to a mouse primed to LCMV some weeks previously (Hotchin 1971; Lehmann-Grube 1971; Doherty and Zinkernagel 1974; Buchmeier et al. 1980). Since virus is eliminated relatively rapidly, the swelling reaction disappears much more quickly when compared to the controls.

The transgenic mice expressing a TCR $\alpha\beta$ for LCMV + D^b and for Mls^a will obviously offer opportunities to study mechanisms and ontogeny of tolerance to viral antigens, to evaluate homing and effector function of antiviral effector T cells, and to analyze what kinds of signals (interleukins, cellular contacts, and triggering via cell-surface determinants) may activate transgenic T8 effector cell precursors in vitro and in vivo.

REFERENCES

Ahmed, R., A. Salmi, L.D. Butler, J.M. Chiller, and M.B.A. Oldstone. 1984. Selection of genetic variants of lymphocytic choriomeningitis virus in spleens of persistently infected mice: Role in suppression of cytotoxic T lymphocyte response and viral persistence. *J. Exp. Med.* **60:** 521.

Andrew, M.E., B.E.H. Coupar, D.B. Boyle, and G.L. Ada. 1987. The roles of influenza virus haemagglutinin and nucleoprotein in protection: Analysis using vaccinia virus recombinants. *Scand. J. Immunol.* **25:** 21.

Baenziger, J., H. Hengartner, R.M. Zinkernagel, and G.A. Cole. 1986. Induction or prevention of immunopathological disease by cloned cytotoxic T cell lines specific for lymphocytic choriomeningitis virus. *Eur. J. Immunol.* **16:** 387.

Bennink, J.R. and J.W. Yewdell. 1988. Murine cytotoxic T lymphocyte recognition of individual influenza virus proteins. High frequency of nonresponder MHC class I alleles. *J. Exp. Med.* **168:** 1935.

Bianchi, L. 1981. The immunopathology of acute type B hepatitis. *Springer Semin. Immunopathol.* **3:** 421.

Bishop, D.H.L. and D.D. Auperin. 1987. Arenavirus gene structure and organization. *Curr. Top. Microbiol. Immunol.* **133:** 5.

Bjorkman, P.J., M.A. Saper, B. Samraoui, W.S. Bennett, J.L. Strominger, and D.C. Wiley. 1987. The foreign antigen binding site and T cell recognition regions of class I histocompatibility antigens. *Nature* **329:** 512.

Buchmeier, M.J. and B.S. Parekh. 1987. Protein structure and expression among arenaviruses. *Curr. Top. Microbiol. Immunol.* **133:** 41.

Buchmeier, M.J., R.M. Welsh, F.J. Dutko, and M.B.A. Oldstone. 1980. The virology and immunobiology of lymphocytic choriomeningitis virus infection. *Adv. Immunol.* **30:** 275.

Burnet, F.M. and F.J. Fenner. 1949. *The production of antibody.* Macmillan, Melbourne, Australia.

Buus, S., A. Sette, S.M. Colon, C. Miles, and H.M. Grey. 1987. The relation between major histocompatibility complex (MHC) restriction and the capacity of Ia to bind immunogenic peptides. *Science* **235:** 1353.

Chakrabati, S., K. Brechling, and B. Moss. 1985. Vaccinia virus expression vector: Coexpression of galactosidase provides visual screening of recombinant virus plaques. *Mol. Cell Biol.* **5:** 3403.

Cole, G.A., N. Nathanson, and R.A. Prendergast. 1972. Requirement for thetabearing cells in lymphocytic choriomeningitis virus-induced central nervous system disease. *Nature* **238:** 335.

Doherty, P.C. and R.M. Zinkernagel. 1974. T-cell-mediated immunopathology in viral infection. *Transplant. Rev.* **19:** 89.

Earl, P.L., B. Moss, R.P. Morrison, K. Wehrly, J. Nishio, and B. Chesebro. 1986. T-lymphocyte priming and protection against leukemia by vaccinia-retrovirus *env* gene recombinant. *Science* **234:** 728.

Guillet, J.G., M.-Z. Lai, Th.J. Briner, S. Buus, A. Sette, H.M. Grey, J.A. Smith, and M.L. Gefter. 1987. Immunological self, nonself discrimination. *Science* **235:** 865.

Hany, M., S. Oehen, M. Schulz, H. Hengartner, M. Mackett, D.H.L. Bishop, and R.M. Zinkernagel. 1989. Anti-viral protection and prevention of lymphocytic choriomeningitis or of the local footpad swelling reaction in mice by immunisation with vaccinia-recombinant virus expressing LCMV-WE nucleoprotein or glycoprotein. *Eur. J. Immunol.* **19:** 417.

Hedrick, S.M., D.I. Cohen, E.A. Nielsen, and M.M. Davis. 1984. Isolation of cDNA clones encoding T cell-specific membrane-associated proteins. *Nature* **308:** 149.

Hirsch, M.S., F.A. Murphy, H.P. Russe, and M.D. Hicklin. 1967. Effects of antithymocyte serum on lymphocytic choriomeningitis (LCM) virus infection in mice. *Proc. Soc. Exp. Biol. Med.* **125:** 980.

Hotchin, J. 1962. The biology of lymphocytic choriomeningitis infection: Virus induced immune disease. *Cold Spring Harbor Symp. Quant. Biol.* **27:** 479.

———. 1971. Persistent and slow virus infections. *Monogr. Virol.* **3:** 1.

Jonjic, S., M. Val del, G.M. Keil, M.J. Reddehase, and U.H. Koszinowski. 1988. A nonstructural viral protein expressed by a recombinant vaccinia virus protects against cytomegalovirus infection. *J. Virol.* **62:** 1653.

Kappler, J.W., U.D. Staerz, J. White, and P. Marrack. 1988. Self tolerance eliminates T cells specific for Mls-modified products of the major histocompatibility complex. *Nature* **332:** 35.

King, A.M., Stott, E.J., S.J. Langer, K.K.Y. Young, L.A. Ball, and G.W. Wertz. 1987. Recombinant vaccinia virus carrying the N gene of human respiratory syncytial virus: Studies of gene expression in cell culture and immune response in mice. *J. Virol.* **61:** 2885.

Kisielow, P., H. Blüthmann, U.D. Staerz, M. Steinmetz, and H. von Boehmer. 1988. Tolerance in T cell receptor transgenic mice involves deletion of nonmature CD4[+]8[+] thymocytes. *Nature* **333:** 742.

Lehmann-Grube, F. 1971. Lymphocytic choriomeningitis virus. *Virol. Monogr.* **10:** 1.

Leist, T.P., M. Eppler, E. Rüedi, and R.M. Zinkernagel. 1988. Virus triggered AIDS in mice is a T cell mediated immunopathology caused by virus-specific cytotoxic T cells: Prevention by tolerance or by treatment with anti-CD8 antibodies. *J. Exp. Med.* **167:** 1749.

Mackett, M., G.L. Smith, and B. Moss. 1985. The construction and characterization of vaccinia virus recombinants expressing foreign genes. In *DNA cloning* (ed. D. Glover), p. 191. IRL Press, Oxford.

Marker, O. and M. Volkert. 1973. Studies on cell-mediated immunity to lymphocytic choriomeningitis virus in mice. *J. Exp. Med.* **137:** 1511.

Martin, S. and B.T. Rouse. 1987. The mechanisms of antiviral immunity induced by a vaccinia virus recombinant expressing Herpes simplex virus type I glycoprotein D: Clearance of local infection. *J. Immunol.* **138:** 3431.

Mims, C.A. and S. Wainwright. 1968. The immunodepressive action of lymphocytic choriomeningitis virus in mice. *J. Immunol.* **101:** 717.

Mondelli, M. and A.L.W.F. Eddleston. 1984. Mechanisms of liver cell injury in acute and chronic hepatitis B. *Semin. Liver Dis.* **4:** 47.

Möller, G. 1983. HLA and disease susceptibility. *Immunol. Rev.* **70:** 5.

Notkins, A.L. 1975. *Viral immunology and immunopathology.* Academic Press, New York.

Oldstone, M.B.A. and F.J. Dixon. 1967. Lymphocytic choriomeningitis: Production of anti-LCM antibody by "tolerant" LCM-infected mice. *Science* **158:** 1193.

———. 1970. Tissue injury in lymphocytic choriomeningitis viral infection: Virus-induced immunologically specific release of a cytotoxic factor from immune lymphoid cells. *Virology* **42:** 805.

Oldstone, M.B.A., J.L. Whitton, H. Lewicki, and A. Tishon. 1988. Fine dissection of a nine amino acid glycoprotein epitope, a major determinant recognized by lymphocytic choriomeningitis virus-specific class-1-restricted H-2Db cytotoxic T lymphocytes. *J. Exp. Med.* **168:** 559.

Panicali, D., S.W. Davis, R.L. Weinberg, and E. Paoletti. 1983. Construction of live vaccines by using genetically engineered poxviruses: Biological activity of recombinant vaccinia virus expressing influenza virus hemagglutinine. *Proc. Natl. Acad. Sci.* **80:** 5364.

Pfau, C.J., J.K. Valenti, D.C. Pevear, and K.D. Hunt. 1982. Lymphocytic choriomeningitis virus killer T cells are lethal only in weakly disseminated infections. *J. Exp. Med* **156:** 79.

Pircher, H.P., T.W. Mak, R. Lang, W. Ballhausen, E. Rüedi, H. Hengartner, R.M. Zinkernagel, and K. Bürki. 1989. T cell tolerance to Mls[a] encoded antigens in T cell receptor β-chain transgenic mice. *EMBO J.* **8:** 719.

Romanowski, V., Y. Matsuura, and D.H.L. Bishop. 1985. Complete sequence of the S RNA of lymphocytic choriomeningitis virus (WE strain) compared to that of Pichinde arenavirus. *Virus Res.* **3:** 101.

Rowe, W.P. 1954. Studies on pathogenesis and immunity in lymphocytic choriomeningitis infection of the mouse. *Navy Res. Rep.* **12:** 167.

Rupprecht, C.E., T.J. Wiktor, D.V. Johnston, A.N. Hamir, B. Dietzschold, W.H. Wunner, L.T. Glickman, and H. Koprowski. 1986. Oral immunization and protection of raccoons (*Procyon lotor*) with a vaccinia-rabies glycoprotein recombinant virus vaccine. *Proc. Natl. Acad. Sci.* **83:** 7947.

Schulz, M., P. Aichele, M. Vollenweider, F.W. Bobe, F. Cardinaux, H. Hengartner, and R.M. Zinkernagel. 1989. MHC dependent T cell epitopes of LCMV nucleoprotein and their protective capacity against viral disease. *Eur. J. Immunol.* (in press).

Sha, W.C., C.A. Nelson, R.D. Newberry, D.M. Kranz, J.H. Russel, and D.Y. Loh. 1988a. Selective expression of an antigen receptor on CD8-bearing T lymphocytes in transgenic mice. *Nature* **334:** 271.

Southern, P.J and D.H.L. Bishop. 1987. Sequence comparison among arena viruses. *Curr. Top. Microbiol. Immunol.* **133:** 19.

Teh, H.S., P. Kisielow, B. Scott, H. Kishi, Y. Uematsu, H. Blüthmann, and H. von Boehmer. 1988. Thymic major histocompatibility complex antigens and the α β T cell receptor determine the CD4/CD8 phenotype of T cells. *Nature* **335:** 229.

Townsend, A.R.M., J. Rothbard, F.M. Gotch, G. Bahadur, D. Wraith, and A.J. McMichael. 1986. The epitopes of influenza nucleoprotein recognized by cytotoxic T lymphocytes can be defined with short synthetic peptides. *Cell* **44:** 959.

Toyonaga, B., Y. Yanagi, N. Suciu-Foca, M. Minden, and T.W. Mak. 1984. Rearrangements of T-cell receptor gene YT35 in human DNA from thymic leukemia T-cell lines and functional T-cell clones. *Nature* **311:** 385.

Traub, E. 1936. Persistence of lymphocytic choriomeningitis virus in immune animals and its relation to immunity. *J. Exp. Med.* **63:** 847.

Whitton, J.L., P.J. Southern, and M.B.A. Oldstone. 1988a. Analyses of the cytotoxic T lymphocyte responses to glycoprotein and nucleoprotein components of lymphocytic choriomeningitis virus. *Virology* **163:** 321.

Whitton, J.L., J.R. Gebhard, H. Lewicki, A. Tishon, and M.B. Oldstone. 1988b. Molecular definition of a major cytotoxic T-lymphocyte epitope in the glycoprotein of lymphocytic choriomeningitis virus. *J. Virol.* **62:** 687.

Yewdell, J.W., J.R. Bennink, G.L. Smith, and B. Moss. 1985. Influenza A virus nucleoprotein is a major target antigen for cross-reactive anti-influenza A virus cytotoxic T lymphocytes. *Proc. Natl. Acad. Sci.* **82:** 1785.

Zinkernagel, R.M. and P.C. Doherty. 1974. Restriction of in vitro T cell mediated cytotoxicity in lymphocytic choriomeningitis within a syngeneic or semiallogeneic system. *Nature* **248:** 701.

Zinkernagel, R.M., G.N. Callahan, A. Althage, S. Cooper, J.W. Streilein, and J.J. Klein. 1978. The lymphoreticular system in triggering virus-plus-self-specific cytotoxic T cells: Evidence for T help. *J. Exp. Med.* **147:** 897.

Zinkernagel, R.M., E. Haenseler, T.P. Leist, A. Cerny, H. Hengartner, and A. Althage. 1986. T cell mediated hepatitis in mice infected with lymphocytic choriomeningitis virus. *J. Exp. Med.* **164:** 1075.

Evolution, Function, and Utilization of Major Histocompatibility Complex Polymorphism in Autoimmune Disease

H.O. McDevitt,[*][†] D.C. Wraith,[*] D.E. Smilek,[*] A.S. Lundberg,[*] and L. Steinman[‡]

Departments of Microbiology and Immunology and †Medicine; ‡Departments of Neurology, Pediatrics, and Genetics, Stanford University School of Medicine, Stanford, California 94305

Initiation of the immune response to foreign protein antigens and, presumably, to self-protein antigens in the case of autoimmunity is the result of an initial interaction with a peptide fragment of the protein antigen and a major histocompatibility complex (MHC) class II molecule. Following binding of a degraded peptide fragment of the protein in the active binding site of the class II molecule, recognition of this complex by T cells with complementary T-cell receptors initiates the development of memory helper T cells and triggers the proliferation of both T-cell and B-cell immune responses to the degraded fragments of the antigen and to the intact three-dimensional protein (Moller 1987).

The immunogenicity of a particular protein and the selection of the immunodominant peptide fragments of that protein in a given individual are determined, in large part, by the amino acid sequences of the α and β chains making up the class II molecules of the individual (Schwartz 1986). Thus, the ability to generate a specific immune response to a particular peptide and susceptibility to a variety of autoimmune diseases in mouse and humans are, in part, functions of the allelic polymorphism of class II MHC molecules (Schwartz 1986; Todd et al. 1988).

Nucleotide Sequence Comparisons

Allelic comparison of class II molecules in mouse and man indicates that this polymorphism is strongly selected for, as indicated by a very high replacement to silent substitution ratio in compared nucleotide sequences (Benoist et al. 1983; Figueroa et al. 1988). Allelic comparisons within a species show that much of the polymorphism within the species is generated by genetic interchange between alleles of the same locus, as well as some instances of genetic interchange between alleles at two closely related loci (e.g., $DR_\beta I$ and $DR_\beta III$). This genetic interchange almost always involves an en bloc exchange of the complete allelic hypervariable region sequence of one or more of the three/four allelic hypervariable region sequences in the first domain of class II α and β chains (Bell et al. 1987).

The extraordinary polymorphism of class I and II MHC loci, and their remarkable sequence divergence, have raised the issue of whether MHC polymorphism is initiated anew within each species following the specia-

tion event or is inherited from preceding species. Recent studies have shown that polymorphisms found in the mouse are also found in species diverging from *Mus musculus* 3–5 million years ago (Figueroa et al. 1988). Similarly, chimpanzees have many of the same class I polymorphisms found in humans (Lawlor et al. 1988).

A comparison of amino acid sequences for several alleles of homologous murine and human class II α and β chains shows considerable sequence homology in the framework regions but marked sequence divergence in the allelic hypervariable regions encoding the polymorphic residues lining the floor and sides of the peptide-binding site of class II molecules (Brown et al. 1988).

When comparisons of single allelic hypervariable region sequences are made, however, striking similarities can be observed between the sequences from DR β chains and the corresponding sequences of particular alleles of the I-E β chains in the mouse. Several of these allelic hypervariable region sequence similarities are presented in Table 1. Thus, when comparisons are made at the level of individual allelic hypervariable regions, several examples can be identified in which the sequence is nearly identical in the two species.

To test the hypothesis that individual allelic hypervariable region sequences in man are directly descended from the same sequences in the mouse, we compared codon usage for each of the allelic hypervariable region pairs in which the sequences were identical in four or five residues of the hypervariable region. Similar comparisons were made for an immediately adjacent stretch of framework (constant region) amino acid sequence of length similar to the length of the allelic hypervariable region sequence. Table 2 presents

Table 1. Allelic Hypervariable Region Sequence Similarities between Murine and Human Class II β Chains

Region[a]	Position	DR_β[b]	E_β[c]
HVR$_1$	9–13	EYSTS[3]	EYVTS[d]
HVR$_2$	26–30	FLERY[3]	FLERF[d]
HVR$_3$	67–71	LLEQR[4,1]	FLEQR[s]

[a](HVR) Hypervariable region.
[b]The number next to a sequence indicates the HLA-$DR_\beta I$ or -$DR_\beta III$ alleles in which the sequence occurs.
[c]The lowercase letter next to the sequence indicates the I-A$_\beta$ allele in which the sequence occurs.

Table 2. Codon Usage Comparison for Similar Murine and Human Allelic Hypervariable Region Sequences

Region[a]	#[b]	Nucleotide differences[c]		Codon match[d]	
		observed average	expected average	observed	expected
HVR$_1$	3	3.6	4.6	0.4	0.147
Const$_1$	2	1.5	4	0.7	0.157
HVR$_2$	1	1	4	0.833	0.28
Const$_2$	1	1	5	0.833	0.229
HVR$_3$	2	2	3	0.5	0.178
Const$_3$	1	0	3	1.0	0.489
HVR$_4$	4	3.75	7.75	0.687	0.14
Const$_4$	2	3	6	0.625	0.222

[a](HVR) Hypervariable region; (Const) constant region.

[b]Number of comparisons made between mouse and human sequences for a particular hypervariable or constant region adjacent to it.

[c]Number of nucleotides differing between compared sequences.

[d]Frequency of codon identity for each amino acid in a compared sequence for those positions in which amino acids were identical between mouse and human. (Observed) The frequency of identical codons/sequence length; (expected) $1/\text{len.seq.} \sum_{m=1}^{\text{len.seq}} (1/\text{degen} \sum_{n=1}^{\text{aa deference}} \text{freq1 (aa}_m, \text{codon}_n) \text{freq2 (aa}_m, \text{codon}_n))$.

an analysis of these nucleotide sequence comparisons. The observed codon match is compared with the expected frequency of codon identity if the murine and human sequences were not related by direct descent but, instead, arose by convergent evolution. In the latter case, allowing for codon usage, all possible combinations of codons could be expected. As Table 2 shows, the frequency of codon matching is uniformly higher than expected on the basis of random codon usage to generate the second sequence. Codon match frequency is similar when comparing either hypervariable region sequences or adjacent constant region sequences and exceeds the expected frequency based on random codon usage by the same amount for allelic hypervariable regions and constant region sequences.

When these values are subjected to a chi-square test, $0.01 > p > 0.005$ for identical codon usage at positions where the amino acid is identical. These results clearly indicate that when comparison is made between human and mouse allelic hypervariable region sequences, codon usage shows that the human sequence is a direct descendant of the murine sequence. Thus, although much of the polymorphism within a species is generated by genetic interchange between alleles of the species, the interchangeable units (the allelic hypervariable regions) have been conserved in evolution over much longer periods of time than would have been suspected previously. This, in turn, indicates that there is strong selection for the maintenance in the population of particular allelic hypervariable region sequences and for generation of polymorphism by generating alternate combinations by genetic interchange. Examination of hypervariable sequences indicates that they are rich in charged and hydrophobic amino acids. Because their position in the class II peptide-binding site places them on the floor or along the sides of the peptide-binding groove, these residues play a critical role in the nature of the peptides that can be bound in a particular peptide-binding site.

These findings have considerable significance for the role of MHC class II polymorphisms in susceptibility to autoimmune disease. Analysis of MHC susceptibility haplotypes in patients with type-1 insulin-dependent diabetes mellitus (IDDM), rheumatoid arthritis (RA), and pemphigus vulgaris (PV) indicates that these short allelic hypervariable region sequences play a major role in susceptibility to each of these autoimmune diseases (Todd et al. 1987, 1988; Scharf et al. 1988; Sinha et al. 1988). In each of these diseases, susceptibility and, in some cases, resistance to a particular autoimmune disease is associated with a particular allelic hypervariable region sequence that is shared by several HLA-DR or -DQ alleles. Thus, it seems likely that by conferring the ability to bind a particular self-peptide with a high affinity, a particular allelic hypervariable region sequence confers susceptibility to a particular autoimmune disease. Clearly, other polymorphic residues lining the peptide-binding groove of a class II molecule may also play a role, so it is likely that the allelic hypervariable region sequences associated with disease susceptibility in population studies may have their effects modified by other parts of the α- and/or β-chain sequences.

Knowledge of the alleles and allelic hypervariable region sequences that predispose to autoimmune disease can be used in strategies designed to prevent or treat these diseases. In these strategies, the three-way interaction between MHC molecules, peptides, and T-cell receptors (TCRs) can be attacked at several points. For those situations in which TCR V_α or V_β gene usage is restricted to one or several V genes, antibodies to the V_α or V_β gene product can be used to treat or prevent the autoimmune disease (Acha-Orbea et al. 1988; Owhashi and Heber-Katz 1988; Urban et al.

1988). However, in many diseases, the T cells capable of inducing the autoimmune disease may use multiple V_α and V_β genes (Sakai et al. 1988). In this case, an alternative approach to preventing or treating the autoimmune disease relies on developing blocking peptides with a high affinity for the peptide-binding site of the MHC susceptibility allele but with no cross-reactivity with the peptides responsible for inducing the autoimmune disease. This type of competitive inhibition has been demonstrated at two levels. Gefter and co-workers have shown that it is possible to inhibit T-cell activation in vitro through the addition to the system of peptides that compete with the specific T-cell antigen for MHC binding (Guillet et al. 1987). Furthermore, Adorini and co-workers have successfully blocked the in vivo priming of murine I-A^k-restricted T cells, specific for an epitope of hen egg white lysozyme, by coinjection of an excess of the homologous I-A^k-binding mouse (self) lysozyme peptide (Adorini et al. 1988).

One experimental model in which dominant peptide epitopes, TCR gene usage, and MHC susceptibility alleles have been clearly identified is experimental autoimmune encephalomyelitis (EAE) in the mouse. EAE can be induced by immunization with myelin basic protein (MBP) or with peptide fragments from MBP and is characterized by lymphocyte infiltration into the CNS resulting in demyelination and paralysis (for summary of the encephalitogenic peptides of MBP, see Fig. 1).

Our primary goal is to dissect T-cell recognition of the acetylated amino-terminal peptide (Ac1-11) from rat MBP. This peptide shares the first 9 amino acids with mouse MBP and is therefore able to induce encephalitogenic T cells in mice expressing I-A^u antigens. T-cell recognition of Ac1-11 is an important model for immune intervention in autoimmune disease, since this epitope is immunodominant for disease induction in both PL/J (H-2^u) and (PL/J × SJL) F$_1$ (H-2^{uxs}) mice,

even though the latter mounts a T-cell response to both Ac1-11 and 89-101. The ultimate goal of this work is to define MHC and TCR interaction determinants to design peptides that might inhibit the autoimmune response leading to EAE.

It has been shown previously that encephalitogenic T-cell clones from PL/J and (PL/J × SJL) F$_1$ mice use only four TCR types for recognition of Ac1-11. Nevertheless, these clones all displayed similar recognition patterns when tested on a panel of peptide analogs constructed by single amino acid substitution of the first 9 amino acids of Ac1-11. These data are summarized in Table 3. Most of the substituted peptides relative to the original Ac1-11 peptide stimulated encephalitogenic T-cell clones at the same concentration as the original Ac1-11 peptide. This showed that these peptides were still capable of binding to I-A^u and implied that substitution of residues 2, 7, 8, and 9 with alanine did not affect interaction with TCRs of the encephalitogenic T-cell clones. Substituting alanine for lysine at position 4, however, generated a heteroclitic peptide, Ac1-11[4A], which stimulated the T-cell clones much better than Ac1-11. On the other hand, substituting alanine for glutamine at position 3 (Ac1-11[3A]) or proline at position 6 (Ac1-11[6A]) abolished the response of the clones to the peptide analogs.

To distinguish whether these differences in T-cell clone responsiveness to the analogs were based on MHC/peptide or TCR/peptide interactions, an MHC-binding assay was developed (Wraith et al. 1989). A radiolabeled, photoaffinity probe was designed that would bind and cross-link directly to I-A^u. The ability of an unlabeled peptide to inhibit binding of the probe then provided a measure of the peptide's ability to bind to I-A^u. Using this approach, Ac1-11[4A] was found to bind to I-A^u with an affinity greater than 10-fold higher relative to Ac1-11, providing an explanation for its heteroclitic stimulation of the T-cell clones. Ac1-

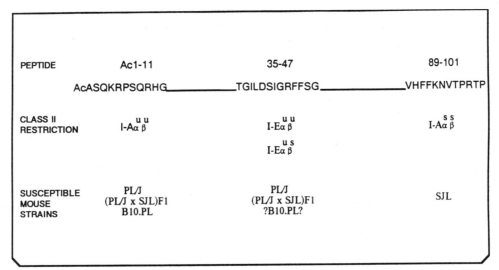

Figure 1. Amino acid sequences of MBP encephalitogenic peptides are listed with their corresponding restriction elements and susceptible mouse strains.

Table 3. In Vitro I-A Binding and T-cell Activation Properties of Ac1-11-substituted Peptides

		T-cell activation[a]	I-A^u binding[b]
Ac1-11	A S Q K R P S Q R H G	++	++
Ac1-11[1S]	S S Q K R P S Q R H G	+	n.d.
Ac1-11[2A]	S A Q K R P S Q R H G	++	n.d.
Ac1-11[3A]	A S A K R P S Q R H G	−	+
Ac1-11[4A]	A S Q A R P S Q R H G	++++	++++
Ac1-11[5A]	A S Q K A P S Q R H G	+	n.d.
Ac1-11[6A]	A S Q K R A S Q R H G	−	++
Ac1-11[7A]	A S Q K R P A Q R H G	++	n.d.
Ac1-11[8A]	A S Q K R P S A R H G	++	n.d.
Ac1-11[9A]	A S Q K R P S Q A H G	++	n.d.
1-11[4A]		++	++
1-11[3A, 4A]		−	++
Ac1-11[3A, 4A]		−	++++

Data for T-cell activation by substituted peptides [1A]–[9A] are summarized from Acha-Orbea et al. (1988).

[a]Sensitivity of H-2^u-restricted T-cell clone to different substituted peptides relative to the original Ac1-11 peptide.

[b]n.d. indicates not determined.

11[3A] and Ac1-11[6A] also bound to I-A^u, despite their inability to activate the encephalitogenic T-cell clones (Table 3). Subsequent lymph node proliferation studies showed that these two latter peptides activated T cells that were specific for the immunizing peptide and were not cross-reactive with the original Ac1-11 peptide. Further I-A^u binding experiments revealed the importance of the N-acetyl group for MHC interaction. Thus, nonacetylated peptide 1-11[4A] displayed reduced levels of binding relative to the heteroclitic Ac1-11[4A] peptide and was correspondingly less effective in T-cell activation (Table 3). Taken together, these data define the N-acetyl group and residue 4 as determinants important in I-A^u binding and residues 3 and 6 as determinants important in TCR interactions (Fig. 2).

In an extension of these findings, it has been possible to design a peptide with predictable properties. A peptide with substitutions at both positions 3 and 4 (Ac1-11[3A,4A]) retains the I-A^u-binding properties of the heteroclitic peptide Ac1-11[4A] and yet fails to activate encephalitic T cells (Table 3). This confirms the assignment of function to individual residues of Ac1-11 (Fig. 2). As a result of its increased affinity for I-A^u and its inability to activate encephalitogenic T-cell clones, peptide Ac1-11[3A,4A] should compete for recognition of the amino-terminal mouse MBP peptide and any other, as yet unidentified, I-A^u-binding encephalitogenic epitopes. Ac1-11[3A,4A] is currently being used to design strategies for therapy of established EAE to test whether or not competitive peptide binding to MHC is a feasible approach to immune intervention in human autoimmune diseases.

Ac1-11[4A] is heteroclitic both for I-A^u binding and T-cell activation (Table 3). Surprisingly, this peptide was a poor immunogen when tested in lymph node T-cell activation experiments in (PL/J × SJL) F$_1$ mice. Subsequent experiments have suggested that the

Determinants for TcR interactions

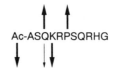

Ac-ASQKRPSQRHG

Determinants for MHC interactions

Figure 2. Arrows point from each amino acid residue of Ac1-11 to its role as either a T cell or an MHC interaction determinant.

heteroclitic analog induces a state of specific unresponsiveness in potentially encephalitogenic, Ac1-11-specific T cells in vivo. We have shown that on coimmunization with an encephalitogenic dose of Ac1-11, Ac1-11[4A] significantly inhibits the disease induced by injection of Ac1-11 alone (Wraith et al. 1989). Further experiments are required to establish whether the use of heteroclitic analogs will provide an alternative means of immune intervention through the use of synthetic peptides.

In summary, it is clear that definition of T-cell recognition at the molecular level will provide novel approaches to immune intervention in autoimmune disease. Detailed characterization of disease-associated T-cell epitopes may well provide a way of predictably designing MHC blocking peptides, as shown here for the amino-terminal peptide of MBP. Furthermore, through the use of heteroclitic analogs, it may be possible to modulate the immune response to self-peptides and thus reduce the severity of autoimmune disease.

ACKNOWLEDGMENT

This research was supported by grants from the National Institutes of Health.

REFERENCES

Acha-Orbea, H., D.J. Mitchell, L. Timmermann, D.C. Wraith, G.S. Tausch, M.K. Waldor, S.S. Zamvil, H.O. McDevitt, and L. Steinman. 1988. Limited heterogeneity of T cell receptors from lymphocytes mediating autoimmune encephalomyelitis allows specific immune intervention. *Cell* **54:** 263.

Adorini, L., S. Muller, F. Cardinaux, P.V. Lehmann, F. Falcioni, and Z.A. Nagy. 1988. *In vivo* competition between self peptides and foreign antigens in T-cell activation. *Nature* **334:** 623.

Bell, J.I., D. Denney, L. Foster, T. Belt, J.A. Todd, and H.O. McDevitt. 1987. Allelic variation in the DR subregion of the human major histocompatibility complex. *Proc. Natl. Acad. Sci.* **84:** 6234.

Benoist, C.O., D.J. Mathis, M.R. Kanter, V.E. Williams, and H.O. McDevitt. 1983. Regions of allelic hypervariability in the murine Aα immune response gene. *Cell* **34:** 169.

Brown, J.H., T. Jardetzky, M.A. Saper, B. Samraoui, P.J. Bjorkman, and D.C. Wiley. 1988. A hypothetical model of the foreign antigen binding site of Class II histocompatibility molecules. *Nature* **332:** 845.

Figueroa, F., E. Gunther, and J. Klein. 1988. MHC polymorphisms predating speciation. *Nature* **335:** 265.

Guillet, J.-G., M.Z. Lai, T.J. Briner, S. Buus, A. Sette, H.M.

Grey, J.A. Smith, and M.L. Gefter. 1987. Immunological self non-self discrimination. *Science* **235**: 865.

Lawlor, D.A., F.E. Wared, P.D. Ennis, A.P. Jackson, and P. Parham. 1988. HLA-A and B polymorphisms predate the divergence of humans and chimpanzees. *Nature* **335**: 268.

McCaldon, P. and P. Argos. 1988. Oligopeptide biases in protein sequences and their use in predicting protein coding regions in nucleotide sequences. *Proteins Struct. Funct. Genet.* **4**: 99.

Moller, G. 1987. Antigenic requirements for activation of MHC restricted responses. *Immunol. Rev.* **9**: 1.

Owhashi, M. and E. Heber-Katz. 1988. Protection from experimental allergic encephalomyelitis conferred by a monoclonal antibody directed against a shared idiotype on rat T cell receptors specific for myelin basic protein. *J. Exp. Med.* **168**: 2153.

Sakai, K., A.A. Sinha, D.J. Mitchell, S.S. Zamvill, J.B. Rothbard, H.O. McDevitt, and L. Steinman. 1988. Involvement of distinct murine T cell-receptors in the autoimmune encephalitogenic response to nested epitopes of myelin basic protein. *Proc. Natl. Acad. Sci.* **85**: 8608.

Scharf, S.J., A. Friedman, C. Brautbar, F. Szafer, L. Steinman, G. Horn, U. Gyllensten, and H.A. Erlich. 1988. HLA Class II allelic variation and susceptibility to pemphigus vulgaris. *Proc. Natl. Acad. Sci.* **85**: 3504.

Schwartz, R.H. 1986. Immune response (Ir) genes of the murine histocompatibility complex. *Adv. Immunol.* **38**: 31.

Sinha, A.A., C. Brautbar, F. Szafer, A. Friedmann, E. Tzfoni, J.A. Todd, L. Steinman, and H.O. McDevitt. 1988. A newly characterized HLA DQ β allele associated with pemphigus vulgaris. *Science* **239**: 1026.

Todd, J.A., J.I. Bell, and H.O. McDevitt. 1987. HLA-DQ B gene contributes to susceptibility and resistance to insulin-dependent diabetes. *Nature* **329**: 599.

Todd, J.A., H. Acha-Orbea, J.I. Bell, N. Chao, Z. Fronek, C.O. Jacob, M. McDermott, A.A. Sinha, L. Timmerman, L. Steinman, and H.O. McDevitt. 1988. A molecular basis for MHC class II-associated autoimmunity. *Science* **240**: 1003.

Urban, J.L., V. Kumar, D.H. Kono, C. Gomez, S.J. Horvath, J. Clayton, D.G. Ando, E.E. Sercarz, and L. Hood. 1988. Restricted use of T cell receptor V genes in murine autoimmunity encephalomyelitis raises possibilities for antibody therapy. *Cell* **54**: 577.

Wraith, D.C., D.E. Smilek, D.J. Mitchell, L. Steinman, and H.O. McDevitt. 1989. Antigen recognition in autoimmune encephalomyelitis and the potential for peptide mediated immunotherapy. *Cell* (in press).

Autoimmune Disease and T-cell Immunologic Recognition

L. Hood,* V. Kumar,* G. Osman,* S.S. Beall,* C. Gomez,*
W. Funkhouser,* D.H. Kono,† D. Nickerson,*
D.M. Zaller,* and J.L. Urban*

*Division of Biology, California Institute of Technology, Pasadena, California 91125; †Scripps Clinic
and Research Foundation, La Jolla, California 92037

The immune system has evolved T-cell receptors (TCRs) and B-cell receptors with exquisite specificity to distinguish self from nonself. On occasion, the immune system will attack self-components leading to autoimmune disease (for review, see Kumar et al. 1989). Approximately 4 years ago, we initiated studies of autoimmune responses based on several general concepts. First, it is clear that an understanding of the molecular features of immune recognition will be a key to understanding autoimmune responses since helper T (T_H) cells are pivotal in initiating most immune responses. Specifically, we focused our efforts on the trimolecular complex responsible for T_H-cell activation: (1) the TCR for antigen, (2) the antigen-presenting class II molecules encoded by the major histocompatibility complex (MHC), and (3) the peptide antigen (Fig. 1). Second, it is likely that the primary response to self-antigens may be limited, both with regard to the number of peptide epitopes employed for T_H-cell activation and in the diversity of the TCRs used for these responses. This hypothesis was based on our earlier studies on nonself-antigens and on the relatively limited receptor repertoire used for T-cell immune recognition of these antigens (Winoto et al. 1986). Finally, we felt that a detailed knowledge of the peptide determinants initiating a particular autoimmune disease along with the TCRs employed in triggering the autoimmune disease would lead to strategies for the elimination of the T_H-cell subsets responsible for autoimmunity. To examine these concepts in detail, we chose an autoimmune disease model in mice, experimental allergic encephalomyelitis (EAE). Although we will generally only discuss our own findings in detail here, many other laboratories have contributed to our understanding of EAE (e.g., Banerjee et al. 1988; see Fritz et al. 1983; Cohen 1986; Owhashi and Heber-Katz 1988; Burns et al. 1989; Wraith et al. 1989).

Experimental Allergic Encephalomyelitis

When certain inbred mouse or rat strains are immunized with myelin basic protein (MBP), they develop a chronic, relapsing demyelinating disease, EAE, (Pettinelli and McFarlin 1981; Fritz et al. 1985) that resembles multiple sclerosis (MS) in certain histological and pathological features (Raine et al. 1974; Wisniewski

and Keith 1977; Lassman and Wisniewski 1979). Disease transfer from afflicted animals to naive recipients can be accomplished by the transfer of cloned T_H cells in both rodent systems (Ortiz-Ortiz and Weigle 1976; Richert et al. 1979; Hold et al. 1980; Pettinelli and McFarlin 1981; Ben-Nun and Lando 1983; Houser et al. 1984; Mokhtarian et al. 1984; Zamvil et al. 1985; Sakai et al. 1986). Therefore, cloned T_H cells clearly

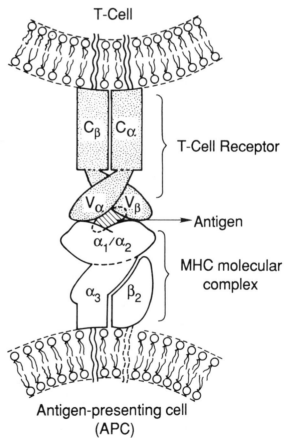

Figure 1. A diagrammatic representation of the trimolecular T-cell activation complex comprised of the TCR molecule, antigen, and MHC molecule. The V_α, V_β, C_α, and C_β symbols represent variable and constant regions, respectively, of α and β chains of the TCR. The α_1, α_2, and α_3 symbols represent the three heavy-chain domains, and β_2 denotes β_2-microglobulin of the class I MHC complex. (Reprinted, with permission, from Kumar et al. 1989.)

initiate EAE. Even more striking, in rats it is possible to give individual animals irradiated cloned disease-causing T_H cells that vaccinate and protect the animals not only against disease initiation by MBP but also against disease transfer by T_H cells (Ben-Nun et al. 1981; Lider et al. 1988). This latter observation suggested to us that the TCRs employed by the T_H cells initiating disease were highly restricted because the disease could be blocked, presumably as a consequence of immune response manipulation by the TCRs from a single irradiated T_H clone. Thus, the relative ease of disease inducibility, its simple identification, and the suggestions for a highly restricted T-cell response made EAE an ideal model for studying the molecular basis of autoimmune disease (Fig. 2).

MHC Restriction and EAE

Early studies of EAE established that only mice with particular MHC haplotypes are capable of responding to MBP (Gasser and Silvers 1974; Bernard 1976; Lando et al. 1976; Fritz et al. 1985). Experiments using pepsin fragments of MBP established that among these responder strains, mice of differing MHC haplotypes respond to distinct MBP epitopes (Fig. 3) (Pettinelli et al. 1982; Fritz et al. 1983). For example, mice of the H-2^u and H-2^k haplotypes respond to an amino-terminal pepsin fragment, whereas mice of the H-2^s and H-2^q haplotypes respond to a carboxy-terminal pepsin fragment (Fig. 3). These early studies were consistent with the notion that the ability of a particular peptide antigen to stimulate T_H cells depends at least in part on its

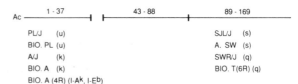

Figure 3. Pepsin cleavage fragments of MBP that induce EAE in mice. The susceptible mouse strains (H-2 haplotype in parentheses) are listed with the corresponding fragments that induce EAE on injection.

ability to interact with a particular class II MHC molecule. Furthermore, they demonstrated that EAE could be induced not only by immunization with the intact MBP protein, but also with the appropriate peptide fragments alone.

MBP Determinants Recognized by Encephalitogenic T_H Cells

To define more precisely the number and location of pathogenic MBP epitopes in mice, we synthesized a series of 16 overlapping peptides that together encompassed the entire MBP molecule. Each peptide overlapped with the preceding peptide by ten residues. These peptides were then injected individually into B10.PL and SJL/J mice to determine which fragments could (1) activate T cells and (2) induce EAE. In B10.PL mice, we found that four discrete peptides had the capacity to both activate MBP-specific T cells and induce EAE (D. Kono, unpubl.). In SJL/J mice only two peptide epitopes, each distinct from their B10.PL counterparts, activated MBP-specific T_H cells and induced disease (Fig. 4) (D. Kono et al. 1988; D. Kono, unpubl.) In contrast with the results with the synthetic peptides, virtually the entire T-cell response was directed against a single amino-terminal peptide fragment (MBP[1–20]) when B10.PL animals were immunized with the intact rat MBP (Urban et al. 1988). Similarly, responses in SJL/J mice were directed against only one of the two disease-causing peptide fragments from MBP (MBP[81–100]) (D. Kono, unpubl.). The explanation for the dominance of these epitopes is unknown, but it could arise from higher binding affinity of the dominant epitopes to MHC molecules, antigen processing which destroys subdominant epitopes, or a T-cell repertoire that produces higher-affinity receptors for dominant rather than subdominant epitopes. It is interesting to note that the total number of T-cell epitopes correlates with the number of class II MHC molecules expressed in each mouse strain. Thus, B10.PL mice with four MBP epitopes express two class II MHC molecules (I-A^u and

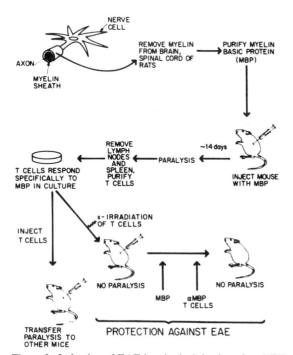

Figure 2. Induction of EAE in mice by injection of rat MBP, adoptive transfer of the disease with MBP-specific T_H cells, and vaccination against EAE with irradiated MBP-specific T cells.

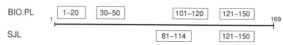

Figure 4. Synthetic peptides of MBP that both stimulate T-cell responses and induce EAE in B10.PL and SJL/J mice.

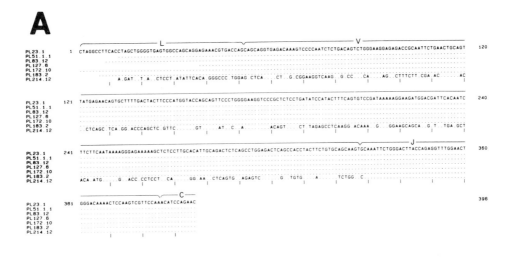

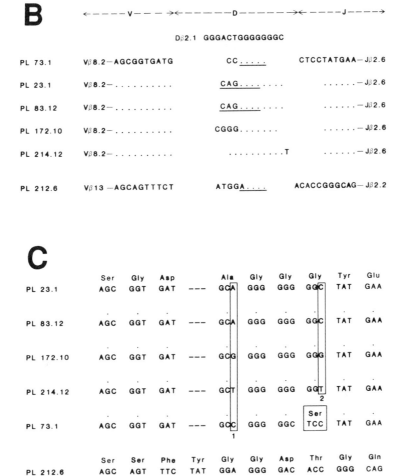

Figure 5. (*A*) Nucleotide sequences of TCRα cDNA clones derived from seven T_H hybridomas specific for the amino-terminal MBP peptide. The leader (L), variable (V), joining (J), and constant (C) regions are indicated. Dots indicate identity to the PL23.1 sequence. (*B*) The V_β junctional sequences from six T_H cells specific for the amino-terminal MBP peptide. Only nucleotides in and around the diversity (D) gene segment are shown. Dots in the V and J regions indicate identity to the PL73.1 sequence and in the D region to the D_β2.1 sequence. (*C*) Nucleotide sequences from *B* with their amino acid translations. Dots indicate identity to the β-chain sequence of T_H cell PL23.1. Vertical boxes indicate positions of degeneracy in the codons for amino acids flanking D-region-encoded residues. The square surrounds the only nonidentical amino acid among the five V_β8 sequences. (Reprinted, with permission, from Urban et al. 1988.)

I-E^u), and SJL/J mice with two MBP epitopes express a single class II MHC molecule (I-A^s). The important observation is that despite the existence of multiple peptide epitopes only a single epitope is primarily recognized upon injection of the whole MBP protein (Zamvil et al. 1986; Urban et al. 1988).

TCR Usage in EAE

After immunizing B10.PL mice with MBP, we generated 59 MBP-specific T$_H$ hybridomas (Urban et al. 1988). Consistent with the principle of immunodominance, we found that each of these hybridomas was specific for the amino-terminal MBP peptide epitope. The nucleotide sequences of seven (variable) V$_\alpha$ genes and six V$_\beta$ genes were determined (Fig. 5) and revealed three intriguing observations. First, V gene usage in MBP responses appears limited. Only two V$_\alpha$ and two V$_\beta$ gene segments are employed in this set of TCRs. Second, junctional regions (third hypervariable regions) that probably play a central role in antigen binding appear to be extremely conserved within a V subfamily. For the six V$_\alpha$2.3 genes derived from clonally distinct T cells, the junctional regions are identical. For the five V$_\beta$8.2 genes, despite considerable nucleotide variability, amino acid sequences are highly conserved with just a single glycine-to-serine substitution. Lastly, the V$_\alpha$ and V$_\beta$ regions are used in a combinatorial fashion with each α chain joining with either β chain. A more extensive analysis of 33 clonally distinct MBP-specific T$_H$ hybridomas supports the conclusion that only two V$_\alpha$ and two V$_\beta$ gene segments are used in these MBP responses. Once again, they are employed in a combinatorial fashion (Table 1). Thus, there appear to be four distinct types of MBP-specific T$_H$ cells in B10.PL mice (Fig. 6).

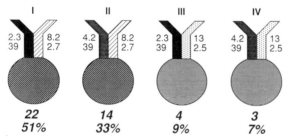

22   14   4   3
51%   33%   9%   7%

Figure 6. Schematic representation of the four different types of MBP-specific T$_H$ cells in B10.PL mice that are reactive with the amino-terminal immunodominant epitope of MBP. The types are defined on the basis of the combinations of α and β TCR chains (Urban et al. 1988). Bars represent TCR heterodimers with α chains on the left and β chains on the right. Numbers beside each bar indicate V and J gene segments (V on top, J on the bottom) constituting complete rearranged genes encoding each chain (D gene segments for the β chain are not shown). Circles with different shading represent T cells with different profiles of antigen fine specificity. (Reprinted, with permission, from Urban et al. 1989.)

Table 1. Summary of Gene Segment Use by T$_H$ Recognizing the MBP (1–9)NAc Encephalitogenic Peptide

α chain	
V$_\alpha$2.3	V$_\alpha$4.2
19	14
(58%)	(42%)
J$_\alpha$39 = 33(100%)	

β chain	
V$_\beta$8.2	V$_\beta$13
26	7
(79%)	(21%)
J$_\beta$2.6	J$_\beta$2.2
26	7
(79%)	(21%)

(Reprinted, with permission, from Urban et al. 1988.)

Molecular Dissection of an MBP Encephalitogenic Determinant

Of the amino-terminal peptide epitope, 39 variants were used to evaluate the key structural features crucial for binding to the MHC and TCR molecules (Table 2). Several conclusions have been reached from these studies (Urban et al. 1989).

First, MBP residues 1–6 constitute an antigenic core of the amino-terminal peptide determinant in H-2^u mice. We synthesized amino-terminal peptides for mouse MBP that were 5, 6, 7, 8, 9, 11, 16, 20, or 25 residues in length and then tested them for their ability to stimulate a representative B10.PL T$_H$ hybridoma 172.10 specific for the amino-terminal MBP epitope (Fig. 7). A progressive 11,000-fold increase in reactivity was seen between the 6-mer, the minimal length

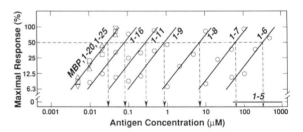

Figure 7. The effect of peptide length on the ability of synthetic amino-terminal MBP peptides to stimulate MBP-specific B10.PL T$_H$ cells. Numbers above the lines indicate the residues of native mouse MBP included in each peptide. T$_H$ cells from the B10.PL hybridoma 172.10 were incubated with varying concentrations of antigen and irradiated B10.PL spleen cells as a source of antigen-presenting cells. After 18 hr of culture, supernatants were transferred to the interleukin-2 (IL-2)-dependent cell line HT-2, and the [^{3}H]thymidine ([^{3}H]TdR) incorporation was determined as a measure of IL-2 release into the supernatant. [^{3}H]TdR incorporation was plotted on a logarithmic scale as a percentage of the maximal response. The maximal response for each stimulatory peptide ranged from 200,000 to 280,000 cpm. Each value represents the mean for six to eight individual experiments with in all cases the S.E.M. less than 10% of the mean. (Reprinted, with permission, from Urban et al. 1989.)

Table 2. Amino Acid Sequences of Synthetic Amino-terminal MBP Peptides

No.	Name	Sequence[a]
1	MBP(1–25)	Ac A S Q K R P S Q R S K Y L A T A S T M D H A R H G
2	MBP(1–5)	– – – – –
3	MBP(1–6)	– – – – – –
4	MBP(1–7)	– – – – – – –
5	MBP(1–8)	– – – – – – – –
6	MBP(1–9)	– – – – – – – – –
7	MBP(1–11)	– – – – – – – – – – –
8	MBP(1–16)	– – – – – – – – – – – – – – – –
9	MBP(1–20)	– – – – – – – – – – – – – – – – – – – –
10	MBP(1–9)Ala-1	– – – – – – – – –
11	MBP(1–9)Ala-2	– – A – – – – – –
12	MBP(1–9)Ala-3	– – – A – – – – –
13	MBP(1–9)Ala-4	– – – – A – – – –
14	MBP(1–9)Ala-5	– – – – – A – – –
15	MBP(1–9)Ala-6	– – – – – – A – –
16	MBP(1–9)Ala-7	– – – – – – – A –
17	MBP(1–9)Ala-8	– – – – – – – – A
18	MBP(1–9)Ala-9	– – – – – – – – A
19	MBP(1–20)Ala-1	– – – – – – – – – – – – – – – – – – – –
20	MBP(1–20)Ala-2	– – A – – – – – – – – – – – – – – – – –
21	MBP(1–20)Ala-3	– – – A – – – – – – – – – – – – – – – –
22	MBP(1–20)Ala-4	– – – – A – – – – – – – – – – – – – – –
23	MBP(1–20)Ala-5	– – – – – A – – – – – – – – – – – – – –
24	MBP(1–20)Ala-6	– – – – – – A – – – – – – – – – – – – –
25	MBP(1–9)Ala-3, 4	– – – A A – – – –
26	MBP(1–9)Ala-4, 5	– – – – A A – – –
27	MBP(1–20)Ala-1, 4	– – – A – – – – – – – – – – – – – – – –
28	MBP(1–20)Ala-3, 4	– – – A A – – – – – – – – – – – – – – –
29	MBP(1–20)Ala-4, 5	– – – – A A – – – – – – – – – – – – – –
30	MBP(1–20)Ala-4, 6	– – – – A – A – – – – – – – – – – – – –
31	MBP(1–9)Glu-3	– – – E – – – – –
32	MBP(1–9)Asn-3	– – – N – – – – –
33	MBP(1–9)Lys-5	– – – – – K – – –
34	MBP(87–98)	F K N I V T P R T P P P
35	MBP(10–20)	– – – – – – – – – – –
36	MBP(1–9:87–98)	– – – – – – – – – F K N I V T P R T P P P
37	rat MBP(1–11)	– – – – – – – – – H G
38	MBP[1–6:Ala(14)]	– – – – – – A A A A A A A A A A A A A A
39	MBP(1–6:8–25)	– – – – – – ( ) – – – – – – – – – – – – – – – – –

[a]Amino acid sequences are given in single letter code with the amino-terminal end of the peptide on the left. (Ac) Amino-terminal acetylation of Ala-1. Dashes indicate identity to the MBP(1–25) sequence. The sequences shown are those for murine MBP with the exception of the rat MBP(1–11) peptide (no. 37). (Reprinted, with permission, from Urban et al. 1989.)

stimulatory peptide, and the 20- and 25-mers, the maximal length stimulatory peptides. Identical results were obtained with seven other MBP-specific B10.PL hybridomas representing each of the four distinct T_H-cell types (see Fig. 6). Therefore, the 6-mer defines the "antigenic core region" (Reddehase et al. 1989) of the amino-terminal epitope of MBP.

Second, individual replacement of residues 1–6 with alanine, a structurally simple amino acid that should not affect the conformation of the main chain, affected the stimulatory ability of the MBP(1–9) peptide in one of three ways (Fig. 8). (1) Alanine substitutions at residues 3 or 5 completely abrogated the stimulatory capacity of these variant peptides, indicating that the corresponding side chains of the wild-type peptide are critical for interaction with the TCR, the I-A^u molecule, or both. (2) Substitution of residues 1, 2, or 6 rendered the variant peptides less stimulatory than the parent peptide. Therefore, the side chains of these residues are important but not essential for proper peptide interactions with the MHC and TCR mole-

cules. (3) Alanine substitution at position 4 increased the stimulatory ability of the variant peptide 500-fold over its wild-type lysine counterpart. Thus, the wild-type amino-terminal peptide can be further optimized regarding the activation of MBP-specific T_H cells.

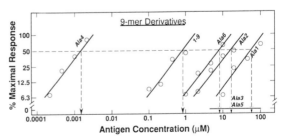

Figure 8. Single alanine replacement at positions 1–6 affects the stimulatory ability of the MBP(1–9) peptide. The maximal response for the Ala-4 peptide ranged from 300,000 to 360,000 cpm; the maximal response for the other stimulatory peptides ranged from 200,000 to 260,000 cpm. (For other details, see Fig. 7). (Reprinted, with permission, from Urban et al. 1989.)

Third, many amino acid substitutions at positions beyond the amino-terminal residue 6 serve to increase the stimulatory capacity of the core determinant. For example, maximal stimulation of the 172.10 hybridoma was induced when MBP residues 10–20 were substituted with MBP residues 87–98 that contain no sequence similarity to residues in the parent peptide at positions 10–20 (Fig. 9). Neither the MBP(10–20) peptide nor the MBP(87–98) peptide alone were stimulatory for MBP-specific T_H hybridoma cells. We also found that alanine substitution of residues 7, 8, or 9 of the MBP(1–9) peptide had only a modest effect on reactivity (Fig. 10). These residues appear similar to residues 10–20 in increasing the stimulatory capacity of the amino-terminal six residues in a manner that is partially independent of the specific amino acid side-chain interactions. Presumably, these residues, which we denote as the tail (e.g., residues beyond position 6), in some manner change the conformation of the core residues that exhibit specific interaction with TCRs and/or the I-A^u molecule.

Several lines of evidence indicate that this stimulatory effect is not totally independent of the primary amino acid sequence of the tail. (1) A deletion of residue 7 in the MBP(1–25) peptide totally abrogates its stimulatory ability (Fig. 11). (2) Addition of a 14-mer alanine tail onto the hexameric core determinant did not result in maximal activity (Fig. 11). (3) Rat and mouse MBP(1-11) peptides, which differ at positions 10 and 11, have different stimulatory abilities (compare Fig. 11 with Fig. 7).

Fourth, amino acid substitutions at position 4 of the amino-terminal epitope demonstrate that a single residue can dramatically affect T-cell activation (V. Kumar et al., in prep.). Lysine is the fourth residue of the wild-type epitope and has four methyl groups and a positively charged amino group. Substitutions of lysine with negatively charged smaller side chains (aspartic and glutamic acids) or with no side chain (glycine) have similar peptide activation properties to the wild-type peptide (Fig. 12), whereas substitutions with residues containing neutral side chains are more effective in T-cell activation than the wild-type lysine (glutamine, alanine, tryptophan, methionine, and valine). The MBP(1–9)Trp-4 peptide is also five- to tenfold better than the wild-type peptide in MBP-specific T_H hybrid-

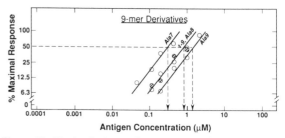

Figure 10. Single alanine replacement at positions 7–9 has a minimal effect on the stimulatory ability of the MBP(1–9) peptide. Cross-hatched data circles are for the unsubstituted MBP(1–9) peptide. For other details see Fig. 8. (Reprinted, with permission, from Urban et al. 1989.)

oma activation. The MBP(1–9)Val-4 and MBP(1–9)Met-4 peptides are 10-fold better than the MBP(1–9)Ala-4 peptide that is 500-fold greater in its stimulatory ability for T-cell activation than the wild-type peptide. These data suggest that the side chain at position 4 of the MBP(1–9) peptide contacts a hydrophobic region in the MHC or TCR molecule. It is interesting to note that eight of the nine position-4-substituted peptides can activate T cells equal to or better than the wild-type peptide. Since MHC molecules must accommodate a broad spectrum of peptides, it seems reasonable that the changes that result from side-chain diversity may arise from changes in interactions with the MHC molecule rather than the TCR with its exquisite specificity. In fact, competition experiments discussed below suggest that the variant peptides that have higher T-cell stimulatory capacities bind more effectively than their wild-type counterpart to the MHC molecule. As we shall see later, there is also evidence that side chains at position 4 can directly or indirectly affect interactions with the TCR.

Fifth, T-cell recognition of the MBP(1–20) peptide is qualitatively different from that of the shorter MBP(1–9) peptide. To assess these different activities of the 9-mer and 20-mer peptides, we tested the stimulatory abilities of derivatives of the MBP(1–20) peptide by introducing single alanine substitutions at positions 1–6 with the T-cell hybridoma 172.10. Similar to the results from MBP(1–9) derivatives, alanine substitution at residue 2 uniformly reduced activity, alanine replacement of residue 4 dramatically increased reactivity, and the

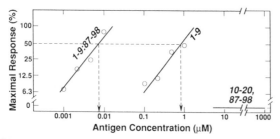

Figure 9. The MBP(1–9:87–98) peptide is highly stimulatory for MBP-specific T_H cells. For other details see Fig. 7. (Reprinted, with permission, from Urban et al. 1989.)

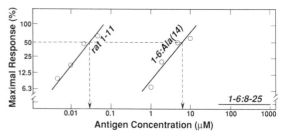

Figure 11. Effect of various tail sequences on the ability of the amino-terminal peptide to stimulate MBP-specific T_H cells. For other details see Fig. 7. (Reprinted, with permission, from Urban et al. 1989.)

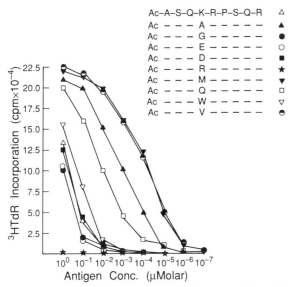

Figure 12. Effect of amino acid substitution at position 4 of the MBP(1–9) peptide on the stimulation of MBP-specific T_H cells. Peptide sequences are shown using single letter code. Horizontal lines indicate sequence identity to the wild-type MBP(1–9) peptide. For other details see Fig. 8. (Reprinted, with permission, from V. Kumar et al., in prep.).

alanine substitutions at residues 3 or 5 completely abrogated activity (Fig. 13). However, alanine replacement of residues 1 or 6 in the 20-mer peptide completely eliminated reactivity in contrast with findings with the 9-mer peptide (see Fig. 8). Moreover, fixed antigen-presenting cells present 9-mer and 20-mer peptides as described above, suggesting that antigen processing does not play a role in generating these differences. This suggests that the 20-mer peptide is presented differently within the MHC antigen-binding cleft than the shorter 9-mer peptide, so that some different side chains of the core region are more critical for TCR interactions and hence T-cell stimulation.

Sixth, altered MBP peptides, which apparently bind to the I-A^u molecule but do not stimulate MBP-specific T cells, can competitively inhibit T-cell reactivity in vitro. Nonstimulatory peptides when tested in a functional competition assay for T-cell stimulation may compete, implying that the peptide still binds to the I-A^u molecule and thus that the wild-type residue is

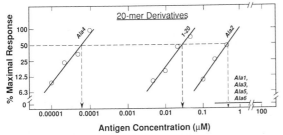

Figure 13. The ability of alanine-substituted derivatives of the MBP(1–20) peptide to stimulate MBP-specific T_H cells. For other details see Fig. 8. (Reprinted, with permission, from Urban et al. 1989.)

involved directly or indirectly in contacting the TCR, or fail to compete, implying that the peptide does not bind to the I-A^u molecule and thus that the substituted residue is involved directly or indirectly in contacting the I-A^u molecule. To categorize residues 3 or 5 of the 9-mer peptide and residues 1, 3, 5, or 6 of the 20-mer peptide in this manner, we tested their corresponding alanine-substituted derivatives for the ability to inhibit the T_H-cell response to the MBP(1–20) peptide in a functional competition assay. Using the 172.10 hybridoma, we first found that neither of the nonstimulatory derivatives of the 9-mer peptide were effective inhibitors. However, by replacing both positions 3 and 4 with alanine (MBP[1–9]Ala-3,-4), we found that the substituted 9-mer peptide could act as an effective inhibitor of T-cell reactivity to either the wild-type 9-mer or the 20-mer peptides (9-mer, not shown; Fig. 14A,B, 20-mer). In a similar fashion, we found that all four 20-mer derivatives with single alanine substitutions (positions 1, 3, 5, or 6) were capable of inhibiting T-cell reactivity (Fig. 14C,D). Some competitors are more effective than others. For example, the MBP(1–20)Ala-3,-4 peptide is roughly tenfold more effective as an inhibitor than the MBP(1–20)Ala-3 derivative (Fig. 14C,D). Two additional sets of experiments suggest that peptide inhibition is mediated at least partially through MHC binding. We have demonstrated that the MBP(1–20)Ala-3 peptide can block the stimulation of other T_H cells that also employ the I-A^u molecule for antigen presentation (Urban et al. 1989). McDevitt et al. (this volume) demonstrated direct binding of amino-terminal MBP peptides to the I-A^u molecule. Interestingly, no single residue of the MBP(1–20) peptide was found to be absolutely critical for binding to the I-A^u molecule (Urban et al. 1989). This observation is compatible with the idea that MHC molecules must bind a large number of different peptides.

Competitor peptides that are nonstimulatory but retain the ability to bind to class II molecules can be used to determine the relative binding affinity of stimulatory peptides for the same class II molecule. This affinity evaluation is based on their relative ability to inhibit the T-cell response in vitro. The data show a close correlation between the relative amount of competitor required for 50% inhibition (Fig. 15) and the stimulatory ability of each peptide (see Figs. 7, 8, and 10). This suggests that the ability of each peptide to bind to the I-A^u molecule is a major factor influencing T_H-cell stimulation.

Peptide and Antibody Therapy

Since we could effectively inhibit the in vitro B10.PL T_H-cell responses with variant peptides, we attempted to use such peptides as competitors during the priming of T-cells in vivo. The MBP(1–20)Ala-3 peptide was capable of suppressing the induction of T-cell responses to the MBP(1–9) peptide in both B10.PL and PL/J mice (Table 3). The degree of inhibition was dependent on the molar ratio of the competitor to the priming

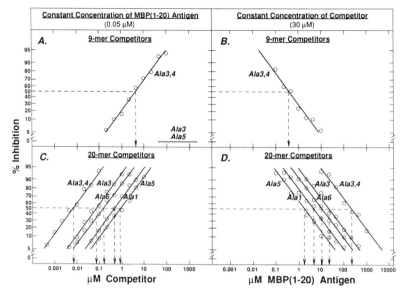

Figure 14. Dose-dependent competitive inhibition of the response to the MBP(1–20) peptide by nonstimulatory alanine-substituted derivatives of the MBP(1–9) peptide (A and B) or of the MBP(1–20) peptide (C and D). T_H cells from the B10.PL hybridoma 172.10 were exposed to varying antigen-to-competitor molar ratios under conditions where either the concentration of antigen (A and C) or that of the competitor (B and D) was held constant. Reactivity was plotted as a percentage of the maximal response on a probability grid that was calculated as follows: % inhibition = 100 × ([cpm without competitor − cpm with competitor]/cpm without competitor). Each value represents the mean for five to seven individual experiments with the S.E.M. always less than 10% of the mean. (Reprinted, with permission, from Urban et al. 1989.)

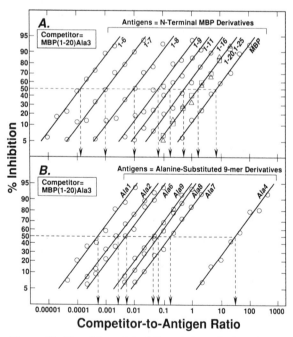

Figure 15. The differential ability of the MBP(1–20)Ala-3 peptide to inhibit competitively the B10.PL T_H cell response to stimulatory MBP antigens. (A) Native mouse MBP and synthetic amino-terminal derivatives encompassing the indicated residues of murine MBP. (B) Alanine-substituted derivatives of the MBP(1–9) peptide. Peptide antigens were used at twice the concentration required for half-maximal stimulation: peptides in A, see Fig. 7; peptides in B, see Figs. 8 and 10. For other details see Fig. 14. (Reprinted, with permission, from Urban et al. 1989.)

peptide and as noted earlier in vitro, the MBP(1–20)Ala-3,-4 derivative was more effective in blocking on a molar basis than the same peptide with a single alanine substitution at position 3. No inhibition was observed by the peptides MBP(31–50) or MBP(81–98), which are restricted to the I-E^u and I-A^s molecules, respectively (Kono et al. 1988; Zamvil et al. 1988). Furthermore, the MBP(1–20)Ala-3 peptide did not suppress T-cell responses to these peptides (Urban et al. 1989). This is consistent with earlier in vitro results that suggested inhibition is specific for the I-A^u molecule.

Since T-cell reactivity to MBP is key in initiating EAE, we tested whether inhibitory peptides could prevent EAE. Induction of EAE by the MBP(1–9) synthetic peptide was abrogated by the coinjection of the MBP(1–20)Ala-3 or MBP(1–20)Ala-3,-4 peptide derivatives (Urban et al. 1989) and the MBP(1–9)Ala-3, -4 or MBP(1–9)Ala-3,Met-4 peptides (V. Kumar et al., in prep.). Similarly, EAE induced by the intact mouse MBP protein was completely prevented by coinjection of the MBP(1–20)Ala-3,-4 peptide (Table 4).

Since approximately 80% of the MBP-specific T_H cells employ the $V_\beta 8.2$ gene segment (Fig. 6), we determined whether or not antibodies against the $V_\beta 8$ chain can be used to block EAE induction. The antibodies were given simultaneously with the MBP antigen. We observed a significant reduction in the incidence of EAE (93–57%) (Urban et al. 1988). It is possible that a complete abrogation of the disease could not be achieved because we did not have an antibody

Table 3. Nonstimulatory Amino-terminal Alanine Derivatives of MBP Inhibit the Induction of a T-cell Response to MBP In Vivo in B10.PL and PL/J mice.

Mouse strain[a]	Priming antigen			Competitor			[3H]TdR incorporation (Δ cpm ± s.e.m.)[b]	Inhibition (%)[c]
	peptide	MHC	nmole	peptide	MHC	nmole		
B10.PL	MBP(1–9)	I-A^u	80	none	—	—	54766 ± 6998	—
				MBP(1–20)Ala-3	I-A^u	80	19942 ± 4218	64
						320	4392 ± 2046	92
						1280	352 ± 525	99
				MBP(1–20)Ala-3,-4	I-A^u	80	1962 ± 1370	96
				MBP(31–50)	I-E^u	1280	52966 ± 3808	3
				MBP(81–98)	I-A^s	1280	57731 ± 11933	<0
	MBP(31–50)	I-E^u	80	none	—	—	68096 ± 10965	—
				MBP(1–20)Ala-3	I-A^u	1280	65280 ± 13806	4
PL/J	MBP(1–9)	I-A^u	80	none	—	—	83383 ± 15816	—
				MBP(1–20)Ala-3	I-A^u	1280	984 ± 1920	99
SJL/J	MBP(81–98)	I-A^s	80	none	—	—	48234 ± 6054	—
				MBP(1–20)Ala-3	I-A^u	1280	51866 ± 17050	<0
B10.PL	mouse MBP	I-A^u	8	none	—	—	35747 ± 5152	—
				MBP(1–20)Ala-3	I-A^u	1280	6434 ± 3560	82
				MBP(1–20)Ala-3,-4	I-A^u	1280	663 ± 448	98
				MBP(31–50)	I-E^u	1280	39892 ± 2454	<0
				MBP(87–98)	I-A^s	1280	34686 ± 7183	3

[a] Mice were immunized subcutaneously with the indicated amounts of MBP peptide or intact mouse MBP, alone or in combination with the indicated doses of MBP competitor peptides. The MHC restriction of each peptide is shown.

[b] Lymphocyte proliferation was determined 10 days after immunization by restimulating draining lymph node cells in vitro with an optimal concentration of the priming antigen (80 μM for MBP peptides and 4 μM for mouse MBP). Later (4 days) the cultures were pulsed for 18 hr with [3H]thymidine ([3H]TdR). The results are expressed as the difference in cpm between cultures with and without antigen, measured by [3H]TdR incorporation in triplicate cultures and expressed as the mean ±s.e.m. for six individual animals per group. The background incorporation for cultures without antigen ranged from 1500–9000 cpm. Responses to purified protein derivative of turberculin served as controls for the success of the immunization and ranged from 60,000 to 150,000 cpm for each individual mouse.

[c] The percentage of inhibition in [3H]TdR incorporation because of each competitor peptide was calculated as in Fig. 14. (Reprinted, with permission, from Urban et al. 1989.)

Table 4. Nonstimulatory Amino-terminal Alanine Derivatives of MBP Suppress the Induction of EAE in B10.PL and PL/J Mice

Mouse strain	Priming antigen			Competitor			EAE incidence[a]
	peptide	MHC	nmoles	peptide	MHC	nmoles	
B10.PL	MBP(1–9)	I-A^u	80	none	—	—	8/10
				MBP(1–20)Ala-3	I-A^u	80	5/8
						320	1/8
						1280	0/8
				MBP(1–20)Ala-3,-4	I-A^u	80	0/7
				MBP(31–50)	I-E^u	1280	6/7
				MBP(81–98)	I-A^s	1280	6/7
	MBP(31–50)	I-E^u	80	none	—	—	3/4
				MBP(1–20)Ala-3	I-A^u	1280	4/5
PL/J	MBP(1–9)	I-A^u	80	none	—	—	7/10
				MBP(1–20)Ala-3	I-A^u	1280	0/10
SJL/J	MBP(81–98)	I-A^s	80	none	—	—	5/6
				MBP(1–20)Ala-3	I-A^u	1280	5/6
B10.PL	mouse MBP	I-A^u	8	none	—	—	7/10
				MBP(1–20)Ala-3	I-A^u	1280	2/10
				MBP(1–20)Ala-3,-4	I-A^u	1280	0/7
				MBP(31–50)	I-E^u	1280	5/7
				MBP(87–98)	I-A^s	1280	5/7

[a] EAE was induced in separate groups of mice by injecting with MBP protein or peptides as above, except *Bordetella pertussis* was used as an additional adjuvant (10^{10} heat-killed organisms given intravenously 24 and 72 hr after the antigen). The data are expressed as the number of mice developing EAE/number of mice challenged. The mice were observed daily and graded on a 5-point scale. The average maximal severity and average day of onset of EAE (mean for mice that developed disease) ranged from 1.5 to 2.8 and 9 to 14 days, respectively, for each susceptible group. For other details, see Table 3. (Reprinted, with permission, from Urban et al. 1989.)

against the second minor V_β chain, $V_\beta 13$, that is also employed in the MBP-specific T cells (Fig. 6). An antibody to $V_\beta 13$ chains is now available, and experiments using both anti-$V_\beta 8.2$ and anti-$V_\beta 13$ antibodies are in progress.

The experiments described above suggest that either high-affinity Ia-blocking peptide variants or antibodies against the TCR may be useful in preventing the onset of autoimmune disease. However, we believe that ultimately antibody therapy against TCRs offer several significant advantages over peptide therapy. First, the antibody therapy uses the exquisite specificity of the immune system to delete only a small subset of antigen-specific T cells from the entire repertoire. Indeed, in humans, antibodies against particular TCR V_α or V_β subfamilies may delete up to several percent of the T cells present, and the hope is that antibodies against particular V segments can be raised (as has been done with the $V_\beta 8.2$ segment in mice), thus providing even greater specificity. The antibody therapy approach is thus a far more specific deletion process than is achieved by the current methods using steroids, cyclosporin, or cytotoxic reagents that suppress or kill nonspecifically very large numbers of lymphocytes. Indeed, the antibody therapy has an additional advantage in that specific antibodies to the α and β chains can be used concurrently as independent reagents to remove the autoimmune effector cells. Furthermore, antibodies to TCRs appear to delete the corresponding cells for long periods of time. Initial studies in mice suggest that these reactive T_H-cell populations can be completely deleted for up to 6 weeks after a single antibody treatment (J. Urban, unpubl.). Thus, antibody-mediated attempts to remove the offending subset of lymphocytes may be very long term. Antibodies may also have the capacity, at least in some cases, to reverse ongoing disease (Acha-Orbea et al. 1988). Therefore, antibod-

ies may be useful in the reversal of active on-going disease as well as prevention. Finally, systems are now being developed for the generation of human monoclonal antibodies that should circumvent at least some of the difficulties in repeated injection of xenogeneic antibodies (McCune et al. 1988).

The major objection to peptides blocking class II molecules is that they lack the specificity of antibodies. Our own data (Urban et al. 1989; V. Kumar et al., in prep.) and those of other investigators (Buus et al. 1987) suggest that such peptides nonspecifically block presentation of other antigens restricted to the same MHC molecule. Because of the limited number of MHC molecules present in each individual and the large number of peptide fragments they must interact with, this may present a significant restraint on peptide therapy. Second, our results indicate that treatment with blocking peptides, like anti-class-II antibodies, have limited efficiency. This therapy is restricted to early stages of the disease, particularly the inductive phase when pathogenic T_H cells are first stimulated and before they have triggered the subsequent autoimmune process (Urban et al. 1989; V. Kumar et al., in prep.). Finally, it is expected that comparatively high concentrations of class-II-blocking peptides may be required on a routine basis to prevent disease. Several approaches could be used to counteract, at least in part, these limitations. Dextrorotary (D) amino acids can be used in the synthetic process to prevent proteolytic degradation and to prolong the peptide half-life. Furthermore, as we have shown previously (Urban et al. 1989; V. Kumar et al., in prep.), derivatives with a higher affinity for the Ia molecule can be synthesized, and, accordingly, lower concentrations can be used to achieve the same therapeutic effect. It should be noted that peptides are relatively nontoxic, less immunogenic, and are easily manufactured synthetically. We are now exploring the possibility that peptide blocking agents may be effective in more acute situations such as those found in organ graft rejection. For example, in the future, transplantation surgeons may use blocking peptides to circumvent or restrict the T-cell response to a foreign graft.

Analysis of EAE in B10.PL versus SJL/J and PL/J Mice

The SJL/J mouse differs from the B10.PL mouse not only in its MHC haplotype (H-2^s versus H-2^u), but also in its TCR haplotype (the SJL/J mouse has a deletion of about half of its V_β gene segments with respect to the B10.PL mouse [Behlke et al. 1986]). EAE can be readily induced in SJL/J mice, but the peptide epitope to which the MBP-specific T cells respond is different from that of the B10.PL mice (Fig. 3), and the nature of the TCRs employed is quite distinct (Sakai et al. 1988; J. Urban et al., unpubl.). These differences are not surprising considering that the major components of the trimolecular complex, the TCRs and MHC molecules, are distinct in these two strains.

Perhaps a more interesting comparison is that of B10.PL versus PL/J mice. These mice have the same MHC haplotype, but Southern blot analyses suggest that there are limited but distinct differences in their TCR haplotypes (J. Urban, unpubl.). We have examined the MBP response in these two strains of mice and found that they differ in several ways: (1) The MBP-specific TCR gene segments employed by these two strains are in some cases closely related but in every case quite distinct (Table 5). For example, although both strains use the V_β8.2 gene segment, an extra codon is always included in the junctional region of TCRs from the B10.PL mice. Indeed, if one looks at the sequences of these TCR chains in the junctional region (Fig. 16), it is clear that significant differences exist. (2) MBP-specific T_H cells in B10.PL and PL/J mice display strain-specific reactivity. Both strains pos-

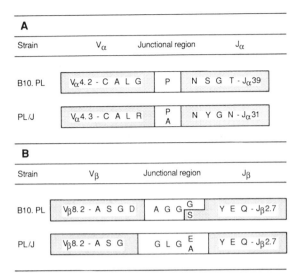

Figure 16. Different B10.PL and PL/J TCR V_α and V_β-chain junctional sequences in MBP-specific T_H cells expressing similar V region genes (see Fig. 6). The junctional (nonstippled) residues in the α chain (A) are presumably encoded by amino-region nucleotides randomly inserted during the process of V-J joining. Junctional nucleotides in the β chain (B) are derived from amino-region insertions and from one to two germ-line D_β gene segments. B10.PL data are from Urban et al. (1988), and PL/J data are from Acha-Orbea et al. (1988) and Urban et al. (1989).

sess four distinct types of MBP-specific T_H cells (Fig. 6, B10.PL; Fig. 17, PL/J). Although the different types of T cells within each strain respond similarly to our panel of amino-terminal MBP peptides, there are subtle strain-specific differences (Fig. 18, B10.PL; Fig. 19, PL/J). In particular, the ability of the two strains to respond to the MBP(1–20)Ala-4,-6 peptide variant is quite distinct (Fig. 20) (Urban et al. 1989). In addition, the response to the MBP(1–9)Ala-4 peptide in vivo is different for the two strains. When used as an immunogen, this peptide induces an effective lymph node proliferative response in the B10.PL mouse that cross-reacts extensively with the wild-type amino-terminal peptide, whereas the same peptide is a very poor immunogen in PL/J mice (Fig. 21). As noted earlier, this suggests that substitutions at position 4 in the amino-

Table 5. Comparisons of TCR Gene Segment Usage by MBP-specific T_H Cells from B10.PL and PL/J Mice

	B10.PL[a] (%)	PL/J[b] (%)
V_α2.3	60	—
V_α4.2	40	—
V_α4.3	—	100
V_β8.2	84	82
V_β4	—	18
V_β13	16	—
J_α39	100	—
J_α31	—	73
J_α11	—	9
J_α12	—	18
J_β2.7	84	45
J_β2.3	—	27
J_β2.5	16	27

[a] Derived from data in Fig. 6.
[b] Derived from data in Fig. 17.

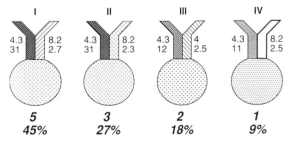

Figure 17. The four different types of MBP-specific T_H cells in PL/J mice that are reactive with the amino-terminal MBP determinant. The types are defined on the basis of the different combinations of α and β TCR chains (Acha-Orbea et al. 1988). For other details, see Fig. 6. (Reprinted, with permission, from Urban et al. 1989.)

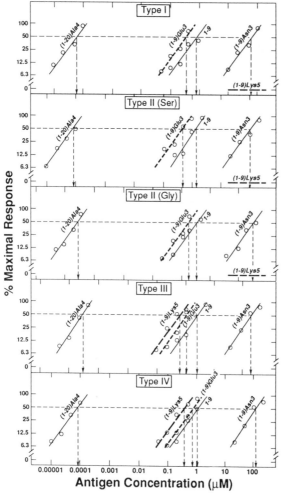

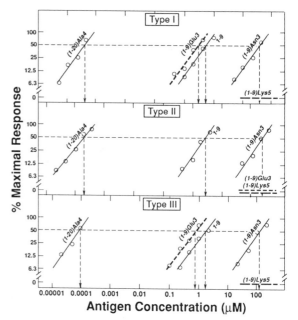

Figure 19. The antigenic fine specificity of PL/J T$_H$ cells responding to the amino-terminal MBP determinant. The hybridomas are representative of three of the four cell types responding to the amino-terminal MBP determinant based on their expressed TCR V$_\alpha$ and V$_\beta$ genes (see Fig. 17). Responses to all 39 peptides listed in Table 2 were tested; of those not shown, all except the response to the MBP(1–20)Ala-4,-6 peptide shown in Fig. 20 were essentially identical to those of the B10.PL hybridoma 172.10 (see Figs. 7–11 and 13). (Adapted from Urban et al. 1989.)

Figure 18. The antigenic fine specificity of B10.PL T$_H$ cells responding to the amino-terminal MBP determinant. The indicated peptide derivatives of MBP were tested for their ability to stimulate each of five B10.PL hybridomas in an IL-2-release assay. The hybridomas are representative of the four cell types responding to the amino-terminal MBP determinant based on their expressed TCR V$_\alpha$ and V$_\beta$ genes (see Fig. 6). Two B10.PL hybridomas were from the same V$_\alpha$4.2/V$_\beta$8.2 type (type II) but possessed a single amino acid difference in their β junctional regions (glycine or serine: see Fig. 5C for position). The responses to all 39 peptides listed in Table 2 were tested; of those not shown, all were essentially identical to those of the hybridoma 172.10 (type I) (see Figs. 7–11 and 13). (Adapted from Urban et al. 1989.)

terminal epitope can also modify in vivo interactions with the TCR in a strain-specific manner. Hence, in several ways it appears that the T-cell responses against MBP in the two strains are quite distinct from one another.

An important point that emerges from these data is that given the knowledge of the MHC TCR haplotypes in these two strains, we can accurately predict the types of T cells that will respond to MBP and induce EAE. Accordingly, if the appropriate therapeutic regimes can be instituted, an autoimmune disease can be prevented by ablating or blocking the reactivity of these T-cell subsets. The key question is, of course, whether or not

this strategy can be extended to human autoimmune diseases.

Approaches to Human Autoimmune Disease

Since the antigen has not been identified in the majority of human autoimmune diseases, the approach that we have taken above to study EAE in mice is not yet practical. Thus, alternative methods are required to define the human MHC and TCR haplotypes that correlate with autoimmune disease. This approach has been carried out extensively with the human leukemia

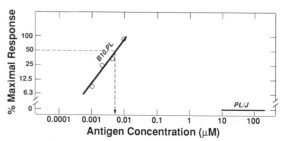

Figure 20. B10.PL and PL/J T$_H$ cells respond differently to the MBP(1–20)Ala-4, -6 peptide. The B10.PL response is representative for all five T$_H$ cells profiled in Fig. 18 (actual response is for the type I T$_H$ cell). Likewise, the PL/J response is representative for all three T$_H$ cells profiled in Fig. 19 (the actual response is for the type I T$_H$ cell). (Adapted from Urban et al. 1989.)

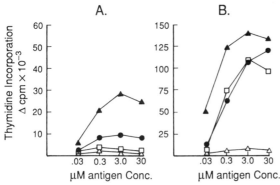

Figure 21. Proliferative lymph role responses of PL/J (*A*) and B10.PL (*B*) mice to challenge with MBP or MBP peptides after primary immunization with the MBP(1–9)Ala-4 peptide. (□) MBP, (●) MBP(1–9), (▲) MBP(1–9)Ala-4, and (△) MBP(87–98).

Table 6. Comparison of the Haplotype Frequencies Defined by $V_\beta 8$ and $V_\beta 11$ Alleles in DR2$^+$ MS Patients and DR2$^+$ Normal Subjects

Haplotypes ($V_\beta 8/V_\beta 11$)	Observed MS	Observed normal[a]	Frequencies MS	Frequencies normal
23/25	2	2	0.05	0.06
2/25	7	16	0.18	0.50[c]
23/20	25	14	0.63	0.44
2/20	6	0	0.15	0.00

$$\chi^2 = 9.45, \ p = 0.009 \ (2 \ df)^b$$

[a] Caucasian individuals from control population no. 2.
[b] χ^2 analysis of the haplotype frequency distributions between the normal population and the MS patient population. Data for the two rarest haplotypes (23/25 and 2/20) were combined so that small expected cell numbers would not degrade the accuracy of the χ^2 test. (Reprinted, with permission, from Beall et al. 1989).
[c] Corrected p value = 0.013

A antigen (HLA) haplotypes, and there are clear correlations between particular HLA haplotypes and a variety of different autoimmune diseases (Howell et al. 1988; Scharf et al. 1988; Sinha et al. 1988; Todd et al. 1988). Several years ago, we began to define human TCR haplotypes (Concannon et al. 1987) and have recently started to identify correlations between particular TCR haplotypes and susceptibility to particular autoimmune diseases. Our initial studies have focused on the human V_β locus. Studies on 30 different individuals using a variety of TCR V region polymorphisms defined at least 27 distinct TCR haplotypes (Concannon et al. 1987). These studies demonstrated a modest linkage disequilibrium between a polymorphism detected with a $V_\beta 11$ probe and one detected with a constant (C_β) probe. In contrast, alleles at $V_\beta 8$ and $V_\beta 11$ loci are in strong linkage disequilibrium.

Recently, we have examined the TCR haplotypes defined by these three polymorphisms in patients with MS (Beall et al. 1989). We have determined that certain TCR haplotypes confer an increased susceptibility to MS if they are coinherited with the genes coding for the HLA-DR2 molecule (Table 6). These data suggest a coordinated action between these two susceptibility genes, the first an MHC gene, and the second, one or more V_β gene segments, that predispose one to develop MS. The question remains how one can identify the particular V_β gene involved in disease predisposition. We are now undertaking several different approaches to analyze this question. We have developed a rapid and automated diagnostic method for discriminating DNA sequence polymorphisms (Landegren et al. 1988a,b). We are now in the process of defining polymorphic sites every 100 kb or so across the human α and β TCR loci to define a series of haplotypes that may be examined in individuals with and without a particular autoimmune disease. This will enable us to focus on specific regions of the TCR loci that correlate with increased susceptibility to disease. Also, we are attempting to sequence all of the human V_α and V_β gene segments. Once a particular region of disease association (e.g., MS) has been identified, V gene seg-

ments in these regions can be sequenced and compared in normal and patient populations. If differences are found between the patient and normal populations, one could then isolate T cells from the cerebral spinal fluid of MS patients, for example, and determine whether or not there is an unusually high expression of the candidate V gene segment. Finally, perhaps one of the most exciting approaches comes from the ability to place a human immune system in a mouse. SCID-hu animals are mutant mice that lack an immune system and into which fetal human thymus, liver, and lymph nodes have been transplanted (McCune et al. 1988; also see Moiser et al. 1988). These mice appear to reconstitute the human immune system at least in part. This raises the possibility of being able, in an animal system, to search for antigens that can induce human autoimmune disease and to characterize the nature of the human TCR responses in these diseases. Any results from the SCID-hu mouse model system can then be checked against appropriate autoimmune patients for verification. Thus, together with the automated DNA diagnostic techniques and our increasing knowledge of the TCR V region sequences in humans, we hope to be in a powerful position to identify the antigens that cause human autoimmune disease and the nature of the TCR responses to these antigens to thus design effective therapeutic strategies using immunologic specificity.

CONCLUSIONS AND FUTURE PROSPECTS

Many of our early concepts concerning the nature of autoimmune disease have now been verified in the case of one model autoimmune disease, EAE. The intriguing question is whether the same generalizations, given below, will apply to other mouse model autoimmune diseases (Banerjee et al. 1988) and at least some human autoimmune diseases.

1. T_H cells are the key factors in mediating autoimmune diseases.
2. The initial T-cell responses to self-antigens may be highly restricted, perhaps in some cases to a single peptide epitope.
3. TCR usage in these initial responses is restricted in

that relatively limited numbers of V_α and V_β gene segments are used.

4. Knowledge of the specific MHC and TCR haplotypes that correlate with disease susceptibilities may allow us to predict which limited sets of TCRs will be employed in a particular autoimmune response. Once the disease-susceptibility TCR and HLA haplotypes have been well-defined in man, it may be possible to use automated DNA diagnostic techniques at birth to predict a particular individual's propensity for a variety of different autoimmune diseases. This view argues that various environmental factors merely activate and render effective preexisting T_H subsets causing disease. Moreover, given the knowledge of the TCR and MHC haplotypes, it also may be possible to predict which TCR molecules will be employed by the autoimmune-inducing T cells.

5. If such TCR V segment predisposition to autoimmune disease can be identified, therapies using either antibodies against the TCR or modified peptides may be employed to ablate or paralyze the small subpopulation of T cells that can cause the autoimmune disease. In this manner, it may be possible to design preventive strategies for avoiding autoimmune disease, rather than trying to deal with the disease after its onset.

The attractiveness of this strategy is that it uses the specificity of the immune response to dissect out the small subset of offending lymphocytes rather than destroying a significant fraction of immune potential of an individual as is done currently by other therapies such as steroids, cyclosporin, or cytotoxic reagents. It is important to emphasize that the strategy cited above will be successful even if a multiplicity of different TCRs is employed in the autoimmune response. Since SJL/J mice have lost up to 50% of their V_β genes and still appear to be viable (Behlke et al. 1986), it would seem possible to delete very significant fractions of the human T-cell repertoire and still maintain appropriate immune responses to most antigens.

It is worth pointing out that each pathogenic lymphocyte has two distinct targets for therapy, the TCR α and β chains. In time, we predict that a battery of antibodies will be available to many V regions from both α and β families, and appropriate double therapies can be initiated, perhaps in an altering fashion to avoid any propensity to generate immune responses against the human antibodies employed. One other interesting possibility for the future is that in time we will be able to design very small agents that are complementary to particular targets. Thus, very small peptides could be designed that are complementary to the V_β chains and perhaps, if necessary, made dimeric so that appropriate T-cell removal could be achieved or coupled to small cytotoxic moieties. Theoretically, TCRs should serve as much better targets for therapy than their antibody counterparts in that (1) they are always directly attached to the cell surface and hence serve as a target for destroying the cell that synthesizes them; (2) there is no somatic hypermutation in the TCR genes, and accordingly antibodies directed against the V_α or V_β regions should be effective throughout the lifetime of the individual; (3) the germ-line repertoires of the V_α and V_β gene segments are far more limited than their antibody light- and heavy-chain counterparts; and (4) T-cell responses for individual antigens appear to be more lim-

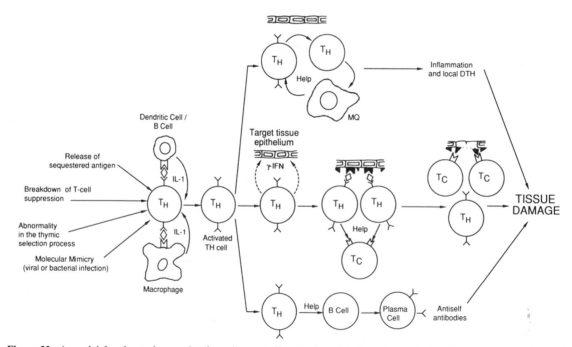

Figure 22. A model for the pathogenesis of autoimmune disease. (Reprinted, with permission, from Kumar et al. 1989.)

ited with regard to epitope interaction, and accordingly a more limited number of antigen receptors should be employed.

It is clear that insights into the nature of the tri-molecular complex, i.e., the TCR, the antigenic peptide, and the MHC molecule, can in theory lead to the design of peptides that are far more effective in binding to the MHC molecule and failing to bind to the TCR molecule and thus activate T cells. Accordingly, these peptides will be ideal blocking components for immunologic recognition. As noted above, perhaps peptide therapy will be useful in acute situations such as organ transplantation or when used in conjunction with antibody therapy for certain autoimmune conditions.

The attractive aspect of this strategy is that it is independent of the initiating cause of the disease (Fig. 22). Autoimmune diseases may be induced by the release of a sequestered antigen, molecular mimicry against bacteria or viruses, or the abrogation of control mechanisms. Moreover, T_H cells play a key role in controlling both cellular and humoral immune responses (Fig. 22). Thus, through manipulation of the key pathogenic T_H cells, it may be possible to circumvent the autoimmune disease by the strategy outlined above. In humans, the first step will be the identification of antigens that initiate autoimmune diseases and, in particular, the peptide epitopes that are responsible for this process. The next step will be the identification of the corresponding TCRs in lymphocyte subpopulations that cause the disease. These appear to be feasible strategies to explore over the next 10–15 years.

As we come to a better understanding of the nature of immune recognition and activation, we will undoubtedly gain the ability to expand particular subpopulations of lymphocytes to facilitate responses to infections or cancers. Therefore, our ability to manipulate the immune response may either lead to the highly selective removal or expansion of particular lymphocyte populations. Thus, a new era of medical opportunities will be created by using the specificity of the immune response to manipulate (e.g., expand, contract, activate, and suppress) specific lymphocyte subpopulations.

ACKNOWLEDGMENTS

We thank the Seaver Foundation for generous support for this project. J.L.U. is supported by a Leukemia Society of America Fellowship and V.K. by a Multiple Sclerosis Society of America Fellowship. D.H.K. is a recipient of The Arthritis Investigator Award.

REFERENCES

Acha-Orbea, H., D.J. Mitchell, L. Timmermann, D.C. Wraith, G.S. Tausch, M.K. Waldor, S.S. Zamvill, H.O. McDevitt, and L. Steinman. 1988. Limited heterogeneity of T-cell receptors from lymphocytes mediating autoimmune encephalomyelitis allows specific immune interventions. *Cell* **54:** 263.

Banerjee, S.J., T.M. Haggi, H.S. Luthra, J.M. Stuart, and C.S. David. 1988. Possible role of V_β T-cell receptor genes in susceptibility to collagen-induced arthritis in mice. *J. Exp. Med.* **167:** 832.

Beall, S.S., P. Concannon, P. Charmley, H.F. McFarland, R.A. Gatti, L.E. Hood, D.E. McFarlin, and W.E. Biddison. 1989. The germline repertoire of T-cell receptor β-chain genes in patients with chronic progressive multiple sclerosis. *J. Neuroimmunol.* **21:** 59.

Behlke, M.A., H.S. Chou, K. Huppi, and D.Y. Loh. 1986. T-cell receptor mutants with deletions of β-chain variable region genes. *Proc. Natl. Acad. Sci.* **83:** 767.

Ben-Nun, A. and Z. Lando. 1983. Detection of autoimmune cells proliferating to myelin basic protein and selection of T-cell lines that mediate experimental autoimmune encephalomyelitis (EAE) in mice. *J. Immunol.* **130:** 1205.

Ben-Nun, A., H. Wekerle, and I.R. Cohen. 1981. Vaccination against autoimmune encephalomyelitis with T-lymphocyte line cells reactive against myelin basic protein. *Nature* **292:** 60.

Bernard, C.C.A. 1976. Experimental autoimmune encephalomyelitis in mice: Genetic control of susceptibility. *J. Immunogenet.* **3:** 263.

Burns, F.R., X. Li, N. Shen, H. Offner, Y.K. Chou, A. Vandenbark, and E. Heber-Katz. 1989. Both rat and mouse T-cell receptors specific for the encephalitogenic determinants of myelin basic protein use similar V_α and V_β chain genes. *J. Exp. Med.* **169:** 27.

Buus, S., A. Sette, S. Colon, C. Miles, and H.M. Grey. 1987. The relation between major histocompatibility complex (MHC) restriction and the capacity of Ia to bind immunogenic peptides. *Science* **235:** 1353.

Cohen, I.R. 1986. Regulation of autoimmune disease physiological and therapeutic. *Immunol. Rev.* **94:** 5.

Concannon, P., R.A. Gatti, and L.E. Hood. 1987. Human T-cell receptor V_β gene polymorphism. *J. Exp. Med.* **165:** 1130.

Fritz, R.B., C.-H. Jen-Chou, and D.E. McFarlin. 1983. Induction of experimental allergic encephalomyelitis in PL/J and (SJL/J x PL/J)F$_1$ mice by myelin basic protein and its peptides: Localization of a second encephalitogenic determinant. *J. Immunol.* **130:** 191.

Fritz, R.B., M.J. Skeen, C.-H. Jen-Chou, J. Garcia, and I.K. Egorov. 1985. Major histocompatibility complex-linked control of the murine response to myelin basic protein. *J. Immunol.* **134:** 2328.

Gasser, D.L. and W.K. Silvers. 1974. Genetic determinants of immunological responsiveness. *Adv. Immunol.* **18:** 1.

Hold, J.H., A.M. Welch, and R.H. Swanborg. 1980. Autoimmune effector cells. I. Transfer of experimental allergic encephalomyelitis with lymphoid cells cultured with antigen. *Eur. J. Immunol.* **10:** 657.

Houser, S.L., H.L. Weiner, A.K. Bhan, M.E. Shapiro, M. Che, W.I.R. Aldrich, and N.L. Letvin. 1984. Lyt-1 cells mediate acute murine experimental allergic encephalomyelitis. *J. Immunol.* **133:** 2288.

Howell, M.D., J.A. Smith, R.K. Austin, D. Kelleher, G.T. Nepon, B. Volk, and M.F. Kagnoff. 1988. An extended HLA-D region haplotype associated with celiac disease. *Proc. Natl. Acad. Sci.* **85:** 222.

Kono, D.H., J.L. Urban, S.J. Horvath, D.G. Ando, R.A. Saavedra, and L. Hood. 1988. Two minor determinants of myelin basic protein induce experimental allergic encephalomyelitis in SJL/J mice. *J. Exp. Med.* **168:** 213.

Kumar, V., D.H. Kono, J.L. Urban, and L. Hood. 1989. The T-cell receptor and autoimmune diseases. *Annu. Rev. Immunol.* **7:** 657.

Landegren, U., R. Kaiser, C.T. Caskey, and L. Hood. 1988a. DNA diagnostics—Molecular techniques and automation. *Science* **242:** 229.

Landegren, U., R. Kaiser, J. Sanders, and L. Hood. 1988b. A ligase-mediated gene detection technique. *Science* **241:** 1077.

Lando, Z., D. Teitelbaum, and R. Arnon. 1976. Genetic control of susceptibility to experimental allergic encephalomyelitis in mice. *Immunogenetics* **9:** 435.

Lassman, H.K. and H.M. Wisniewski. 1979. Chronic relapsing experimental allergic encephalomyelitis. Clinicopathological comparison with multiple sclerosis. *Arch. Neurol.* **36:** 490.

Lider, O., T. Reshef, E. Beraud, A. Ben-Nun, and I.R. Cohen. 1988. Anti-idiotypic network induced by T cell vaccination against experimental autoimmune encephalomyelitis. *Science* **239:** 181.

McCune, J.M., R. Namikawa, H. Kaneshima, L.D. Shultz, M. Lieberman, and I.L. Weissman. 1988. The SCID-hu mouse: Murine model for the analysis of human hematolymphoid differentiation and function. *Science* **241:** 1632.

Mokhtarian, F., D.E. McFarlin, and C.S. Raine. 1984. Adoptive transfer of myelin basic protein-sensitized T cells produce chronic relapsing demyelinating disease in mice. *Nature* **309:** 356.

Mosier, D.E., R.J. Gulizia, S.M. Baird, and D.B. Wilson. 1988. Transfer of a functional human immune system to mice with severe combined immunodeficiency. *Nature* **335:** 256.

Ortiz-Ortiz, L. and W.O. Weigle. 1976. Cellular events in the induction of experimental allergic encephalomyelitis in rats. *J. Exp. Med.* **144:** 604.

Owhashi, M. and E. Heber-Katz. 1988. Protection from experimental allergic encephalomyelitis conferred by a monoclonal antibody directed against a shared idiotype on rat T-cell receptors specific for myelin basic protein. *J. Exp. Med.* **168:** 2153.

Pettinelli, C.B. and D.E. McFarlin. 1981. Adoptive transfer of experimental allergic encephalomyelitis in SJL/J mice after in vitro activation of lymph node cells by myelin basic protein: Requirement of Lyt1$^+$2$^-$-T lymphocytes. *J. Immunol.* **127:** 1420.

Pettinelli, C.B., R.B. Fritz, C.-H. Jen-Chou, and D.E. McFarlin. 1982. Encephalitogenic activity of guinea pig myelin basic protein in the SJL mouse. *J. Immunol.* **129:** 1209.

Raine, C.S., D.H. Snyder, M.P. Valsamis, and S.H. Stone. 1974. Chronic experimental allergic encephalomyelitis in guinea pigs. An ultrastructural study. *Lab. Invest.* **31:** 369.

Reddehase, M., J.B. Rothbard, and H.K. Ulrich. 1989. A pentapeptide as minimal antigenic determinant for MHC class-I-restricted T lymphocytes. *Nature* **337:** 651.

Richert, J.R., B.F. Driscoli, M.W. Kies, and E.C. Alvord, Jr. 1979. Adoptive transfer of experimental allergic encephalomyelitis: Incubation of rat spleen cells with specific antigen. *J. Immunol.* **122:** 494.

Sakai, K., T. Namikawa, T. Kunishita, K. Yamonouchi, and T. Tabira. 1986. Studies of experimental allergic encephalomyelitis by using encephalitogenic T-cell lines and clones in euthymic and athymic mice. *J. Immunol.* **137:** 1527.

Sakai, K., S.S. Zambil, D.J. Mitchell, N. Lim, J.B. Rothbard, and L. Steinman. 1988. Characterization of an encephalitogenic T-cell epitope in SJL/J mice with synthetic oligopeptides of myelin basic protein. *J. Neuroimmunol.* **19:** 21.

Scharf, S.J., A. Friedmann, C. Brautbar, F. Szater, L. Steinman, G. Horn, U. Gyllensten, and H.A. Erlich. 1988. HLA class II allelic variation and susceptibility to pemphigus vulgaris. *Proc. Natl. Acad. Sci.* **85:** 3504.

Sinha, A.A., C. Brautbar, F. Szafer, A. Friedmann, E. Tztomi, J.A. Todd, L. Steinman, and H.O. McDevitt. 1988. A newly characterized HLA DQ $_\beta$ allele associated with pemphigus vulgaris. *Science* **239:** 1026.

Todd, J.A., J.I. Bell, and H.O. McDevitt. 1988. A molecular basis for genetic susceptibility to insulin dependent diabetes mellitus. *Trends Genet.* **4:** 129.

Urban, J.L., S.J. Horvath, and L. Hood. 1989. Autoimmune T cells: Immune recognition of normal and variant peptide epitopes and peptide-based therapy. *Cell* **59:** 257.

Urban, J.L., V. Kumar, D.H. Kono, C. Gomez, S.J. Horvath, J. Clayton, D.G. Ando, E.E. Sercarz, and L. Hood. 1988. Restricted use of T-cell receptor V genes in murine autoimmune encephalomyelitis raises possibilities for antibody therapy. *Cell* **54:** 577.

Winoto, A., J.L. Urban, N.C. Lan, J. Goverman, L. Hood, and D. Hansburg. 1986. Predominant use of a V_α gene segment in mouse T-cell receptors for cytochrome c. *Nature* **324:** 679.

Wisniewski, H.M. and A.B. Keith. 1977. Chronic relapsing experimental encephalomyelitis: An experimental model of multiple sclerosis. *Ann. Neurol.* **1:** 144.

Wraith, D.C., H.O. McDevitt, L. Steinman, and H. Acha-Orbea. 1989. T-cell recognition as a target for immune intervention in autoimmune disease. *Cell* **57:** 709.

Zamvil, S., D.J. Mitchell, A.C. Moore, K. Kitamura, L. Steinman, and J.B. Rothbard. 1986. T-cell epitope of the autoantigen myelin basic protein that induces encephalomyelitis. *Nature* **324:** 258.

Zamvil, S.S., D.J. Mitchell, M.B. Powell, K. Sakai, J.B. Rothbard, and S. Steinman. 1988. Multiple discrete encephalitogenic epitopes of the autoantigen myelin basic protein include a determinant for I-E class II restricted T cells. *J. Exp. Med.* **168:** 1181.

Zamvil, S., P. Nelson, J. Trotter, D. Mitchell, R. Knobler, R. Fritz, and L. Steinman. 1985. T-cell clones specific for myelin basic protein induce chronic relapsing paralysis and demyelination. *Nature* **317:** 355.

A New Hierarchy of TCR Specificity: Autoimmune Diseases Are Defined by Particular $V_\alpha V_\beta$ Combinations and Not by Antigen Specificity

E. HEBER-KATZ

The Wistar Institute of Anatomy and Biology, Philadelphia, Pennsylvania 19104

It is widely believed that the identified α and β chains of the T-cell receptor (TCR) are directly involved in the recognition of protein antigen in the form of a peptide bound to a major histocompatibility complex (MHC) gene product (Hedrick et al. 1984; Dembic et al. 1986; Saito and Germaine 1987). An idealized model for such an interaction has been proposed (Davis and Bjorkman 1988), and the ability of these molecules in soluble form to bind to the antigen/MHC complex is presented in this volume (Davis et al.). The TCR displays limited gene usage for particular antigen/ MHC combinations as was first shown in the T-cell response to pigeon cytochrome c (Fink et al. 1986) and generalized to other antigenic systems (Winoto et al. 1986; Hochgeschwender et al. 1987; Tan et al. 1988).

TCR gene usage in T-cell-mediated autoimmune disease states has begun to be examined only recently (Acha-Orbea et al. 1988; Banerjee et al. 1988; Hafler et al. 1988; Kono et al. 1989; Sakai et al. 1988; Urban et al. 1988; Zamvil et al. 1988; Beall et al. 1989; Burns et al. 1989; Chluba et al. 1989; Oksenberg et al. 1989). In principal, the presence of restricted gene usage is compatible with regulation of an antiself-response both at the cellular and humoral level. Our studies have utilized the rat T-cell repertoire in the autoimmune disease experimental allergic encephalomyelitis (EAE). Besides the examination of rat T-cell fine specificities to myelin basic protein (MBP), the disease-inducing antigen, we made a monoclonal antibody (MAb) against a Lewis rat T-cell hybridoma specific for the major encephalitogenic determinant of Lewis (residues 68–88 of MBP) with high affinity for self (rat)-MBP. This antibody immunoprecipitated the rat TCR and bound to most, if not all, of the T cells in disease-inducing, MBP-68–88-specific, long-term T-cell lines (Owhashi and Heber-Katz 1988). The T cells in this population, however, when individually analyzed were all found to be different from one another (7 of 7 analyzed) by TCR β-chain rearrangements (Happ et al. 1988), thus indicating that these cells were derived not from a single progenitor but rather from multiple cells and must share an idiotypic TCR determinant. The antibody was tested for its ability to protect animals from disease by injecting it along with the disease-inducing MBP. The antibody was protective although in certain circumstances it could also enhance disease. Similar results were obtained in the mouse where two anti-TCR variable (V_β) antibodies were tested (Acha-Orbea et al. 1988; Urban et al. 1988; Zamvil et al. 1988). Taken together, these results indicate the ability to intervene in such an autoimmune process.

EAE TCRs from both the rat and the mouse were also analyzed at the molecular level. In the Lewis rat, TCR mRNA from the same T-cell hybridoma used for making the antiidiotype was found to have V regions, when compared with known mouse sequences, that were most closely homologous to the murine $V_\beta 8.2$ and $V_\alpha 2.1$. Using those V regions as probes to examine a panel of MBP-68–88-specific encephalitogenic clones and T-cell hybridomas, we found 100% $V_\beta 8$ usage and a 70% $V_\alpha 2$ usage with normal and third-party antigen controls being negative (Burns et al. 1989).

It was to our great surprise when we compared our data with that of the mouse and found that the TCR V gene usage was similar. Thus, the B10.Pl/J mouse in its T-cell response to the encephalitogenic determinant of MBP used $V_\alpha 2 V_\beta 8.2$ 51% of the time and $V_\alpha 4 V_\beta 8.2$ 33% of the time (Urban et al. 1988). In the Pl/J mouse at least 88% of the T-cell response utilized $V_\alpha 4 V_\beta 8.2$ (Acha-Orbea et al. 1988). Besides the fact that these results come from two different species, the B10.Pl mouse and the Lewis rat also recognize different antigenic determinants (although both are encephalitogenic) and different MHC molecules. One possible explanation was cross-reactivity between the two peptide/MHC combinations. However, antigen cross-presentation experiments proved to be negative (Heber-Katz and Acha-Orbea 1989). Thus, there appeared to be no correlation between the V regions being used and the antigen/MHC being recognized. We thought it might be telling to examine encephalitogenic T-cell populations that recognized other antigenic determinants and MHC molecules. This was the motivation for the experiments described below.

METHODS

T-cell populations. Cell lines: Animals were immunized in hind footpads with guinea pig MBP or ovalbumin (OVA) in complete Freund's adjuvant. Cells from popliteal lymph nodes were cultured with antigen for 3 days. Blasts were then separated on a Ficoll gradient and rested. Cells were restimulated with thymocytes as antigen-presenting cells (APC) and then treated as before (Owhashi and Heber-Katz 1988).

T-cell hybridomas: MBP-specific lymph node T cells from ACI and BUF rats were cultured for 3 days in vitro with antigen. These activated cells were then fused to BW5147 as described previously (Happ and Heber-Katz 1988). Hybridomas that produced interleukin-2 in response to antigen plus APC were then subcloned and analyzed for V gene usage.

Northern blot analysis. Total cellular RNA was isolated from both conconavalin-A (Con A)-stimulated and MBP-specific T cells. RNA (20 μg) was run on 1% agarose/2% formaldehyde gels, and the gels were blotted onto Nytran membranes (Schleicher and Scheull). The blots were prehybridized and hybridized in 50% formamide, 5× SSPE (sodium chloride, sodium phosphate, and ethylenediaminetrichloroacetic acid) buffer, 100 μg of salmon sperm DNA, 0.1% SDS, and 5× Denhardt's solution. Hybridization was performed using $V_\beta 510$ and $V_\alpha 510$ and constant region probes as described previously (Burns et al. 1989). The filters were first hybridized with V region probes, and then they were rehybridized with the corresponding constant region probes.

Adoptive transfer of disease. T-cell lines were harvested 3 days after antigen stimulation, and blasts were separated on a Ficoll gradient and transferred intraperitoneally at a dose of 2×10^6 cells into 350 rads X-irradiated recipients. The recipient rats were examined daily for signs of disease (Owhashi and Heber-Katz 1988).

Fluorescence-activated cell-sorter analysis of antiidiotype. T cells (10^5) were first incubated with the murine anti-rat MAb 10.18 then incubated with fluorescein-isothyocynate-labeled sheep $F(ab)_2$ anti-mouse immunoglobulin G as described previously (Owhashi and Heber-Katz 1988). The cells were analyzed on an Ortho 50 mHH Cytofluorograf.

RESULTS

TCR V Gene Usage by Encephalitogenic T Cells

In the context of the observation that the B10.Pl/J mouse and the Lewis rat choose the same TCR V gene families in their response to the encephalitogenic determinant of MBP, although the antigenic determinant is different, we predicted that different rat strains that recognize encephalitogenic determinants of MBP other than the 68–88 (72–84) antigenic determinant would use the same $V_\alpha 2V_\beta 8$ combination used by the Lewis rat and B10.Pl/J mouse. T-cell lines were generated from five strains of rat: Lewis and Fischer, which share the same class II determinants and recognize the same encephalitogenic determinant, ACI having a second MHC and recognizing a second determinant, BUF with a third MHC and a third determinant, and BN with a fourth MHC and recognizing a fourth encephalitogenic

determinant. The five rat strains were immunized with MBP, and long-term T-cell lines from these animals were analyzed for their antigen specificity and ability to cause EAE. All of the lines induced paralysis when adoptively transferred into normal syngeneic recipients, and each line except Lewis and Fischer responded to a distinct antigenic determinant of MBP. As control T cells, Con-A-stimulated T-cell blasts from normal spleens of all of the rat strains were generated. These were nonencephalitogenic and non-MBP reactive. RNA was derived from these lines, and the Lewis MBP-68–88-specific V_α ($V_\alpha 510$ or $V_\alpha 2$) and V_β ($V_\beta 510$ or $V_\beta 8.2$) probes were used to hybridize Northern blots with constant region probes as controls. In all cases, the encephalitogenic T-cell lines derived from different strains and each recognizing unique MBP determinants were positive for both Lewis $V_\alpha 2$ and $V_\beta 8$. In all cases, Con A blasts from the same rat strains were negative. Although the presence of this V_α and V_β was indicated in all encephalitogenic populations, it was important to show that the $V_\alpha V_\beta$ existed in combination. We thus generated T-cell hybridomas specific for the encephalitogenic determinant from the BUF and ACI strains and used mRNA from cloned populations to analyze V region usage. Approximately 40% of the T-cell hybrids from both strains were double-positive for $V_\alpha 2$ and $V_\beta 8$. Furthermore, none of the hybridomas were single-positive for either of the probes. It appears then that in all strains tested, the encephalitogenic T-cell response uses this $V_\alpha 2V_\beta 8$ gene combination irrespective of the antigenic and MHC fine specificity.

Idiotype Usage by Encephalitogenic T Cells

Since we have shown above that the TCR V gene usage was similar in T cells specific for unique antigen/MHC class II combinations from five separate rat strains, we thought that the idiotype defined by the MAb 10.18 (Owhashi and Heber-Katz 1988) might also be present on encephalitogenic T cells from the different stains tested above. MBP-specific T cells were those used above and compared with OVA-specific T cells made from each of the five strains. MBP-specific T cells from Lewis, Fischer, and BUF were 10.18 positive, and ACI and BN were negative. OVA-specific cells from all strains were 10.18 negative. The differences in the results with 10.18 and the V region probes could indicate that different members of the $V_\alpha 2$ and $V_\beta 8$ families are being used.

Functional Cross-reactivity

As previously tested for Pl/J and Lewis rat T-cell antigenic determinants (Heber-Katz and Acha-Orbea 1989), the functional cross-reactivity of the various rat MHC peptides was also tested. MBP-specific T-cell lines from the five rat strains were tested with APC from all five different rat strains plus MPB. The only significant response above background was seen with syngeneic APC, which supported the idea that these antigen/MHC complexes were not functionally cross-reactive. However, to eliminate any possibility of artifacts because of residual alloreactivity, these experiments must be carried out using cloned T cells.

DISCUSSION

We have analyzed sets of T cells that are interesting in both their differences and their similarities. These T cells are derived from two strains of mouse and five strains of rat. These T cells recognize different antigenic determinants in association with different MHC-encoded class II molecules that yield functionally noncross-reactive peptide/MHC combinations. These T cells, on the other hand, all respond to MBP and are all encephalitogenic. Furthermore, these cells all use similar or the same $V_\alpha 2 V_\beta 8$ combinations to respond to antigen and for three of five rat strains tested bear the 10.18-defined idiotype.

These observations have held up in almost all situations we have examined (see Table 1):

1. *T cells from different strains that are susceptible to disease but recognize different antigens and different MHC molecules even within the same strain use this $V_\alpha V_\beta$* (Table 1a). One example, the Lewis T-cell response to MBP 87–99, is an I-E-restricted response that appears late after immunization with syngeneic rat MBP as opposed to guinea pig MBP (the early dominant response is to MBP 68–88, which is I-A restricted) (Offner et al. 1989).

2. *T cells from animals that are EAE resistant* (Table 1b). It is possible to generate T cells from these animals that upon adoptive transfer can cause disease. This is true for the BN rat in which such a T-cell line utilizes $V_\alpha 2 V_\beta 8$, or, in the case of the LeR (Lewis resistant) rat, from which en-

cephalitogenic T-cell clones utilize $V_\alpha 4 V_\beta 8$ (this combination has been seen in PL/J and B10.PL; E. Blankenhorn and W. Hickey, in prep.).

3. *Other experimental diseases* (Table 1c). Interestingly, our findings have recently been extended to the experimental allergic neuritis (EAN) disease model in Lewis rats, which is also a T-cell-mediated disease but involves the peripheral nervous system (E. Heber-Katz and M. Rostami, in prep.). Here, the antigen is not MBP and the disease is not central nervous system (CNS) encephalitis, but the T cells use the same $V_\alpha V_\beta$ combination.

In attempting to explain this lack of correlation of antigenic specificity and V gene usage in the light of the definitive correlation between this $V_\alpha V_\beta$ gene usage and disease, we proposed the *V region disease hypothesis* (Heber-Katz and Acha-Orbea 1989), which attributes two functions to the TCR: one involved in the recognition of distinct antigen/MHC determinants and the other involved in the association of such V region combinations with the encephalitogenicity induced by these cells. The most likely locus of the first function is in the CDR3 or junctional region. The proposed location of the second function is within the V region, involving the recognition of a ligand other than antigenic peptide/MHC. Thus, there would be a hierarchy of function above antigen plus MHC, a selection based on the recognition of a self-molecule that would at least be found in the CNS. However, given the fact that a second experimental disease, EAN, displays the same usage of TCR V regions, we must extend this to an additional site in vivo. Is it possible then that there is a general autoimmune TCR, or are we looking at an experimentally induced set of receptors? We are in the process of attempting to extend these findings to other autoimmune phenomena, both induced and spontaneous, to test this possibility.

Table 1. Autoimmune T-cell Populations in Which the $V_\alpha 2 V_\beta 8$ or $V_\alpha 4 V_\beta 8$ Combinations Are Used

Species-strain	MHC	Antigen	$V_\alpha V_\beta$[a]	Idiotype[b]	References[c]
(a) EAE					
Rat-Lewis	RT-1^l(I-A)	MBP 72–84	$_\alpha 2_\beta 8$ (clonal)	+	1, 2
Rat-Lewis	RT-1^l(I-E)	MBP 87-99	$_\alpha 2_\beta 8$ (clonal)	n.d.	3
Rat-Fischer	RT-1^l(I-A)	MBP 68–88	$_\alpha 2_\beta 8$ (line)	+	4
Rat-ACI	RT-1^a(I-A)	MBP 34–54	$_\alpha 2_\beta 8$ (clonal)	−	4
Rat-BUF	RT-1^b(I-A)	MBP (?)	$_\alpha 2_\beta 8$ (clonal)	+	4
Mouse-PL/J	I-A^u	MBP 1–9	$_\alpha 4_\beta 8$ (clonal)	n.d.	5
Mouse-B10.PL	I-A^u	MBP 1–9	$_\alpha 2,4_\beta 8$ (clonal)	n.d.	6
(b) Resistant EAE					
Rat-BN	RT-1^n(I-A)	MBP 43–68	$_\alpha 2_\beta 8$ (line)	−	4
Rat-LeR	RT-1^l(I-A)	MBP 68–88	$_\alpha 4_\beta 8$ (clonal)	n.d.	7
(c) Other autoimmune diseases					
Rat-Lewis (EAN)	RT-1^l(I-A)	P$_2$ 53–78	$_\alpha 2_\beta 8$ (line)	+	8

n.d. indicates not determined.

[a]The V region are as described in Materials and Methods (Burns et al. 1989).

[b]The MAb 10.18 was used as described in Materials and Methods (Owhashi and Heber-Katz 1988).

[c]References: (1) Burns et al. 1989; (2) Chluba et al. 1989; (3) Offner et al. 1989; (4) Heber-Katz and Acha-Orbea 1989; X. Li et al., in prep.; (5) Acha-Orbea et al. 1988; (6) Urban et al. 1988; (7) E. Blankenhorn and W. Hickey, in prep.; (8) E. Heber-Katz and M. Rostami, in prep.

ACKNOWLEDGMENTS

This work was funded through the generous support of National Multiple Sclerosis Society grant NMS-RG-1593A and U.S. Public Health Service grant NS-11036. I am thankful to all of my collaborators: Mary Pat Happ who started this project, provided all of the T-cell hybridomas, and analyzed their fine specificity; Halina Offner and Art Vandenbark who generously provided T-cell clones to all specificities at any time; Frank Burns, Xioapin Li, and Ning Shen who cloned and sequenced everything; Makoto Owhashi who carried out the antibody work; and Mohammed Rostami with whom I have collaborated on EAN.

REFERENCES

Acha-Orbea, H., D.J. Mitchell, L. Timmerman, D.C. Wraith, G.S. Taich, M.K. Waldor, S. Zamvil, H. McDevitt, and L. Steinman. 1988. Limited heterogeneity of TcRs from lymphocytes mediating autoimmune encephalomyelitis allows specific immune intervention. *Cell* **54:** 263.

Banerjee, S.J., T.M. Haqqi, H.S. Luthra, J.M. Stuart, and C.S. David. 1988. Possible role of Vβ T cell receptor genes in susceptibility to collagen-induced arthritis in mice. *J. Exp. Med.* **167:** 832.

Beall, S.S., P. Concannon, P. Charmley, H.F. McFarland, R.A. Gatti, L.E. Hood, D.E. McFarlin, and W.E. Biddison. 1989. The germline repertoire of T cell receptor β chain genes in patients with chronic progressive multiple sclerosis. *J. Neuroimmunol.* **21:** 59.

Burns, F., X. Li, N. Shen, H. Offner, Y.K. Chou, A.A. Vandenbark, and E. Heber-Katz. 1989. Both rat and mouse TcRs specific for the encephalitogenic determinant of MBP use similar Vα and Vβ chain genes even though the MHC and encephalitogenic determinants being recognized are different. *J. Exp. Med.* **169:** 27.

Chluba, J., C. Steeg, A. Becker, H. Wekerle, and J.T. Epplen. 1989. TcR β chain usage in MBP specific rat T lymphocytes. *Eur. J. Immunol.* **19:** 279.

Davis, M.M. and P.J. Bjorkman. 1988. T cell antigen receptor genes and T cell recognition. *Nature* **334:** 395.

Dembic, Z., H. von Boehmer, and M. Steinmetz. 1986. The role of T cell receptor α and β genes in MHC restricted antigen recognition. *Immunol. Today* **7:** 308.

Fink, P.J., L. Matis, D.L. McElliott, M. Bookman, and S. Hedrick. 1986. Correlations between T cell specificity and the structure of the antigen receptor. *Nature* **312:** 219.

Hafler, D.A., A.D. Duby, S.J. Lee, D. Benjamin, J.G. Seidman, and H.L. Weiner. 1988. Oligoclonal T lymphocytes in the cerebrospinal fluid of patients with multiple sclerosis. *J. Exp. Med.* **167:** 1313.

Happ, M.P. and E. Heber-Katz. 1988. Differences in the repertoire of the Lewis rat T cell response to self and non-self MBPs. *J. Exp. Med.* **167:** 502.

Happ, M.P., A.S. Kiraly, H. Offner, A. Vandenbark, and E. Heber-Katz. 1988. The autoreactive T cell population in experimental allergic encephalomyelitis: T cell receptor β chain rearrangements. *J. Neuroimmunol.* **19:** 191.

Heber-Katz, E. and H. Acha-Orbea. 1989. The V-region hypothesis: Evidence from autoimmune encephalomyelitis. *Immunol. Today* **10:** 164.

Hedrick, S.M., D.I. Cohen, E.A. Nielson, and M.M. Davis. 1984. Isolation of cDNA clones encoding T-cell specific membrane associated proteins. *Nature* **308:** 149.

Hochgeschwender, U., H.G. Simon, H.U. Weltsien, F. Bartles, A. Becker, and J.T. Epplen. 1987. Dominance of one T cell receptor in the H-2K^b/TNP response. *Nature* **326:** 307.

Kono, D.H., J.L. Urban, S.J. Horvath, D.G. Ando, R.A. Saavedra, and L. Hood. 1988. Two minor determinants of myelin basic protein induce experimental allergic encephalomyelitis in SJL/J mice. *J. Exp. Med.* **168:** 213.

Offner, H., G.A. Hashim, B. Celnick, A. Galang, X. Li, F.R. Burns, N. Shen, E. Heber-Katz, and A.A. Vandenbark. 1989. T cell determinants of myelin basic protein include a unique encephalitogenic I-E restricted epitope for Lewis rats. *J. Exp. Med.* **170:** 355.

Oksenberg, J.G., M. Sherritt, A.B. Begovich, H.A. Erlich, C.C. Bernard, L.L. Cavalli-Sforza, and L. Steinman. 1989. T cell receptor Vα and Cα alleles associated with multiple sclerosis and myasthenia gravis. *Proc. Natl. Acad. Sci.* **86:** 988.

Owhashi, M. and E. Heber-Katz. 1988. Protection from EAE conferred by a monoclonal antibody against a shared idiotype on rat TcRs specific for MBP. *J. Exp. Med.* **168:** 2153.

Saito, T. and R.N. Germaine. 1987. Predictable acquisition of a new MHC recognition specificity following expression of a transfected T cell receptor β chain gene. *Nature* **329:** 256.

Sakai, K., A.A. Sinha, D.J. Mitchell, S.S. Zamvil, J.B. Rothbard, H.O. McDevitt, and L. Steinman. 1988. Involvement of distinct T cell receptors in the autoimmune encephalitogenic response to nested epitopes of myelin basic protein. *Proc. Natl. Acad. Sci.* **85:** 8608.

Tan, K.-N., B.M. Datlot, J.A. Gilmore, A.C. Kronman, J.H. Lee, M.M. Maxam, and A. Rao. 1988. The T cell receptor Vα3 gene segment is associated with reactivity to azobenene-arsonate. *Cell* **54:** 247.

Urban, J., V. Kumar, D. Kono, C. Gomez, S.J. Horvath, J. Clayton, D.G. Ando, E.E. Sercarz, and L. Hood. 1988. Restricted use of Tcr V genes in murine autoimmune encephalomyelitis raises possibilities for antibody therapy. *Cell* **54:** 577.

Winoto, A., J.L. Urban, N.C. Lan, J. Governman, L. Hood, and D. Hansburg. 1986. Predominant use of a Vα gene segment in mouse T cell receptors for cytochrome c. *Nature* **324:** 679.

Zamvil, S.S., D.J. Mitchell, N.E. Lee, A.C. Moore, M.K. Waldorf, K. Saki, J.B. Rothbard, H.O. McDevitt, L. Steinman, and H. Acha-Orbea. 1988. Predominant expression of a T cell receptor Vβ gene subfamily in autoimmune encephalomyelitis. *J. Exp. Med.* **167:** 263.

Physiological Basis of T-cell Vaccination against Autoimmune Disease

I.R. COHEN

Department of Cell Biology, The Weizmann Institute of Science, 76100 Rehovot, Israel

T-cell vaccination denotes a procedure whereby autoimmune T cells are administered to individuals in a way that induces active resistance to a specific autoimmune disease, the disease with which the T cells are associated (Ben-Nun et al. 1981a; Cohen 1986). T-cell vaccination is analogous to the use of attenuated or avirulent microbes to specifically immunize individuals against the disease caused by the particular virulent microbe, except that here the vaccine is a population of T cells and the pathogens to be controlled are not foreign microbes but endogenous clones of autoimmune lymphocytes.

In T-cell vaccination, the antigens are specific T cells and, as I discuss here, the responders are T cells. The vaccination phenomenon thus is a special case of T cells recognizing T cells or, more specifically, autoimmune T cells recognizing autoimmune T cells.

The aim of this paper is to review the results of experiments, particularly those not yet published or about to be published, that document the effectiveness of T-cell vaccination in treating autoimmune diseases (that it works) and shed light on the mechanisms of resistance mobilized by T-cell vaccination (how it works). Finally, I discuss new observations relating to the physiological basis of T-cell vaccination (why it works).

EXPERIMENTAL PROCEDURES

T-cell lines and clones. Autoimmune lines and clones of the $CD4^+$ $CD8^-$ phenotype were raised and maintained as described previously (Ben-Nun et al. 1981b; Ben-Nun and Cohen 1982a; Holoshitz et al. 1984; Vandenbark et al. 1986).

T-cell vaccination. Cells activated by incubation with specific antigen or with the T-cell mitogen, concanavalin A (Con A) (Naparstek et al. 1983), were inoculated (10×10^6 to 20×10^6) subcutaneously or intraperitoneally into recipient Lewis rats after treatment with gamma radiation (2500 rads) (Ben-Nun et al. 1981a) or the chemical cross-linker glutaraldehyde (0.3%) (Lider et al. 1987). Vaccination was also done using subpathogenic doses (10^2–10^4) of virulent T cells (Lider et al. 1988, 1989; Beraud et al. 1989).

Autoimmune diseases. Acute monophasic experimental autoimmune encephalomyelitis (EAE) was induced actively in Lewis rats by immunization to myelin basic protein (BP) emulsified in complete Freund's adjuvant (Ben-Nun and Cohen 1982b) or by intravenous inoculation of 1×10^6 to 10×10^6 activated, virulent anti-BP T cells (Ben-Nun et al. 1981b). Adjuvant arthritis was induced in Lewis rats by active immunization to 1 mg of pulverized, killed *Mycobacterium tuberculosis* organisms (H37Ra) (MT) in oil (Holoshitz et al. 1983b). Insulin-dependent diabetes mellitus (IDDM) occurs spontaneously in mice of the NOD strain, beginning at about 4 months of age and reaching a peak incidence at about 8 months of 90% in females and 50% in males (Rossini et al. 1985).

RESULTS

Therapeutic Effectiveness of T-cell Vaccination

Investigation of T-cell vaccination has taken two divergent but complementary routes. One path of research is utilitarian; it is directed to exploiting its potential as a specific therapy for clinical autoimmune disease. The other path of research can be called basic; it aims at elucidating the cellular and molecular basis for the phenomenon and to see what the process can tell us about the physiology of immune regulation. Neither path is a detour.

The utilitarian path has led to a number of empirical observations. It was discovered that no T cell would induce resistance to an autoimmune disease unless it was activated before inoculation into the recipient. Activation is accomplished by incubating the particular T cells with their specific antigen or with a T-cell mitogen, such as Con A (Naparstek et al. 1983). The changes resulting from activation critical for vaccination are yet unknown but require about 6–8 hours of culture in vitro.

Even after activation, not all CD4 T cells appear to be capable of vaccinating. However, it was discovered, again empirically, that the effectiveness of vaccination can be enhanced considerably by treating the activated T cells with agents that cause aggregation of components of the cell membrane (Cohen 1986). At present, the simplest way to produce this aggregation is to treat the activated T cells with chemical cross-linkers such as glutaraldehyde or formaldehyde (Lider et al. 1987). Cross-linking is useful clinically because as it improves their ability to vaccinate; the treatment kills the autoimmune cells and inactivates any virus or oncogene that might inadvertently be expressed in them.

The utilitarian aim has two components: safety and effectiveness, both of which can be related to immunological specificity. T-cell vaccination is relatively specific; the vaccine is most effective when it contains the T cells to be controlled. It was seen, for example, that two T-cell lines responding to two different BP molecules, bovine or guinea pig, each vaccinated rats against EAE induced by immunization with the specific type of BP (Holoshitz et al. 1983a). This early observation was compatible with a mechanism of anti-idiotype immunity. The T-cell vaccine, however, was effective even if the specific autoimmune T cells were only a small part of the administered cells; antigen-primed lymph node cells, not only defined lines or clones, were found to vaccinate effectively against disease (Lider et al. 1987; Cohen 1988).

Since only activated T cells serve as effective vaccines, a relatively specific T-cell vaccine can be formulated from a mixed population of T cells by using the specific antigen to activate primarily the desired autoimmune T cells. The nonresponding T cells specific for other antigens, T cells whose functions might be best left intact, would not effectively arouse an anti-idiotypic response because they would not be activated by the autoantigen. Nevertheless, the specific autoantigen in many human autoimmune diseases is not known. How, then, can one construct a specific vaccine without the specific autoantigen?

This question was studied by F. Mor in our laboratory (F. Mor et al., in prep.). Mor was able to exploit the fact that T cells already having been activated in vivo transiently enjoy a growth advantage over naive T cells upon culture in vitro with a T-cell mitogen. Using a limiting dilution analysis, Mor found that the frequency of MT-specific T cells obtained from arthritic rats increased about 40-fold after one cycle of activation in vitro with Con A (from ~1:1000 to 1:25). Similarly, activation with Con A increased the frequency of BP-specific T cells obtained from rats with EAE.

Drawing on this information, D. Elias and A. Lohse (D. Elias et al., in prep.) were able to vaccinate therapeutically NOD mice against autoimmune diabetes, a disease whose target antigen is unknown. We reasoned that the spleen cells of 4-month-old NOD mice, a period of marked insulitis preceding clinical diabetes, would contain specific autoimmune T cells since such cells can transfer disease (Bendelac et al. 1987). We therefore cultured the spleen cells with Con A in the manner of Mor, hoping to augment the concentration of the unidentified autoimmune T cells while activating them. The cell population was then treated with a chemical cross-linker to attenuate the cells and aggregate their membrane components. Groups of 12–14 NOD mice, males or females, were sham-vaccinated or vaccinated with the treated spleen cells (5×10^6) at 6 weeks of age, the onset of insulitis, and three more times at monthly intervals. At the age of 8 months, the sham-vaccinated mice showed the expected incidence of diabetes, approximately 50% for males and 90% for females. In contrast, the T-cell-vaccinated males had no diabetes, and only 25% of the treated females were ill.

These results indicate that T-cell vaccination can be therapeutic in spontaneous autoimmune disease, using a vaccine made from the T cells of autoimmune animals without specific antigen. Results such as these, combined with a lack of toxicity, suggest that the T-cell vaccination might indeed have utilitarian value in clinical disease.

Mechanisms of Resistance: Anti-idiotypic T Cells

T-cell vaccination raises many difficult questions about underlying mechanisms responsible for the observations. What are the molecular signals borne by the vaccine? What does cell activation contribute? Why do some T clones require treatment with chemical cross-linkers, whereas others vaccinate without membrane aggregation? How are the vaccinating signals processed, presented, and received?

The immunologically specific resistance resulting from T-cell vaccination seems to involve anti-idiotypic T cells. O. Lider et al. (1988, 1989) demonstrated that T-cell vaccination with lines or clones led to recipient T-cell proliferative responses that were much greater to the vaccinating T cells than they were to syngeneic CD4 T clones of unrelated specificity. To analyze this anti-T-cell response, we vaccinated rats in the hind footpads with anti-BP T cells and studied the response of the draining lymph nodes. Anti-idiotypic proliferative responses appeared in the popliteal lymph nodes about 5 days after vaccination and then spread systemically several days later (Lider et al. 1989). Removal of the anti-idiotypic lymph nodes before systemic spread robbed vaccinated rats of their protection to EAE, whereas transfer of the lymph node cells to naive recipients transferred protection. Thus, resistance to EAE appeared to be a function of the anti-idiotypic lymph node population. Cloning of the anti-idiotypic cells yielded CD4 anti-idiotypic T cells that stimulated the anti-BP T cells in vitro and CD8 anti-idiotypic T cells that suppressed the anti-BP T cells in vitro (Lider et al. 1988). Sun et al. (1988) have shown that CD8 anti-anti-BP T cells can actually suppress EAE in vivo. Thus, anti-idiotypic T cells, stimulated by T-cell vaccination, might indeed contribute to resistance to disease.

How anti-idiotypic T cells regulate autoimmune effector T cells is not clear. The CD8 anti-idiotypic T cells studied by Sun et al. (1988) were specifically cytotoxic to the anti-BP T cells in vitro, suggesting that resistance to EAE might involve cytotoxicity in vivo (Sun et al. 1988). Killing of the autoimmune T cells, however, cannot explain the observation that virulent anti-BP T cells persist in rats that have acquired resistance to EAE (Ben-Nun and Cohen 1982b; Naparstek et al. 1982). It seems that anti-BP T cells can survive in rats in a quiescent or suppressed state (Cohen 1986).

W. van Eden (unpubl.) has found in cell-culture experiments that the lymph node cells of vaccinated rats suppress the proliferation to antigen of idiotype-positive T cells but do not suppress syngeneic T-cell clones responding to other irrelevant antigens. However, adding the idiotype-specific T cells to the cultures induces the anti-idiotypic lymph node cells to suppress the responses of unrelated syngeneic T cells to their antigens. Thus, a specific idiotype can activate anti-idiotypic T cells to produce a suppressive effect on adjacent T cells that is not immunologically specific.

Specific triggering of a nonspecific effect could also account for the surprising fact that vaccination with a single T clone can induce resistance to adjuvant arthritis caused by immunization to MT (Lider et al. 1987). Clone A2b, recognizing a 9-amino-acid peptide in the sequence of the MT 65-kD heat-shock protein (hsp65) (van Eden et al. 1988), can be used to either prevent arthritis or induce remission of established arthritis (Lider et al. 1987). Recently, D. Markovits (unpubl.) has isolated a new T-cell line specific for the hsp65 molecule, designated M1. M1 recognizes a peptide sequence other than that recognized by A2b. In addition, M1 and A2b do not share idiotypes; anti-idiotypic T cells responding to either A2b or M1 do not recognize the other clone. Nevertheless, M1 can vaccinate rats against arthritis at least as efficiently as clone A2b does, implying that the same autoimmune disease can be regulated by different anti-idiotypic T cells.

It is conceivable that both A2b and M1 represent common idiotypes that appear together in lesions of arthritic rats. Therefore, an anti-idiotype specific for either one could affect all of the T cells in the lesion by releasing the putative nonspecific suppressor lymphokine.

Anti-ergotypic T Cells

In addition to the evidence for anti-idiotypic T cells outlined above, A. Lohse and other investigators in the laboratory have detected a second type of T-cell response that could contribute to the effect of T-cell vaccination. We have termed this type of response anti-ergotypic (ergon = activity or work) because it seems to recognize the state of activation of the target T cell not the idiotype (Lohse et al. 1989). These studies were initiated by the observation that along with the specific proliferative response to the T clone used for vaccination, the T cells of vaccinated rats often showed a lesser degree of proliferation when stimulated by syngeneic T cells of diverse unrelated specificities (Lider et al. 1989). Lohse isolated the nonspecific T blasts and found that they responded to any activated syngeneic CD4 T cell, regardless of its specificity, but not to resting syngeneic T cells. In contrast with anti-ergotypic T cells, anti-idiotypic T cells respond to both resting and activated T cells. Anti-ergotypic T cells, which include CD4 and CD8 T cells, seem to be important because they are capable of suppressing autoimmune diseases upon inoculation into recipients.

For example, an intraperitoneal injection of 10^7 isolated anti-ergotypic T blasts can protect syngeneic Lewis rats against either adoptive EAE produced by intravenously transferred anti-BP T clones or active EAE induced by immunization to BP (Lohse et al. 1989). The response of T cells to syngeneic-activated T cells has been noted by other investigators in the past (Damle and Gupta 1982). The present findings indicate that such cells can regulate an autoimmune response in vivo. It is conceivable that anti-ergotypic T cells might function physiologically as negative feedback on immune responses generally. Nevertheless, the efficiency of idiotype-specific T-cell vaccination is clearly much greater than nonspecific anti-ergotypic vaccination. Anti-BP T cells vaccinate strongly against EAE but negligibly against arthritis, and anti-hsp65 T cells vaccinate strongly against arthritis but negligibly against EAE (Lider et al. 1986). The relative weakness of vaccination with immunologically nonspecific, activated T cells may be because the anti-ergotypic response, unlike the anti-idiotypic response, does not persist beyond several days and does not appear to have a memory (A. Lohse et al., unpubl.). Indeed, to observe suppression of EAE, the anti-ergotypic T cells had to be amplified in vitro and transferred to recipients as a concentrated cell population. However, as idiotype-specific T-cell vaccines mobilize both anti-idiotypic and anti-ergotypic mechanisms, some nonspecific effects of T-cell vaccination might be detectable, at least transiently. The significance of this in clinical T-cell vaccination remains to be seen.

Physiological Basis of T-cell Vaccination

In T-cell vaccination, does the autoimmune T cell merely serve as a conventional immunogen or is it a signal for implementation of a naturally prearranged program? Is T-cell vaccination pharmacology or physiology?

A number of observations suggest that the immune system is preprogrammed to receive the autoimmune T-cell vaccine. The mass of vaccinating T-cell antigen can be remarkably small: As few as 10^4, 10^3, or even 10^2 anti-BP T-clone cells can induce resistance to an otherwise lethal dose of millions of virulent anti-BP T cells (Beraud et al. 1989). The lag time for the anti-idiotypic response may be as short as 4 or 5 days (Lider et al. 1989). A de novo immune response to a conventional antigen might be expected to require more antigen and more time to produce such marked effects.

Another indication that the autoimmune idiotype may be a signal and not merely an antigenic structure is the requirement for cell activation; 5×10^7 nonactivated T cells do not induce a detectable anti-idiotypic response, whereas 10^4 activated T cells do. Apparently, it is not the amount of the idiotypic structure alone that triggers the system but its combination with additional signals. Perhaps the system is built to deal with activated autoimmune T cells that require attention, not with quiescent ones that cause no harm.

Direct evidence for the preexistence of selected anti-idiotypic networks has been obtained in our laboratory by N. Karin et al. (in prep.). Karin induced adjuvant arthritis by immunizing rats to whole MT and investigated the evolution of T-cell proliferative responses in the draining lymph nodes to the hsp65 molecule and to other MT antigens and to various clones of syngeneic T cells. Remarkably, Karin found that 4 days after immunization to MT, the lymph node cells responded strongly to the M1 anti-hsp65 T-cell line. This anti-anti-hsp65 response was all the more striking because the response to hsp65 and to other MT antigens was barely detectable. By day 10, the responses to MT antigens became greater than the response to the M1 line although the anti-M1 response continued to rise.

More experiments must be done to document the details of the evolution of the T-cell response to hsp65 and to the M1 T-cell line. Nevertheless, it seems that an anti-idiotypic response to M1 might actually precede, at least in its magnitude, the response to the hsp65 antigen itself.

Karin found that the anti-anti-hsp65 response was selective; it was directed to M1 T cells but not to A2b T cells, which recognize a different epitope on the hsp65 molecule (N. Karin et al., in prep.). Thus, the arthritogenic hsp65 antigen may actually impinge on a preformed anti-idiotypic network.

In addition to the networks associated with the BP and hsp65 molecules described here, we have detected a natural, preexisting network related to the autoimmune response to insulin (Shechter et al. 1982, 1988; Cohen et al. 1984). Autoimmune networks related to acetylcholine (Cleveland et al. 1983) and to thyroid-stimulating hormone (Farid 1988) also have been described.

These immune networks and, in fact, any network may be viewed as a ready-made system for channeling information into prearranged categories. Antigens for which anti-idiotypic networks exist will be dealt with in ways different than other antigens. The system seems to anticipate such antigens, i.e., the existence of a preformed anti-idiotypic network constitutes a representation of the antigen already encoded in the system. Elsewhere, I have referred to the set of network-encoded antigens as the immunological homunculus (Cohen 1989). The term is derived from the neurological homunculus, the representative of the body mapped onto the motor and sensory cortices of the brain, which allows the nervous system to organize and structure neurological experience and activity related to self. So, too, might the immunological homunculus of preformed networks serve as a reference library directing the attention of the immune system to selected self-antigens.

The long-standing belief that self-tolerance is based on deletion of the T-cell receptor repertoire has now been demonstrated experimentally, at least for some self-antigens (von Boehmer et al. 1989). However, major histocompatibility complex (MHC) restriction in or out of the thymus cannot account for the immunological dominance of some self-antigens, a dominance that cuts across individuals and species. For example, BP is the dominant antigen in the central nervous system for mice and rats, dogs and cats, and monkeys and humans. The MHC appears to determine which peptides will be chosen for the T-cell response, but the dominance of the BP molecule seems to be independent of the MHC. Likewise is the immunological dominance of the hsp65 molecule (Young et al. 1988) or the array of lupus antibodies shared by mice and humans (Mendlovic et al. 1989). Perhaps these particular self-antigens are dominant across MHC alleles and species because preformed networks have already encoded them in the various immune systems. The systems are therefore compelled to give these antigens undivided attention. MHC gene products will only restrict the response to particular segments of the antigen; the dominance of the molecule as a whole, irrespective of peptide restrictions, is apparently not the business of the MHC.

Obviously, to say that preformed networks are responsible for the uniformity of autoimmune responses merely prompts the question of why some autoantigens have dominating networks and others do not. Recently, it has become apparent that the major autoantigens monotonously chosen for autoimmune attack are functional molecules: receptors (myasthenia gravis, Grave's disease), hormones (type 1 diabetes), or enzymes (autoimmune thyroiditis, autoimmune liver disease). Regrettably, a function for BP has yet to be defined. However, heat-shock proteins, now beginning to be associated with autoimmunity (Minota et al. 1988; Res et al. 1988; van Eden et al. 1988), must have very important functions because they are highly conserved throughout biological evolution from prokaryotes to humans (McMullin and Hallberg 1988). These observations suggest that the dominant autoantigens may achieve their status by virtue of their functions. How the physiological functions of various self-antigen molecules might influence the network organization of the immune system is an open question.

Irrespective of how self-antigen networks may arise, their malfunction may produce disease. For example, Mendlovic et al. (1988, 1989) found that administering the 16/6 human idiotypic anti-DNA antibody to some strains of mice can unleash full-blown systemic lupus erythematosus with all of its attendant autoantibodies. These mice with idiotype-induced lupus are not of strains that develop lupus spontaneously and do not respond to immunization to DNA itself. Thus, an idiotype interacting with its network can generate a more powerful response than the putative antigen itself does.

Antibodies to the insulin receptor may arise through anti-idiotypic networks in both mice (Cohen et al. 1984) and humans (Shoelson et al. 1986). Moreover, the human and mouse antibodies share idiotypes (Elias et al. 1987). Thus, dysfunction of a network might produce a particular autoimmune disease and also account for the characteristic dominance of its target antigen. A healthy network ideally should prevent disease.

The fact that T-cell vaccination can be effective in preventing or inducing remission of established autoimmune disease is valid, irrespective of whether natural networks are involved in autoimmunity in the real world. Nevertheless, it would be fortunate if T-cell vaccination derived its effectiveness from its ability to exert control through manipulation of preexisting T-cell networks. The network whose malfunction was responsible for initiating the disease might be the most efficient network to control the disease, once its regulatory anti-idiotypic T cells have been augmented by T-cell vaccination. Physiology should promote utility.

ACKNOWLEDGMENTS

I thank Ms. Malvine Baer for preparing the manuscript. The experiments have been supported in part by grants NS-23372 and AM-32192 from the National Institutes of Health. I am the incumbent of the Mauerberger Chair in Immunology.

REFERENCES

Ben-Nun and I.R. Cohen. 1982a. Experimental autoimmune encephalomyelitis (EAE) mediated by T cell lines. Process of selection of lines and characterization. *J. Immunol.* **129:** 303.

———. 1982b. Spontaneous remission and acquired resistance to autoimmune encephalomyelitis (EAE) are associated with suppression of T cell reactivity: Suppressed EAE effector T cells recovered as T cell lines. *J. Immunol.* **128:** 1450.

Ben-Nun, A., H. Wekerle, and I.R. Cohen. 1981a. Vaccination against autoimmune encephalomyelitis with T lymphocyte line cells reactive against myelin basic protein. *Nature* **292:** 60.

———. 1981b. The rapid isolation of clonable antigen-specific T lymphocyte lines capable of mediating autoimmune encephalomyelitis. *Eur. J. Immunol.* **11:** 195.

Bendelac, A.C., C. Carnaud, C. Boitard, and J.F. Bach. 1987. Syngeneic transfer of autoimmune diabetes from diabetic NOD mice to healthy neonates. *J. Exp. Med.* **166:** 1987.

Beraud, E., O. Lider, E. Baharav, T. Reshef, and I.R. Cohen. 1989. Vaccination against experimental autoimmune encephalomyelitis using a subencephalitogenic dose of autoimmune effector cells. I. Characteristics of vaccination. *J. Autoimmun.* **2:** 75.

Cleveland, W.L., N.H. Wasserman, R. Sarangarajan, A.S. Penn, and B.F. Erlanger. 1983. Monoclonal antibodies to the acetylcholine receptor by a normally functioning auto-anti-idiotypic mechanism. *Nature* **305:** 56.

Cohen, I.R. 1986. Regulation of autoimmune disease: Physiological and therapeutic. *Immunol. Rev.* **94:** 5.

———. 1988. The self, the world and autoimmunity. *Sci. Am.* **258:** 52.

———. 1989. Natural Id-anti-Id networks and the immunological homunculus. In *Theories of immune networks* (ed. H. Atlan and I.R. Cohen). Springer-Verlag, Berlin. (In press.)

Cohen, I.R., D. Elias, R. Maron, and Y. Shechter. 1984. Immunization to insulin generates anti-idiotypes that behave as antibodies to the insulin hormone receptor and cause diabetes mellitus. In *Idiotypy* (ed. H. Kohler et al.), vol. 20, p. 385. Academic Press, New York.

Damle, N.K. and S. Gupta. 1982. Autologous mixed lymphocyte reaction in man. V. Functionally and phenotypically distinct human T-cell subpopulations respond to non-T and activated T-cells in AMLR. *Scand. J. Immunol.* **16:** 59.

Elias, D., I.R. Cohen, Y. Shechter, Z. Spirer, and A. Golander. 1987. Antibodies to insulin receptor followed by anti-idiotype antibodies to insulin in a child with hypoglycemia. *Diabetes* **36:** 348.

Farid, N.R. 1988. Anti-idiotypic antibodies approach to the study of the TSH receptor. In *Anti-idiotypes, receptors, and molecular mimicry* (ed. D.S. Linthicum and N.R. Farid), p. 61. Springer-Verlag, New York.

Holoshitz, J., A. Matitiau, and I.R. Cohen. 1984. Arthritis induced in rats by cloned T lymphocytes responsive to mycobacteria but not to collagen type II. *J. Clin. Invest.* **73:** 211.

Holoshitz, J., A. Frenkel, A. Ben-Nun, and I.R. Cohen. 1983a. Autoimmune EAE mediated or prevented by T lymphocyte lines directed against diverse antigenic determinants of myelin basic protein. Vaccination is determinant specific. *J. Immunol.* **131:** 2810.

Holoshitz, J., Y. Naparstek, A. Ben-Nun, and I.R. Cohen. 1983b. Lines of T lymphocytes mediate or vaccinate against autoimmune arthritis. *Science* **219:** 56.

Lider, O., M. Shinitzky, and I.R. Cohen. 1986. Vaccination against experimental autoimmune diseases using T lymphocytes treated with hydrostatic pressure. *Ann. N.Y. Acad. Sci.* **457:** 267.

Lider, O., N. Karin, M. Shinitzky, and I.R. Cohen. 1987. Therapeutic vaccination against adjuvant arthritis using autoimmune T lymphocytes treated with hydrostatic pressure. *Proc. Natl. Acad. Sci.* **84:** 4577.

Lider, O., E. Beraud, T. Reshef, A. Friedman, and I.R. Cohen. 1989. Vaccination against experimental autoimmune encephalomyelitis using a subencephalitogenic dose of autoimmune effector T cells. II. Induction of a protective anti-idiotypic response. *J. Autoimmun.* **2:** 87.

Lider, O., T. Reshef, E. Beraud, A. Ben-Nun, and I.R. Cohen. 1988. Anti-idiotypic network induced by T cell vaccination against experimental autoimmune encephalomyelitis. *Science* **239:** 181.

Lohse, A.W., F. Mor, N. Karin, and I.R. Cohen. 1989. Control of experimental autoimmune encephalomyelitis by T cells responding to activated T cells. *Science* **244:** 820.

McMullin, T.W. and R.L. Hallberg. 1988. A highly evolutionarily conserved mitochondrial protein is structurally related to the protein encoded by the *Escherichia coli* groEL gene. *Mol. Cell. Biol.* **8:** 371.

Mendlovic, S., H. Fricke, Y. Shoenfeld, and E. Mozes. 1989. The role of anti-idiotypic antibodies in the induction of experimental systemic lupus erythematosus in mice. *Eur. J. Immunol.* **19:** 729.

Mendlovic, S., S. Brocke, Y. Shoenfeld, M. Ben-Bassat, A. Meshorer, R. Bakimer, and E. Mozes. 1988. Induction of a systemic lupus erythemetosus-like disease in mice by a common human anti-DNA idiotype. *Proc. Natl. Acad. Sci.* **85:** 2260.

Minota, S., S. Koyaso, K.I. Yahara, and J. Winfield. 1988. Autoantibodies to the heat-shock protein hsp90 in systemic lupus erythematosus. *J. Clin. Invest.* **81:** 106.

Naparstek, Y., A. Ben-Nun, J. Holoshitz, T. Reshef, A. Frenkel, M. Rosenberg, and I.R. Cohen. 1983. T lymphocyte lines producing or vaccinating against autoimmune encephalomyelitis (EAE): Functional activation induces PNA receptors and accumulation in the brain and thymus of line cells. *Eur. J. Immunol.* **13:** 418.

Naparstek, Y., J. Holoshitz, S. Eisenstein, T. Reshef, S. Rappaport, J. Chemke, A. Ben-Nun, and I.R. Cohen. 1982. Effector T lymphocyte line cells migrate to the thymus and persist there. *Nature* **300:** 262.

Res, P.C.M., C.G. Schaar, F.C. Breedveld, W. van Eden, J.D.A. van Embden, I.R. Cohen, and R.R.P. de Vries. 1988. Synovial fluid T cell reactivity against 65 kD heat shock protein of mycobacteria in early chronic arthritis. *Lancet* **II:** 478.

Rossini, A.A., J.P. Mordes, and A.A. Like. 1985. Immunology of insulin-dependent diabetes mellitus. *Annu. Rev. Immunol.* **3:** 289.

Shechter, Y., R. Maron, D. Elias, and I.R. Cohen. 1982. Autoantibodies to the insulin receptor spontaneously arise as anti-idiotypes in mice immunized with insulin. *Science* **216:** 542.

Shechter, Y., D. Elias, R. Bruck, R. Maron, and I.R. Cohen. 1988. Mice immunized to insulin develop anti-idiotypic antibody to the insulin receptor. In *Anti-idiotypes, receptors, and molecular mimicry* (ed. D.S. Linthicum and N.R. Farid), p. 73. Springer-Verlag, New York.

Shoelson, S.E., S. Marshall, H. Horikoshi, O.G. Kalterman, A.H. Rubinstein, and J.M. Olefsky. 1986. Anti-insulin receptor antibodies in an insulin-dependent diabetic may arise as autoantibodies. *J. Clin. Endocrinol. Metab.* **63:** 56.

Sun, D., Y. Qin, J. Chluba, J.T. Epplen, and H. Wekerle.

1988. Suppression of experimentally induced autoimmune encephalomyelitis by cytolytic T-T interactions. *Nature* **332:** 843.

Vandenbark, A.A., H. Offner, T. Reshef, R. Fritz, C.-H.J. Chou, D. Bernard, and I.R. Cohen. 1986. Specificity of T lymphocyte lines for peptides of myelin basic protein. *J. Immunol.* **135:** 229.

van Eden, W., J.E.R. Thole, R. van der Zee, A. Noordzij, J.D.A. Embden, E.J. Hensen, and I.R. Cohen. 1988. Cloning of the mycobacterial epitope recognized by T lymphocytes in adjuvant arthritis. *Nature* **331:** 171.

von Boehmer, H., H.S. Teh, and P. Kisielow. 1989. The thymus selects the useful, neglects the useless and destroys the harmful. *Immunol. Today* **10:** 57.

Young, D., R. Lathigra, R. Hendrix, D. Sweetser, and R.A. Young. 1988. Stress proteins as immune targets in leprosy and tuberculosis. *Proc. Natl. Acad. Sci.* **85:** 4267.

Tolerance Induction in the Adult Using Monoclonal Antibodies to CD4, CD8, and CD11a (LFA-1)

H. Waldmann, S.P. Cobbold, S. Qin, R.J. Benjamin, and M. Wise
Immunology Division, Department of Pathology, University of Cambridge, Cambridge CB2 1QP, United Kingdom

A major challenge in immunology has been to find a means of selectively abolishing an individual's potential to mount an immune response to certain antigens while preserving responsiveness to others. If this were possible, there would be major therapeutic implications for organ and marrow transplantation, the control of allergy, and the treatment of autoimmune diseases. The fact that transplantation tolerance could be achieved by injection of foreign donor hematopoietic cells into the neonatal mouse (Billingham et al. 1953) suggested that the same might be possible in the adult animal if a comparable state of immunological naiveté could be recreated. An array of different immunosuppressive regimes that destroyed lymphocytes (e.g., irradiation, antilymphocyte globulin, and thoracic duct drainage) could all facilitate tolerance induction (for review, see Weigle 1973) in mature animals. With the development of monoclonal antibodies to cells of the immune system, a new means of producing immunosuppression was possible. Cobbold et al. (1985) observed that certain rat antibodies to the mouse CD4 and CD8 T-cell subsets were capable of depleting their target cells in vivo as part of their profound immunosuppressive effect. We subsequently noticed that the immunosuppressive effect of a short course of CD4 and CD8 monoclonal antibody therapy far outlived the period of lymphocyte deficiency. This was the case even in mice previously primed to donor transplantation antigens (Cobbold and Waldmann 1986). These observations led us to ask what record the immune system had kept of antigens that had been administered under cover of monoclonal antibody immunosuppressants. We found that CD4, CD8, and CD11a monoclonal antibodies can create a tolerogenic milieu in mice, allowing specific unresponsiveness to certain soluble proteins and to marrow and skin allografts. Although our work began with selected rat IgG2b-depleting antibodies, it has since become apparent that cell depletion is not always sufficient or even essential. This paper reviews our work so far. We describe the range of models in which we have achieved immunological tolerance in the adult mouse, and we provide some evidence on the mechanisms that may be responsible. The findings suggest that comparable strategies may be used to achieve immunological unresponsiveness for therapeutic purposes.

EXPERIMENTAL PROCEDURES

Most of the experimental procedures were described extensively in the following publications: Cobbold and Waldmann (1986); Cobbold et al. (1986a,b); Qin et al. (1987, 1989); Benjamin et al. (1988). Only experimental procedures that are crucial to understanding the new data are documented here.

Monoclonal antibodies. The synergistic pair of rat IgG2b (rIgG2b) CD4 monoclonal antibodies were YTS 191 and YTA 3.1. The two rIgG2b CD3 monoclonal antibodies were YTS 169 (anti-Lyt-2) and YTS 156 (anti-Lyt-3) (Cobbold et al. 1986a; Qin et al. 1989). The rIgG2a monoclonal antibodies were YTS 177 (CD4) and YTS 105 (CD8). All antibodies were obtained from (DA × LOU)F$_1$ rat ascitic fluid, purified by ammonium sulfate precipitation, and dialyzed against phosphate-buffered saline (PBS). Anti-Thy-1.1 and anti-Thy-1.2 monoclonal antibodies were kind gifts from D. Thomas (Thomas et al. 1986). The V$_\beta$6 MAbs 44-22-1 and 46-6B5 were kind gifts from H. Hengartner and R. MacDonald (Payne et al. 1988; MacDonald et al. 1989). The CD3 MAb 145-2C11 was obtained from the hybridoma kindly provided by J. Bluestone.

Bone marrow transplantation. Marrow cells were flushed from donor femoral and tibial bones and washed with cold Eagle's HEPES medium. T-cell-depleted marrow was obtained from donors that had been pretreated with CD4- and CD8-depleting rIgG2b antibodies (2 mg/mouse; 0.5 mg of each antibody).

Skin grafting. Skin grafts were performed as reported previously (Cobbold and Waldmann 1986). In short, donor tail skin grafts (0.5 × 0.5 cm) were transplanted onto the lateral thoracic wall of the recipient and covered with clean gauze and plaster for 7 days. The graft survival was documented regularly thereafter.

Measurement of lymphocyte proliferative responses. Spleen cells (2×10^6/ml) were incubated with mitomycin-C-treated stimulator cells in Iscove's modified Dulbecco's medium (MDM) containing 5% heat-inactivated human AB serum. Microplates precoated with the anti-V$_\beta$6 MAb 46-6B5 or the hamster CD3 MAb 145-2C11 provided alternative forms of stimulation of test populations. Responses were measured by IUdR incorporation (see Qin et al. 1989). All samples were performed in triplicate.

Measurement of chimerism. Measurement of chimerism was performed as described by Qin et al. (1989). Two-color flow cytometry mouse spleen or lymph node cells were incubated with biotinylated anti-Thy-1.1 or anti-Thy-1.2 and stained with avidin/ phycoerythrin. $V_\beta 6^+$ cells were detected by staining with the rIgG2a MAb 44-22-1 followed by fluorescein-isothiocyanate (FITC)-labeled anti-rat IgG2a mono-clonal antibody.

RESULTS

Tolerance to Human and Rat Gamma Globulins

Benjamin and Waldmann (1986) and Gutstein et al. (1986) observed that rIgG2b CD4 monoclonal antibodies given at high doses could produce tolerance to other rIgG2b immunoglobulins. Benjamin and Waldmann (1988; Benjamin et al. 1988) also showed that CD4 therapy would allow tolerance to human (HGG) and rabbit immunoglobulins if they were given simultaneously. Tolerance to HGG could be so induced and also expressed in the absence of CD8 cells, was not transferred on adoptive transfer with normal cells, and could be very long-lived if antigen (HGG) was reinjected at regular intervals. Adoptive transfer studies also demonstrated that tolerance was expressed at the T helper cell but not the B-cell level. Qin et al. (1987) showed that pairs of CD4 antibodies, at doses too low

to deplete CD4 cells, could also permit tolerance. Carteron et al. (1988) and Benjamin et al. (1988) went on to show that F(ab)$_2$ fragments were also effective, although large doses were needed (probably to compensate for rapid clearance).

Recently, we have observed (S.-X. Qin et al., in prep.) that a particular rIgG2a CD4 monoclonal antibody (YTS 177) was also capable of producing tolerance to both rIgG2a and HGG (Fig. 1A,B), yet was extremely inefficient at depletion of CD4 cells even after prolonged therapy (see below). This antibody has proved to be a valuable alternative to antibody fragments where CD4 blockade, rather than depletion, has been required. Tolerance to soluble proteins without cell depletion is not unique to CD4 monoclonal antibodies but was also observed with CD11a rIgG2b MAb FD441.8 (Benjamin et al. 1988).

Our findings that CD4 monoclonal antibodies enabled tolerance to rat and human immunoglobulins led us to wonder whether there might be some broader applicability of antibody tolerance therapy to other modalities of immunity. We demonstrate below that it has been possible to extend these initial observations to achieving specific unresponsiveness to both bone marrow and skin allografts, even in primed recipients.

Classic-type Transplantation Tolerance

Basic observations. Billingham et al. (1953) demonstrated that the injection of hematopoietic cells into the newborn mouse could produce donor-specific tolerance. If it were possible to smuggle allogeneic bone

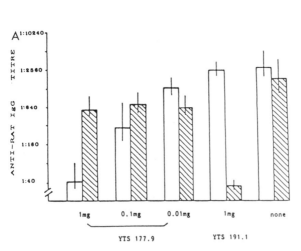

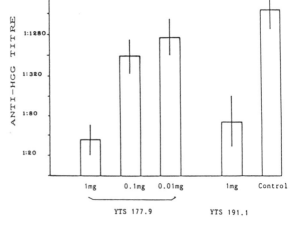

Figure 1. (*A*) Injection of the nondepleting rIgG2a CD4 MAb YTS 177 induces tolerance to rIgG2a. Normal CBA/Ca mice were given three injections of rIgG2a CD4 MAb YTS 177 (open bar) or rIgG2b CD4 MAb YTS 191 (hatched bar) on 3 consecutive days at the doses shown. Six weeks later, mice were rechallenged with weekly injections of 0.5 mg of an irrelevant rIgG2a or rIgG2b, first in complete Freund's adjuvant and later in incomplete Freund's adjuvant. On the tenth week, they were bled, and mouse anti-rat IgG2a or IgG2b titers were measured with an enzyme-linked immunosorbent assay (ELISA). (1B) Tolerance to HGG induced by rIgG2a CD4 MAb YTS 177. CBA/Ca mice were injected with YTS 177 or YTS 191 at doses indicated on days −1, 0, and 1. On day zero (0), 1 mg of heat-aggregated HGG was injected. The mice were rechallenged with 0.5 mg of HGG on days 28 and 35. Control mice received antibody but were not given HGG until days 28 and 35. Serum titers were measured on day 45 by an ELISA.

marrow grafts into adult animals, classic-type transplantation tolerance (CTTT) might be achieved for organ grafts transplanted at the same time.

Of the many attempts to graft bone marrow into adult animals at the experimental level, the most successful have used irradiation, ablative chemotherapy, and antilymphocytic sera (Wood et al. 1971; Rappaport 1977; Slavin et al. 1977; Thomas et al. 1983; Ilstad and Sachs 1984; Mayumi et al. 1986). In essence, the common theme of these strategies was to establish some level of hematopoietic chimerism. The ubiquitous distribution of chimeric hematopoietic cells clearly favors them as vehicles to present donor antigens for tolerance, regardless of the mechanisms involved.

We have recently shown that CTTT can be achieved in a number of mouse strain combinations with a very short course of monoclonal antibodies (CD4 and CD8) as the only therapeutic modality (Qin et al. 1989). Where the short course of antibody, itself, proved insufficient (e.g., for the complete major histocompatibility complex [MHC] and minor mismatched combination BALB/c into CBA/Ca), additional sublethal irradiation (300 rads) and the addition of a CD11a monoclonal antibody permitted long-term mixed chimerism and donor hyporesponsiveness (R.J. Benjamin et al., in prep.). Previously, Cobbold et al. (1986b) showed that a short course of CD4 and CD8 monoclonal antibody therapy could prevent marrow rejection in recipients irradiated with 600 rads. However, the chimerism obtained was wholly donor rather than mixed. Recently, Sharabi and Sachs (1989) used CD4 and CD8 antibodies combined with thymic irradiation to achieve the mixed chimerism across complete MHC plus minor differences.

The most informative of our attempts to achieve CTTT in the adult has been with the H-2-matched, but multiple, minor mismatch combinations (Qin et al. 1989). We have shown that both CD4 and CD8 cells reject donor marrow. The combination of CD4 and CD8 antibodies—but neither alone—was needed to obtained tolerance and chimerism. Although our initial work used depleting rIgG2b antibodies, we subsequently showed that the rIgG2a nondepleting CD4 monoclonal antibody could adequately replace the rIgG2b in the tolerizing regimen. Similarly, nondepleting antibody fragments were able to replace the rIgG2b

Table 1. $V_\beta 6^+$ Cells in Mls Unresponsive Mice Are of Recipient, Not Donor, Origin

	Tolerant CBA/Ca	Normal CBA/Ca
Thy-1.1$^+$	2.6 ± 1.7	0.3 ± 0.6
Thy-1.2$^+$	31.0 ± 8.6	40.1 ± 4.7
$V_\beta 6^+$	5.3 ± 2.0	6.2 ± 0.6
Thy-1.1$^+$ $V_\beta 6^+$	0.1 ± 0.1	0.2 ± 0.1
Thy-1.2$^+$ $V_\beta 6^+$	4.3 ± 1.1	6.1 ± 2.7

CBA/Ca mice were rendered tolerant to AKR/J by CD4 and CD8 monoclonal antibody treatment and donor BMT. Recipient spleen cells were analyzed by 6–8 weeks later by two-color flow cytometry.

CD8 monoclonal antibody. Clearly, this tells us that tolerance and donor chimerism were possible without the need to deplete recipient T cells of either of the two major subsets.

In another minor mismatch combination (AKR into CBA/Ca), we demonstrated that the majority of T cells that reconstituted chimeras after depleting antibody therapy were largely of recipient (Thy-1.2) type, although donor T-cell chimerism was detectable. Recipient T cells must therefore have been rendered tolerant of AKR antigens. As CBA/Ca and AKR differ in the Mls locus, we were able to investigate whether CBA/Ca T cells were tolerized to the Mls^a of the chimeric AKR cells. We found the spleen cells of these tolerant animals to be unresponsive to AKR stimulators in vitro.

Mechanisms of tolerance. In the AKR-to-CBA/Ca combination, all tolerant animals expressed virtually normal levels of $V_\beta 6^+$ cells. Previous work (Kappler et al. 1988; MacDonald et al. 1989) suggested that central tolerance induced in the thymus would be associated with loss of T cells expressing particular V specificities. It emerges that the $V_\beta 6^+$ cells in these antibody-induced chimeras, however, are all of recipient (CBA/Ca) origin (Table 1). This contrasts with data from single or double marrow irradiation chimeras derived by injection of either AKR or both CBA/Ca and AKR bone marrow cells into lethally irradiated CBA/Ca recipients, where none of the animals developed $V_\beta 6^+$ T cells (Table 2).

Although the spleen cells of the antibody-derived chimeras were unresponsive to AKR stimulators, four

Table 2. Absence of $V_\beta 6^+$ Cells in Irradiation Chimeras

Group	Fluorescence staining (%)			
	Thy-1$^+$	Thy-1.1$^+$	Thy-1.2$^+$	$V_\beta 6^+$
1	47.4 ± 6.3	28.2 ± 5.4	23.3 ± 4.7	1.6 ± 1.1
2	50.1 ± 8.7	48.7 ± 4.5	3.4 ± 5.7	1.1 ± 0.8
CBA/Ca	50.7 ± 3.3	1.5 ± 4.6	52.2 ± 5.5	10.2 ± 3.1
AKR/J	37.3 ± 4.2	35.3 ± 5.8	0.8 ± 0.8	1.2 ± 0.9

Two experimental groups of CBA/Ca mice were given total body irradiation of 850 rads on the first day and three injections of CD4 and CD8 monoclonal antibodies during the next 5 days. Then, 8 hrs after irradiation, they were given a mixture of 10^7 AKR/J and 10^7 syngeneic CBA/Ca bone marrow cells (group 1) or 2×10^7 AKR/J cells only (group 2). The mice were bled and PBL stained with biotinylated monoclonal antibodies to the surface antigens 12 weeks after irradiation. The results were obtained by flow cytometry and presented as means of four mice in each group.

Table 3. $V_\beta 6^+$ T Cells Are Present in Mice Rendered Unresponsive to Mls[a]

Mice	Fluorescent staining (%)			Proliferation to (cpm)			
	Thy-1.1$^+$	Thy-1.2$^+$	VB6$^+$	AKR/J	anti-V_β6	anti-CD3	−ve
1	4.2	16.4	2.1	n.d.	621	25702	725
2	3.8	38.6	7.1	695	13975	16503	607
3	1.3	31.7	4.8	1567	23352	19189	496
4	3.2	33.9	6.8	583	18732	21923	576
5	2.2	34.5	5.8	798	15787	22125	785
CBA/Ca	0.3 ± 0.6	40.1 ± 4.7	6.2 ± 0.6	22531*1.2	34702*1.1	15416*1.4	617*1.6
AKR/J	22.0 ± 1.1	1.1 ± 0.8	0.6 ± 0.5	1101*1.4	1086*1.2	8600*1.2	1105*1.4

CBA/Ca mice were treated with rat anti-mouse CD4 and CD8 monoclonal antibodies for 5 days after infusion of 2×10^7 AKR/J bone marrow cells. Then, 6 (mouse 1) to 8 weeks (mice 2–5) later, the spleen cells from these mice were stained with monoclonal antibodies to the surface antigens. The results were analyzed by two-color flow cytometry. Meanwhile, cells from the same mice were stimulated with mitomycin-treated AKR/J spleen cells, an anti-V_β6 monoclonal antibody (46–6B5, 2.5 μg/ml on plastic), and an anti-mouse CD3 monoclonal antibody (145-2C11, 2 μg/ml in solution). Then 3 to 4 days later, the proliferation was measured by 6-hr incorporation of ^{135}IUR. n.d. indicates not determined.
(*) Standard error of geometric mean. (−ve) indicates negative control.

of five sets of spleen cells were capable of proliferating when stimulated with the anti-V_β6 MAb 46-6B5, and all responded to a hamster CD3 monoclonal antibody (Table 3). A subsequent experiment showed 4/5 tolerant mice unreactive to stimulation with anti-V_β6 MAb. To explain these data, we must assume that the V_β-6$^+$ cells detected are all derived from CBA/Ca peripheral T cells that have survived the antibody therapy. Insofar as these cells had expanded to normal numbers, they could not have been deleted at the time of marrow infusion. Unless the V_β6$^+$ cells were derived from a small number of postthymic cells that were Mls[a] unreactive themselves, the data would be inconsistent with simple clonal deletion models. We must therefore conclude that the V_β6$^+$ cells have somehow increased their triggering threshold (so that they could only be stimulated by mitogenic antibody in four of five cases) or were blocked by nonstimulatory forms of antigen or other regulatory cells.

The possibility that regulatory (veto/suppressive) influences are contributing to the state of tolerance to skin grafts is suggested by experiments where we have failed to break tolerance by the transfer of large numbers of normal spleen cells into tolerant animals (Table 4). The adoptive transfer of spleen cells from primed mice did, however, break tolerance and the state of chimerism in four of six mice.

Tolerance to Skin Grafts

Tolerance across multiple minor mismatch combinations. Figure 2 shows skin graft survival, using three different monoclonal antibody treatment protocols (S.P. Cobbold et al.; S.-X. Qin et al.; both in prep.). The short course of three injections of IgG2b monoclonal antibodies (1.2 mg/mouse total antibody on days 0, 2, and 4 of the synergistic pairs of CD4 and CD8 antibodies) was insufficient to produce tolerance to skin grafts in the absence of marrow. The pair of rIgG2a CD4 and CD8 monoclonal antibodies given over a similar period were more immunosuppressive although all grafts were eventually rejected (S.-X. Qin et al., in prep.). However, the same monoclonal antibodies given over 3 weeks (three doses per week; 9 mg total antibody) produced tolerance in all mice grafted (eight of eight). Second grafts were all accepted, and

Table 4. Resistance of Tolerant Mice to In Vivo Challenge

Animals	Cell injection[a]	Graft survival[b]	Chimerism[c] (%)
Tolerant[d] CBA/Ca	B10.BR	>100 (n = 6)	2.1, 1.5, 1.3, 1.9, 2.3, 1.1
Tolerant CBA/Ca	CBA/Ca	>100 (n = 5)	1.1, 1.2, 1.5, 1.9, 2.2, 2.5
Tolerant CBA/Ca	B10.BR-primed[e] CBA/Ca	9, 10, 12, 13, >100, >100	0, 0, 0, 0.2, 1.5, 1.9
ATX CBA/Ca	B10.BR-primed CBA/Ca	7, 7, 8, 9, 9	n.d.
ATX CBA/Ca	none	>100 (n = 5)	n.d.

[a] Spleen cells 5×10^7 were injected intraperitoneally into CBA/Ca mice that had been tolerized to B10.BR and carried B10.BR skin for >60 days or into thymectomized CBA/Ca mice that had been T-cell depleted with 4 mg CD4 and CD8 monoclonal antibodies 4 weeks prior.
[b] Days after spleen cell injection.
[c] Percentage of IgH-1b immunogloblin 4 weeks after cell injection. n.d. indicates not determined.
[d] CBA/Ca mice rendered tolerant to B10.BR, carrying B10.BR skin for 60 days.
[e] CBA/Ca mice primed with B10.BR spleen 2 weeks previously.

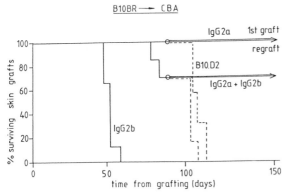

Figure 2. Tolerance of CBA/Ca mice to B10.BR skin grafts transplanted under cover of CD4 and CD8 monoclonal antibodies. Antibodies were injected into groups of eight mice that were grafted on day 0 with tail skin under cover of various antibody regimens (see text). One group received three injections of synergistic rIgG2b CD4 and CD8 monoclonal antibodies (1.2 mg/mouse total) around the time of grafting; two other groups received 3 weeks of therapy with the rIgG2a CD4 and CD8 monoclonal antibodies only (9 mg/mouse total) or 1 week of rIgG2b, followed by 2 weeks of rIgG2a monoclonal antibodies (see text). Second grafts were transplanted after 3 months (○). These grafts were from the original B10.BR strain (solid lines) or B10.D2 strain (dashed lines).

third-party B10.D2 grafts were promptly rejected. The substitution of depleting antibodies in the first week gave comparable results although some animals in this group exhibited delayed rejections.

CD4 cells are not depleted following 3 weeks of rIgG2a therapy. Figure 3 shows the peripheral blood lymphocyte (PBL) counts from mice 1 week following the cessation of rIgG2a CD4 and CD8 monoclonal antibody therapy. The number of Thy-1[+] cells is similar to that of untreated controls. Similarly, the percentage of CD4 cells remains unchanged although the population shows reduced fluorescence intensity (consistent

with modulation). However, the CD8 population appears to have been depleted. Of the Thy-1[+] cells, 10% were negative for CD4 and CD8. These are either an expanded population of double-negative T cells or may represent CD4 or CD8 cells that remain modulated. The important point is that at no time in the course of the rIgG2a CD4 therapy did we see depletion rather than modulation of CD4 cells. We must conclude that the immunosuppressive/tolerizing effects of this monoclonal antibody are related to its capacity to bind to, but not to kill, CD4[+] cells.

Prolonged graft survival across MHC and minor mismatch combinations. Figures 4 and 5 show the skin-graft survival data in two strain combinations that represent completely mismatched grafts. In Figure 4, neither the 3-week course of the rIgG2a (9 mg total antibody) nor the 5-week course of synergistic pairs of CD4 and CD8 rIgG2b antibodies (6 mg total antibody) was able to delay graft survival of BALB/c skin grafts on CBA/Ca recipients (H-2[d] into H-2[k]) beyond 2 months. However, a combination of two depleting doses of rIgG2b, followed by 3 weeks of rIgG2a, was able to produce prolonged graft survival in this combination. Regrafting at 3 months was followed by a gradual loss of nearly all grafts (mean survival time [MST] of second grafts was 43 days). A third-party (B10) graft was rejected at a much faster rate (MST, 17 days). Clearly, there must have been some level of specific tolerance to the BALB/c donor antigens. The same therapy administered over the B10-to-CBA/Ca combination (Fig. 5; H-2[b] into H-2[k]) resulted in prolonged survival of nearly all grafts for over 4 months (14/15 mice). Tolerance was assessed by regrafting one group of mice at 4 months. The MST of the third-party graft (BALB/c) was 13 days and that of the B10 graft was >200 days for the first graft and 44 days for the second.

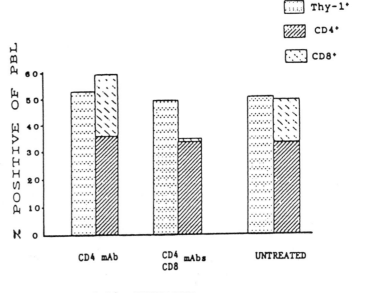

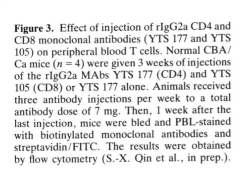

Figure 3. Effect of injection of rIgG2a CD4 and CD8 monoclonal antibodies (YTS 177 and YTS 105) on peripheral blood T cells. Normal CBA/Ca mice (*n* = 4) were given 3 weeks of injections of the rIgG2a MAbs YTS 177 (CD4) and YTS 105 (CD8) or YTS 177 alone. Animals received three antibody injections per week to a total antibody dose of 7 mg. Then, 1 week after the last injection, mice were bled and PBL-stained with biotinylated monoclonal antibodies and streptavidin/FITC. The results were obtained by flow cytometry (S.-X. Qin et al., in prep.).

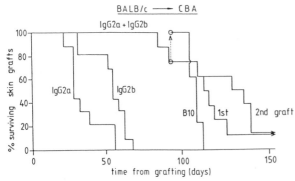

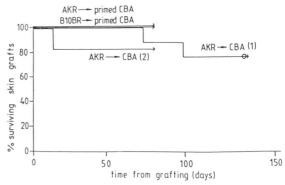

Figure 4. CD4 and CD8 antibodies produce prolonged skin-graft survival across H-2 differences in BALB/c grafts to CBA/Ca recipients. Various groups of CBA/Ca mice (H-2^k) were grafted with BALB/c (H-2^d) skin under cover of different antibody regimens, as described in the text. The groups receiving rIgG2b (5 weeks) or rIgG2a (3 weeks) only rejected their grafts within 2 months. Animals receiving a combined regimen of rIgG2b (two injections, total 800 μg/mouse of synergistic CD4 and CD8 monoclonal antibodies) followed by rIgG2a for 3 weeks (total 9 mg/mouse) held their grafts and were regrafted at 3 months (O) with a second graft of donor tail skin or skin from a third party (B10).

Figure 6. CD4 and CD8 monoclonal antibodies can produce prolonged graft survival in primed mice. CBA/Ca mice were primed to irradiated (2500 rads) B10.BR or AKR spleen cells and grafted with tail skin from the same donors under cover of the rIgG2b/rIgG2a CD4 + CD8 monoclonal antibody combination 2 weeks later (as in Fig. 5). Data from first-set grafts subject to the same antibody therapy or to rIgG2a monoclonal antibodies alone are also shown (2 and 1, respectively).

Prolonged survival of second-set grafts. As mentioned previously, prolonged survival of second-set grafts was observed in the multiple minor mismatch combination B10.BR to CBA/Ca, given rIgG2b CD4 and CD8 antibodies (Cobbold and Waldmann 1986). In view of the potent immunosuppressive effects of the rIgG2b and rIgG2a combination, we analyzed second-set graft survival in two groups of CBA/Ca mice previously primed to B10.BR and AKR, respectively (seven of seven for each group). As shown in Figure 6, graft survival in primed animals is 100% at 3 months. In comparison, first-set graft survival in the AKR-to-CBA/Ca combination has now extended to 5 months in five of seven mice.

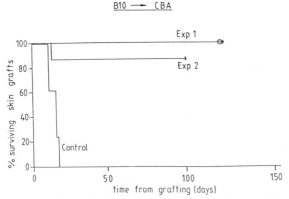

Figure 5. CD4 and CD8 antibodies produce prolonged skin-graft survival across H-2 differences in B10 grafts to CBA/Ca mice. CBA/Ca mice (H-2^k) received tail skin from B10 mice (H-2^b) under cover of CD4 and CD8 monoclonal antibody therapy. The test groups received an antibody regiment of two depleting doses of rIgG2b monoclonal antibodies, followed by the rIgG2a antibodies for 3 weeks (as in Fig. 4). Controls received no antibody (S.P. Cobbold et al., in prep.).

DISCUSSION

Here, we have documented many different models of tolerance induction with monoclonal antibody therapy. These models have embraced specific unresponsiveness to xenogeneic immunoglobulins: first-set multiple minor mismatched and major mismatched marrow and skin grafts and, more recently, second-set minor mismatched skin grafts. Following our initial demonstration of CD4 monoclonal antibodies as agents to promote tolerance induction (Benjamin and Waldmann 1986), as well as prolonged graft survival (Cobbold and Waldmann 1986; Mottram et al. 1987; Shizuru et al. 1987), we and other investigators have asked whether the same principles could be applied to produce tolerance to allografts (Herbert and Roser 1988; Madsen 1988; Qin et al. 1989). In both mouse and rat, it has proved reasonably straightforward to induce tolerance to vascularized heart grafts (Madsen et al. 1988) or to fetal heart grafts transplanted to the ear (Herbert and Roser 1988). The major challenge has been to produce tolerance to skin grafts since these are perhaps the most immunogenic of all rodent grafts. Our work suggests that this is possible without the need for other immunosuppressive agents. Recently, Roser (1989) reported failure to obtain skin-graft tolerance in rats with CD4 monoclonal antibody, unless the antibody was combined with cyclosporin A. Our findings suggest that there is a general principle that can be extrapolated from our earlier work extending monoclonal antibody therapy (particularly with CD4, CD8, and CD11a) over a broad spectrum of situations. The observation of extended graft survival in second-set situations provides some optimism for monoclonal antibody treatment of autoimmunity where T cells are already primed to peptide-self-MHC. In that sense, the situation is no different from the model above where animals are primed to minor transplantation antigens.

The particularly exciting prospect for tolerance therapy is the fact that a substantial effect can be obtained by CD4 antibodies that deplete poorly. In clinical practice, this would allow a minimum interference approach to tolerance induction, especially if synergistic combinations could be found. In terms of understanding tolerance mechanisms, the data show that mature T cells must be able to decide between switching on or off. There are three possible explanations of how they might do this, none of which are mutually exclusive. First, it is possible that the T-cell receptor (TCR) and CD4, CD8, and possibly CD11a somehow interact to provide the required on signal. Interference with this process might render the T cells refractory, inept, or suicidal. This idea embraces negative signaling and cross-linking mechanisms among the possibilities. The second explanation (see Waldmann et al. 1989) is a T-cell frequency argument, which is based on the assumption that all on responses require a minimal cooperative unit of multiple cells (T cells and others). If T cells have been depleted or blocked by antibody, any TCR occupancy by antigen may occur without help from collaborating cells. Consequently, antigen-binding T cells would be turned off. The third explanation is that regulatory mechanisms (suppressive or veto) come into play if immunity has been prevented. Note that these mechanisms must have been spared selectively by antibody therapy.

Our observation that peripheral T cells were unreactive to Mls^a in the antibody-facilitated AKR-to-CBA/Ca chimeras yet some mice could respond normally (four of five mice) to a mitogenic V$_\beta$6 antibody suggests that the T cells in question may be refractory (have raised their triggering thresholds). Alternatively, they are under some form of regulation. If raised thresholds were the means by which postthymic T cells normally became unresponsive to peripheral tissue-specific antigens, then breakdown of self-tolerance might arise if this triggering threshold was overcome. This could occur, for example, through a strong stimulus from mimicry or from exposure to an appropriate superantigen (White et al. 1989).

Our failure to break tolerance in antibody-facilitated bone marrow chimera by the transfer of normal cells implies that a regulatory mechanism is (also) operating. There is clear precedent for the existence of such peripheral failsafes in the two thymus experiments of Zamoyska et al. (1988). Both model systems require additional work to identify mechanisms.

In conclusion, we have demonstrated that simple protocols of CD4, CD8, and CD11a monoclonal antibody therapy may allow tolerance to be obtained in the adult mouse. In clinical terms, our findings suggest that there is much to be gained by judicious attempts at tolerance therapy with monoclonal antibodies in the clinical arena. At the fundamental level, we have available numerous examples of tolerance induced in the peripheral immune system, which should provide fertile ground for identification of tolerance mechanisms; this may, in turn, lead to clues as to how peripheral tolerance can break down in autoimmunity and may find application in tolerance therapy in humans.

ACKNOWLEDGMENTS

This work was supported by grants from the Medical Research Council of Great Britain, from the Arthritis and Rheumatism Council, the Oliver Bird Trust, and Wellcome Biotech, Ltd. We thank Gilly Martin and Mark Frewin for their assistance.

REFERENCES

Benjamin, R.J. and H. Waldmann. 1986. Induction of tolerance by monoclonal antibody therapy. *Nature* **320**: 449.

Benjamin, R.J., S.P. Cobbold, M.R. Clark, and H. Waldmann. 1986. Tolerance to rat monoclonal antibodies. Implications for serotherapy. *J. Exp. Med.* **163**: 1539.

Benjamin, R.J., S.-X. Qin, M.P. Wise, S.P. Cobbold, and H. Waldmann. 1988. Mechanisms of monoclonal antibody-facilitated tolerance induction: A possible role for the CD4 (L3T4) and CD11a (LFA-1) molecules in self-non-self discrimination. *Eur. J. Immunol.* **18**: 1079.

Billingham, R.E., L. Brent, and P. Medawar. 1953. Actively acquired tolerance of foreign cells. *Nature* **172**: 603.

Carteron, N.L., D. Wofsy, and W.E. Seaman. 1988. Induction of immune tolerance during administration of monoclonal antibody to L3T4 does not depend upon depletion of L3T4 cells. *J. Immunol.* **140**: 703.

Cobbold, S.P. and H. Waldmann. 1986. Skin allograft rejection by L3T4 and Lyt2 T-cell subsets. *Transplantation* **41**: 634.

Cobbold, S.P., G. Martin, and H. Waldmann. 1986a. Monoclonal antibodies for the prevention of graft versus host disease. The depletion of T-cell subsets in-vitro and in-vivo. *Transplantation* **42**: 239.

Cobbold, S.P., G. Martin, S.-X. Qin, and H. Waldmann. 1986b. Monoclonal antibodies to promote marrow engraftment and tissue graft tolerance. *Nature* **323**: 164.

Cobbold, S.P., A. Jayasuriya, A. Nash, T. Prospero, and H. Waldmann. 1985. Therapy with monoclonal antibodies by elimination of T-cell subsets in-vivo. *Nature* **312**: 548.

Gutstein, N.L., W.E. Seaman, J.H. Scott, and D. Wofsy. 1986. Induction of immune tolerance by administration of monoclonal antibody to L3T4. *J. Exp. Med.* **164**: 911.

Herbert, J. and B. Roser. 1988. Strategies of monoclonal antibody therapy which induce permanent tolerance of organ transplants. *Transplantation* **46**: 128.

Istad, S.T. and D.H. Sachs. 1984. Reconstitution with syngeneic plus allogeneic or xenogeneic bone-marrow leads to specific acceptance of skin allografts or xenografts. *Nature* **307**: 168.

Kappler, J.W., U. Staerz, J. White, and P. Marrack. 1988. Self tolerance eliminates T-cell specific for Mls-modified products of the major histocompatibility complex. *Nature* **332**: 35.

MacDonald, H.R., A.L. Glasebrook, R. Schneider, R.K. Lees, H. Pircher, T. Pedrazzini, O. Kanagawa, J.-F. Nicolas, R.C. Howe, R.M. Zinkernagel, and H. Hengartner. 1989. T-cell reactivity and tolerance to Mls^a-encoded antigens. *Immunol. Rev.* **107**: 89.

Madsen, J.C., W.N. Peugh, K.J. Wood, and P.J. Morris. 1988. The effect of anti-L3T4 antibody treatment on the first set rejection of murine cardiac allografts. *Transplantation* **44**: 849.

Mayumi, H.K., K. Himeno, N. Tanaka, J. Tokuda, J.-L. Fan, and K. Nomoto. 1986. Drug induced tolerance to allografts in mice. *Transplantation* **42**: 417.

Mottram, P.L., J. Wheelan, I.F.C. MacKenzie, and G.J.A. Clunie. 1987. Murine cardiac allograft survival following treatment of recipients with monoclonal anti-L3T4 or Lyt2 antibodies. *Transplant Proc.* **19**: 2898.

Payne, J., B.T. Huber, M.A. Cannon, R. Schneider, M.W. Schilham, H. Acha-Orbea, H.R. MacDonald, and H. Hengartner. 1988. Two monoclonal rat antibodies with specificity for the beta chain variable chain region $V_\beta 6$ of the murine T-cell receptor. *Proc. Natl. Acad. Sci.* **85**: 7695.

Qin, S.-X., S.P. Cobbold, R.J. Benjamin, and H. Waldmann. 1989. Induction of classical transplantation tolerance in the adult. *J. Exp. Med.* **169**: 779.

Qin, S.-X., S.P. Cobbold, H. Tighe, R. Benjamin, and H. Waldmann. 1987. CD4 Mab pairs for immunosuppression and tolerance induction. *Eur. J. Immunol.* **18**: 495.

Rappaport, F.T. 1977. Immunological tolerance: Irradiation and bone-marrow transplantation induce canine allogeneic unresponsiveness. *Transplant Proc.* **9**: 981.

Roser, B. 1989. Cellular mechanisms in neonatal and adult tolerance. *Immunol. Rev.* **107**: 179.

Sharabi, Y. and D.H. Sachs. 1989. Mixed chimerism and permanent specific transplantation tolerance induced by a non-lethal preparative regimen. *J. Exp. Med.* **169**: 439.

Shizuru, J.A., A.K. Gregory, C.B. Chao, and G.C. Fathman. 1987. Islet cell allograft survival after a single course of treatment with antibody to L3T4. *Science* **237**: 738.

Slavin, S., S. Strober, Z. Fukes, and H.S. Kaplan. 1977. Induction of specific tissue transplantation tolerance using fractionated total lymphoid irradiation in adult mice. Long term survival of allogeneic bone-marrow and skin grafts. *J. Exp. Med.* **146**: 34.

Thomas, D.B., V. Giguere, C.M. Graham, and O.L.P. Oliviera. 1986. Autoimmunity to Thy-1. *Eur. J. Immunol.* **16**: 10.

Thomas, J.M., F.M. Carver, M.B. Foil, W.R. Hall, C. Adams, G.C. Fahrenbruch, and F.T. Thomas. 1983. Renal allograft tolerance induced with ATG and donor bone-marrow in outbred rhesus monkeys. *Transplantation* **38**: 152.

Waldmann, H., S.P. Cobbold, R.J. Benjamin, and S.-X. Qin. 1989. A theoretical framework for self-tolerance and its relevance in the therapy of autoimmune disease. *J. Autoimmun.* **2**: 127.

Weigle, W.O. 1973. Immunological unresponsiveness. *Adv. Immunol.* **16**: 61.

White, J., A. Herman, A. Pullen, R. Kubo, J.W. Kappler, and P. Marrack. 1989. The V-beta specific superantigen staphylococcal enterotoxin B: Stimulation of mature T-cells and clonal deletion in neonatal mice. *Cell* **56**: 27.

Wood, M.L., A.P. Monaco, J.J. Gozzo, and A. Liegeois. 1971. Use of homozygous allogeneic bone-marrow for induction of tolerance with ALS. *Transplant. Proc.* **3**: 676.

Zamoyska, R., H. Waldmann, and P. Matzinger. 1988. Peripheral tolerance mechanisms prevent the development of autoreactive T-cells in chimeras grafted with two minor incompatible thymuses. *Eur. J. Immunol.* **19**: 111.

Immunologic Tolerance within the B-lymphocyte Compartment: An Adult Tolerance Model

G.J.V. NOSSAL, M. KARVELAS, AND P.A. LALOR

The Walter and Eliza Hall Institute of Medical Research, Royal Melbourne Hospital,
Victoria 3050, Australia

For some years, the main interest of our laboratory has been in the field of B-lymphocyte tolerance (Nossal 1983; Pike et al. 1987). We have shown that the virgin, preimmune B-cell repertoire can be functionally purged of anti-hapten B lymphocytes through the injection of hapten-human gamma globulin conjugates during uterine or newborn life. Although large doses of toleragen do cause a reduction in the number of hapten-binding B cells in the spleens of tolerant mice (clonal abortion), smaller doses chosen to be on the sensitive portion of the antigen-dose:tolerance-response curve do not. Thus, B cells remain within the spleen that are hapten-specific but functionally nonresponsive to normally immunogenic stimuli. We have used the term clonal anergy to describe this state. Recent elegant experiments involving transgenic mice have confirmed that indeed clonal abortion (Nemazee and Bürki 1989) and clonal anergy (Goodnow et al. 1988) can be demonstrated as valid tolerance mechanisms within the B-cell compartment.

It is evident that the median affinity of the anti-hapten immunoglobulin M (IgM) responses that have been the focus of this work, as well as that of many autoimmune responses studied through clonal techniques (reviewed in Nossal 1987), is quite low. For example (McHeyzer-Williams and Nossal 1988), when spleen cells from unimmunized mice are polyclonally activated in limiting dilution microculture, 3% of the B-cell repertoire can score as "antiself" when syngeneic, methanol-fixed cells are used as the capture reagent in an enzyme-linked immunosorbent assay (ELISA), but when an interleukin-4 (IL-4)-induced switch to IgG1 secretion permits examination of a bivalent, rather than a decavalent, antibody product, the vast majority of these clonotypes fail to register. Similarly, when a protein antigen such as keyhole-limpet hemocyanin (KLH) acts as the capture layer, 98% of clones forming anti-KLH IgM fail to register as anti-KLH when their IgG product is examined (Nossal and Riedel 1989). Following immunization with alum-precipitated KLH and *Bordetella pertussis* organisms, substantial numbers of anti-KLH IgG1-antibody-forming cell precursors (AFCP) appear suddenly on day 5 after immunization. Because of the sharpness of the rise in their numbers (a 350-fold increase between day 3 and day 7 after immunization) and the higher amount of antibody bound from clonal supernatants, the pos-

sibility exists that these cells are not just the direct progeny of the few anti-KLH IgG1-AFCP seen during preimmunization. They may include the first products of the immunoglobulin variable (V) gene hypermutation that characterizes active immune responses (McKean et al. 1984; Berek and Milstein 1987; Rajewsky et al. 1987).

This possibility raises interesting issues with respect to B-cell tolerance. The V gene mutation rate during an immune response may be as high as 10^{-3} bp/division. Given the large number of self-epitopes, it seems inevitable that sooner or later in a normal (antiforeign) immune response B cells with V gene mutations that confer antiself reactivity will arise fortuitously. Is there a way of silencing or eliminating such cells? Admittedly, in the absence of helper T cells reactive to peptides from the self-antigen in question, such mutants would not pose an immediate threat. However, their continuance in the memory B-cell pool could create an undesirable population, subject to induction by bacterial mitogens or lymphokines. Linton et al. (1988) have produced evidence to suggest that a second window of tolerance susceptibility exists shortly after B cells are activated that are the precursors of a secondary response. This could represent a mechanism for censoring mutant forbidden clones of the above type.

In this paper, we present some further characteristics of anti-KLH IgG1-AFCP, and we also describe an adult tolerance model following intraperitoneal injection of human serum albumin (HSA). In the latter, anti-HSA IgG1-AFCP fail to appear after immunization with HSA.

METHODS

These were essentially as described previously (McHeyzer-Williams and Nossal 1989; Nossal and Riedel 1989). Briefly, adult CBA or C57BL mice were immunized intraperitoneally with 100 µg of alum-precipitated KLH or HSA plus 10^9 *B. pertussis* organisms. Some mice also received intraperitoneally soluble, freshly deaggregated HSA, KLH, or ovalbumin (OVA) at various doses and times. Spleen cells from immunized or unimmunized mice were cultured for 7 days in 200 µl of microcultures in the presence of 5000 3T3 filler cells. They were stimulated with 30 µg/ml *Escherichia coli* lipopolysaccharide (LPS) and either a supernatant from stimulated EL-4 thymoma cells or a mixture of molecularly cloned lymphokines, namely 100 units/ml IL-4, 10 units/ml IL-2, and an optimal amount (1% of a transfected cell supernatant) of IL-5. Care was taken to ensure that the B-cell density was low enough to permit optimal antibody production per input B cell and never higher than 5000 splenocytes/well. Aliquots of culture supernatants, as well as serum samples from immunized mice, were examined for IgG1 anti-KLH or anti-HSA antibody by ELISA. In some experiments, spleen cell preparations were depleted of T cells by the use of a mixture of anti-CD4, anti-CD8, and anti-Thy-1 antibodies and complement. In others, B-cell populations with particular densities of surface IgM, IgD, or IgG1 were prepared by standard fluorescence-activated cell sorting using a Becton-Dickinson FACStar Plus instrument.

RESULTS

Cell-surface Phenotype of Anti-KLH IgG1-AFCP in Spleen 7 Days after Immunization with KLH

After immunization (1 week), the spleens of KLH-immunized mice contain 4×10^5 to 8×10^5 B cells, which have the capacity to be stimulated by LPS plus lymphokines to form a clone of antibody-forming cells secreting IgG1 capable of binding to KLH. This represents about 1 splenocyte/400 within the grossly enlarged spleen. In contrast, the spleens from unimmunized mice contained only 1×10^3 to 2×10^3 of such cells, and moreover their antibody usually bound to KLH with poor avidity. To characterize the phenotype of the greatly enlarged anti-KLH IgG1-AFCP population in immunized mice, B cells were sorted into three populations as shown in Figures 1 and 2. These were high-density surface IgM, low-density surface IgD (which has been referred to as "population III" by

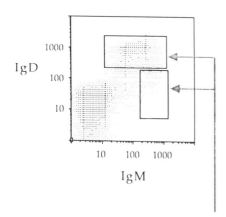

>99% of IgM anti KLH precursors

~5% of IgG1 anti KLH precursors

Figure 1. Flow cytometric profile of B lymphocytes 7 days after challenge with KLH plus pertussis. The upper box represents cells classified as IgM^{low} or ^{high}IgD^{high}. The lower box represents cells classified as IgM^{high}IgD^{low}.

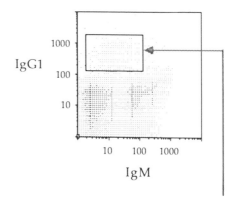

No IgM anti KLH precursors

~95% of IgG1 anti KLH precursors

Figure 2. Appearance of surface IgG1$^+$ B cells 7 days after challenge with KLH plus pertussis. The boxed area is virtually empty in the unimmunized spleen. Note that the majority of IgG1$^+$ cells are IgM$^-$. Given their low frequency, it is difficult to be certain that the few IgM$^+$IgG1$^+$ signals represent double-positive cells.

Hardy et al. [1982]), high-density IgD, and low- or high-density IgM (a mixture of "populations I and II"), and a small population of cells positive for surface IgG1 and negative or very low for surface IgM. It turned out that virtually all the cells capable of forming IgM antibody against KLH were in the former two populations, which, however, contained very few IgG1 precursors. In contrast, the IgG1 surface-positive subset contained no IgM anti-KLH precursors and about 95% of the IgG1 anti-KLH precursors.

The essential independence of these populations is further illustrated by Table 1. Of 48-well samples examining the three B-cell populations, 4 lots were surveyed for their content of anti-KLH IgM, IgG1, or both. Although for each population the number of negative wells considerably exceeded the number of positive wells, clonal overlap has to be taken into account, especially for the IgD^{low} population. The cleanest results were obtained for the IgM$^-$ IgG1$^+$ cells. These were absolutely restricted to IgG1 production and contained no anti-KLH IgM-AFCP. Of 35 positive wells, 2 in the 192 wells from IgM^{low}IgD^{high} B cells formed either IgG1 only or IgG1 plus IgM. It is difficult to exclude the possibility that the only double-producing well (Table 1) by chance included one of each type of precursor. The majority, IgD^{high} B-cell population, could have been somewhat contaminated with other cells, e.g., surface IgG1$^+$ cells. The observed number of IgM plus IgG1$^+$ wells certainly does not exceed the number expected on the basis of two independent populations by a statistically significant margin. However, it is also possible that some B cells retained the IgM$^+$IgD$^+$ surface phenotype in vivo, made some IgM in vitro, but then switched to IgG1 production in vitro. This phenotype, of course, is frequent in unimmunized spleen, but its antibody product usually cannot bind to

Table 1. Independence of Clones Making IgM or IgG1
Anti-KLH Antibody

Sorted B cells	No. of wells containing anti-KLH antibodies of tested isotype[a]			Expected M + G
	IgM	IgG1	IgM + IgG1	
IgM$^{low \ or \ high}$IgD^{high}	33	1	1	0.34
IgM^{high}IgD^{low}	59	8	7	4.6
IgM$^-$IgG1$^+$	0	30	0	0

Spleens were harvested 7 days after immunization with KLH.
[a]192 wells in limit dilution cultures sampled per B-cell population.

KLH as an IgG1 (Nossal and Riedel 1989). It is possible that, at 7 days immunization, some B cells of adequate affinity have accumulated and have retained a surface IgM$^+$IgD$^+$ phenotype. Be that as it may, the majority of the effective anti-KLH IgG1-AFCP have clearly switched to the IgG1$^+$ surface phenotype in vivo and can, as a consequence, synthesize IgG1 but not IgM in vitro. It is tempting to speculate that these have already undergone some V gene mutations that have raised their affinity for KLH. It remains to be determined whether the majority of cells were the (mutated) progeny of cells that had previously been anti-KLH IgM-AFCP, or whether, as Linton et al. (1988) have proposed, they constitute a separate subpopulation that proliferates in response to antigen to create secondary B cells that only give rise to antibody-producing cells on secondary antigenic or mitogenic stimulation.

Induction of Hyporeactivity to HSA by Injection of Freshly Deaggregated Antigen

Mice were injected intraperitoneally with alum-precipitated HSA plus pertussis, or with 5 mg of KLH 4 days before and then HSA plus pertussis, or with 5 mg of freshly deaggregated HSA without adjuvant. Figure

3 shows the resulting serum anti-HSA IgG1 antibody titers as determined by ELISA. Preinjection of an irrelevant protein did not affect the anti-HSA titers, which, as expected for an antigen injected as a depot together with a strong adjuvant, rose progressively for several weeks. Next, 5 mg of HSA was administered prior to alum-precipitated HSA plus pertussis. As Figure 4 shows, serum titers were significantly reduced, more so in this experiment by an injection 4 days prior to challenge rather than 1 day prior to challenge. Mice given soluble HSA 7 days prior to challenge gave titers comparable with the -4 day group (data not shown). Next, mice were given various doses of soluble HSA 4 days prior to challenge (Fig. 5). The serum titers at day 14 show the considerable interanimal variation common in tolerance experiments, but a significant lowering of serum anti-HSA IgG was achieved at all doses down to 40 μg. In a further experiment (Table 2), the timing of the soluble HSA antigen injection was varied widely, and in this experiment 5 mg of antigen plus adjuvant given even 3 days after challenge succeeded in lowering the 14-day antibody titer.

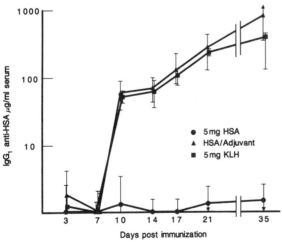

Figure 3. Serum anti-HSA antibody levels following challenge with HSA plus pertussis; means ± S.D. of groups of 4 mice. (▲) Challenge only; (■) challenge but preinjection of 5 mg of KLH 4 days previously; (●) no challenge but only 5 mg of freshly deaggregated HSA on day 0.

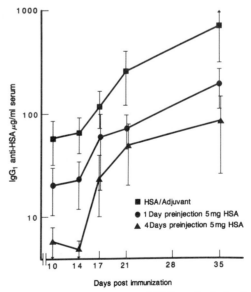

Figure 4. Reductions in serum anti-HSA antibody levels by preinjection of 5 mg of freshly deaggregated HSA; means ± S.D. of groups of 4 mice. (■) No preinjection; (●) preinjection day -1; (▲) preinjection day -4.

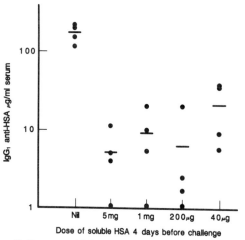

Figure 5. Serum anti-HSA antibody levels 14 days after challenge following preinjection of various doses of freshly deaggregated HSA 4 days prior to challenge. (●) One mouse; (—) the mean.

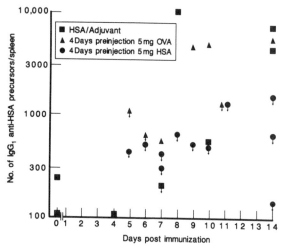

Figure 6. Number of clonable anti-HSA IgG1-AFCP/spleen at various times after challenge with HSA and pertussis. (■) No preinjection; (●) preinjection with 5 mg of freshly deaggregated HSA 4 days before challenge; (▲) preinjection with 5 mg of freshly deaggregated OVA 4 days before challenge.

Numbers of Anti-HSA IgG1-AFCP at Various Times after Challenge and the Effect of Preinjection of Soluble HSA

Figure 6 shows the results of clonotype analysis of B cells from spleens of mice immunized with alum-precipitated HSA plus pertussis with or without an injection of 5 mg of HSA or OVA 4 days before challenge. Unimmunized mice showed very few cells that could act as anti-HSA IgG1-AFCP. In immunized mice, the numbers rose but not before 8 days after immunization. As expected for an antigen that is much less immunogenic than KLH, the numbers detected were lower than noted for KLH. However, in all experiments except one, the control mice (either immunized without preinjection or preinjected with OVA) showed significant numbers (up to 10^4/spleen) of the desired AFCP, provided that more than 1 week was allowed to elapse between challenge and killing. In contrast, not one single, positive clone has yet been identified in cultures from spleens of mice that had been preinjected with HSA. This was an immunologically specific phenomenon, since such mice produced substantial numbers of IgG1-forming AFCP if the capture layer on the ELISA was an anti-murine immunogobulin antibody (data not shown).

Despite the fact that the B-cell stimulus used in culture was a "T-independent" polyclonal activator together with a lymphokine mixture, the formal possibility remained that the tolerant mice produced large numbers of T cells that could somehow suppress the LPS-driven anti-HSA IgG1 response in vitro. Accordingly, splenocyte populations were depleted of T cells by the combined use of antibodies against CD4, CD8, and Thy-1. As shown in Table 3, this did not affect the failure of the appearance of anti-HSA IgG1-AFCP caused by preinjection of deaggregated HSA.

DISCUSSION

The serum antibody data of the present study do not by themselves constitute convincing evidence of a tolerance model because the large amount of antigen injected could mask a considerable amount of formed antibody. This objection has less force if further work confirms that 40 μg or even less of antigen can lower

Table 2. IgG1 Anti-HSA Antibody Titers 14 Days after Challenge with HSA/Adjuvant

Timing of soluble HSA (5 mg)	Antibody μg/ml serum[a]
Nil	280 ± 20
Day −4	9.1 ± 4.1
Day −2	128 ± 140
Day 0	100 ± 18
Day +3	50 ± 5

100 μg of alum-precipitated HSA plus 10^9 *B. pertussis* organisms.

[a]Mean ±S.D. of groups of 4 mice.

Table 3. Clonal Studies of Anti-HSA IgG1 Precursors following T-cell Removal

Preinjection (day −4)	Precursor frequency[a] ($\times 10^{-6}$)
5 mg of OVA	87 ± 42
5 mg of HSA	<8

Splenocytes were treated with a mixture of antibodies against CD4, CD8, and Thy-1 antigens plus complement.

[a]As determined by limiting dilution analysis; B cells were stimulated with LPS and EL-4-conditioned medium in the presence of 3T3 filler cells. After 7 days culture, ELISA determinations were made on culture supernatants.

the IgG1 response to challenge. Some antibody was detected in all tolerant animals, which should not have been the case if all formed antibody had complexed with antigen in the zone of antigen excess. Nevertheless, it is possible that complexes partially dissociated in vitro and that some previously complexed antibody rebound to the ELISA plates. Studies on antigen half-life and immune clearance are currently in progress to illuminate this issue. As far as they go, they do not support antibody masking as the reason for lower serum titers.

Far more important results are those that show a failure of B cells from immunized mice to form anti-HSA IgG1 antibody in vitro after a strong polyclonal, T-cell-independent challenge. This failure is unlikely to have been due to the in vitro effects of suppressor T cells since T-cell-depleted B-cell populations were equally inactive in limiting dilution cultures. It is difficult to escape the conclusion that for whatever reason the challenge injection failed to elicit the appearance of the B-cell population characteristic of the 8–14-day postchallenge control spleens.

Three explanations for this failure require discussion. Since the in vivo isotype switch, which precedes the appearance of the majority of the IgG1-AFCP, requires helper T cells, the defect may be in the T-cell population. Either tolerance may have been induced in helper T-cell precursors, or suppressor T cells may have been induced. A few years ago, the latter would have been the preferred explanation, but recently the suppressor T-cell concept has been less popular. If T-cell suppression represents the true explanation, the system may offer the possibility of exact exploration of what the mechanism of suppression is, provided the requisite adoptive transfer model can be generated.

Secondly, injection of soluble antigen into mice prior to the immunogenic precipitated form of the antigen could interfere with the development of antibody responses by some form of immune deviation. Immediately following injection of T-dependent antigens (such as the alum-precipitated HSA we use), newly produced, IgM$^+$, virgin B cells can be activated by antigen, presumably on extrafollicular dendritic cells, and can subsequently migrate into the follicular areas of lymphoid organs (MacLennan and Gray 1986; Lortan et al. 1987). As a consequence of this selection, the clones are engaged within the follicles in a characteristic set of responses, namely T-cell help, isotype switch, germinal center formation, differentiation and antibody secretion, and generation of long-lived recirculating B-cell clones. The fate of virgin B cells, however, if they should not gain entry to the follicles through the initial, antigen-selected mechanism, is rapid death. It is therefore possible that high levels of soluble circulating antigen interfere with recruitment into secondary lymphoid organs of specific B-cell precursors. Interference could be envisaged by a receptor blockade of virgin B-cell precursors that leave the bone marrow or by blocking B-cell clonal activation on extrafollicular dendritic cells.

The third explanation is that Linton et al. (1988) have correctly identified a second window of tolerance susceptibility in B cells shortly after their triggering. The putative precursor of the anti-HSA IgG1-AFCP indeed starts proliferating shortly after challenge, perhaps as part of a T-cell/B-cell conjugate. So activated, the B cell moves toward the germinal center to enter the compartment where hypermutation occurs (MacLennan and Gray 1986). However, during the process the cell encounters soluble antigen and is silenced or eliminated. It is too early to regard this as the most likely explanation, but further exploration of the model from this perspective should be rewarding.

The postulate that the anti-KLH and anti-HSA IgG1-AFCP are the results of somatic V gene mutations can only be proven by analysis of the amino-acid sequence or nucleotide sequence of the relevant gene product or gene. The polymerase chain reaction makes it more feasible to entertain such an approach. It may be advantageous to test the hypothesis using antigen and strain combinations where the primary response involves only a restricted B-cell population with a common idiotype.

ACKNOWLEDGMENTS

Dr. F.L. Battye and Mr. Mark Cozens gave valuable help in cell sorting. Dr. A.P. Kyne designed the computer software for processing of ELISA results. This work was supported by the National Health and Medical Research Council, Canberra, Australia; by grant AI-03958 from the National Institute of Allergy and Infectious Diseases, U.S. Public Health Service; and by the generosity of a number of private donors to The Walter and Eliza Hall Institute.

REFERENCES

Berek, C. and C. Milstein. 1987. Mutation drift and repertoire shift in the maturation of the immune response. *Immunol. Rev.* **96:** 23.

Goodnow, C.C., J. Crosbie, S. Adelstein, T.B. Lavoie, S.J. Smith-Gill, R.A. Brink, H. Pritchard-Briscoe, J.S. Wotherspoon, R.H. Loblay, K. Raphael, R.J. Trent, and A. Basten. 1988. Altered immunoglobulin expression and functional silencing of self-reactive B lymphocytes in transgenic mice. *Nature* **334:** 676.

Hardy, R.R., K. Hayakawa, J. Haaijman, and L.A. Herzenberg. 1982. B-cell subpopulations identified by two-colour fluorescence analysis. *Nature* **297:** 589.

Linton, P.-J., G.L. Gilmore, and N.R. Klinman. 1988. The secondary B cell lineage. In *B cell development* (ed. O. Witte et al.), p. 75. Alan R. Liss, New York.

Lortan, J.E., C.A. Roobottom, S. Oldfield, and I.C.M. MacLennan. 1987. Newly produced virgin B cells migrate to secondary lymphoid organs but their capacity to enter follicles is restricted. *Eur. J. Immunol.* **17:** 1311.

MacLennan, I.C.M. and D. Gray. 1986. Antigen-driven selection of virgin and memory B cells. *Immunol. Rev.* **91:** 61.

McHeyzer-Williams, M.G. and G.J.V. Nossal. 1988. Clonal analysis of autoantibody-producing cell precursors in the preimmune B cell repertoire. *J. Immunol.* **141:** 4118.

———. 1989. Inhibition of antibody production at high cell

density following mitogen stimulation and isotype switching in vitro. *J. Immunol. Methods* **119**: 9.

McKean, D., K. Huppi, M. Bell, L. Staudt, W. Gerhard, and M. Weigert. 1984. Generation of antibody diversity in the immune response of BALB/c mice to influenza virus hemagglutinin. *Proc. Natl. Acad. Sci.* **81**: 3180.

Nemazee, D.A. and K. Bürki. 1989. Clonal deletion of B lymphocytes in a transgenic mouse bearing anti-MHC class I antibody genes. *Nature* **337**: 562.

Nossal, G.J.V. 1983. Cellular mechanisms of immunological tolerance. *Annu. Rev. Immunol.* **1**: 33.

———. 1987. Bone marrow pre-B cells and the clonal anergy theory of immunologic tolerance. *Int. Rev. Immunol.* **2**: 321.

Nossal, G.J.V. and C. Riedel. 1989. Sudden appearance of anti-protein IgG$_1$-forming cell precursors early during primary immunization. *Proc. Natl. Acad. Sci.* **86**: 4679.

Pike, B.L., M.R. Alderson, and G.J.V. Nossal. 1987. T-independent activation of single B cells: An orderly analysis of overlapping stages in the activation pathway. *Immunol. Rev.* **99**: 119.

Rajewsky, K., I. Förster, and A. Cumano. 1987. Evolutionary and somatic selection of the antibody repertoire in the mouse. *Science* **238**: 1088.

Models of B-cell Unresponsiveness

D.W. Scott, J.-E. Alés-Martínez, J.H. Chace, N.J. LoCascio, L. Silver, and G.L. Warner

Immunology Unit, University of Rochester Cancer Center and Department of Microbiology and Immunology, University of Rochester School of Medicine and Dentistry, Rochester, New York 14642

Self-nonself discrimination is one of the basic tenets of immunology. Earlier suggestions that clonal elimination completely limited anti-self reactivity have been challenged by the observation that potentially auto-recognizing clones of B and T cells exist. However, recent data supporting the deletion of at least some of the T-cell anti-self repertoire have been confirmed (Kappler et al. 1987; Teh et al. 1988); evidence for a similar elimination of B cells in self-tolerance has been lacking. Our laboratory has pursued the mechanisms of tolerance at the B- and T-cell levels for many years (Scott et al. 1979, 1980, 1987b). We recently described alternative approaches for exploring this process in B cells, the results of which extended our earlier reports made with hapten-specific B cells from normal and tolerant mice. Our data suggest that control of B-cell responsiveness occurs at several levels, including deletion (cell death), anergy, and suppression of differentiation to antibody secretion. Commitment to one of these mechanisms is dependent not only on the maturity of the target cell population and the nature of the antigen/tolerogen, but also on whether T cells are activated in this process.

Hapten-specific B Cells from Normal and Tolerant Mice

Following our initial observation that fluorescein (FL)-labeled conjugates of heterologous immunoglobulins were tolerogenic for both the FL-hapten and the immunoglobulin (Ig) carrier, we followed the fate of cells labeled in vivo with FL-sheep immunoglobulin and found that they persisted as tolerogen-bearing cells for several days after systemic injection and that cells with free receptors were detectable 1 week after the administration of tolerogen (Venkataraman and Scott 1979). These observations suggested that tolerant B cells might persist in animals that were clearly unresponsive to epitopes on the tolerogen. Isolation of these cells was attempted using affinity chromatography, as described by G.J.V. Nossal and initiated during a sabbatical at the Hall Institute by one of us (D.W.S.).

To summarize, we have found that FL-hapten-binding B lymphocytes (antigen-binding cells, or ABCs) can be isolated from normal, as well as tolerogen-injected, mice by adsorption to and elution from haptenated gelatin dishes (Haas and Layton 1975; Scott et al. 1979). Similar numbers of ABCs (1/2500) are recovered from naive mice and from animals injected 7 days earlier with FL-conjugated tolerogen. However, limiting dilution analysis showed that the precursor frequency of ABCs from tolerant mice was reduced three- to sixfold and the total plaque-forming cells (pfc) response was less than 25% of FL-binding B cells from control mice (Pillai and Scott 1983). Thus, tolerant B cells exist, but they are anergic to antigen-driven stimuli leading to antibody formation. Extensive analyses have led to the conclusion that these tolerant B cells are able to increase surface class 2 (Ia) antigens via a number of stimuli to the same extent as normal cells (Chace and Scott 1988). When exposed to antigen, they enlarge and enter G_1 normally but fail to efficiently enter the S phase of the cell cycle and divide. This proliferation defect accounts for the deficit in pfc (Scott et al. 1987b). Table 1 summarizes these results. Hence, these cells are anergic at a critical point in the cell cycle, as reported previously for B-lymphoma cells that are growth inhibited by anti-Ig reagents (see below and Pennell and Scott 1986a).

B-lymphoma Cell Death Induced by Anti-Ig as Model for Clonal Deletion

Studies with hapten-specific B cells are limited by their rare frequency and the inability to derive cloned B-cell lines. In an effort to obtain clonal populations representing B-cell subsets, we began to utilize several unique B lymphomas. Several years ago, Boyd and Schrader (1981) reported that the growth of the WEHI-231 B-lymphoma line was dramatically inhibited by anti-μ antibodies. Our laboratory has examined

Table 1. Properties of Hapten-binding B Cells from Tolerant Mice

B-cell activation step	Occurrence in tolerant B cells
Calcium mobilization	?
c-*myc* transcription	?
Class-2 transcription (induced by anti-Ig, antigen, LPS, IL-4)	normal
$G_0 \rightarrow G_1$ entry	normal
$G_1 \rightarrow S$ progression	diminished
DNA synthesis	diminished
Maturation to IgM synthesis	?[a]

[a] Absolute numbers of PFC are reduced, however, because those clones that are able to divide go on to form antibody (with normal burst size), the primary defect is presumed to be at division. Because one cannot measure the responses of G_1 blocked B cells, a defect in IgM synthesis (e.g., J-chain transcription) is still possible.

WEHI-231, as well as two other murine B-cell lymphomas, CH31 and CH33, to form the focus of our work. The origins and properties of these cells are noted in our previous publications (Scott et al. 1985, 1987b; Pennell and Scott 1986a,b). These B-cell lymphomas, which resemble immature B cells by surface markers and functional responsiveness, can be growth regulated by exposure to anti-Ig reagents, including polyclonal and monoclonal antibodies against any domain of μ heavy or light chains or idiotype (Scott et al. 1985, 1987b; Pennell and Scott 1986a,b). Indeed, these anti-Ig inhibitable lymphomas die within 48 hours of anti-Ig exposure, perhaps representing a clonal deletion event.

Cell-cycle dependence of anti-Ig-mediated negative signaling. Initially, we found that all three lines are blocked by anti-Ig cross-linking at a point late in G_1, on the basis of acridine orange staining (Scott et al. 1986; Pennell and Scott 1986a). Using a simple protocol of overnight exposure with the microtubule-disrupting drug nocodazole, we found that WEHI-231, CH31, and CH33 could all be synchronized at nocodazole concentrations of 0.05-1 μg/ml. When such cells are released by washing, most will divide within 1–2 hours and move into G_1. At this point (and only during the next 2 hours), they are susceptible to growth inhibition by anti-Ig cross-linking and do not progress into the first S phase after release (Scott et al. 1987c). Preliminary studies indicate that DNA breakdown may occur as an early event in these cells (J.E. Alés-Martínez and R.P. Phipps, unpubl.). Significantly, lymphomas that are not sensitive to anti-μ (such as CH12 and NBL) are not inhibited by this treatment protocol. This suggests that either this growth-inhibitable period is unique to the immature B lymphomas or that noninhibitable lymphomas are able to overcome the negative signal (perhaps by an autocrine growth factor pathway) later in G_1.

Biochemical signals during growth inhibition in B lymphomas. Previously, we established that an initial calcium signal, as well as phosphatidyl inositol hydrolysis (and presumptive protein kinase C [PKC] activation), occurred upon cross-linking IgM in WEHI-231 and CH33, but no Ca^{++} mobilization could be elicited in CH31. Overall, the bulk of our data suggested that this process was neither sufficient nor necessary for regulation of growth to occur, because growth inhibition could be induced in calcium-free medium, in the presence of EGTA, and in Quin-2-loaded cells (whose intracellular calcium would be quenched [Scott et al. 1987c]). Furthermore, exposure of lymphoma cells (synchronized or not) to the PKC/protein kinase A (PKA) inhibitors H-7 and H-8 had no effect on the negative signal (Warner and Scott 1988). As noted below, cross-linking of membrane IgD receptors will induce calcium mobilization and also cause a desensitization (blunting) of a subsequent anti-μ-mediated calcium signal. Because pretreatment with anti-δ has no

effect on growth inhibition by anti-μ (Alés-Martínez et al. 1988), these results also suggest that the initial calcium signal is not required for negative signaling for growth.

We demonstrated further that growth inhibition could be overcome by phorbol esters, such as PMA or PDB, with cells synchronized at G_2/M, although such tumor promoters, themselves, could cause growth retardation with slower kinetics in all cell lines (Scott et al. 1987c; Warner and Scott 1988; J.E. Alés-Martínez, unpubl.). This is an important result, because it emphasizes that protein phosphorylation at different points in the cell cycle could have opposite consequences. If WEHI-231 cells were exposed to PMA or PDB during the 16 hours of synchronization, they had a severely reduced Ca^{++} signal to anti-Ig but retained sensitivity to the down-regulation of growth by anti-Ig. Thus, direct PKC activation (and presumably phosphorylation of available proteins) after anti-Ig has different consequences compared to PKC activation prior to anti-Ig.

Cholera toxin (CT) and forskolin, both of which elicit a rise in cAMP (Phipps et al. 1989; Warner and Scott 1989; G.L. Warner, unpubl.), have no effect on the negative signal for growth in the WEHI-231 B-cell lymphoma. Negative signaling in the CH31 and CH33 lymphomas is also not inhibited by CT. However, CT effects a greater sensitivity to anti-Ig treatment in CH31 and CH33 cells, suggesting that there are differences in the biochemical signaling pathways for growth inhibition in CH31 and CH33 cells, on the one hand, and in WEHI-231 cells, on the other.

We also determined that CT would completely block the entry of normal B cells into cycle, as determined by cell enlargement (Warner and Scott 1989). However, in the presence of IL-4, CT-pretreated B cells progressed into S phase, albeit with a slight retardation in kinetics. Hence, CT dramatically inhibits anti-Ig-positive signaling of normal B cells, whereas it does not inhibit negative signaling of WEHI-231, CH31, and CH33 cells.

Failure of immobilized anti-Ig to cause negative signaling. Interestingly, insolubilized anti-Ig reagents (coupled to Sepharose beads, adsorbed to microtiter plates or conjugated to dextran) were less efficient at inducing growth inhibition compared to the soluble forms of these antibodies (i.e., dose response curves differed by two orders of magnitude [Fig. 1]). The possibility that these differences reflect the importance of both the internalization process and persistent membrane signaling in the regulation of growth or differentiation is currently being investigated. It should be noted that soluble anti-IgM is internalized in all of the B-cell lymphomas we have studied, whether or not they are growth inhibitable. Thus, we believe that internalization may be necessary but not sufficient for growth inhibition (D.W. Scott et al., in prep.). Although both IgM and IgD cap in δ^+ lymphomas, it is not yet known whether differences exist in terms of the internalization

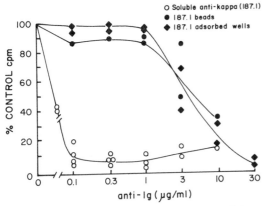

Figure 1. Effect of soluble vs. immobilized anti-κ 187.1 on the growth of WEHI-231 cells. Titration of increasing numbers of beads (at one density) or increasing concentrations of plate adsorbed anti-κ gave identical results to those obtained with dextran-coupled anti-μ (Fig. 2). Thus, the physical form and not the epitope density is critical for this effect. Data are from two to four experiments at each anti-κ concentration.

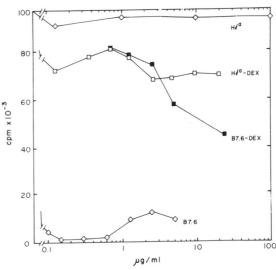

Figure 2. Effect of soluble vs. dextran-bound anti-δ (or anti-μ) on the growth of CH33 transfectant ECH408.1. Lymphoma cells were cultured for 48 hr with indicated doses of soluble or dextran-coupled Hδ1ᵃ or b7.6 anti-μ.

of these isotypes, as reported earlier in the case of human B-cell lymphomas (Roth et al. 1982). This is important because of different functional responses to cross-linking these receptors, as discussed below.

Role of cell-surface isotype in negative signaling. To determine whether membrane IgM and membrane IgD deliver similar signals within the same B-cell lymphoma, the prototype cell lines WEHI-231, CH31, and CH33 were transfected (Alés-Martínez et al. 1988) with a δ-chain construct, originally prepared in P. Tucker's laboratory. These constructs possessed the S107 (T15⁺) V_H, the remainder of which was an IgD heavy chain. The first stable transfectant arose from CH33 lymphoma cells. Because these constructs contain known idiotype but are of a different allotype than the CH33 recipient cell line, we would distinguish signals delivered by endogenous versus transfected immunoglobulins.

Our data (Fig. 2) (Alés-Martínez et al. 1988) demonstrate that IgD-transfected cell lines retain their sensitivity to negative signaling by cross-linking with anti-μ antibodies but are resistant to negative signaling via anti-δ, a result that was confirmed by Tisch et al. (1988) in a similar transfection system. As shown in Figure 2, neither soluble nor immobilized anti-δ inhibited these cells, whereas only soluble anti-μ was effective at growth inhibition. This suggests that the IgD receptor cannot overcome a negative signal nor can it mediate growth inhibition per se. Alternatively, there may be functional defects in the transfected IgD molecules. However, we have demonstrated that these molecules cap normally and mediate the increase in intracellular calcium normally seen when IgM receptors are cross-linked and are able to cause immediate desensitization for the calcium signal stimulated by the alternative isotype (Warner et al. 1989). Moreover, we have now isolated several CH33 clones that express high concen-

trations of endogenous IgD (of the b allotype); anti-δ does not inhibit their growth, whereas anti-μ, anti-CH31 idiotype, or anti-κ still are active (Alés-Martínez et al. 1988 and unpubl.). This is important because it means that endogenous IgD and transfected IgD deliver similar messages to the cell.

Identification of lymphokines capable of preventing the negative signal. Metcalf and Klinman (1976) showed previously that neonatal B-cell precursors were exquisitely sensitive to tolerance induction and that primed T-helper-cell activity would overcome negative tolerogenic signals. We reasoned that we could replace T-cell help and prevent negative signaling with recombinant lymphokines. With Dr. Gerry Klaus at Mill Hill, we initially established that certain T-cell lymphokines can prevent growth inhibition in these B-lymphoma cells. IL-4 and, to a small extent, IL-5 were effective; more recently, we found that tumor necrosis factor (TNF)α and TNFβ both prevented negative signaling (Scott et al. 1987a; N. LoCascio and D.W. Scott, unpubl.). Moreover, preincubation with IL-4 or TNF resulted in greater protection from the negative signal (Fig. 3), and this effect was reversed by γ-interferon (IFN-γ). It is important to note that anti-κ, as well as IL-4, treatment will induce hyperexpression of Ia on CH33 clones (R. Lifrak and D.W. Scott, unpubl.). Thus, Ia transcription can be induced by ligands that have opposite biological consequences. We have not determined whether TNF will induce Ia transcription. These results form the basis of our hypothesis that the pathway to Ia hyperexpression is a critical event in both positive and negative signaling and that lymphokine-mediated Ia induction occurs via signals that override the anti-Ig negative pathway. It is interesting in this regard that we have recently found an anti-CD3-activated CD4⁺ T cell clone of the T_H2 phenotype to

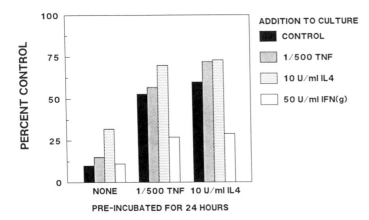

Figure 3. WEHI-231 cells were preincubated overnight with the indicated lymphokines, washed, and then treated with 0.3 μg/ml Bet-2 anti-μ for 44 hr, followed by a 4-hr pulse with titrated thymidine. Data are presented as percentage of control cpm. Lymphokine treatment did not affect control cpm. Doses of lymphokines chosen were suboptimally protective in a standard assay (black bars). Note that IFN-γ, which prevents IL-4-induced Ia induction, diminished the protective effects of both IL-4 and TNF.

completely reverse the negative signaling of CH33 cells (J.-E. Alés-Martínez et al., unpubl.).

Regulation of Immunoglobulin Synthesis in Mature B Cells by Anti-Ig

Treatment of neonatal B cells with anti-μ can lead either to an anergic population or to deletion of the B-cell lineage (Lawton et al. 1972; Pike et al. 1982), depending on the dose and duration of treatment. In contrast to its effect on neonatal B cells, cross-linking of mIg causes mature normal splenic B cells to progress into the cell cycle through a cascade of events that include Ca^{++} mobilization and PKC activation (Cambier and Ransom 1987; Klaus et al. 1987). When mature, normal B cells are simultaneously exposed to anti-Ig and lipopolysaccharide (LPS) in vitro, antibody secretion is dramatically inhibited, although the cells proliferate normally (Andersson et al. 1974; Flahart and Lawton 1987; Yuan 1987). We wished to determine whether this in vitro inhibition of antibody secretion was analogous to that seen in our in vivo adult B-cell tolerance model. B cells are pretreated with anti-μ reagents for up to 24 hours, washed and then stimulated with either specific antigen or LPS for 3 days. In this way, the induction phase (with anti-Ig) is separated from the challenge phase, as is typical in models of

tolerance. As shown in Figure 4, an overnight preincubation led to a profound inhibition of LPS-driven antibody secretion, as measured by our modified spot enzyme-linked immunosorbent assay (ELISA). This reflects a decrease in total IgM synthesis and does not involve a shift in either kinetics or isotype, as determined by analysis of accumulated supernatants (data not shown).

One might predict that anti-Ig pretreatment would inhibit antigen-driven responsiveness by artifactually blocking or modulating mIg receptors (Pierce et al. 1972). Thus, it was surprising to observe that the FL-*Brucella*-induced (Ig receptor-mediated) responses were consistently less sensitive to anti-Ig-mediated inhibition of antibody formation (60–70% vs. 90% for LPS) and that F(ab)$_2$ anti-Fab was usually ineffective in causing nonresponsiveness. Interestingly, the antibody response to FL, coupled to LPS, was as sensitive to inhibition in this model as the polyclonal response to LPS. This suggests that different subsets of B cells vary in their sensitivity to inhibition, as suggested earlier for B-cell tolerance (Cambier et al. 1977). Indeed, recent data suggest that thymus-dependent responsiveness (to sheep red blood cells) is minimally affected by this protocol (not shown). Thus, this form of regulation may be unique to thymus-independent-responding cells. Alternatively, the mode of triggering may be able to override negative signals.

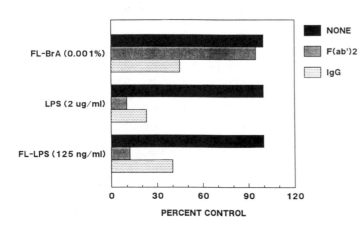

Figure 4. Effect of anti-Ig pretreatment on specific or polyclonal antibody formation. T-depleted B cells were treated with the indicated doses of intact or F(ab)$_2$ anti-Ig for 24 hr, washed, and challenged with FL-*Brucella abortus* (*top*), LPS (*middle*) or FL-LPS (*bottom*). Numbers of AFCs were measured by spot ELISA 3 days later. Similar dose response curves were obtained when AFCs were assayed on days 2–4, thus ruling out a shift in kinetics.

It should also be noted that surface IgM and IgD receptors are modulated by pretreatment with anti-Fab but that IgD returns to near normal levels at 24–48 hours (G. Warner, unpubl.). Indeed, unresponsive adult B cells are IgM^{lo}, IgD^{med}, and J11d^{lo}, as reported recently for tolerant B cells in transgenic mice (Goodnow et al. 1988).

Kinetics of Unresponsiveness and Role of Cycle Entry

Previous results in a coculture system suggested that a 1-hour incubation of B cells with LPS and anti-Ig was sufficient to down-regulate differentiation to antibody synthesis (Flahart and Lawton 1987); however, both LPS and anti-Ig need to be present for this effect to occur. We therefore determined the kinetics for the induction of nonresponsiveness in our preculture protocol. B cells were incubated with anti-Fab for 1, 2, 4, 8, 12, or 18 hours, washed, and then challenged with either LPS or antigen. Our results (G.L. Warner and D.W. Scott, in prep.) indicate that an 8-hour incubation is necessary before nonresponsiveness is induced. This suggests that mere blocking of receptors does not mediate this effect; in fact, our data imply that exit from G_0 and entry into the cell cycle may be required for negative signaling, as suggested previously (Scott and Klinman 1987).

Suppression of Antibody Synthesis by Anti-CD3-Activated T Cells: A Role in Tolerance?

Although the CD4 surface antigen is commonly associated with murine T cells of the helper phenotype, there are several reports of CD4$^+$ T cells that have suppressive activity on B-cell responses (Asano and Hodes 1983; Bottomly et al. 1983; Kim et al. 1985; Boom et al. 1988). Indeed, we have found that anti-CD3-activated normal T cells and T-cell clones will suppress LPS-induced IgM and IgG antibody secretion by B cells. When T and B cells are in direct contact, total thymidine incorporation often decreases significantly, suggesting that B-cell cytolysis or cytostasis may be occurring. However, when the T and B cells are separated by a porous membrane (Table 2), suppression is seen with no significant effect on B-cell proliferation. Thus, this system provides another model for B-cell unresponsiveness, where B cells are blocked in their differentiation toward antibody secretion.

We have also examined the effect of anti-CD3-activated T-cell clones on LPS-stimulated B cells. Two CD4$^+$ clones of the T_H1 phenotype and at least one T_H2 clone suppressed LPS-induced antibody secretion in a major histocompatibility complex-unrestricted fashion, with no significant effect on B-cell proliferation. It is not yet clear whether suppression occurs via similar mechanisms in each of these cases. Further kinetic studies are needed to evaluate isotype switching after long periods of culture and to determine the ultimate fate of these unresponsive B cells.

Table 2. Effect of Anti-CD3-activated T Cells on LPS-induced Antibody Secretion

(a) Normal T and B cells separated by a porous membrane[a]

LPS	2C11	AFCs
−	+	0 ± 0
+	−	595 ± 44
+	+	168 ± 20

(b) T-cell clones and B cells in direct contact[b]

	LPS	2C11	AFCs
BK2.43 (T_H1)	−	−	15 ± 9
	−	+	0 ± 1
	+	−	168 ± 37
	+	+	43 ± 7
AE.7 (T_H1)	−	−	0 ± 0
	−	+	0 ± 0
	+	−	59 ± 15
	+	+	8 ± 3
D10.G4 (T_H2)	−	−	0 ± 0
	−	+	51 ± 12
	+	−	31 ± 10
	+	+	4 ± 0

LPS and the anti-CD3 monoclonal antibody 145-2C11 were added to final concentrations of 10 μg/ml and 2% hybridoma supernatant, respectively. FL-specific IgM and IgG antibody-forming cells (AFCs) were assayed on day 4 by a spot ELISA. In some experiments, ELISAs were also done on 4-day culture supernatants and gave very similar results.
[a]In experiment a, 5×10^5 B6D2 F$_1$ spleen cells were separated from 5×10^5 T-depleted spleen cells (B cells) by a 0.4 μM porous membrane. AFCs per 5×10^5 cells are presented, $\pm$s.e.m.
[b]In experiments b, each well received 2×10^4 T cells and four to ten times as many B cells. AFCs per 10^5 B cells are presented, $\pm$s.e.m. These data were compiled from L. Silver et al. (in prep.).

DISCUSSION

The mechanisms by which B cells become unresponsive remain controversial; indeed, one view is that B cells do not *need* to become unresponsive because T-cell tolerance ensures a lack of autoreactivity (P. Marrack, public comm.). We believe that Nature never finds a single mechanism satisfactory. In fact, our studies and those of Nossal et al. and Goodnow et al. (both this volume) provide convincing evidence for the levels at which B-cell responsiveness can be regulated: namely, deletion of a portion of potentially autoreactive immature cells, anergy (especially with regard to entry into the S phase of the cell cycle for some mature B cells), down-regulation of differentiation via anti-Ig or immune complexes, and finally, T-cell control of humoral responses.

All but the last mechanism are the result of antigen or surrogate antigen binding to Ig(M) ± Fc receptors on B-cell subsets of various maturational ages. Cross-linking of mIg is known to stimulate a series of biochemical events, including the activation of PKC and the elevation of $[Ca^{++}]_i$. Using our immature lymphoma model, we have previously demonstrated that the delivery of a negative proliferative signal by mIg cannot be precisely reproduced by agents that are able to mimic a positive proliferative signal such as PKC activators and calcium ionophores (Scott et al. 1987c; Warner and Scott 1988). Moreover, the ability of phorbol esters to reduce the growth of our prototype B-cell lymphomas is not affected by inhibitors such as H-7 and H-8 (J.-E. Alés-Martínez, unpubl.); thus, the role of PKC (or even PKA) activation in the inhibition of B-lymphoma growth is doubtful.

In addition, we have recently demonstrated that the positive and negative signals mediated by mIg can be differentiated on the basis of their susceptibility to inhibition by CT. That is, positive signaling by antigen or anti-Ig is mediated by a CT-sensitive pathway, whereas negative signaling is not sensitive to such inhibition (Warner and Scott 1989). Taken together, these data indicate the anti-Ig induction of B-cell nonresponsiveness and the induction of B-cell activation (as measured by cell-cycle progression) involve differing, or at least divergent, intracellular signaling pathways.

Although the biochemical pathways for unresponsiveness in mature versus immature B cells are not clear, several features are shared. First, interaction with bivalent ligand appears critical from our studies and those of Metcalf and Klinman (1976). One wonders whether such an interaction is physiologically relevant, because self-protein epitopes are not likely to be multivalent; however, we must remember that most antigens are seen on the surfaces of other cells in vivo and that repeated epitopes are likely to be perceived on the surface of a macrophage. Moreover, recent data of Schad and Phipps (1989) suggest that macrophage-presented antigen is more tolerogenic and that this is mediated, in part, by prostaglandins released in the local milieu by such professional antigen-presenting cells.

A second feature in common is the apparent requirement for certain early events in cell-cycle entry. Interestingly, evidence from B lymphomas supports the notion that early G_1 is a critical period for growth control (Scott et al. 1986). Data from our and Nossal's laboratory suggest that defects in cell-cycle progression also exist for hapten-specific B cells and may be forthcoming in the powerful transgenic models (Goodnow et al. 1988). Several years ago, Teale and Klinman (1984) demonstrated that inhibitors of cell-cycle progression prevented tolerance in neonatal B cells in a splenic focus system. This led Scott and Klinman to propose (1987) that G_1 (as well as G_2/M) are critical periods for signal delivery in the life of a B cell. It is noteworthy that in the surrogate antigen (anti-Ig) polyclonal tolerance model in our laboratory, we find that 4–8 hours are required before unresponsiveness is induced in mature B cells. This time frame and the dose response requirement fit with egress of normal B cells from G_0 into G_1 expected from anti-Ig treatment. However, the failure of CT to prevent negative signaling in this system (Warner and Scott 1989) and the ability of intact IgG anti-μ to induce unresponsiveness would suggest that complete entry into G_1 is not required for negative signaling. Instead, we propose that the remaining common pathway required is (or is coincidental with) induction of class-2 transcription.

Finally, one must consider the role of T cells as the final failsafe mechanism ensuring the down-regulation of excess or undesirable B cell responses. Our data indicate that anti-CD3, which engages the T-cell receptor as surrogate antigen, can activate T-cell clones to act as suppressors of IgM synthesis. Thus, a broader question raised by these data is what determines whether the immune response will be up-regulated or down-regulated upon antigenic stimulation. Does the mode of activation or the dose determine whether $CD4^+$ cells exhibit a helper or suppressor phenotype? We do not believe that suppression represents excess T-cell help, because the same concentration of anti-CD3 stimulated one T_H2 clone for help or suppression in the absence or presence of LPS, respectively (data not shown). Further work is necessary with T-cell subsets, as well as with more T_H1 and T_H2 clones, to investigate the possible pathways of suppression in more detail. Nonetheless, our data clearly indicate that normal T cells are capable of becoming suppressive via a CD3-associated activation. The extent of involvement of this suppressive pathway in self-tolerance is unknown.

ACKNOWLEDGMENTS

The work reported herein has been supported in part by U.S. Public Health Service research grants AI-20757, CA-41363, core grant CA-11198, and National Institutes of Health training grants CA-09363 and AI-07285. In addition, support was also provided by grants from the American Cancer Society (IM-495) and the Council for Tobacco Research (1840 and 1883). J.A.M. is a Wilmot Cancer Research Fellow. We thank Daniella Livnat, Susan Davies, Nina Birnbaum, and Louise Levy for help with various aspects of these projects, and our former colleagues, Drs. Subramonia Pillai and Helen Quill, for initiating some of the work. This is publication no. 50 from the Immunology Unit, University of Rochester Cancer Center.

REFERENCES

Alés-Martínez, J.-E., G. Warner, and D.W. Scott. 1988. IgD and IgM mediate signals that are qualitatively different in B cells with an immature phenotype. *Proc. Natl. Acad. Sci.* **85:** 6919.

Andersson, J., W.W. Bullock, and F. Melchers. 1974. Inhibition of mitogenic stimulation of mouse lymphocytes by anti-mouse immunoglobulin antibodies. *Eur. J. Immunol.* **4:** 715.

Asano, Y. and R.J. Hodes. 1983. T cell regulation of B cell activation. Cloned Lyt-1^+2^- T suppressor cells inhibit the major histocompatibility complex-restricted interaction of T helper cells with B cells and/or accessory cells. *J. Exp. Med.* **158:** 1178.

Boom, W.H., D. Liano, and A.K. Abbas. 1988. Heterogeneity of helper/inducer T lymphocytes. II. Effects of interleukin 4- and interleukin 2-producing T cell clones on resting B lymphocytes. *J. Exp. Med.* **167:** 1350.

Bottomly, K., J. Kaye, B. Jones, F. Jones III, and C.A. Janeway, Jr. 1983. A cloned, antigen-specific, Ia-restricted

Lyt-1$^+$,2$^-$ T cell with suppressive activity. *J. Mol. Cell. Immunol.* **1**: 42.

Boyd, A.W. and J.W. Schrader. 1981. The regulation of growth and differentiation of a murine B cell lymphoma. *J. Immunol.* **126**: 2466.

Cambier, J.T. and J.T. Ransom. 1987. Molecular mechanisms of transmembrane signaling in B lymphocytes. *Annu. Rev. Immunol.* **5**: 175.

Cambier, J.T., E.S. Vitetta, J.R. Kettman, G.M. Wetzel, and J.W. Uhr. 1977. B-cell tolerance. III. Effect of papain-mediated cleavage of cell surface IgD on tolerance susceptibility of murine B cells. *J. Exp. Med.* **146**: 107.

Chace, J.H. and D.W. Scott. 1988. Activation events in hapten-specific B cells from tolerant mice. *J. Immunol.* **141**: 3258.

Flahart, R.E. and A.R. Lawton. 1987. Mechanism of suppression of lipopolysaccharide-driven B cell differentiation by anti-μ antibodies. *J. Exp. Med.* **166**: 864.

Goodnow, C.C., J. Crosbie, S. Adelstein, T.B. Lavoie, S.J. Smith-Gill, R.A. Brink, H. Pritchard-Briscoe, J.S. Wotherspoon, R.H. Loblay, K. Raphael, R.J. Trent, and A. Basten. 1988. Altered immunoglobulin expression and functional silencing of self-reactive B lymphocytes in transgenic mice. *Nature* **334**: 676.

Haas, W. and J.E. Layton. 1975. Separation of antigen-specific lymphocytes. I. Enrichment of antigen-binding cells. *J. Exp. Med.* **141**: 1004.

Kappler, J.W., N. Roehm, and P. Marrack. 1987. T cell tolerance by clonal elimination in the thymus. *Cell* **49**: 273.

Kim, J., A. Woods, E. Becker-Dunn, and K. Bottomly. 1985. Distinct functional phenotypes of cloned Ia-restricted helper T cells. *J. Exp. Med.* **162**: 188.

Klaus, G.G.B., M.K. Bijsterbosch, A. O'Garra, M.M. Harnett, and R. Rigley. 1987. Receptor signalling and cross-link in B lymphocytes. *Immunol. Rev.* **99**: 19.

Lawton, A., R. Asofsky, M. Hylton, and M. Cooper. 1972. Suppression of immunoglobulin class synthesis in mice. I. Effects of treatment with antibody to μ chain. *J. Exp. Med.* **135**: 277.

Metcalf, E.S. and N.R. Klinman. 1976. In vitro tolerance induction of neonatal murine B cells. *J. Exp. Med.* **143**: 1327.

Pennell, C. and D. Scott. 1986a. Models and mechanisms for signal transduction in B cells. *Immunol. Res.* **5**: 61.

———. 1986b. Lymphoma models for B cell activation and tolerance. IV. Growth inhibition by anti-Ig of CH31 and CH33 B lymphoma cells. *Eur. J. Immunol.* **16**: 1577.

Phipps, R.P., D. Lee, V. Schad, and G. Warner. 1989. E-series prostaglandins are potent growth-inhibitors for B lymphomas. *Eur. J. Immunol.* **19**: 995.

Pierce, C., S.M. Solliday, and R.J. Asofsky. 1972. Immune responses in vitro. IV. Suppression of primary γM, γG, and γA plaque-forming cell responses in mouse spleen cell cultures by class-specific antibody to mouse immunoglobulins. *J. Exp. Med.* **135**: 675.

Pike, B.L., A.W. Boyd, and G.J.V. Nossal. 1982. Clonal anergy: The university anergic B lymphocyte. *Proc. Natl. Acad. Sci.* **79**: 2013.

Pillai, P.S. and D.W. Scott. 1983. Cellular events in tolerance. IX. Maintenance of immunological tolerance in the presence of normal B cell precursors and in the absence of demonstrable suppression. *Cell. Immunol.* **77**: 69.

Roth, P., P. Tonda, and B. Pernis. 1982. Membrane IgD expression and dynamics in clones of human B-lymphoblastoid cells. *Ann. N.Y. Acad. Sci.* **399**: 175.

Schad, V. and R.P. Phipps. 1989. The role of the B cell antigen and Fc receptors in prostaglandin mediated negative signaling. *J. Immunol.* **143**: (in press).

Scott, D.W. and N.W. Klinman. 1987. Is tolerance the result of engaging surface Ig of B cells in cycle? *Immunol. Today* **8**: 105.

Scott, D.W., M. Venkataraman, and J. Jandinski. 1979. Multiple pathways of B cell tolerance. *Immunol. Rev.* **43**: 241.

Scott, D., C. Livnat, C. Pennell, and P. Keng. 1986. Lymphoma models for B cell activation and tolerance III. Cell cycle dependent for negative signalling of WEHI-231 B lymphoma cells by anti-Ig. *J. Exp. Med.* **164**: 156.

Scott, D.W., C. Long, J.J. Jandinski, and J.T.C. Li. 1980. Role of self MHC carriers in tolerance and the immune response. *Immunol. Rev.* **50**: 275.

Scott, D.W., A. O'Garra, D. Warren, and G.G.B. Klaus. 1987a. Lymphoma models for B cell activation and tolerance VI. Reversal of anti-Ig-mediated negative signalling. *J. Immunol.* **139**: 3924.

Scott, D., J. Chace, G. Warner, A. O'Garra, G. Klaus, and H. Quill. 1987b. Role of T-cell derived lymphokines in two models of B-cell tolerance. *Immunol. Rev.* **99**: 152.

Scott, D.W., D. Livnat, J. Whitin, S. Dillon, R. Snyderman, and C.A. Pennell. 1987c. Lymphoma models for B cell activation and tolerance. *J. Mol. Cell. Immunol.* **3**: 109.

Scott, D., J. Tuttle, D. Livnat, W. Haynes, J. Cogswell, and P. Keng. 1985. Lymphoma models for B-cell activation and tolerance. II. Growth inhibition by anti-μ of WEHI-231 and the selection and properties of resistant mutants. *Cell. Immunol.* **93**: 124.

Teale, J.M. and N.R. Klinman. 1984. Membrane and metabolic requirements for tolerance induction of neonatal B cells. *J. Immunol.* **133**: 1811.

Teh, H.S., P. Kisielow, B. Scott, H. Kishi, Y. Uematsu, H. Bluthmann, and H. von Boehmer. 1988. Thymic major histocompatibility complex antigens and the $\alpha\beta$ T-cell receptor determine the CD4/CD8 phenotype of T cells. *Nature* **335**: 229.

Tisch, R., C. Roifman, and N. Hozumi. 1988. Functional differences between immunoglobulins M and D expressed on the surface of an immature B-cell line. *Proc. Natl. Acad. Sci.* **85**: 6914.

Venkataraman, M. and D.W. Scott. 1979. Cellular events in tolerance VII. Decrease in tolerance spleens of clonable precursors stimulatable *in vitro* by specific antigens or LPS. *Cell. Immunol.* **47**: 323.

Warner, G.L. and D.W. Scott. 1988. Lymphoma models for B cell activation and tolerance. VII. Pathways in anti-Ig-mediated growth inhibition and its reversal. *Cell. Immunol.* **115**: 195.

———. 1989. Cholera toxin sensitive and insensitive signalling via surface immunoglobulin. *J. Immunol.* **143**: 458.

Warner, G.L., D.W. Scott, and J.-E. Alés-Martínez. 1989. Delivery of growth inhibitory signals to B-cell lines is independent of Ca^{++} mobilization from intracellular stores. *FASEB J.* **3**: A1090.

Yuan, D. 1987. Molecular basis for the inhibition of LPS induced differentiation by anti-immunoglobulin. *J. Mol. Cell. Immunol.* **3**: 133.

Clonal Silencing of Self-reactive B Lymphocytes in a Transgenic Mouse Model

C.C. Goodnow,* J. Crosbie,* S. Adelstein,* T.B. Lavoie,†
S.J. Smith-Gill,† D.Y. Mason,§ H. Jorgensen,* R.A. Brink,*
H. Pritchard-Briscoe,* M. Loughnan,‡ R.H. Loblay,*
R.J. Trent,* and A. Basten*

*Centenary Institute of Cancer Medicine and Cell Biology, University of Sydney, New South Wales,
Australia 2006; †Laboratory of Genetics, National Cancer Institute, National Institutes of Health,
Bethesda, Maryland 20892; ‡Walter and Eliza Hall Insitute, P.O. Royal Melbourne Hospital, Victoria,
Australia 3050; §Nuffield Department of Pathology, John Radcliffe Hospital, Oxford, United Kingdom OX3 9DU

The ability of the immune system to distinguish between self-antigens and foreign antigens is a remarkable process. As a feat of developmental biology, immunological self-tolerance is all the more remarkable even when one considers the diversity of self-antigens that must be tolerated, including carbohydrates, lipids, nucleic acids, and approximately 40,000 different self-proteins, and the diversity of potentially self-reactive lymphocytes that must be tolerized. Among the possible cellular mechanisms for ensuring tolerance to self-antigens, irreversible deletion of self-reactive T lymphocytes has recently been shown to play a major role in maintaining self-tolerance within the helper and cytotoxic T-cell subsets (Kappler et al. 1987, 1988; Kisielow et al. 1988; MacDonald et al. 1988; Pullen et al. 1988; Sha et al. 1988; Davis et al., this volume). Self-tolerance in B lymphocytes expressing immunoglobulin M (IgM) antigen receptors only may also be brought about through clonal deletion of self-reactive cells (Nemazee and Bürki 1989). However, in comparison with T-cell tolerance, the development of self-tolerance within the B-lymphocyte compartment poses a number of unique problems to the immune system and consequently may involve altogether different mechanisms for silencing self-reactive cells. The purpose of this paper is to review some of the unique problems of B-cell tolerance in order to place our own studies of a transgenic mouse model into a broader perspective.

Tolerance and the Developmental Stage of Antigen Receptor Diversification

Clonal deletion of thymocytes expressing self-reactive receptors appears to involve a mechanism of self/nonself discrimination identical to that originally proposed for B lymphocytes by Lederberg (1959); immature thymocytes expressing self-reactive T-cell receptors (TCRs) fail to complete their development apparently because TCR/antigen interaction at an early stage of lymphocyte differentiation activates programmed death of the cell (Smith et al. 1989). Deletion at the thymocyte stage of development is an effective

mechanism for maintaining self-tolerance in the T-cell repertoire because the sequence and specificity of TCRs remains constant after receptor gene rearrangement (Chien et al. 1984; Ikuta et al. 1985; Fink et al. 1986). B lymphocytes, however, continue to mutate and diversify their immunoglobulin genes after they have left the primary lymphoid organ and developed into functionally mature, antigen-reactive cells (Berek and Milstein 1988; French et al. 1989). As a consequence of this peripheral diversification of the B-cell repertoire, self-reactive variants are generated from expanding clones of nonself-reactive B cells at a detectable frequency (Diamond and Scharff 1984; Radic et al., this volume). If these self-reactive mature B cells are to be prevented from giving rise to autoantibodies, a non-Lederberg mechanism for distinguishing self-antigens from foreign antigens (i.e., dependent on some other variable than the developmental stage of the lymphocyte) would appear to be required.

Is Self-tolerance within the B-cell Compartment Necessary?

B-lymphocytes also differ from helper T cells with respect to tolerance in that they are dependent on helper T cells to mount efficient antibody responses to most antigens (Mitchell and Miller 1968; Mitchison 1971). As illustrated in Figure 1a, a B cell expressing a receptor for a foreign antigen will bind, internalize, and process the foreign antigen, and present peptide fragments of that antigen in association with class II major histocompatibility complex (MHC) molecules for recognition by "antiforeign" helper T cells (Lanzavecchia 1985). The T cell in turn provides signals to the B cell that enable efficient clonal expansion and differentiation into plasma cells, thereby giving rise to an antibody response to the foreign antigen. In contrast, a B cell that expresses receptors for a self-antigen could conceivably bind, process, and present fragments of the self-antigen (Fig. 1b) but will fail to receive the necessary "second signals" for expansion and differentiation because helper T cells capable of recognizing the presented self-antigen are either absent or not functional.

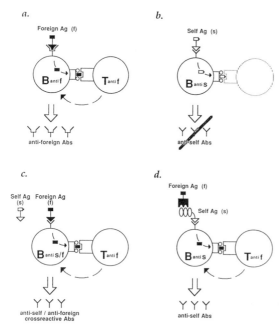

Figure 1. Models for activation of B lymphocytes by self or foreign antigens. (*a*) Collaboration between a B cell with receptor-specificity for a foreign antigen and an antiforeign helper T cell, resulting in an antibody response to the foreign antigen. (*b*) Failure of a self-reactive B cell to mount an antibody response to a self-antigen because of the absence of self-reactive helper T cells. (*c*) Potential development of autoantibodies because of collaboration between a cross-reactive B cell and an antiforeign helper T cell. (*d*) Potential development of autoantibodies through collaboration between a self-reactive B cell and an antiforeign helper T cell, facilitated by formation of complexes between self-antigens and foreign antigens.

On purely theoretical grounds, one could therefore postulate that self-reactive B cells do not, on their own, pose a significant risk to the individual; provided T-cell tolerance is efficient, there may be no need for a Lederberg-type of tolerance mechanism or for that matter any other tolerance mechanism within the B-cell repertoire.

There are, however, two theoretical situations where persistence of self-reactive B cells in a fully responsive form might in theory pose a grave risk of autoimmunity. The first situation, shown in Figure 1c, occurs when a foreign antigen happens to bear one or more surface epitopes that resemble a self-antigen. Any B cell expressing a receptor for one of these cross-reactive surface epitopes can potentially bind, internalize, process, and present the foreign antigen to antiforeign helper T cells. Because the helper T cell cannot distinguish between B cells that have internalized the antigen via a cross-reactive receptor versus a foreign-specific receptor, the necessary second signals are thereby provided to the cross-reactive B cell. If the cross-reactive B cell is competent to respond to these signals, a fraction of the ensuing antibody response will consist of potentially destructive high-affinity IgG autoantibodies. In reality, such a situation would be most likely to occur with foreign antigens that have regions of evolutionarily

conserved surface topology such as the active sites of enzymes and the combining sites of structural proteins or nucleic-acid-binding proteins. It is perhaps intriguing to note that when self-tolerance breaks down the autoantibody response is characteristically directed at these sites precisely (Tan 1989).

A second situation with a similar potential to give rise to autoantibodies results from the formation of complexes between self-antigens and foreign antigens (Fig. 1d). Examples of possible complexes include self-DNA complexed with viral DNA-binding proteins, autologous spliceosomes or ribosomes complexed with viral proteins involved in "hijacking" these functions, viral or bacterial particles associated with cellular receptors, and foreign antigens complexed with self-IgG. In each of these cases, B cells recognizing the self-moiety of the complex will potentially bind, internalize, and process the complex, and present fragments of foreign protein to antiviral or antibacterial helper T cells. Again, it the self-reactive B cell is not itself tolerant, the ensuing antibody response will include high-affinity IgG antibodies to autologous DNA, spliceosomes, ribosomes, cell-surface receptors, or autologous IgG. Moreover, subsequent infections involving entirely different viruses and different DNA-binding proteins or different antigen/IgG complexes will potentially boost the same sets of autoreactive B cells.

Evidence for Self-tolerance in B Lymphocytes

In practice, the two aforementioned situations that might be expected to give rise to autoantibodies are commonplace not only during normal life, but also under experimental conditions. For example, just such a situation is created during the production of species- and allele-specific antisera and monoclonal antibodies by immunizing with xenogeneic or allogeneic cells or proteins, in which some or many of the surface epitopes are common to both the immunogen and the recipient. The assumption that the antibody response will be restricted to the epitopes that *differ* between immunogen and self is fundamental to the entire field of serology and was first stated by Ehrlich over 80 years ago (Ehrlich 1900). Of course, such an assumption depends on the existence of some form of B-cell tolerance since, as highlighted in Figure 1c and d, the simple provision of T-cell help to the foreign moiety of the immunogen would otherwise lead to production of cross-reactive antibodies with specificity for both immunogen and self.

That the antibody response to xenogeneic or allogeneic cells or proteins is restricted to the epitopes that differ between immunogen and self is well documented, not only in terms of the widespread practical use of species- or allele-specific antisera and monoclonal antibodies, but also through a number of detailed experimental studies. The first of these was the analysis of the rabbit antibody response to human hemoglobin by Reichlin (1972) showing clearly that the antibodies were directed only at regions of hemoglobin that differed between rabbit and human. Reichlin's findings with polyclonal antisera from rabbits are borne out by studies of mouse monoclonal antibodies to human hemoglobin (Stamatoyannopoulos et al. 1983); of seven different monoclonal antibodies reactive with hemoglobin from humans and other mammals, none bound significantly to mouse hemoglobin. Studies of the antibody response to cytochrome c yielded equally striking results (for review, see Benjamin et al. 1984); for example, the majority of the rabbit antibody response to guanoco cytochrome c, which differs in only two amino acids from rabbit cytochrome c, was found to be directed only to these two sites on the surface of the molecule (Urbanski and Margoliash 1977). Comparable results to those with cytoplasmic self-proteins were obtained in studies of the antibody response to cell-surface self-proteins, as in the response of Ia^s mice to spleen cells bearing allogeneic Ia^k MHC molecules. Among 35 monoclonal antibodies directed to the I-A or I-E molecules on the immunizing cells, all bound only to the foreign MHC molecules and all were directed to the few regions of difference between Ia^s and Ia^k (Pierres et al. 1981). Finally, perhaps the most illuminating example comes from a comparison of the pathological and normal responses to the SS-B/La autoantigen, which is a nuclear phosphoprotein possibly involved in processing of RNA polymerase III transcripts. Whereas autoantibodies from humans with Sjögren's syndrome cross-react with native SS-B/La from many species including murine and bovine SS-B/La, monoclonal antibodies elicited by immunizing normal mice with bovine SS-B/La either react only with denatured protein or are directed to epitopes found on bovine and human SS-B/La but not on the autologous mouse antigen (Harley et al. 1985; Chan and Tan 1987).

Nevertheless, self-tolerance does not appear to be absolute in either the T- or B-cell compartment. Self-reactive T cells can be elicited to a number of "sequestered" self-antigens such as thyroglobulin and myelin basic protein (Weigle 1973; Cohen 1986), and T cells with low affinity for self-MHC are positively selected in the thymus (Sha et al. 1988; Teh et al. 1988). Thus, some T cells escape tolerance by virtue of either low antigen concentration (Weigle 1973; Howard and Mitchison 1975), low receptor affinity for antigen, or even decreased expression of the CD8 component of the receptor (Kisielow et al. 1988), whereas T cells with high avidity for self-antigen appear to be deleted. With respect to self-tolerance in the B-cell compartment, there is a requirement for higher concentrations of antigen than those needed for T-cell tolerance (Chiller et al. 1971), perhaps because B cells bind native antigen alone in contrast with T cells that recognize processed fragments of antigen on the surface of specialized antigen-presenting cells. As with T cells, low-affinity antiself B cells do not appear to be rendered tolerant; where autoantibodies have been elicited by polyclonal activation or specific immunization, either the antiself-antibodies have been of low affinity and low titer for the self-antigen (Ruoslahti et al. 1975; Primi et

al. 1977; Naysmith et al. 1981; Nemazee and Sato 1983; Benjamin et al. 1984; Holmberg et al. 1986; Ternynck and Avrameus 1986) or alternatively no attempt has been made to quantitate their titer or affinity (Harris et al. 1982).

The tendency for antibodies to recognize conformational epitopes on the surface of proteins poses an additional complication in interpreting apparent failures of B-cell tolerance because although B cells are tolerant to autologous proteins in their native conformation, it is relatively easy to raise high-titer, high-affinity antisera to denatured self-proteins. An elegant example of this problem comes from the comparison of disease-associated autoantibodies and induced autoantibodies to proliferating cell nuclear antigen/cyclin, the auxiliary protein of DNA polymerase δ (Tan 1989). Whereas anticyclin autoantibodies from patients with systemic lupus erythematosus bind strongly to native cyclin and inhibit the function of the protein in in vitro polymerase assays, monoclonal autoantibodies raised by immunizing normal mice with purified rabbit cyclin were able to bind denatured cyclin but not the native conformation of the self-protein (Ogata et al. 1987). In the immunized mice, the antibody response would appear to be confined to epitopes present on a small amount of denatured protein in the original immunizing preparation. Essentially identical findings were obtained when autoantibodies to tRNA synthetases in the sera of patients with polymyositis/dermatomyositis were compared with those obtained by immunizing normal animals (Tan 1989).

Other instances of apparent failures in B-cell tolerance, exemplified by the autoantibody response to the liver protein F (Iverson and Lindenmann 1972; Lane and Silver 1976), may also be related simply to immunization and assay procedures involving partially denatured or proteolysed protein. In the studies of the immune response to F protein, no precautions were taken to avoid proteolysis during preparation of either the immunogen or the purified protein used in the subsequent antibody-binding assays, and all purification steps employed the induced autoantibodies, which may have selectively isolated a denatured or proteolysed fragment. Without structural information or functional assays for native F protein such as those employed in the more detailed studies of immune responses to cytochrome c, cyclin, and tRNA synthetase, any restriction of the antibody response to a proteolysed or denatured moiety of the F-protein preparation would be undetectable. Distinguishing between bona fide autoantibodies and antibodies to "altered self" is a significant pitfall in studies of tolerance in B cells but not in T cells since denaturation or proteolysis generally has little effect on T-cell recognition of protein antigens (Benjamin et al. 1984).

Mechanism of Self-tolerance in B Lymphocytes

Conventional models of B-cell tolerance. Delineation of the mechanism of self-tolerance in B cells depends in particular on the ability to trace the fate of antiself-B cells. However, antigen-specific B cells are generated at low frequency in the preimmune repertoire making it difficult to follow the development of these cells even in the absence of the corresponding self-antigen. Furthermore, nontolerant B cells with low-affinity binding to self-antigen frequently obscure the identification of high-affinity tolerized cells since cells with high affinity for antigen are generated at much lower frequency in the preimmune repertoire (Nossal et al. 1979).

To study the mechanism(s) of B-cell tolerance, four types of conventional model systems have been used. The first type involves the induction of unresponsiveness in B cells in vivo by administration of foreign antigens in an appropriate form or by an appropriate route. These studies showed that B lymphocytes in adult animals could be rendered tolerant to a number of xenogeneic proteins, polysaccharides, and haptens, and established some of the important parameters that may be involved (Katz et al. 1972; Weigle 1973; Rajewsky and Brenig 1974; Howard and Mitchison 1975; Desaymard and Waldmann 1976; Metcalf et al. 1979; Scott et al. 1979; Parks et al. 1982; Nossal 1983). It was difficult, however, to determine the fate of tolerized B cells in these models. Furthermore, the possibility remained that some examples of induced unresponsiveness reflected phenomena that were not directly related to self-tolerance, such as exhaustive differentiation of tolerogen-specific B cells, feedback effects because of immune complexes, and receptor blockade.

To bypass the problem of low frequency of antigen-specific B cells, a second in vivo model system has been developed that employs antiimmunoglobulin antibodies to mimic the effects of antigen by binding to membrane immunoglobulin on the B cell, thus allowing every developing B cell to be equally affected. Exposure of mice to polyclonal anti-IgM antisera during ontogeny resulted in drastic reduction in the number of B cells, suggesting that B-cell tolerance might be brought about by clonal deletion (Lawton and Cooper 1974). More recent studies in this model with a non-complement-fixing IgG1 anti-IgM monoclonal antibody, however, found that B cells were not deleted by cross-linking of membrane IgM per se but that they persisted in an unresponsive state and had reversibly modulated their membrane IgM (Gause et al. 1987). In both studies, parental or neonatal exposure to anti-IgM was necessary to induce unresponsiveness in the B-cell compartment. The significance of early exposure was difficult to interpret since anti-IgM treatment later in development may have failed to induce unresponsiveness either because only immature B cells were susceptible to tolerance induction, because some B cells had already switched to downstream isotypes and were therefore "immune" to the effects of anti-IgM, or because later in ontogeny the T cells had become responsive to the foreign moiety of the anti-IgM antibody and thereby modified the response of the B cells.

In the third type of system for studying B-cell tolerance, polyvalent antigens as well as antiimmunoglobulins have been used to induce B-cell unresponsiveness in vitro (Raff et al. 1975; Sidman and Unanue 1975; Klaus 1979; Metcalf et al. 1979; Scott et al. 1979; Nossal 1983). In many of these studies, receptor cross-linking on immature B cells resulted in either irreversible receptor modulation (clonal abortion) or in a variable degree of unresponsiveness without any apparent change in receptor status (clonal anergy). Mature B cells were not rendered unresponsive by these treatments, supporting the concept of a tolerance-susceptible phase early in B-cell development (Lederberg 1959). Similarly, in the fourth model of B-cell tolerance, proliferation of some B-lymphoma cell lines can be profoundly inhibited by exposure to anti-IgM antibodies in vitro (Boyd and Schrader 1981; DeFranco et al. 1982; Pennell and Scott 1986), raising the possibility of genetic and biochemical dissection of the negative signaling pathway.

There is no doubt that conventional model systems have provided important information on the range of possible mechanisms of B-cell tolerance, but none of them have provided a definitive explanation for B-cell tolerance to autologous antigens in vivo. Perhaps the most controversial issue surrounds the differences between the findings obtained in the in vitro and in vivo models of unresponsiveness. For example, the stage of maturation of the B cell appears critical to susceptibility to tolerance in the in vitro models (Sidman and Unanue 1975; Metcalf et al. 1979; Nossal 1983), whereas B cells at various stages of maturation have been shown to be susceptible in vivo. Secondly, in vitro tolerance in immature B cells is frequently associated with irreversible modulation of membrane IgM (Sidman and Unanue 1975; Raff et al. 1975; Nossal 1983), whereas the in vivo results of Gause et al. (1987) suggest a reversible modulation of membrane IgM. Finally, the antigens that are very effective B-cell tolerogens in vivo are generally ineffective in vitro, and, conversely, antigens that are tolerogenic in vitro are for the most part extremely immunogenic in vivo (Nossal 1983). It is possible that some of the in vitro observations may reflect inadequacies in culture conditions rather than phenomena directly related to tolerance induction since the survival and maintenance of B cells in vitro is very poor compared with their life span in vivo. On the other hand, the complexities involved in the in vivo models make it difficult to distinguish in many cases between induction of B-cell unresponsiveness by clonal deletion, clonal anergy, suppression, or simply exhaustive differentiation of mature B cells.

Transgenic models of B-cell tolerance. To resolve the controversy surrounding the mechanism of self-tolerance in B cells, we have followed a different approach by developing a model system that would enable direct visualization of the fate of self-reactive B

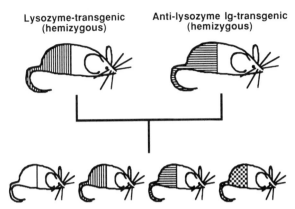

Figure 2. Strategy for a transgenic mouse model of B-cell tolerance. Matings between lysozyme-transgenic mice and antilysozyme immunoglobulin-transgenic mice produce litters of offspring with four possible genotypes. Thus, B cells in the double-transgenic mice can be compared with B cells in age- and sex-matched immunoglobulin-transgenic or nontransgenic littermate controls.

cells with a uniform affinity for a bona fide self-antigen in vivo. The strategy is shown in Figure 2 and involves the generation of two types of transgenic mice. The first type carries the gene for hen egg lysozyme (HEL) and expresses the protein as a neo-self-antigen, rendering both T- and B-cell compartments tolerant. The second type of transgenic mouse carries rearranged immunoglobulin genes encoding a high-affinity antilysozyme antibody, resulting in the production of very high frequencies of antilysozyme B cells in the preimmune repertoire of these mice. By mating the two types of mice, the respective transgenes segregate in a simple Mendelian fashion, and one quarter of the resulting offspring inherit both lysozyme and antilysozyme transgenes. In these "double-transgenic" offspring, tolerance to HEL is maintained, and the development and fate of antilysozyme B cells can be readily followed. This approach has the dual advantage of providing sufficient numbers of cells for functional and biochemical analyses and of allowing precise genetic changes to be made in the two key "players": the self-antigen and the B-cells' receptor for self-antigen.

Lysozyme-transgenic Mice

HEL was chosen as a transgenic self-antigen for several reasons. First, a large body of information has been assembled on the structure and biochemistry of lysozyme and on the normal immune response to lysozyme (Osserman et al. 1974; Smith-Gill and Sercarz 1989). Second, lysozyme is nontoxic and unlikely to alter the general physiological or immunological milieu of the transgenic mice. Finally, large amounts of lysozyme in pure and native form are easily obtained, facilitating immunological analysis of the mice.

To produce transgenic mice that express HEL, gene constructs were prepared by linking a genomic clone of the chicken lysozyme gene (Matthias et al. 1982) to one of two mouse promoter segments. The first promoter used was derived from the mouse metallothionein I gene (Fig. 3) (Palmiter et al. 1982). The metallothionein promoter was an attractive choice because it is expressed in most cells from early in development and because it can be induced to higher levels of expression by exposure to heavy metals (Palmiter and Brinster 1986). The second promoter employed, from the mouse albumin gene (Fig. 3), contrasts with the metallothionein promoter in that the albumin promoter directs gene expression only in hepatocytes (Tilghman and Belayew 1982; Pinkert et al. 1987).

Both gene constructs were excised free of vector sequences and microinjected into fertilized eggs from matings of C57BL/6 mice. Inbred C57BL/6 mice were chosen as the recipient strains for all the transgenes to enable cell transfer experiments between different transgenic mice without graft rejection or allogeneic effects. Furthermore, because C57BL/6 mice are genetic low-responders to HEL (Gammon et al. 1987), one can compare the effects of the transgenes in low-responder mice as well as on high-responder MHC-congenic strain backgrounds.

The metallothionein/lysozyme and albumin/lysozyme transgenes are expressed in many of the transgenic lines established, resulting in secretion of HEL into the serum. The serum levels of lysozyme, as measured by capture enzyme-linked immunosorbent assay (ELISA) using monoclonal antibodies specific for HEL, vary from line to line from as low as 0.5–3 ng/ml in ML3b metallothionein/lysozyme-transgenic mice to as high as 50–100 ng/ml in the AL3 albumin/lysozyme-transgenic line (Fig. 4). Moreover, the concentration of serum lysozyme can be increased from 5- to 100-fold in the metallothionein/lysozyme mice by administering 25 mM zinc sulfate in the drinking water (Fig. 4). The level of expression of the lysozyme transgenes does not appear to correlate with transgene copy number and presumably is influenced primarily by the site of integration as observed for other transgenes (Palmiter and Brinster 1986).

Immunological tolerance to lysozyme was examined in most of the established transgenic mouse lines by immunizing with HEL in one of two forms. In one form of challenge, litters of (CBA × C57BL/6)F₁ hybrid mice (a high-responder background) were bred so that half the mice in the litter were hemizygous for the transgene and the other half would serve as nontransgenic controls. Members of these litters were immunized with lysozyme in complete Freund's adjuvant, thereby requiring both antilysozyme helper T cells and B cells to give rise to an antilysozyme antibody response. By this assay, transgenic mice from all the lines with serologically detectable serum lysozyme were found to be tolerant and failed to mount an antibody response to lysozyme (Goodnow et al. 1988; S. Adelstein et al., in prep.). A more detailed analysis of one line, ML5, showed that antilysozyme helper T-cell

HEN EGG LYSOZYME CONSTRUCTS

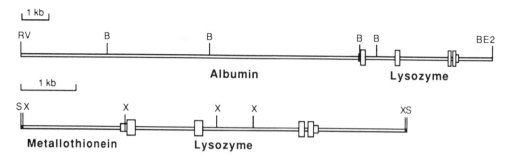

ANTI-LYSOZYME IMMUNOGLOBULIN GENE CONSTRUCTS

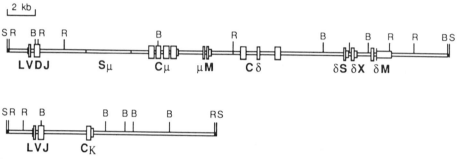

Figure 3. Structure of microinjected gene constructs. Thin bars represent introns or flanking DNA, boxes of intermediate width indicate 5′ or 3′ untranslated regions, and wider boxes indicate coding regions. Relevant restriction sites are indicated: (B) *Bam*HI; (BE2) *Bst*EII; (R) *Eco*RI; (S) *Sal*I; (X) *Xba*I.

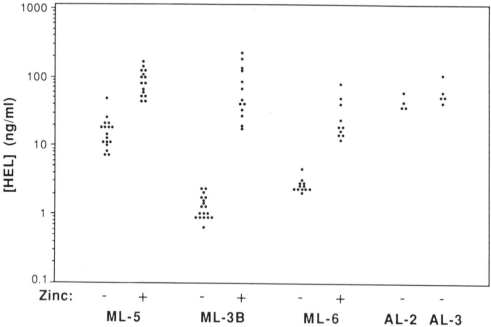

Figure 4. Concentration of HEL in the serum of different lines of lysozyme-transgenic mice. Lysozyme concentrations were determined by capture ELISA (C. Goodnow et al., in prep.) in metallothionein/lysozyme (ML-prefix) transgenic mice or albumin/lysozyme (AL-prefix) mice. Each dot represents the concentration in an individual mouse. The ML mice were either uninduced or exposed to 25 mM zinc in the drinking water for 1 week as indicated.

function was greatly reduced, either when assayed by in vitro proliferation (Goodnow et al. 1988) or by hapten/carrier collaborative responses in adoptive transfer (S. Adelstein, unpubl.).

The second form of immunological challenge has been carried out in C57BL/6 (low-responder) mice to study specifically B-cell responses to lysozyme in a system devoid of complications arising from the presence or absence of antilysozyme helper T cells. C57BL/6 litters containing transgenic mice and nontransgenic littermate controls were immunized with HEL covalently coupled to horse red blood cells (HRBC), the latter acting as a foreign carrier in order to supply potent T-cell help to any available antilysozyme B cells. Tolerance was manifest in the B-cell compartment of all lines of mice with detectable serum lysozyme, resulting in a 50-fold reduction in titers of serum antilysozyme antibody and 10-fold fewer antilysozyme plaque-forming cells in the spleen (Goodnow et al. 1988; S. Adelstein et al., in prep.). As has been observed for tolerance to other antigens (Siskind and Benacerraf 1969; Rajewsky and Brenig 1974; Benjamin et al. 1984), tolerance was not absolute within the B-cell compartment since B cells with low affinity for lysozyme did not appear to be tolerant (Goodnow et al. 1988).

Immunoglobulin-transgenic Mice

Determining the fate of the tolerized high-affinity antilysozyme B cells in the lysozyme-transgenic mice is complicated by the low frequency of these cells (~ 1 in 10^4 B cells) and the presence of greater numbers of low-affinity antilysozyme B cells that are not tolerized, as discussed above. To increase the frequency of high-affinity antilysozyme B cells, functionally rearranged immunoglobulin genes from a high-affinity ($K_a = 2 \times 10^9$ M^{-1}) antilysozyme B-cell hybridoma were introduced into the germ line of transgenic mice. The original hybridoma, HyHEL10, was derived from a hyperimmunized BALB/c mouse, and secretes a highly mutated IgG1 antibody with well-characterized fine specificity (Smith-Gill et al. 1984). The three-dimensional structure of the antibody has been solved as a complex with HEL (Padlan et al. 1989), thereby providing detailed information on the contact residues at the interface between the antigen and the antibody, which will facilitate the design of future experiments in this model system.

Immunoglobulin gene constructs were prepared by linking the productively rearranged (variable, diversity, and joining) VDJ_H and VJ_κ genomic segments from the hybridoma to appropriate (constant) C_H and C_κ segments (Fig. 3). (Goodnow et al. 1988). In the case of the heavy chain, the entire μ to δ constant region locus (including an undeleted switch region) was reconstructed from BALB/c genomic clones to enable developmentally regulated expression of IgM and IgD antigen receptors by the B cells. Amino acid polymorphisms between BALB/c (IgH^a) and C57BL/6 (IgH^b) μ and δ

constant regions allow transgene-encoded heavy chains to be distinguished from endogenous C57BL/6 heavy chains by monoclonal antiallotype antibodies. For the light chain, a genomic clone of the C_κ locus was added, including 3'-flanking DNA that contains the recently identified downstream κ enhancer (K. Meyer and M. Reth, pers. comm.).

Contact residues from both the light and heavy chains of HyHEL10 contribute to high-affinity binding of lysozyme (Smith-Gill et al. 1987; Padlan et al. 1989), thereby requiring both heavy- and light-chain genes to be present for high-affinity antilysozyme B cells to be generated. To ensure that the light- and heavy-chain genes did not segregate during mating, the heavy- and light-chain gene constructs were coinjected at an equimolar ratio into C57BL/6 eggs, since this maneuver has been shown previously to result in cointegration into a single chromosomal locus (Storb et al. 1986). Of seven founder mice, six carried a variable number of copies of both light- and heavy-chain gene constructs integrated together in a single chromosomal location and expressed high-affinity lysozyme-binding antibody (see below). The seventh line carried two copies of the heavy-chain gene only and expressed high concentrations of transgene-encoded (a-allotype) heavy chain, presumably paired with a range of endogenous light chains resulting in only low titers of lysozyme-binding antibody as would be expected.

To determine the frequency of antilysozyme B cells in the immunoglobulin-transgenic mice, lymphoid cell suspensions from various tissues were analyzed by flow cytometry. Lysozyme-binding cells were detected by incubating the cells on ice with biotinylated HEL followed by streptavidin phycoerythrin or by incubating the cells with unlabeled lysozyme followed by a biotinylated antilysozyme monoclonal antibody (HyHEL9), which does not compete for binding with the transgene-encoded HyHEL10 antibody. The results were qualitatively the same with either staining protocol although the latter sandwich technique resulted in five- to tenfold brighter fluorescence without any increase in background. The more sensitive sandwich technique was therefore adopted for routine use. As shown in Figure 5 (extreme top), greater than 90% of spleen B cells bind lysozyme in the immunoglobulin-transgenic mice, compared with less than 0.1% of spleen B cells from nontransgenic littermates. Similar results were obtained in mesenteric lymph node (Fig. 7) and in bone marrow (Goodnow et al. 1988).

Staining with monoclonal antiallotype antibodies revealed that more than 95% of the B cells expressed high levels of transgene-encoded (a-allotype) membrane IgM and a range of levels of a-allotype membrane IgD (Fig. 5, top left). The IgM-bright, IgD$^-$ B cells were primarily seen in the spleen where they were located predominantly in the splenic marginal zones, whereas the IgD$^+$ cells were located in the follicular mantle zones of spleen and lymph node (D.Y. Mason et al., in prep.). The developmental regulation of IgD between marginal zone and follicular mantle zone B

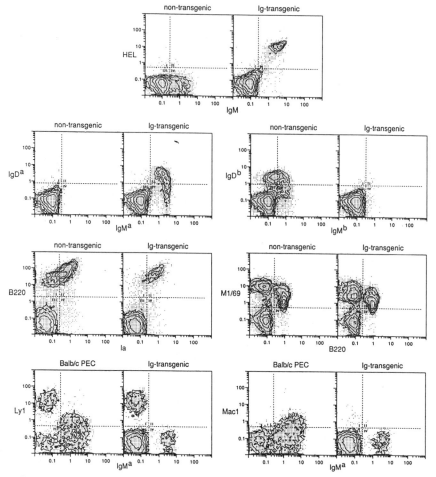

Figure 5. Two-color FACS analysis of spleen cells from antilysozyme immunoglobulin-transgenic mice and nontransgenic littermates. All samples are from MD4 immunoglobulin-transgenic mice, except the staining for Ia, Ly-1, and Mac-1, which was performed on cells from MD3 immunoglobulin-transgenic mice. Antibodies used to detect each marker are indicated. (*Extreme top*) Binding of lysozyme (HEL/HyHEL9-biotin) versus IgM expression (331.12-FITC). (*Top left*) Expression of a-allotype IgD (AMS-15.1-biotin) versus a-allotype IgM (DS1-FITC). (*Top right*) Expression of b-allotype IgD (AF6-122.2-biotin) versus b-allotype IgM (AFS-78.25-FITC). (*Middle left*) Expression of Ia molecules (P7-7/MARK-2-FITC) by B220[+] cells (RA3-6B2-biotin). (*Middle right*) Expression of heat-stable antigen (M1/69-biotin) versus B220 (RA3-6B2-FITC). (*Lower left and right*) Ly-1 expression (*left*) (53-7.8-biotin) or MAC-1 expression (*right*) (M1/70-biotin) versus a-allotype IgM (DS-1-FITC). Immunoglobulin-transgenic spleen cells are compared with BALB/c peritoneal exudate cells (PEC) in the bottom two panels, the latter acting as a positive control for detecting relatively low level expression of Ly-1 or Mac-1 on Ly-1 B cells.

cells therefore appears to occur normally in the immunoglobulin-transgenic mice. Furthermore, the absolute level of IgD expressed by follicular B cells in the transgenic mice is similar to that observed in nontransgenic BALB/c mice (Fig. 8). On the other hand, although the absolute level of membrane IgM on the marginal zone B cells in the immunoglobulin transgenics also appears normal, the level of IgM on follicular B cells is equivalent only to the most IgM-bright subpopulation of follicular B cells found in nontransgenic spleen (Fig. 8). A possible explanation for this interesting difference will be discussed later.

Very few B cells expressing endogenous (b-allotype) heavy chains were detected in spleen (Fig. 5), lymph node (Goodnow et al. 1988), or bone marrow. Rearrangement and therefore expression of endogenous heavy-chain genes are presumably suppressed by the presence of the productively rearranged heavy-chain transgene, as has been observed previously (Weaver et al. 1985). We assume the expression of endogenous light-chain genes is similarly suppressed as has been documented previously (Ritchie et al. 1984). Nevertheless, small numbers of endogenous immunoglobulin-expressing B cells were detectable, particularly in very old mice, and these contribute disproportionately to the plasma cell pool (D.Y. Mason et al., in prep.) and result in almost normal concentrations of serum IgM[b] and IgG in the immunoglobulin-transgenic mice (C.C. Goodnow, unpubl.). The "leakiness" of allelic exclusion would appear therefore to account for the absence of any clinical evidence of immunodeficiency in these mice. The endogenous heavy-chain-expressing B cells carried low levels of transgene-encoded membrane IgM and IgD, suggesting that these cells have down-regulated the transgene at some stage during development, thereby enabling rearrangement of endogenous heavy chains and selective recruitment of these cells in peripheral lymphoid tissue. Similar findings have been described in λ-light-chain transgenic mice (Neuberger et al. 1989; Pettersson et al. 1989).

A comparison of the expression of other B-cell surface markers on spleen cells from immunoglobulin-transgenic mice and nontransgenic littermates was carried out to characterize the developmental state of the B cells. B cells from the spleen of immunoglobulin-transgenic mice expressed high levels of the B220 marker as determined by staining with the antibody RA3-6B2 (Fig. 5, middle left) and did not express the markers Ly-1 (CD5) or Mac-1 (Fig. 5, bottom), indicating that these B cells were not Ly-1 B cells. Immunoglobulin-transgenic B cells expressed Ia molecules at low levels, comparable with the expression of Ia on nontransgenic spleen B cells (Fig. 5, middle left) and had forward and 90° light-scatter characteristics of small resting cells (not shown), indicating that most of the immunoglobulin-transgenic B cells were nonactivated G_0 cells. Finally, the majority of B cells in the spleens of transgenic and nontransgenic mice expressed low levels of heat-stable antigen, a characteristic of mature B cells (Fig. 5, middle right, antibody M1/69) (Hardy et al. 1983). Taken together with the follicular location of the lysozyme-binding B cells (Fig. 6, top) and the normal distribution of T and B cells in the immunoglobulin-transgenic mice (Fig. 6, bottom), it would appear that the extreme skewing of the B-cell repertoire in antilysozyme immunoglobulin-transgenic mice does not disrupt overall lymphoid development and maturation.

Double-transgenic Mice

Double-transgenic mice were prepared initially by matings between one representative line of immunoglobulin-transgenic mice, MD3, and the highest expressing line of metallothionein/lysozyme-transgenic mice, ML5. Analysis of sera from double-transgenic mice and immunoglobulin-transgenic littermate controls revealed an almost complete absence of lysozyme-binding antibody in the double-transgenic mice, whereas high concentrations were spontaneously secreted in the immunoglobulin-transgenic mice. That the absence of antilysozyme antibody in the serum was due to cessation of antibody secretion rather than complexing with circulating lysozyme was demonstrated by the finding of 200-fold fewer or no detectable antilysozyme plaque-forming cells in spleens of MD3 × ML5 double-transgenic mice (Goodnow et al. 1988).

Tolerance to lysozyme was therefore maintained in the double-transgenic mice despite the increased production of antilysozyme B cells in the bone marrow of these mice. The antilysozyme B cells were not clonally deleted, however, since fluorescence-activated cell sorter (FACS) analysis of spleen or lymph node cells (Fig. 7A) or bone marrow (Goodnow et al. 1988) showed little or no reduction in the number of lysozyme-binding B cells in double-transgenic mice. Intriguingly, there was a 10- to 20-fold reduction in the level of membrane IgM expressed on the B cells in the double-transgenic mice (Fig. 7A) but no reduction in the level of IgD (Fig. 8) and no change in expression of other surface markers. The self-reactive B cells also appeared to be functionally altered since B cells from double-transgenic spleen or lymph node responded very poorly in adoptive transfer (Fig. 7B) and did not proliferate in culture with lipopolysaccharide (M. Loughnan, unpubl.), whereas B cells from immunoglobulin-transgenic controls performed well in both these assays.

The phenotypic change in the B cells between immunoglobulin- and double-transgenic mice is provocative. In spleens from adult nontransgenic mice, three phenotypic populations of B cells have been defined on the basis of IgM/IgD expression (Hardy et al. 1983). B cells with high levels of IgD, which are predominantly long-lived recirculating cells found in the follicular mantle zone, constitute two of the subpopulations: "population I", which has low levels of membrane IgM, and "population II", which has high levels of IgM (Fig. 8). The third population, "population III", expresses little or no IgD and high levels of IgM and is primarily composed of sessile long-lived marginal zone B cells in addition to small numbers of immature B cells and Ly-1 B cells.

According to this classification, B cells in the spleen of the antilysozyme immunoglobulin-transgenic mice appear representative of populations II and III, but no cells are observed with the phenotype of population I (Fig. 8). In contrast, in the double-transgenic mice populations II and III are absent and replaced by cells with the phenotype of population I (Fig. 8). Immunohistological analysis of double-transgenic spleens shows that the marginal zone cells (population III) are indeed absent (D.Y. Mason et al., in prep.), whereas the population II cells in the follicular mantle zone appear simply to have down-regulated their membrane IgM to adopt the phenotype of population I. Since this selective change in phenotype can be induced in immunoglobulin-transgenic B cells within 20 hours (see below) and since the decreased expression of membrane IgM in population I cells from nontransgenic mice appears to be a posttranslational phenomenon (Yuan 1984), it is tempting to speculate that population I and II follicular B cells normally represent a continuum of cells: At one extreme, some follicular B cells have high avidity for self antigens (lowest IgM), whereas at the other extreme B cells exist that do not bind appreciably to any self-antigen (highest IgM).

The selective down-regulation of membrane IgM receptors observed on double-transgenic B cells appears to be intimately linked to functional silencing of the B cell. Thus, the same phenotypic and functional changes occurred in double-transgenic mice resulting from matings of the original ML5 line of metallothionein/lysozyme-transgenic mice with four of the five other immunoglobulin-transgenic lines (R. Brink et al., in

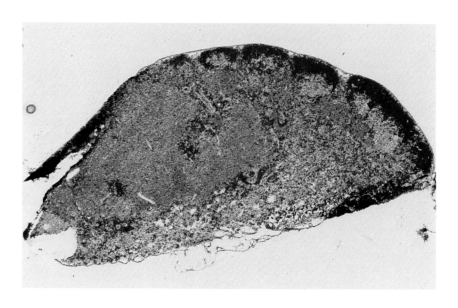

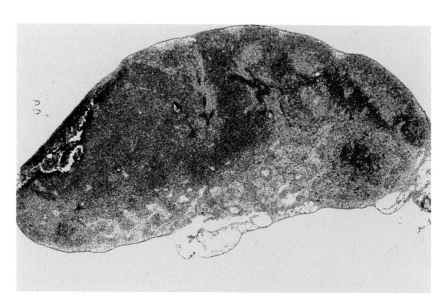

Figure 6. Normal lymphoid architecture in immunoglobulin-transgenic mice. Serial frozen sections of mesenteric lymph node from an MD3 immunoglobulin-transgenic mouse were stained for lysozyme-binding B cells (*top*), or Ly-1-bearing T cells (*bottom*), using the alkaline phosphatase technique (D.Y. Mason et al., in prep.). Lysozyme-binding B cells are concentrated in the mantle zones of secondary follicles, whereas T cells are predominantly found in the paracortex. B-cell blasts in the germinal centers are surface-immunoglobulin-negative as is observed in nontransgenic mice.

prep.), whereas tolerance was not observed in double-transgenic mice from the fifth line, MD5. In parallel with the failure of B-cell silencing in MD5 × ML5 double-transgenic mice, only a slight decrease in membrane IgM occurs on the lysozyme-binding B cells (C.C. Goodnow et al., in prep.). The explanation for the lack of tolerance and membrane IgM down-regulation in MD5 mice is unknown but may be linked to an almost complete failure of allelic exclusion that is also unique to this line of anti-HEL immunoglobulin-transgenic mice.

Similarly, tolerance and membrane IgM down-regulation failed to occur in double-transgenic mice produced by matings of the original MD3 immunoglobulin-transgenic line and a different line of metallothionein/lysozyme-transgenic mice, ML3. The failure of tolerance and IgM down-regulation in MD3 × ML3 double-transgenic mice was shown to be related to a tenfold-lower concentration of lysozyme expressed in ML3 mice compared with ML5 mice, and a consequent tenfold decrease in receptor occupancy on the B cell (C.C. Goodnow et al., in prep.). When MD3 × ML3 low-

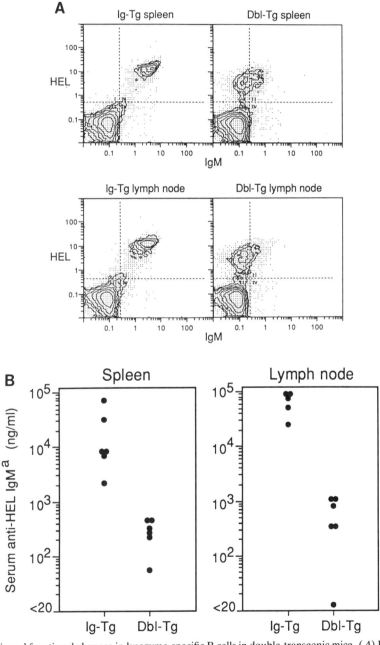

Figure 7. Phenotypic and functional changes in lysozyme-specific B cells in double-transgenic mice. (*A*) Expression of membrane IgM on lysozyme-binding B cells from spleen or lymph node of immunoglobulin-transgenic and double-transgenic mice. (*B*) Antilysozyme antibody responses in adoptive transfer recipients of spleen or lymph node cells from immunoglobulin-transgenic or double-transgenic mice, assayed 7 days after transfer and challenge with lysozyme coupled to HRBC.

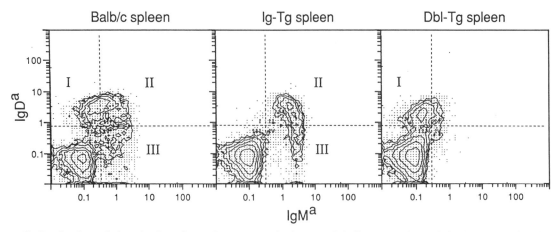

Figure 8. B-cell subpopulations in the spleen of nontransgenic, immunoglobulin-transgenic, and double-transgenic mice, as defined by expression of IgD and IgM. Population I: IgD^{high}, IgM^{low}. Population II: IgD^{high}, IgM^{high}. Population III: IgD^{low}, IgM^{high}.

lysozyme double-transgenic mice were given zinc in the drinking water, the serum lysozyme concentration was increased 50- to 100-fold, and both tolerance and IgM down-regulation were rapidly induced in previously nontolerant peripheral B cells. The same finding, namely rapid induction of tolerance and receptor down-regulation in mature peripheral B cells, was observed after transferring spleen cells from immuno-globulin-transgenic mice into irradiated ML5 (high-lysozyme) recipients.

DISCUSSION

The susceptibility of mature B cells to clonal silencing in this transgenic model is perhaps not surprising since it has been reproducibly found that mature B cells and memory B cells can be rendered unresponsive in vivo by exposure to haptens, serum proteins, and poly-saccharides (Katz et al. 1972; Howard and Mitchison 1975; Desaymard and Waldmann 1976; Metcalf et al. 1979; Scott et al. 1979; Parks et al. 1982; Nossal 1983). The results from the double-transgenic model would tend to support the concept that mature B cells are indeed rendered tolerant by encounter with autologous antigen or tolerogen and are not simply triggered into exhaustive differentiation. As discussed above, somatic hypermutation of immunoglobulin genes in mature B cells results in the generation of a "second wave" of potentially self-reactive B cells (Diamond and Scharff 1984; Radic et al., this volume). Consequently, a mechanism of tolerance that is capable of silencing B cells at multiple stages of development may be a necessary defense against the development of high-affinity, pathogenic autoantibodies.

The fact that self-reactive B cells persist despite their functionally silenced state is curious. Under normal conditions their persistence may be short-lived because of competition with nonself-reactive B cells for "space" in the peripheral lymphoid tissue. On the other hand, the existence of significant numbers of B cells in normal

mice with an identical phenotype to the silenced double-transgenic B cells (Fig. 8) speaks against this conclusion and in favor of a relatively long life span. One possible advantage of a persisting pool of self-reactive B cells is that they could serve as a substrate for hypermutation since hypermutation could generate nonself-reactive variants from initially self-reactive clones (Schwartz 1986).

ACKNOWLEDGMENTS

We thank Dr. S. Tilghman for the gift of the mouse albumin promoter and Dr. P. Lalor for conjugated antibodies to B-cell differentiation antigens. We also thank Tracy Anderson and Pat Gregory for technical assistance and Andrew Cheung for animal husbandry. C.C.G. was supported by a Medical Postdoctoral Fellowship from the Medical Foundation, University of Sydney.

REFERENCES

Benjamin, D.C., J.A. Berzofsky, I.J. East, F.R.N. Gurd, C. Hannum, S.J. Leach, E. Margoliash, J.G. Michael, A. Miller, E.M. Prager, M. Reichlin, E.E. Sercarz, S.J. Smith-Gill, P.E. Todd, and A.C. Wilson. 1984. The antigenic structure of proteins: A reappraisal. *Annu. Rev. Immunol.* **2:** 67.

Berek, C. and C. Milstein. 1988. The dynamic nature of the antibody repertoire. *Immunol. Rev.* **105:** 5.

Boyd, A.W. and J.W. Schrader. 1981. The regulation of growth and differentiation of a murine B cell lymphoma. II. The inhibition of WEHI 231 by anti-immunoglobulin antibodies. *J. Immunol.* **126:** 2466.

Chan, E.K.L. and E.M. Tan. 1987. Human autoantibody-reactive epitopes of SSB/La are highly conserved in comparison with epitopes recognized by murine monoclonal antibodies. *J. Exp. Med.* **166:** 1627.

Chien, Y.-H., N.R.J. Gascoigne, J. Kavaler, N.E. Lee, and M.M. Davis. 1984. Somatic recombination in a murine T-cell receptor gene. *Nature* **309:** 322.

Chiller, J.M., G.S. Habicht, and W.O. Weigle. 1971. Kinetic

differences in unresponsiveness of thymus and bone marrow cells. *Science* **171**: 813.

Cohen, I. 1986. Regulation of autoimmune disease physiological and therapeutic. *Immunol. Rev.* **94**: 5.

DeFranco, A.L., M.M. Davis, and W.E. Paul. 1982. WEHI-231 as a tumor model for tolerance induction in immature B lymphocytes. In *B and T cell tumours* (ed. E.S. Vitetta), p. 445. Academic Press, New York.

Desaymard, C. and H. Waldmann. 1976. Evidence for the inactivation of precursor B cells in high dose unresponsiveness. *Nature* **264**: 780.

Diamond, B. and M.D. Scharff. 1984. Somatic mutation of the T15 heavy chain gives rise to an antibody with autoantibody specificity. *Proc. Natl. Acad. Sci.* **81**: 5841.

Ehrlich, P. 1900. On immunity with special reference to cell life. *Proc. R. Soc. Lond. B. Biol. Sci.* **66**: 424.

Fink, P.J., L.A. Matis, D.L. McElligott, M. Bookman, and S.M. Hedrick. 1986. Correlations between T-cell specificity and the structure of the antigen receptor. *Nature* **321**: 219.

French, D.L., R. Laskov, and M.D. Scharff. 1989. The role of somatic hypermutation in the generation of antibody diversity. *Science* **244**: 1152.

Gammon, G., N. Shastri, J. Cogswell, S. Wilbur, S. Sadegh-Nasseri, U. Krzych, A. Miller, and E. Sercarz. 1987. The choice of T-cell epitopes utilized on a protein antigen depends on multiple factors distant from, as well as at the determinant site. *Immunol. Rev.* **98**: 53.

Gause, A., N. Yoshida, C. Kappen, and K. Rajewsky. 1987. In vivo generation and function of B cells in the presence of a monoclonal anti-IgM antibody: Implications for B cell tolerance. *Eur. J. Immunol.* **17**: 981.

Goodnow, C.C., J. Crosbie, S. Adelstein, T.B. Lavoie, S.J. Smith-Gill, R.A. Brink, H. Pritchard-Briscoe, J.S. Wotherspoon, R.H. Loblay, K. Raphael, R.J. Trent, and A. Basten. 1988. Altered immunoglobulin expression and functional silencing of self-reactive B lymphocytes in transgenic mice. *Nature* **334**: 676.

Hardy, R.R., K. Hayakawa, D.R. Parks, and L.A. Herzenberg. 1983. Demonstration of B cell maturation in X-linked immunodeficient mice by simultaneous three-colour immunofluorescence. *Nature* **306**: 270.

Harley, J.B., M.O. Rosario, H. Yamagata, O.F. Fox, and E. Koren. 1985. Immunologic and structural studies of the lupus/Sjögren's syndrome autoantigen, La/SSB, with a monoclonal antibody. *J. Clin. Invest.* **76**: 801.

Harris, D.E., L. Cairns, F.S. Rosen, and Y. Borel. 1982. A natural model of immunologic tolerance. Tolerance to murine C5 is mediated by T cells, and antigen is required to maintain unresponsiveness. *J. Exp. Med.* **156**: 567.

Holmberg, D., A.A. Freitas, D. Portnoï, F. Jacquemart, S. Avrameas, and A. Coutinho. 1986. Antibody repertoires of normal BALB/c mice: B lymphocyte populations defined by state of activation. *Immunol. Rev.* **93**: 147.

Howard, J.G. and N.A. Mitchison. 1975. Immunological tolerance. *Prog. Allergy* **18**: 43.

Ikuta, K., T. Ogura, A. Shimizu, and T. Honjo. 1985. Low frequency of somatic mutation in β-chain variable region genes of human T-cell receptors. *Proc. Natl. Acad. Sci.* **82**: 7701.

Iverson, G.M. and J. Lindenmann. 1972. The role of a carrier determinant and T cells in the induction of liver-specific autoantibodies in the mouse. *Eur. J. Immunol.* **2**: 195.

Kappler, J.W., N. Roehm, and P. Marrack. 1987. T cell tolerance by clonal elimination in the thymus. *Cell* **49**: 273.

Kappler, J.W., U. Staerz, J. White, and P. Marrack. 1988. Self-tolerance eliminates T cells specific for Mls-modified products of the major histocompatibility complex. *Nature* **332**: 35.

Katz, D.H., T. Hamaoka, and B. Benacerraf. 1972. Immunological tolerance in bone marrow-derived lymphocytes. *J. Exp. Med.* **136**: 1404.

Kisielow, P., H. Blüthmann, U.D. Staerz, M. Steinmetz, and

H. von Boehmer. 1988. Tolerance in T-cell-receptor transgenic mice involves deletion of nonmature CD4$^+$8$^+$ thymocytes. *Nature* **333**: 742.

Klaus, G.G.B. 1979. Irreversible receptor modulation on B lymphocytes and the control of antibody-forming cells by antigen. *Immunol. Rev.* **43**: 97.

Lane, D.P. and D.M. Silver. 1976. Isolation of a murine liver-specific alloantigen, F antigen, and examination of its immunogenic properties by radioimmunoassay. *Eur. J. Immunol.* **6**: 480.

Lanzavecchia, A. 1985. Antigen-specific interaction between T and B cells. *Nature* **314**: 537.

Lawton, A.R. and M.D. Cooper. 1974. Modification of B lymphocyte differentiation by anti-immunoglobulins. *Contemp. Top. Immunobiol.* **3**: 193.

Lederberg, J. 1959. Genes and antibodies. *Science* **129**: 1649.

MacDonald, H.R., R. Schneider, R.K. Lees, R.C. Howe, H. Acha-Orbea, H. Festenstein, R.M. Zinkernagel, and H. Hengartner. 1988. T-cell receptor V$_\beta$ use predicts reactivity and tolerance to Mls^a-encoded antigens. *Nature* **332**: 40.

Matthias, P.D., R. Renkawitz, M. Grez, and G. Schütz. 1982. Transient expression of the chicken lysozyme gene after transfer into human cells. *EMBO J.* **1**: 1207.

Metcalf, E.S., A.F. Schrater, and N.R. Klinman. 1979. Murine models of tolerance induction in developing and mature B cells. *Immunol. Rev.* **43**: 143.

Mitchell, G.F. and J.F.A.P. Miller. 1968. Cell to cell interaction in the immune response. II. The source of hemolysin-forming cells in irradiated mice given bone marrow and thymus or thoractic duct lymphocytes. *J. Exp. Med.* **128**: 821.

Mitchison, N.A. 1971. The carrier effect in the secondary responses to hapten-protein conjugates. II. Cellular cooperation. *Eur. J. Immunol.* **1**: 18.

Naysmith, J.D., M.G. Ortega-Pierres, and C.J. Elson. 1981. Rat erythrocyte-induced anti-erythrocyte autoantibody production and control in normal mice. *Immunol. Rev.* **55**: 55.

Nemazee, D.A. and K. Bürki. 1989. Clonal deletion of B lymphocytes in a transgenic mouse bearing anti-MHC class I antibody genes. *Nature* **337**: 562.

Nemazee, D.A. and V.L. Sato. 1983. Induction of rheumatoid antibodies in the mouse. *J. Exp. Med.* **158**: 529.

Neuberger, M.S., H.M. Caskey, S. Pettersson, G.T. Williams, and M.A. Surani. 1989. Isotype exclusion and transgene down-regulation in immunoglobulin-λ transgenic mice. *Nature* **338**: 350.

Nossal, G.J.V. 1983. Cellular mechanisms of immunologic tolerance. *Annu. Rev. Immunol.* **1**: 33.

Nossal, G.J.V., B.L. Pike, J.M. Teale, J.E. Layton, T.W. Kay, and F.L. Battye. 1979. Cell fractionation methods and the target cells for clonal abortion of B lymphocytes. *Immunol. Rev.* **43**: 185.

Ogata, K., Y. Ogata, Y. Takasaki, and E.M. Tan. 1987. Epitopes on proliferating cell nuclear antigen recognized by human lupus autoantibody and murine monoclonal antibody. *J. Immunol.* **139**: 2942.

Osserman, E.F., R.E. Canfield, and S. Beychok. 1974. *Lysozyme.* Academic Press, New York.

Padlan, E.A., E.W. Silverton, S. Sheriff, G.H. Cohen, S.J. Smith-Gill, and D.R. Davies. 1989. Structure of an antibody-antigen complex: Crystal structure of the HyHEL-10 Fab-lysozyme complex. *Proc. Natl. Acad. Sci.* (in press).

Palmiter, R.D. and R.L. Brinster. 1986. Germline transformation of mice. *Annu. Rev. Genet.* **20**: 465.

Palmiter, R.D., H.Y. Chen, and R.L. Brinster. 1982. Differential regulation of metallothionein-thymidine kinase fusion genes in transgenic mice and their offspring. *Cell* **29**: 701.

Parks, D.E., P.A. Nelson, S.M. Walker, and W.O. Weigle. 1982. Immunological unresponsiveness in primed B lymphocytes. *Ann. N.Y. Acad. Sci.* **392**: 210.

Pennell, C.A. and D.W. Scott. 1986. Lymphoma models for B

cell activation and tolerance. IV. Growth inhibition by anti-Ig of CH31 and CH33 B lymphoma cells. *Eur. J. Immunol.* **16:** 1577.

Pettersson, S., M.J. Sharpe, D.R. Gilmore, M.A. Surani, and M.S. Neuberger. 1989. Cellular selection leads to age-dependent and reversible downregulation of transgenic immunoglobulin light chain genes. *Int. Immunol.* (in press).

Pierres, M., C. Devaux, M. Dosseto, and S. Marchetto. 1981. Clonal analysis of B- and T-cell responses to Ia antigens. I. Topology of epitope regions on I-A^k and I-E^k molecules analyzed with 35 monoclonal alloantibodies. *Immunogenetics* **14:** 481.

Pinkert, C.A., D.M. Ornitz, R.L. Brinster, and R.D. Palmiter. 1987. An albumin enhancer located 10 kb upstream functions along with its promoter to direct efficient, liver-specific expression in transgenic mice. *Genes Dev.* **1:** 268.

Primi, D., L. Hammarström, C.I.E. Smith, and G. Moller. 1977. Characterization of self-reactive B cells by polyclonal B-cell activators. *J. Exp. Med.* **145:** 21.

Pullen, A.M., P. Marrack, and J.W. Kappler. 1988. The T-cell repertoire is heavily influenced by tolerance to polymorphic self-antigens. *Nature* **335:** 796.

Raff, M.C., J.J.T. Owen, M.D. Cooper, A.R. Lawton, M. Megson, and W.E. Gathings. 1975. Differences in susceptibility of mature and immature mouse B lymphocytes to anti-immunoglobulin-induced immunoglobulin suppression in vitro. *J. Exp. Med.* **142:** 1052.

Rajewsky, K. and C. Brenig. 1974. Paralysis to serum albumins in T and B lymphocytes in mice. Dose dependence, specificity, and kinetics of escape. *Eur. J. Immunol.* **4:** 120.

Reichlin, M. 1972. Localizing antigenic determinants in human haemoglobin with mutants: Molecular correlations of immunological tolerance. *J. Mol. Biol.* **64:** 485.

Ritchie, K.A., R.L. Brinster, and U. Storb. 1984. Allelic exclusion and control of endogenous immunoglobulin gene rearrangement in κ transgenic mice. *Nature* **312:** 517.

Ruoslahti, E., H. Pihko, M. Becker, and O. Mäkelä. 1975. Rabbit alpha-fetoprotein: Normal levels and breakage of tolerance with haptenated homologous alpha-fetoprotein. *Eur. J. Immunol.* **5:** 7.

Schwartz, R.S. 1986. Autoantibodies and normal antibodies. In *Progress in immunology* (ed. B. Cinader and R.G. Miller), vol. 6, p. 478. Academic Press, New York.

Scott, D.W., M. Venkataraman, and J.J. Jandinski. 1979. Multiple pathways of B lymphocyte tolerance. *Immunol. Rev.* **43:** 241.

Sha, W.C., C.A. Nelson, R.D. Newberry, D.M. Kranz, J.H. Russell, and D.Y. Loh. 1988. Positive and negative selection of an antigen receptor on T cells in transgenic mice. *Nature* **336:** 73.

Sidman, C.L. and E.R. Unanue. 1985. Receptor-mediated inactivation of early B lymphocytes. *Nature* **257:** 149.

Siskind, G.W. and B. Benacerraf. 1969. Cell selection by antigen in the immune response. *Adv. Immunol.* **10:** 1.

Smith, C.A., G.T. Williams, R. Kingston, E.J. Jenkinson, and J.J.T. Owen. 1989. Antibodies to CD3/T-cell receptor complex induce death by apoptosis in immature T cells in thymic cultures. *Nature* **337:** 181.

Smith-Gill, S.J. and E.E. Sercarz. 1989. *The immune response to structurally defined proteins: The lysozyme model.* Adenine Press, New York.

Smith-Gill, S.J., T.B. Lavoie, and C.R. Mainhart. 1984. Antigenic regions defined by monoclonal antibodies correspond to structural domains of avian lysozyme. *J. Immunol.* **133:** 384.

Smith-Gill, S.J., P.A. Hamel, T.B. Lavoie, and K.J. Dorrington. 1987. Contributions of immunoglobulin heavy and light chains to antibody specificity for lysozyme and two haptens. *J. Immunol.* **139:** 4135.

Stamatoyannopoulos, G., M. Farquhar, D. Lindsley, M. Brice, T. Papayannopoulou, and P.E. Nute. 1983. Monoclonal antibodies specific for globin chains. *Blood* **61:** 530.

Storb, U., C. Pinkert, B. Arp, P. Engler, K. Gollahon, J. Manz, W. Brady, and R.L. Brinster. 1986. Transgenic mice with μ and κ genes encoding antiphosphorylcholine antibodies. *J. Exp. Med.* **164:** 627.

Tan, E.M. 1989. Antinuclear antibodies: Diagnostic markers for autoimmune diseases and probes for cell biology. *Adv. Immunol.* **44:** 93.

Teh, H.S., P. Kisielow, B. Scott, H. Kishi, Y. Uematsu, H. Blüthmann, and H. von Boehmer. 1988. Thymic major histocompatibility complex antigens and the αβ T-cell receptor determine the CD4/CD8 phenotype of T cells. *Nature* **335:** 229.

Ternynck, T. and S. Avrameas. 1986. Murine natural monoclonal autoantibodies: A study of their polyspecificities and their affinities. *Immunol. Rev.* **94:** 99.

Tilghman, S.M. and A. Belayew. 1982. Transcriptional control of the murine albumin/α-fetoprotein locus during development. *Proc. Natl. Acad. Sci.* **79:** 5254.

Urbanski, G.J. and E. Margoliash. 1977. Topographic determinants on cytochrome c. *J. Immunol.* **118:** 1170.

Weaver, D., F. Costantini, T. Imanishi-Kari, and D. Baltimore. 1985. A transgenic immunoglobulin mu gene prevents rearrangement of endogenous genes. *Cell* **42:** 117.

Weigle, W.O. 1973. Immunological unresponsiveness. *Adv. Immunol.* **16:** 61.

Yuan, D. 1984. Regulation of IgM and IgD synthesis in B lymphocytes. II. Translation and post-translational events. *J. Immunol.* **132:** 1566.

Impact of Somatic Mutation on the S107(T15) Heavy-chain V Region of Antibodies Reactive with Self and Nonself

S.M. Behar,* N.C. Chien,* S. Corbet,* B. Diamond,* E.D. Getzoff,†
D. Lustgarten,* V.A. Roberts,† M.D. Scharff,* and S.-U. Shin*
*Department of Cell Biology, Albert Einstein College of Medicine, Bronx, New York 10461; †Department
of Molecular Biology, Research Institute of Scripps Clinic, La Jolla, California 92037

In recent years, we have learned a great deal about how individual B cells use multiple germ-line genetic elements to create a very large repertoire of heavy- (H) and light- (L) chain variable (V) regions each with a unique amino acid sequence (Tonegawa 1983). On the basis of the number of different germ-line V, (diversity) D, and (joining) J region genes for the H chain and V and J region genes for the L chain, the potential for junctional diversity, the introduction of additional sequences during the joining of these elements, and the association of different H and L chains, it has been estimated that at least 10^8 to 10^{10} different antibody molecules can be generated in a single individual (Tonegawa 1983). Even this enormous sequence diversity is apparently not sufficient to provide us with the high-affinity antibodies we need to protect us from agents such as toxins and viruses, which bind with relatively high affinity to target cells. To make large amounts of high-affinity antibodies to compete with target-cell receptors, B cells expressing low-affinity germ-line-encoded immunoglobulin M (IgM) antibodies on their surface are stimulated by antigen and T cells to differentiate and proliferate, undergo somatic diversification and affinity maturation of their V region sequences, and switch from making IgM to secreting IgG (French et al. 1989).

A great deal is known about the cellular and molecular events involved in creating the V region repertoire (Tonegawa 1983; Yancopoulos and Alt 1986) and in class and subclass switching (Cebra et al. 1984; Shimizu and Honjo 1984). In contrast, the mechanisms responsible for the somatic diversification of already rearranged and expressed V regions are less well understood (French et al. 1989; Kocks and Rajewsky 1989). Through the analysis of the sequences of many monoclonal antibodies generated at different times in the immune response, it has been concluded that base changes are introduced into rearranged H- and L-chain V regions at a rate of approximately 10^{-3} to 10^{-4} bp/generation (Clarke et al. 1985; Sablitzky et al. 1985; Berek and Milstein 1987; Manser et al. 1987b). It appears that these base changes occur in a somewhat random fashion although hot spots have been observed previously (Allen et al. 1987; Berek and Milstein 1987, 1988; Blier and Bothwell 1988). The instability of the V region is restricted to the coding sequence and its immediate flanking sequences and probably occurs during a brief period of B-cell differentiation (Berek and Milstein 1987, 1988; Rajewsky et al. 1987). Although the exact mechanisms responsible for V region diversification in mouse and man are unknown, three general mechanisms have received serious consideration: (1) gene conversion (Baltimore 1981), which has been shown to create the V region repertoire in chicken L chains (Reynaud et al. 1987; Thompson and Neiman 1987) and may be responsible for some of the somatic diversification in the mouse (Dildrop et al. 1982; Kocks and Rajewsky 1989); (2) V region replacement in which an upstream V region can replace the expressed V region (Kleinfield et al. 1986; Reth et al. 1986; Kleinfield and Weigert 1989), which has occurred in cultured mouse cells creating diversity in the progeny of a single B-cell clone but has not been proven to occur in vivo; and (3) somatic point mutation. Since Weigert et al. (1970) first reported multiple single amino acid substitutions in different λ-light chains and it was shown that these λ chains were encoded by a single germ-line V region gene (Bernard et al. 1978), somatic point mutation has been considered the most likely mechanism to explain most of the diversity that is generated during B-cell differentiation in the mouse (Tonegawa et al. 1983; Rajewsky et al. 1987; French et al. 1989).

Whatever the underlying mechanism, it is clear that at an early stage in B-cell differentiation, the germ-line V region genes accumulate large numbers of base changes. Subsequently, presumably under the influence of antigen and T cells, those B cells expressing the highest-affinity antibody on their surface are selectively stimulated to proliferate and differentiate (Wysocki et al. 1986; Allen et al. 1987; Berek and Milstein 1987). This explanation of affinity mutation is supported by the work of Berek and Milstein (1987, 1988) and Rajewsky and his colleagues (Allen et al. 1987; Kocks and Rajewsky 1988), who have shown that single amino acid substitutions can result in two- to tenfold increases in affinity although it remains unclear how antigen and T cells can selectively stimulate the proliferation of B cells that express immunoglobulin receptors with only a two- to threefold increase in affinity.

If somatic mutation is a relatively random event, then we would expect that during the course of B-cell differentiation many subclones would also be created that have lost the ability to synthesize the immunoglobulin because of the introduction of nonsense mutations in the coding sequences or mutations in promoters or enhancers or can no longer bind the eliciting antigen because of the introduction of mutations that change the configuration of the antigen-binding site or interfere with the correct assembly of the immunoglobulin molecule. It is also likely that, during the course of random somatic mutation, a particular B-cell clone would generate antibodies that had acquired new specificities including reactivity with self-antigens. In fact, B cells with either nonsense mutations or loss of antigen binding are only rarely recovered in the course of making monoclonal antibodies (Manser et al. 1987a; Kocks and Rajewsky 1989). Although this would be expected if hybridomas were identified only on the basis of the inability to bind antigen, deliberate attempts to identify all products of somatic hypermutation by screening hybridomas for mRNA containing the relevant V region have only revealed a few examples of such "degenerate" B cells (Manser et al. 1987a).

In an attempt to examine the molecular mechanisms and impact of somatic mutation, we have focused on the diversification of the H-chain V regions encoded by the S107 H-chain V region family. We have examined mutant antibodies that arose during the immune response to phosphorylcholine (PC) in vivo and were generated in vitro by the S107 cell line. In addition, we have studied autoantibodies created by the S107 family in autoimmune mice. These studies indicate that the dominant mechanism for generating diversity in this V region family both in vivo and in vitro is somatic point mutation. Antibodies that have lost the ability to bind antigen arose frequently and spontaneously in vitro, and the analysis of these mutant antibodies provides interesting insights into the structure of the antigen-binding site. Finally, we have shown that point mutations can convert the protective S107 antibody into a potentially pathogenic autoantibody and that members of this V region family play an important role in autoimmune mice both in the response to environmental antigens and in the generation of autoantibodies. Highlights of these studies will be summarized below.

METHODS

The methods used in most of the experiments presented below were described previously (Giusti et al. 1987; Behar and Scharff 1988; Chien et al. 1988). We have not described previously our attempts to clone the U10 donor fragment. In these experiments, a genomic DNA library was constructed using the EMBL3 vector and BALB/c liver DNA that had been partially digested with MboI. The library was screened using the MS-9 oligonucleotide (sequence: CCCCAGACAG-CGAAGTACC), which had been end-labeled with [γ-^{32}P]ATP using polynucleotide kinase. Hybridization

was done as described previously (Zeff et al. 1986) at a temperature of 55°C, which is 7°C below the T_m. A piece of DNA was cloned that contained a 4.8-kb BamHI fragment to which MS-9 hybridizes. This fragment is the same size as the fragment identified by Southern blot analysis of liver DNA.

RESULTS

Somatic Point Mutation Is Responsible for the Diversification of the S107 V_H Gene In Vivo

The nature and distribution of the base changes that are introduced into the rearranged V regions during B-cell differentiation suggest that some form of somatic point mutation is responsible (Berek and Milstein 1988; French et al. 1989; Kocks and Rajewsky 1989). However, there continues to be controversy about the mechanisms underlying somatic diversification in mouse and man because of the frequent appearance of two or even three base changes in a single or neighboring codons (Allen et al. 1987; Berek and Milstein 1987; Claflin et al. 1987; Malipiero et al. 1987; Manser et al. 1987b), insufficient information about the true number and sequence of germ-line V region genes (Livant et al. 1986), and the occurrence of V region replacement in vitro (Kleinfield and Weigert 1989) and perhaps of gene conversion in cultured mouse cells (Dildrop et al. 1982). We have attempted to examine the mechanism of somatic diversification in vivo by making oligonucleotides that specifically hybridize to clustered base changes in antibodies that have arisen in the S107 V_H1 early and late in the immune response to PC-keyhole limpet hemocyanin (KLH).

The sequence of the H-chain V region of the P28 IgM antibody that arose early in the immune response to PC-KLH is shown in Figure 1. There are three single-base changes in the P28 V region as compared with the germ-line (S107) sequence. Two of these are A-T changes and are within and just adjoining HV2, the second complementarity-determining region in P28 (Fig. 1). The A-T change in the third codon after HV2 results in the substitution of a phenylalanine for an isoleucine causing a slight change in the relative binding of analogs of PC and loss of reactivity with a monoclonal antiidiotype antibody (Chien et al. 1988). None of these single-base changes are present in the other germ-line genes of the S107 V_H gene family (Crews et al. 1981) or in other V_H1-encoded monoclonal antibodies that have been sequenced (Perlmutter et al. 1984; Malipiero et al. 1987). Oligonucleotides that recognize either both of the A-T base changes or each individually (see Fig. 1) were used to probe the DNA from BALB/c liver and from the P28 hybridoma expressing the mutations. Southern analysis using one of these oligonucleotides is shown in Figure 2. Since digestion with a single restriction enzyme could result in fragments that might be lost to analysis, liver DNA was also digested with a variety of restriction enzymes and hybridized to the oligonucleotides. No cross-hybridizing

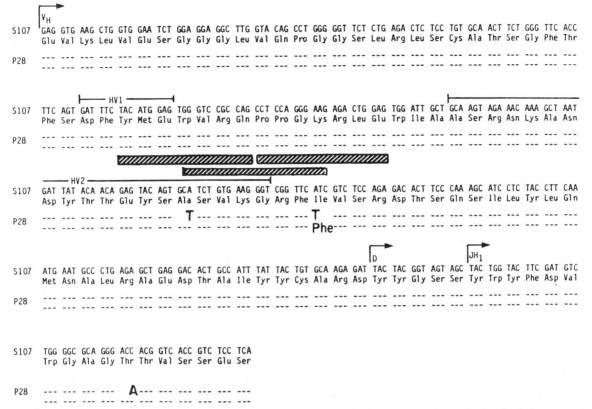

Figure 1. The nucleotide sequence and translated amino acid sequence of the VDJ of the P28 IgM anti-PC antibody is compared with the germ-line V_H1 DFL16.1 J_H1 represented by S107. Dashed lines represent identity. The cross-hatched boxes are the oligonucleotides that were used to look for potential donor sequences. Sequencing was done directly from mRNA as described previously (Chien et al. 1988).

fragments were detected (Chien et al. 1988). These results suggested that no other germ-line V_H gene could have encoded these changes either directly or by V region replacement. Furthermore, we could not detect a potential donor sequence for gene conversion although we could not rule out a donor sequence with less than a 19-bp homology with V_H1. Similar examination of other antibodies from later in the immune response (Chien et al. 1988) and from autoimmune animals (Behar 1989) suggests that, at least in the mouse, somatic point mutation is a major mechanism for the generation of the sequence diversity that arises in antibodies after the formation and expression of mature V regions.

Role of Somatic Mutation in Generating Antibodies That Had Lost Antigen Binding In Vitro

To study the detailed mechanisms underlying the somatic instability of immunoglobulin V regions and to recover all of the products of this process in the absence of selection by antigen, we and other investigators have tried to establish tissue cell culture systems that would mimic the events that occur in vivo (Morrison and Scharff 1981; French et al. 1989). In our studies, we have used the S107 mouse myeloma cell line, which

secretes an IgA anti-PC antibody whose sequence is identical to that of the germ-line V_H1 DFL.16.1 J_H1 H chain and V_K22 J_K5 L chain that dominate the early response to PC-KLH. Although current theories suggest that highly differentiated plasma cells have turned off their somatic mutational process (Berek and Milstein 1988; Kocks and Rajewsky 1989), our early studies with this plasmacytoma cell line revealed V region mutants arising at a spontaneous frequency of 0.1–.01% (Cook and Scharff 1977). Although S107 no longer generates such V region mutants, two mutants that we initially isolated and subsequently characterized have provided important insights on the impact of somatic point mutation.

U10 Mutant

The U10 mutant arose from the S107 cell line through a primary mutation of the rearranged and expressed S107 V_H1 gene (Shin 1987). It had lost the ability to bind PC but was indistinguishable from the parental S107 antibody in the size of its H and L chains and its covalent and noncovalent assembly. Detailed serological analysis of the U10 mutant revealed a complete loss of PC binding and an inability to bind monoclonal and polyclonal antiidiotypic antibinding-site antibodies suggesting local structural changes in the

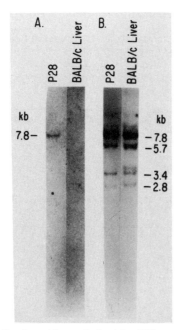

Figure 2. Southern blot analysis with a P28-specific oligonucleotide. The oligonucleotide shown in Fig. 1 that includes the two A-T substitutions was hybridized to DNA from the P28 hybridoma and BALB/c liver. The DNA was digested with *Eco*RI and was hybridized under stringent conditions with the P28-specific oligonucleotide (*A*). The blot was stripped and rehybridized with a V_H1 genomic probe that hybridizes strongly to the S107 V_H1 (7.8 kb) and V_H11 (5.7 kb) and more weakly to the V_H3 (3.4 kb) and V_H13 (2.8 kb) members of the S107 V_H family (*B*). *B* shows that similar amounts of V_H1 were present in both lanes of *A*.

base change resulting in an aspartic acid to alanine substitution at the fifth residue in J_H1 (Fig. 3) (residue 101 based on the Kabat numbering system [Kabat et al. 1987]). No other base changes were found in the H-chain V region, in the adjoining C_H1 domain, or in L-chain V or C region (Chien et al. 1989).

To examine the three-dimensional structure of the binding site of U10, we referred to the McPC603 PC-binding antibody, which uses the same H-chain V, D, and J elements as S107. The three-dimensional structure of McPC603 has been determined with PC or SO_4 in the binding site (Bernstein et al. 1977; Satow et al. 1986). We constructed a model for the S107 V region from the McPC603 structure by appropriate substitutions and one insertion (Chien et al. 1989). In both the McPC603 crystal structure and the S107 model, Asp-101 is distant (11.8 Å) from the PC-binding site and on the outer surface of the molecule (Fig. 4, top). It was therefore surprising that a single substitution at this location would result in the complete loss of antigen binding. However, in McPC603 and our model of S107, the disruption of the interactions between Asp-101 and Arg-94, whose side chain is also extended away from the PC-binding site (Fig. 4, top), could allow the arginine side chain to extend into the negatively charged pocket that in the wild-type molecule binds the trimethylammonium group of choline in PC (Figure 4, middle and bottom). This positioning of the Arg-94 side chain would disrupt the conformation of the binding site and allow Glu-35, which is very important in PC-binding (see below; Davies and Metzger 1983; Giusti et al. 1987), to form a salt bridge with the Arg-94 side chain, preventing it from interacting with PC (Fig. 4, middle). This hypothesis was tested by examining the energetics of models of U10 with the Arg-94 side chain both inside and outside of the binding site as illustrated in Figure 4. The model with the arginine side chain in the binding site is energetically feasible and explains the complete loss of PC binding with little overall conformational change (Chien et al. 1989).

antigen-binding site. Antiidiotypic antibodies that react with epitopes formed by framework residues or by the interaction of H and L chains did not distinguish between the parental and mutant antibodies suggesting that the mutation had not caused a global disruption of the structure of the V region (Chien et al. 1989). Nucleic acid sequence analysis revealed a single A-C

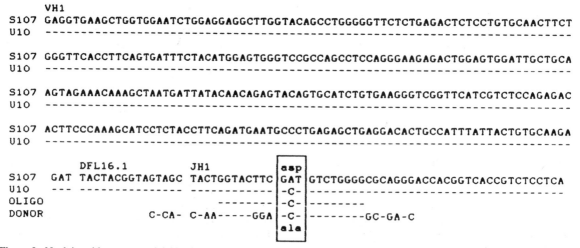

Figure 3. Nucleic acid sequence of the U10 H-chain V region. The location of the A-C substitution is identified by the box. The sequences of the U10-mutant-specific oligonucleotide and the cloned "putative donor" sequences are shown.

These results indicate that amino acid substitutions that are distant from the antigen-binding site can have a dramatic effect on the specificity and affinity of antigen binding. Since such changes must occur frequently and are in fact found in other J_H1-encoded antibodies (Gough and Bernard 1981; Clarke et al. 1985), we imagine that somatic hypermutation frequently generates antibodies like U10 with profound changes in affinity and specificity. Since we were unable to detect binding of U10 to a variety of other antigens, we do not know whether U10-like events represent wastage or useful diversification of the S107-binding site so that it will bind other antigens and increase the antibody repertoire.

We were also interested in whether the single-base change in J_H1 that gave rise to U10 was the result of somatic mutation. We therefore probed liver, S107, and U10 DNA with a U10 mutant-specific oligonucleotide (Fig. 5, left). The mutant gene was identified as a 1.2-kb BamHI fragment (Fig. 5, left). In addition, a novel 4.8-kb fragment hybridized to the mutant but not to the wild-type oligonucleotide (Fig. 5, left). Since this fragment persisted in U10, it could contain a sequence that had donated the U10 mutant sequence in some nonreciprocal fashion. Although we were concerned that the cross-hybridization might be an artifact because the 4.8-kb fragment hybridized better than the mutant gene itself (Fig. 5), we proceeded to clone and sequence the 4.8-kb fragment. The fragment contained a few similar but not identical sequences that were homologous to the oligonucleotide and to U10 at their 5' and 3' ends but which were not identical to J_H1 or to the U10 mutant. Using the mutant oligonucleotide as a primer for sequencing, we were able to identify the sequence that was most homologous to the mutant-specific oligonucleotide. As can be seen in Figure 3, this sequence has a 3-bp mismatch (GGA instead of TTC) adjacent to the mutant C replacement in the U10 oligonucleotide. We concluded that the cross-hybridization was artifactual, probably because of the GC-rich nature of the ends of the probe and of the presence of multiple weakly cross-hybridizing sequences adjacent to each other in this stretch of DNA. Since we could not identify any other potential donor sequence, we concluded that U10 had arisen through somatic hypermutation of the S107 gene in culture. This study shows the importance of sequencing putative donor sequences before suggesting that gene conversion has occurred.

U4 Mutant

Although the U10 mutation did not reveal whether somatic mutation could generate new antibody specificities, U4, a second spontaneous V region mutant of S107, was more informative in this regard. Like U10, U4 was identified as a primary mutant of the S107 cell line that had lost the ability to bind PC but was otherwise indistinguishable from the parent. The U4 H-chain V region contained single A-C transversion in the first CDR that resulted in the substitution of an alanine for glutamic acid at residue 35. The L chain was identical to the parent (Giusti et al. 1987). As already noted, Glu-35 is critical for PC binding and is found in almost all PC-binding antibodies. The three-dimensional structure of McPC603 and the model of S107 presented in Figure 4 suggest that Glu-35 interacts with the choline moiety of PC (Satow et al. 1986). The loss of PC binding in U4 confirms the predictions from statistical (Kabat et al. 1976) and three-dimensional analysis (Davies and Metzger 1983). As with the previous mutants, we were unable to find any donor sequence or other T15 V regions containing the U4 sequence, and we concluded that it had also arisen through somatic mutation (Giusti et al. 1987).

Since the sequence of a DNA-binding antibody from an $(NZB \times NZW)F_1$ mouse was homologous to S107 but had a serine instead of a glutamic acid at residue 35 (Eilat et al. 1984), we examined the U4 protein for its ability to bind to double-stranded (ds)DNA (Table 1). The S107 parental protein did not bind DNA, phosphorylated proteins, or the phospholipid cardiolipin. U4 has not only lost the ability to bind PC but has acquired binding for dsDNA, phosphorylated protamine, and cardiolipin (Diamond and Scharff 1984). Since the glutamic acid substitution in U4 affects the binding of the choline part of PC, we assume that the change in the binding site allows continued interaction with the phosphate but now in the context of DNA, phosphoproteins, and phospholipid as has been described previously for other human and mouse autoantibodies (Andrzejewsky et al. 1980).

U4 shows that a single somatic point mutation could not only result in a change in specificity, but also can convert an antibody that protects the animal from bacterial infections (Briles et al. 1982) to a potentially pathogenic autoantibody. The impact of single somatic mutations, such as those that occurred in U10 and U4, on the PC-binding site raises the question of how fre-

Table 1. Binding of U4 and S107 to Phosphorylated Macromolecules

	PC-KLH	dsDNA ($\times10$)	Protamine	Cardiolipin
S107	4945	280	158	39
U4	781	1388	677	433

These are solid-phase radioimmunoassays except for the binding to dsDNA, which was done by filter assay with radioactive dsDNA. Backgrounds have been subtracted.

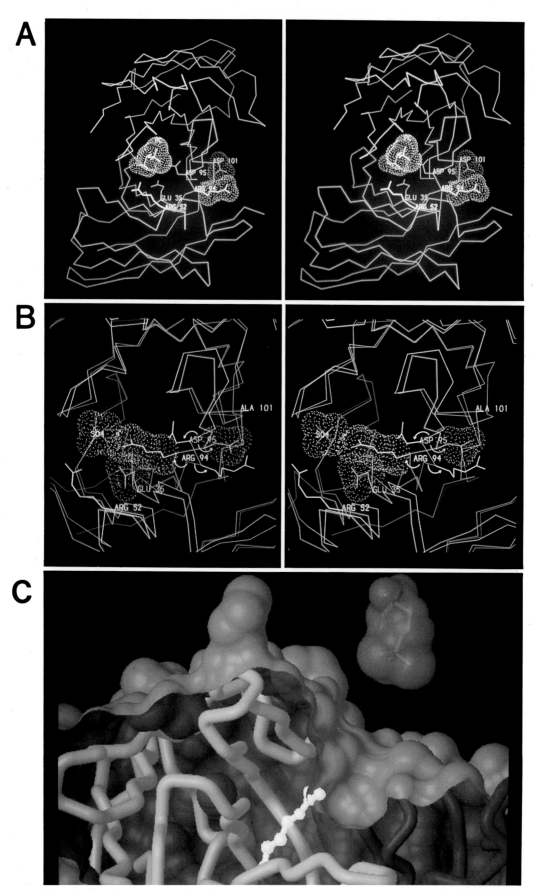

Figure 4. (*See facing page for legend.*)

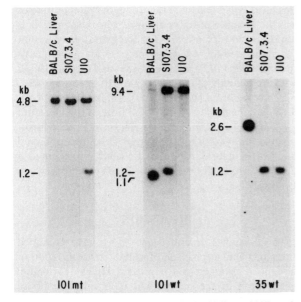

Figure 5. Southern blot analysis of BALB/c liver, S107, and U10 DNA with the U10-specific oligonucleotide. The DNA was digested with *Bam*HI and electrophoresed in a 1.5% agarose gel. The oligonucleotide used is shown in Fig. 3. (*Left*) The DNA was hybridized with the U10-specific (101 mt) oligonucleotide (see Fig. 3); (*middle*) the wild-type (101 wt) oligonucleotide that contained the germ-line sequence; and (*right*) an oligonucleotide (35 wt) that hybridizes with the first HV region of the V_H1 gene. The 1.2-kb fragment includes the rearranged V_H1 and D and J present in both S107 and U10. The unrearranged V_H1 migrates at 2.6 kb (*right*). The rearranged J_H1 is also found at 1.2 kb, but the germ-line J_H1 is on a 1.1 kb (*middle*, liver). The J_H1 hybridizing band at 9.4 kb (*middle*) is associated with the rearranged c-*myc* gene in S107.

quently antibodies with loss of antigen binding or with changes in specificity arise during the normal diversification of B-cell clones. Since the U4 observation suggested that autoantibodies may be routinely generated during the course of the normal immune response, there must also be mechanisms in adult animals to suppress the expression of such autoantibodies (Goodnow et al. 1988).

Autoantibodies Encoded by the S107 V_H Gene Family

The S107-U4 observation provided an opportunity to investigate the role of previous exposure to environmental antigens on the use of certain V_H genes in the subsequent production of autoantibodies and to study the contribution of one V_H family to the production of autoimmunity in lupus-like strains of mice. Since S107-like DNA-binding antibodies had been observed in both (NZB × NZW)F$_1$ (Eilat et al. 1984) and MRL/lpr animals (Trepicchio and Barrett 1987), it seemed likely that members of the S107 V_H family routinely contributed to the autoimmune response. However, it was difficult to identify which genes were involved because none of the S107 V_H germ-line genes from autoimmune strains had been cloned and sequenced at that time.

Since the S107 V_H gene family is a small one, we cloned and sequenced the four strongly cross-hybridizing members of this family from both NZB and NZW. The coding sequences of the V_H1, V_H3, V_H11, and V_H13 germ-line genes are homologous to those reported for BALB/c, C57BL/10, and CBA/J, and do

Figure 4. Computer graphics of the S107 and U10 antibody V region models. (*Top*) A stereo pair showing the location and stereochemistry of critical charged residue side chains in the computationally derived model of the PC-binding antibody S107. The α-carbon backbones for the heavy (blue) and light (light purple) chains are shown together with residue labels and bonds for positive (light blue) and negative (red) side chains and PC (center) moieties. The trimethylammonium portion of PC is shown in light blue (rear center) and the phosphate portion in red (front center). The salt-bridge between Asp-101 (red label, bonds, and surface) and Arg-94 (light blue label, bonds, and surface) occurs on the outside surface of the antibody (right) over 9 Å from the PC-binding site formed at the interface of the H and L chains. (Adapted from Chien et al. 1989.) (*Middle*) A stereo pair showing the two minimized computationally derived models for the single-site U10 mutant of S107. In the ARG-OUT mutant structure as in McPC603 and the S107 model, the Arg-94 side chain points away from the wild-type PC-binding site. In the ARG-IN mutant structure, the Arg-94 side chain extends into the wild-type PC binding site. The α-carbon backbones for the ARG-IN (H chain, light blue, and L chain, pink) and the ARG-OUT models (H chain, light green, and L chain, purple) superimpose closely except for V_H CDR3. The side chains (yellow label, bonds, and surface), binding pocket side chains of Arg-52 (blue label and bonds; lower left), and Glu-35 (red label, bonds, and surface; lower center), and the single site mutation at Ala-101 (light-blue label and bond; right) are shown in the energetically favored ARG-IN model only. The side chains of Arg-94 and Asp-95 are shown in both the ARG-IN and ARG-OUT models. In the ARG-OUT model (yellow bonds and arrows from label), Arg-94 extends out from the wild-type PC-binding site but has lost its charged interaction with residue 101 (Ala in U10), whereas Asp-95 points into the wild-type PC-binding site containing negatively charged Glu-35. In the ARG-IN model, Arg-94 (light blue bonds, label and arrow) extends into the wild-type binding site, and Asp-95 (red bonds, label and arrow) extends to the outside surface and points away from the binding site. (Adapted from Chien et al. 1989.) (*Bottom*) Steric hindrance in the binding site of the U10 mutant. Computational results suggest a mechanism for the loss of PC binding in the single-site U10 mutant in which placement of the Arg-94 side chain in the binding pocket as modeled by ARG-IN causes electrostatic and steric repulsion of the choline moiety of PC. The external molecular surface of McPC603 is shown as a hollow shell that is shaded light purple on the outside and dark purple on the inside. A clipping plane cuts away the front surface of the antibody to reveal simultaneously both inside and outside surface topography. The Arg-94 side chain (bonds and atoms shown as light blue spheres and connections) penetrates the deepest part of the PC-binding pocket, which is an invagination between the H (blue) and L (red) chains (shown as bent tubes). PC (top right, shown with transparent purple molecule surface and red bonds) is shown translated up from its bound position in McPC603. (Computer graphics rendering and photograph by Michael Pique and John Tainer.)

not contain any differences that would make the genes from the autoimmune strains more likely to encode autoantibodies (Behar and Scharff 1988; S. Corbet et al., in prep.).

We then immunized young (NZB × NZW)F$_1$ and MRL/lpr mice that had not yet developed disease with PC-KLH to determine if they, like BALB/c mice, used the S107 V$_H$1 gene to produce anti-PC antibodies. When PC-KLH in saline is injected into young (NZB × NZW)F$_1$ mice and MRL/1pr mice, V$_H$1-encoded antibodies dominate the anti-PC response (Behar et al. 1989; Chien et al. 1988). If the animals are boosted with PC-KLH when they begin to develop autoimmune disease and to produce large amounts of IgG anti-DNA antibodies and their spleen cells are fused to generate monoclonal antibodies, antibodies encoded by the S107 V$_H$ gene family can be identified in most fusions (Behar and Scharff 1988). To recover all of the antibodies expressing any member of the S107 V$_H$ gene family irrespective of their specificity, we screened the hybrids by RNA dot blot with a S107 V$_H$ probe. We expected to reproduce the S107-U4 phenomenon and thought the anti-DNA antibodies would be encoded by V$_H$1. In fact, all of the 17 DNA-binding (NZB × NZW)F$_1$ S107 V$_H$-encoded antibodies from two fusions that we have studied so far express the V$_H$11 gene and none express V$_H$1 (Behar and Scharff 1988; S.M. Behar et al., in prep.).

The differences between the sequences of five V$_H$11-encoded heavy chains that we have reported previously (Behar and Scharff 1988) and the V$_H$11 germ-line gene are summarized in Table 2. They are all derived from a single fusion and, based on criteria set forth previously by Weigert and his colleagues (Shlomchik et al. 1987b), are all the products of a single B-cell clone. Compared with the germ-line sequences of V$_H$11 from NZB and NZW mice, which are identical in their coding and adjacent flanking sequences (Behar and Scharff 1988), there are many base changes in the anti-dsDNA antibodies we have sequenced (Table 2). This leads us to conclude, in agreement with Shlomchik et al. (1987a), that the anti-DNA antibodies are the product of an antigen-driven response. Shlomchik et al. (1987b) have also suggested that a ratio of replacement (R) to silent (S) mutation greater than 1.5/1 in the CDRs suggests that the antigen has selectively stimulated the proliferation of B cells producing antibodies with somatic mutations in their antigen-binding sites. On the basis of

Table 2. H-chain Mutation

Antibody	Total (base changes)	CDR (R/S)	FW (R/S)
N4-1	6	4/0	0/2
N4-19	12	3/2	5/2
N4-10	13	5/1	4/3
N4-2	6	1/1	4/0
N4-18	16	5/3	6/2
Total	53	18/7	19/9
Average (R/S)		2.6	1.9

The ratio of R mutations to S mutations was calculated for CDRs and FWs of the H-chain VDJ sequences of each monoclonal antibody.

this criteria, it is possible that some of these antibodies are the product of an antigen-selected response. It is important to reemphasize that the hybridomas are initially screened for V region expression and subsequently for antigen binding. Since Manser and Gefter (1984), who are the only other investigators to screen this way, have not reported an attempt to organize their antibodies into genealogies, there is still little in the literature to compare with our findings. However, other investigators studying foreign antigens have also observed families of hybridomas each of which represented a different product of the original B-cell clone (Blier and Bothwell 1988).

DISCUSSION

In the studies described above, we have examined the molecular mechanism of somatic diversification of already rearranged and expressed H-chain V region genes both in the animal and in a cultured mouse myeloma cell line. We have focused our attention on the S107 V$_H$1 gene, which dominates the early response of BALB/c and other strains of mice to the PC haptenic group on bacterial polysaccharides or on protein carriers (Kohler 1975). This response is exceptionally well-characterized, and the relevant germ-line genes and other members of the S107 V$_H$1 family have been cloned and sequenced previously (Crews et al. 1981; Clarke and Rudikoff 1984; Ferguson et al. 1988). In addition, the three-dimensional structure of an antibody encoded by one of these genes has been determined previously (Satow et al. 1986).

Three mutant antibodies, P28, U10, and U4, that are the product of somatic diversification of the S107 germ-line V$_H$1 gene have been described here. Each of these mutant antibodies differs from V$_H$1 by one amino acid replacement that results in altered specificity. Examination of these antibodies has led to the conclusion that the major mechanism of somatic diversification of this H-chain gene family both in vivo and in vitro is somatic point mutation. Although it is impossible to rule out gene conversion mediated through very small donor sequences, the highly homologous upstream V regions (Crews et al. 1981) that constitute the S107 V$_H$ family and the large number of monoclonal antibodies and myeloma proteins that have been sequenced (Perlmutter et al. 1984; Claflin et al. 1987; Malipiero et al. 1987) do not contain any of the substitutions present in these three mutant antibodies. Thus, it is unlikely that V region replacement is responsible for the somatic diversification of the V$_H$1 or V$_H$11 genes or that the immediate upstream V regions are providing donor sequences for gene conversion. Although this does not preclude V region replacement or gene conversion in responses utilizing other germ-line families, such as J558, that have more members, it does suggest that point mutation is the major mechanism for generating V region diversity in the mouse.

Although we have used a variety of oligonucleotides probes and restriction enzymes, we have not yet been able to identify donor sequences that could mediate gene conversion. The one potential donor sequence for the U10 mutation of S107 that we did identify differs significantly in its sequence from both the germ-line and mutant V regions and illustrates the need to clone and sequence cross-hybridizing DNA before it can be considered a legitimate candidate for gene conversion. Even if an identical sequence had been identified and located in the genome, it would have been difficult to prove that it was the donor for a particular mutation.

The ease with which we were able to obtain nonantigen-binding mutants from the S107 cell line in culture suggests that B cells producing such "degenerate" antibodies should arise frequently during the normal immune response to T-dependent antigens. The impact of mutations of residues that are quite distant from the binding site, such as the one that occurred in the U10 mutant of S107, suggests that many mutations may lead to major changes in the antigen binding. The rarity of hybridomas producing such antibodies probably reflects the fact that they would not be isolated if antigen binding were used to screen the fusions. However, even when such low- or nonantigen-binding monoclonal antibodies have been specifically looked for, they have been difficult to find (Manser et al. 1987a) suggesting that there are few B cells producing such antibodies, presumably because of the selective outgrowth and proliferation of cells expressing high-affinity antibodies. The U4 mutant is especially informative since it shows that somatic mutation may result in the loss of ability to bind the eliciting antigen and in the acquisition of binding for another antigen. Although there is little evidence for such events during the normal immune response, studies with the response to oxazalone (Berek and Milstein 1987, 1988) and PC (Stenzel-Poore et al. 1988) show that B cells using V regions that dominate the initial response may be partially or completely replaced by B cells utilizing other V regions. The V region combinations expressed by these later arising B cells may have encoded lower-affinity antibodies for the eliciting antigen and, as a result of somatic hypermutation, subsequently achieved higher affinities (Wysocki et al. 1986; Berek and Milstein 1988). It is also possible, however, that they were B cells responding to another common environmental antigen that as a result of somatic mutation, acquired specificity for the eliciting antigen and became incorporated into this new immune response.

In addition, U4 shows that an important protective antibody can, as the result of a single-base change, acquire reactivity with a self-component and become one of the autoantibodies found in autoimmune diseases such as lupus. Our attempt to reproduce a U4-like event in vivo using autoimmune $(NZB \times NZW)F_1$ mice has not yet been successful because we have not found S107 V_H1-encoded anti-DNA antibodies in such mice. We are currently attempting to determine whether this means that V_H1 cannot encode pathogenic antibodies or if we have obscured this event because of the timing of our immunization protocols. It should be noted that R. Shefner and B. Diamond (unpubl.) have been able to identify such V_H1-encoded anti-DNA antibodies in BALB/c mice. However, our finding that S107 V_H11-encoded antibodies arise frequently in PC primed and boosted mice (Behar and Scharff 1988) suggests that the earlier immunological experiences of the individual may influence the V regions used to produce autoantibodies. In addition, the small size of the S107 V_H family has allowed us to clone and sequence the relevant germ-line V region genes. This has made it possible to conclude with certainty that extensive somatic mutation has occurred in the S107-like anti-DNA antibodies that participate in the autoimmune response of lupus-like mice (Behar and Scharff 1988; Behar et al. 1989). Furthermore, we cannot identify any characteristics of the S107 V_H germ-line genes in the $(NZB \times NZW)F_1$ mice that would make them more likely to encode autoantibodies. In contrast with the observations reported previously by Eilat et al. (1988) and Radic et al. (this volume), we have not observed the use of unusual reading frames or inversions in the D region of these autoantibodies.

In summary, an examination of antibodies encoded by the S107 V_H family has led us to conclude the following: (1) point mutation is the major mechanism responsible for the somatic diversification of already rearranged and expressed variable region genes, at least in the S107 V_H family in the mouse; (2) in the course of the immune response to foreign antigens, somatic mutations, both in the antigen-binding sites and at sites distant from it, can generate antibodies that have lost the ability to react with the eliciting antigen. In some cases such antibodies will react with new antigens; (3) antibodies against environmental antigens can as a result of somatic mutation become potentially pathogenic autoantibodies; (4) there may not be inherent differences in the V region genes that encode antibodies to foreign antibodies and those that encode autoantibodies suggesting that autoimmune individuals have defects in the regulation of their immune response; and (5) the autoantibody response in autoimmune mice is antigen driven. However, we do not know in the case described here, whether the antigen is a self-antigen such as dsDNA or a foreign antigen. Furthermore, we believe that these studies show that a combination of in vivo and in vitro analysis can be very useful in dissecting the immune response to foreign and self-antigens.

ACKNOWLEDGMENTS

S.M.B. and D.L. are medical scientist trainees supported by the National Institute of General Medical Sciences (T32-GM7288). N.C.C. and S.-U.S. were supported by a training grant from the National Cancer Institute (5T32-CA09173). S.C. was a recipient of the Miriam and Benedict Wolf Fellowship from the Cancer Research Institute of New York. B.D. is supported by a grant from the National Institute of Health (AR-32371). E.D.G. received support from the Office of

Naval Research (N00014-89-5-1174). M.D.S. is supported by a grant from the National Cancer Institute (CA-05973) and is the occupant of the Harry Eagle Chair in Cancer Research from the National Women's Division of the Albert Einstein College of Medicine.

REFERENCES

Allen, D., A. Cumano, R. Dildrop, C. Kocks, C. Rajewsky, K. Rajewsky, J. Roes, F. Stablitzky, and M. Siekevitz. 1987. Timing, genetic requirements and functional consequences of somatic hypermutation during B cell development. *Immunol. Rev.* **96:** 5.

Andrzejewsky, C., Jr., J. Rauch, E. Lafer, B.D. Stollar, and R.S. Schwartz. 1980. Antigen-binding diversity and idiotypic cross-reactions among hybridoma autoantibodies to DNA. *J. Immunol.* **126:** 226.

Baltimore, D. 1981. Gene conversion: Some implications for immunoglobulin genes. *Cell* **24:** 592.

Behar, S.M. 1989. "The impact of somatic mutation and environmental antigens on the origin of anti-dsDNA autoantibodies." Ph.D. thesis. Albert Einstein College of Medicine, New York.

Behar, S.M. and M.D. Scharff. 1988. Somatic diversification of the S107 (T15) VH11 germ-line gene that encodes anti-dsDNA antibodies in (NZB × NZW) F1 mice. *Proc. Natl. Acad. Sci.* **85:** 3970.

Behar, S.M., S. Corbet, B. Diamond, and M.D. Scharff. 1989. The molecular origin of anti-DNA antibodies. *Int. Rev. Immunol.* **5:** 23.

Berek, C. and C. Milstein. 1987. Mutational drift and repertoire shift in the maturation of the immune response. *Int. Rev. Immunol.* **96:** 23.

———. 1988. The dynamic nature of the antibody repertoire. *Immunol. Rev.* **105:** 5.

Bernard, O., N. Huzumi, and S. Tonegawa. 1978. Sequences of mouse immunoglobulin light chain genes before and after somatic changes. *Cell* **15:** 1133.

Bernstein, F.C., T.F. Koetzle, G.J.B. Williams, E.F. Meyer, Jr., M.D. Brice, J.R. Rodgers, O. Kennard, T. Shirmanouchi, and M. Tasomi. 1977. The protein data bank: A computer based archival file for macromolecular structures. *J. Mol. Biol.* **112:** 535.

Blier, P.R. and A.L.M. Bothwell. 1988. The immune response to the hapten NP in C57Bl/6 mice: Insight into the structure of the B cell repertoire. *Immunol. Rev.* **105:** 27.

Briles, D.E., C. Forman, S. Hudak, and J.L. Claflin. 1982. Anti-phosphorylcholine antibodies of the T15 idiotype are optimally protective against *Streptococcus pneumoniae*. *J. Exp. Med.* **156:** 1177.

Cebra, J.J., J.L. Komisar, and P.A. Schweitzer. 1984. CH isotype "switching" during normal B-lymphocyte development. *Annu. Rev. Immunol.* **2:** 493.

Chien, N.C., R.R. Pollock, C. Desaymard, and M.D. Scharff. 1988. Point mutations cause the somatic diversification of IgM and IgG anti-phosphorylcholine antibodies. *J. Exp. Med.* **167:** 954.

Chien, N.C., V.A. Roberts, N.M. Giusti, M.D. Scharff, and E.G. Getzoff. 1989. Significant structural and functional change of an antigen binding site by a distant amino acid substitution: Proposal of a structural mechanism. *Proc. Natl. Acad. Sci.* **86:** 5532.

Claflin, J.L., J. Berry, D. Flaherty, and W. Dunnick. 1987. Somatic evolution of diversity among anti-phosphocholine antibodies induced with *Proteus morganii*. *J. Immunol.* **138:** 3060.

Clarke, S.H. and S. Rudikoff. 1984. Evidence for gene conversion among immunoglobulin heavy chain variable region genes. *J. Exp. Med.* **159:** 773.

Clarke, S.H., K. Huppi, D. Ruezinsky, L. Staudt, W. Ger-

hard, and M. Weigert. 1985. Inter- and intraclonal diversity in the antibody response to influenza hemagglutinin. *J. Exp. Med.* **161:** 687.

Cook, W.D. and M.D. Scharff. 1977. Antigen binding mutants of mouse myeloma cells. *Proc. Natl. Acad. Sci.* **74:** 5687.

Crews, S., J. Griffin, H. Huang, K. Calame, and L. Hood. 1981. A single VH gene segment encodes the immune response to phosphorylcholine: Somatic mutation is correlated with the class of the antibody. *Cell* **25:** 59.

Davies, D.R. and H. Metzger. 1983. Structural basis of antibody function. *Annu. Rev. Immunol.* **1:** 87.

Diamond, B. and M.D. Scharff. 1984. Somatic mutation of the T15 heavy chain gives rise to an antibody with autoantibody specificity. *Proc. Natl. Acad. Sci.* **81:** 5841.

Dildrop, R., M. Bruggerman, A. Radbruch, K. Rajewsky, and K. Beyreuther. 1982. Immunoglobulin V region variants in hybridoma cells. II. Recombination between V genes. *EMBO J.* **1:** 635.

Eilat, D., D.M. Webster, and A.R. Rees. 1988. V regions of anti-DNA and anti-RNA autoantibodies from NZB/NZW F1 mice. *J. Immunol.* **141:** 1745.

Eilat, D., M. Hochberg, J. Pumphrey, and S. Rudikoff. 1984. Monoclonal antibodies to DNA and RNA from NZB/NZW F1 mice: Antigenic specificities and NH2 terminal amino acid sequences. *J. Immunol.* **133:** 489.

Ferguson, S.E., S. Rudikoff, and B.A. Osborne. 1988. Interaction and sequence diversity among T15 VH genes in CBA/J mice. *J. Exp. Med.* **168:** 1339.

French, D.L., R. Laskov, and M.D. Scharff. 1989. The role of somatic hypermutation in the generation of antibody diversity. *Science* **244:** 152.

Giusti, A.M., N.C. Chien, D.J. Zack, S.-U. Shin, and M.D. Scharff. 1987. Somatic diversification of S107 from an antiphosphocholine to an anti-DNA autoantibody is due to a single base change in its heavy chain variable region. *Proc. Natl. Acad. Sci.* **84:** 2926.

Goodnow, C.D., J. Crosbie, S. Adelstein, T.B. Lavoie, S.J. Smith-Gill, R.A. Brink, H. Pritchard-Briscoe, J.S. Wotherspoon, R.H. Loblay, K. Raphael, R.J. Trent, and A. Bastern. 1988. Altered immunoglobulin expressions and functional silencing of self-reactive B-lymphocytes in transgenic mice. *Nature* **334:** 676.

Gough, N.M. and O. Bernard. 1981. Sequences of the joining region genes and their role in the generation of antibody diversity. *Proc. Natl. Acad. Sci.* **78:** 508.

Kabat, E.A., T.T. Wu, and H. Bilofsky. 1976. Attempts to locate residues in the complementarity determining regions of antibody combining sites that make contact with antigen. *Proc. Natl. Acad. Sci.* **73:** 617.

Kabat, E.A., T.T. Wu, H. Bilofsky, M. Reid-Miller, H.M. Perry, and K.S. Gottesman. 1987. *Sequences of proteins of immunological interest*. U.S. Department of Health and Human Services, Washington, D.C.

Kleinfield, R. and M. Weigert. 1989. Analysis of V_H gene replacement events in B cell lymphoma. *J. Immunol.* **142:** 4475.

Kleinfield, R., R.R. Hardy, D. Tarlington, J. Dangl, L.A. Herzenberg, and M. Weigert. 1986. Recombination between an expressed immunoglobulin heavy-chain gene and a germline variable gene segment in a Ly1 + B-cell lymphoma. *Nature* **322:** 843.

Kocks, C. and K. Rajewsky. 1988. Stepwise intraclonal maturation of antibody affinity through somatic hypermutation. *Proc. Natl. Acad. Sci.* **85:** 8206.

———. 1989. Stable expression and somatic hypermutation of antibody V regions in B-cell developmental pathways. *Annu. Rev. Immunol.* **7:** 537.

Kohler, H. 1975. The response to phosphorylcholine—Dissecting an immune response. *Transplant Rev.* **27:** 24.

Livant, P., C. Blatt, and L. Hood. 1986. One heavy chain variable region gene segment subfamily in the BALB/c mouse contains 500–1000 or more members. *Cell* **47:** 461.

Malipiero, U.V., N.S. Levy, and P.J. Gearhart. 1987. Somatic mutation in anti-phosphorylcholine antibodies. *Immunol. Rev.* **96:** 59.

Manser, T. and M.L. Gefter. 1984. Isolation and hybridomas expressing a specific heavy chain variable gene segment by using a screening technique that detects mRNA sequences in whole cell lysates. *Proc. Natl. Acad. Sci.* **81:** 2470.

Manser, T., B. Parhami-Seren, M.N. Margolies, and M.L. Gefter. 1987a. Somatically mutated forms of a major anti-p-azophenylarsonate antibody variable region with drastically reduced affinity for p-azophenarsonate. *J. Exp. Med.* **166:** 1456.

Manser, T., L.J. Wysocki, M.N. Margolies, and M.L. Gefter. 1987b. Evolution of antibody variable region structure during the immune response. *Immunol. Rev.* **96:** 141.

Morrison, S.L. and M.D. Scharff. 1981. Mutational events in mouse myeloma cells. *CRC Crit. Rev. Immunol.* **3:** 1.

Perlmutter, R.M., S.T. Crews, R. Douglas, G. Sorensen, N. Johnson, N. Nivera, P.J. Gearhart, and L. Hood. 1984. The generation of diversity in phosphorylcholine antibodies. *Adv. Immunol.* **35:** 1.

Rajewsky, K., I. Förster, and A. Cumano. 1987. Evolutionary and somatic selection of antibody repertoire in the mouse. *Science* **238:** 1088.

Reth, M., P. Gehrmann, E. Petrac, and P. Wiese. 1986. A novel V_H to $V_H D_H$ joining mechanism in heavy-chain-negative (null) pre-B cells results in heavy chain production. *Nature* **322:** 840.

Reynaud, C.A., V. Anquez, H. Grimal, and J.C. Weill. 1987. A hyperconversion mechanism generates the chicken light chain preimmune repertoire. *Cell* **48:** 379.

Sablitzky, F., G. Wildner, and K. Rajewsky. 1985. Somatic mutation and clonal expansion of B cells in an antigen driven immune response. *EMBO J.* **4:** 345.

Satow, Y., G.H. Cohen, E.A. Padlan, and D.R. Davis. 1986. Phosphocholine binding immunoglobulin Fab: McPC603, an X-ray diffraction study at 2.7 Å. *J. Mol. Biol.* **190:** 593.

Shimizu, A. and T. Honjo. 1984. Class switching. *Cell* **36:** 801.

Shin, S.U. 1987. "Molecular basis of the somatic instability of S107 immunoglobulin genes." Ph.D. thesis. Albert Einstein College of Medicine, New York.

Shlomchik, M.J., A.H. Aucoin, D.S. Pisetsky, and M.G. Weigert. 1987a. Structure and function of anti-DNA autoantibodies derived from a single autoimmune mouse. *Proc. Natl. Acad. Sci.* **84:** 9150.

Shlomchik, M.J., A. Marshak-Rothstein, C.B. Wolfowicz, T.L. Rothstein, and M.G. Weigert. 1987b. The role of clonal selection and somatic mutation in autoimmunity. *Nature* **328:** 805.

Stenzel-Poore, M.P., U. Bruderer, and M.B. Rittenberg. 1988. The adaptive potential of the memory response: Clonal recruitment and epitope recognition. *Immunol. Rev.* **105:** 113.

Thompson, C.B. and P.E. Neiman. 1987. Somatic diversification of the chicken immunoglobulin light chain gene is limited to the rearranged variable gene segment. *Cell* **48:** 369.

Tonegawa, S. 1983. Somatic generation of antibody diversity. *Nature* **302:** 575.

Trepicchio, W., Jr. and K.J. Barrett. 1987. Eleven MRL-*lpr/lpr* anti-DNA autoantibodies are encoded by genes from four V_H gene families: A potentially biased usage of **VH** genes. *J. Immunol.* **138:** 2323.

Weigert, M.G., I.M. Cesari, S.J. Yonkovich, and M. Cohn. 1970. Variability in lambda light chain sequences of mouse antibody. *Nature* **228:** 1045.

Wysocki, L., T. Manser, and M. Gefter. 1986. Somatic evolution of variable region structures during the immune response. *Proc. Natl. Acad. Sci.* **83:** 1847.

Yancopoulos, G.D. and F.W. Alt. 1986. Regulation of the assembly and expression of variable origin genes. *Annu. Rev. Immunol.* **4:** 339.

Zeff, R.A., J. Gopas, E. Steinhauser, T.V. Rajan, and S.G. Nathenson. 1986. Analysis of somatic cell H-2 variants to define the structural requirements for class I antigen expression. *J. Immunol.* **137:** 897.

Structural Patterns in Anti-DNA Antibodies from MRL/*lpr* Mice

M.Z. Radic, M.A. Mascelli, J. Erikson, H. Shan, M. Shlomchik, and M. Weigert

Institute for Cancer Research, Fox Chase Cancer Center, Philadelphia, Pennsylvania 19111

Antibodies that bind native DNA (anti-dsDNA) are a characteristic of the human autoimmune disease, systemic lupus erythematosus (SLE) and a mouse model for this disease, the MRL/Mp-*lpr/lpr* (MRL/*lpr*) strain (Tan et al. 1966; Arana and Seligmann 1967; Dixon et al. 1971; Notman et al. 1974; Pisetsky et al. 1982). High titers of anti-dsDNA are correlated with disease activity, and these autoantibodies may account for certain SLE symptoms such as renal lesions (Tan et al. 1966; Harbeck et al. 1973; Winfield et al. 1977; Morimoto et al. 1982; Datta et al. 1986; Pankewycz et al. 1987; Raz et al. 1989).

How such antibodies are elicited has been of interest. Our surveys of both rheumatoid factors (Shlomchik et al. 1987a) and anti-DNA (Shlomchik et al. 1987b) from individual MRL/*lpr* mice have shown that these autoantibodies are of oligoclonal origin. Moreover, these autoantibodies are highly mutated, and the patterns of mutations show evidence for antigen selection (Shlomchik et al. 1987a,b). In this regard, autoantibodies are similar to antibodies to foreign antigens, as originally observed in the secondary immune response to influenza hemagglutinin. These similarities argue that autoantibodies are also elicited by antigens, and we presume these antigens to be self components in autoimmune disease.

Our extensive surveys of anti-DNA have revealed several features that account for dsDNA and ssDNA binding. These features include somatic mutations to arginine and asparagine that can interact with DNA and V_H regions with unusually high frequencies of arginine in their third complementarity determining region (CDR3). In addition, a wide variety of V_H and V_κ genes are used, yet certain V_H genes recur (Shlomchik et al. 1989).

These spontaneously arising clones of anti-DNA from the diseased MRL/*lpr* provide a rich source of information on how an antibody specificity, anti-dsDNA, is derived. This has encouraged us to extend our survey. As described here, further study of anti-dsDNA reinforces our earlier conclusions and reveals additional ways by which this specificity is determined.

METHODS

Generation of hybridomas. Spleen cells from an unstimulated 4-month-old female MRL/*lpr* mouse (no. 34) were fused to the SP2/0 fusion partner. We designate this as mouse 6 for the continuity of our anti-DNA survey. Limiting dilution plating at 15 hours postfusion in hypoxanthine/aminopterin/thymidine (HAT) medium yielded 96 hybridomas, of which ~6 were biclonal. Further subcloning ensured monoclonality among cell lines used in this study. Cells were grown in OPTI-MEM medium (GIBCO) supplemented with 4% FCS, and supernatants were collected and stored in the presence of 0.02% Na azide at 4°C.

Southern analysis. Genomic DNA was isolated from Sarkosyl-lysed nuclei by phenol extraction, digested with restriction endonucleases (Promega), and electrophoresed through 0.8% agarose (National Diagnostics). DNA fragments were transferred by Southern blotting with 0.4 N NaOH (Reed and Mann 1985) onto Zeta Probe membrane (Bio-Rad) and hybridized with pJ11 (heavy chain; Marcu et al. 1980) and pECK (light chain; Coleclough et al. 1980) probes labeled by random primed DNA synthesis (Boehringer) with ^{32}P-labeled deoxynucleotide triphosphates (New England Nuclear).

mRNA sequencing. Poly(A)$^+$ RNA was isolated according to the method of Badley et al. (1988), using oligo(dT) cellulose (Collaborative Research), and converted into cDNA using avian reverse transcriptase (Life Sciences). A kinase-labeled κ constant region primer was used in a modified Maxam and Gilbert sequencing protocol (Shlomchik et al. 1986), whereas the Sanger method was adapted for reverse transcription initiating at isotype or J_κ-specific primers (Geliebter et al. 1986). Ambiguities in RNA sequences were minimized by performing reverse transcriptions at 42°C, and/or treating duplicates of Sanger reactions with terminal deoxynucleotide transferase (U.S. Biochemicals), and reading each sequence on more than one gel.

DNA-binding assay. The details of this technique will be published separately (M.Z. Radic and M. Weigert, in prep.). Briefly, sonicated salmon sperm DNA (Sigma) was treated with nuclease S1, phenol-extracted, EtOH precipitated, *Hae*III restriction cut, and covalently modified using photobiotin (Vector), according to manufacturer's suggestions. Dilutions of hybridoma supernatants and biotinylated DNA were made in phosphate-buffered saline (PBS) (GIBCO) containing 1% bovine serum albumin (BSA), 0.5 mM

Na EDTA, and 0.02% Na azide. To measure ssDNA binding, biotinylated DNA was denatured by incubation at 95°C for 5 minutes and rapid chilling with ice-cold dilution buffer. Complexes of DNA and antibodies were allowed to form by mixing various amounts of monoclonal antibodies with a fixed amount of biotinylated DNA (2 μg/ml final concentration). These mixtures were incubated in preblocked microtiter wells at 37°C. After 2 hours, mixtures were transferred to goat anti-mouse κ-coated microtiter plates (Dynatech) and incubated for an additional hour. Material bound in the wells after washing was reacted with alkaline phosphatase conjugated either to streptavidin or to antisera directed against heavy chain constant regions. Binding was quantitated by measuring absorbance at 405 nm.

RESULTS

Anti-DNA B Cells from MRL/lpr Mice Are Oligoclonal

Of the 96 hybridomas derived from the mouse 6 fusion, 11 (12%) are anti-DNA. The clonal composition of these anti-DNA hybridomas was evaluated using our standard criteria for relatedness (McKean et al. 1984; Clarke et al. 1985; Shlomchik et al. 1987b, 1989). The first is the context of rearranged heavy and light chain alleles, particularly that of the nonproductive alleles (H$^-$, κ^-). These alleles rearrange independently of the productive alleles, but by the same mechanism. Thus, the contexts of the H$^-$ and κ^- alleles are highly variable, and nonproductive alleles are rarely of the same restriction fragment size in surveys of independently derived B-cell lines. On the basis of these surveys we have determined that the likelihood of the context of the H$^-$ or κ^- allele being the same in two lines by chance is low ($p = 0.05$ for H and $p = 0.07$ for κ), and it is much lower in three or more lines (S. Litwin and M. Shlomchik, in prep.). Of the 11 anti-DNA hybridomas, the context of the H$^-$ (and κ^-; data not shown) is the same in six lines (H^2; Fig. 1). These must represent one clone (designated clone H). This analysis was uninformative for the two cell lines that segregated H$^-$ after somatic cell hybridization. The rest of the anti-DNA hybridomas that retained an H$^-$ allele are unrelated to clone H and to each other.

The second criterion for relatedness that we have applied to these anti-DNA hybridomas is nucleotide sequence identity in CDR3 of V$_H$. Because of the variety of ways by which this sequence is formed, the V$_H$ CDR3 of independently derived hybridomas, even of similar specificity, is rarely the same. On the basis of sequence surveys of anti-arsonate antibodies (Wysocki et al. 1986; T. Manser, pers. comm.), we have determined that the likelihood of finding two identical CDR3 sequences by chance is low ($p = 0.06$) (S. Litwin and M. Shlomchik, in prep.). By this criterion, six lines (3-1, 5-1, 10-3, 15-1, 23-9, and 44-3, clone H) are related (Fig. 2A), confirming the conclusion reached by comparing H$^-$ context. This method identifies a second

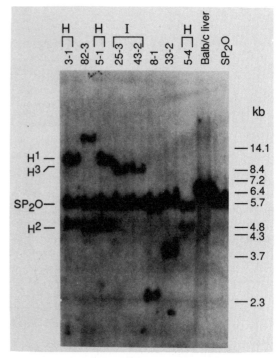

Figure 1. Southern blot analysis of mouse 6 hybridomas. Genomic DNA from representatives of clone H (3-1, 5-1, and 5-4), clone I (25-3 and 43-2), and single isolates (82-3, 8-1, and 33-2) was digested with *Eco*RI and analyzed by Southern blotting and hybridization to pJ11 (Marcu et al. 1980). DNA rearrangements are shared only among clone members. Subclones 5-1 and 5-4 are from the same hybrid. Subclone 5-4 no longer produces antibody, thus identifying the productive allele of clone H as H^1 and the nonproductive allele as H^2. Clone I members have retained only their productive allele, H^3. The slight molecular-weight difference between one of the fragments from 82-3 and the H^2 allele from clone H has been confirmed by digestion with *Xba*I (data not shown).

clone (clone I) that we failed to detect by the context of H$^-$, because this allele was not retained in either line (Fig. 1). The rest of the anti-DNA hybridomas each have a unique CDR3 sequence, confirming their independent origin.

In addition to two clones, there are three single isolates, which could represent clones smaller than H and I or just single B cells. In favor of the former interpretation, the singlets 33-2 and 8-1 have (as do the clones) the characteristics of classic SLE autoantibodies—they are IgG and bind dsDNA. One singlet, 82-3, is different; it is IgM and has no measurable affinity for dsDNA. This anti-DNA hybridoma is akin to those that can be elicited in healthy mice by lipopolysaccharide treatment (Sourouion et al. 1988). Regardless of their interpretation, the singlets comprise a minority of anti-DNA hybridomas in the MRL/lpr strain.

Applying these criteria for relatedness shows that the majority of anti-DNA hybridomas (8 of 11) from this mouse are derived from just two B-cell clones. These clones (H and I) extend our earlier findings on 31 anti-DNA hybridomas from four MRL/lpr mice in which we found seven clones (A–G). Thus, oligo-clonality is a general feature of the spontaneous anti-DNA response of MRL/*lpr* mice.

V Gene Use in Anti-DNA Hybridomas

Table 1 summarizes V gene use in these anti-DNA hybridomas. Of 11 hybridomas, 10 express members of the V_H J558 family, whereas the remaining anti-DNA hybridoma is encoded by a member of the V_H 7183 family (Fig. 2). We find high V_H sequence homology (96–100%) among members of clones H and I, as expected from the clone assignments described above. We also find that the V_H homology between clone H and clone I members is high, between 95% and 97%, suggesting that they use the same gene (Fig. 2A). This is supported by the fact that members of the two anti-DNA clones share identity of leader sequences (data not shown). Additional support for a shared V_H gene comes from the restriction fragment sizes of the productive alleles found in the two clones. These alleles, H^1 of clone H and H^3 of clone I (Fig. 1), differ by $\sim$0.9 kb. This is consistent with the same V_H joining to J_H2 (clone H) or J_H4 (clone I) (Newell et al. 1980). Therefore, in addition to high V_H homology and identity of leader sequence, the V_H of clone H and clone I share the same upstream *Eco*RI site.

Anti-DNA V_κ genes are more diverse than anti-DNA V_H genes (Fig. 2,C,D). In this survey, five different V_κ groups are represented, and each independent isolate uses a unique V_κ group. This finding extends our earlier survey of anti-DNA V_κ groups to 14.

Gene Segment Use in Anti-DNA Antibodies

The J_H, J_κ, and D_H genes used by these anti-DNA antibodies are summarized in Table 1. In this sample, we cannot detect a J_H, J_κ, or D_H preference; however, there are some common themes. Whereas the majority of D_H genes in other antibodies use a reading frame that is characterized by a high frequency of tyrosine residues (Kaartinen and Makela 1985), out-of-frame reading of a DFL 16-2 gene occurs in antibody 33-2 and leads to arginine codons (Fig. 3). This feature, high arginine CDR3 composition, is characteristic of a large fraction of anti-DNA antibodies (Shlomchik et al. 1989) and is due, in part, to the peculiar reading frame of D_H, as originally noted by Eilat et al. (1988). Two additional mechanisms have formed arginine codons in 33-2 CDR3: N nucleotide addition and a presumed somatic mutation (Fig. 3). As a result of these mechanisms, three contiguous arginine codons are produced adjacent to the canonical arginine codon at the end of framework region 3 (FR3). The CDR3 of 33-2 is also unusual in that it may be the product of D_H-D_H fusion involving a DFL 16-2 and an SP2-2 gene. The homology of the CDR3 sequence with the DFL 16-2 gene is six of seven nucleotides, whereas the homology with the SP2-2 gene is seven of seven nucleotides. Five nucleotides separate the two D_H genes, which are probably encoded by N sequence addition.

Analysis of Binding Specificity

Antibodies to dsDNA are diagnostic of autoimmunity (Notman et al. 1974; Tan 1982), and most of the

Table 1. Summary of Anti-DNA Sequences from Mouse 6 Hybridomas

Clone	Hybridoma	Isotype	V_κ	J_κ	V_H	D_H	J_H	Length of CDR3
H	3-1	IgG3	3	1	J558	DFL16-2	2	6
H	5-1	IgG3	3	1	J558	DFL16-2	2	6
H	10-3	IgG3	3	1	J558	DFL16-2	2	6
H	15-1	IgG3	3	1	J558	DFL16-2	2	6
H	23-9	IgG3	3	1	J558	DFL16-2	2	6
H	44-3	IgG3	3	1	J558	DFL16-2	2	6
I	25-3	IgG2a	23	4	J558	SP2[a]	4	7
I	43-2	IgG2a	23	4	J558	SP2[a]	4	7
	8-1	IgG3	10	1	J558	SP2-8	4	13
	82-3	IgM	5	4	J558	SP2-3	4	11
	33-2	IgG2b	9	5	7183	DFL16-2/SP2-2	2	12

Hybrids were assigned to clones by the criteria outlined in the text. Clones were assigned the letters H and I, as they are the eighth and ninth anti-DNA clones characterized in this laboratory (Shlomchik et al., 1989). Clone names were not given to single isolates. V_H and V_κ were assigned to homology groups on the basis of >80% sequence identity to known prototypes. The nomenclature for V_κ group members is described by Potter et al. (1982), and that for V_H families is described by Brodeur and Riblet (1984). D_H designations are by homology to the closest known BALB/c gene (Kurosawa and Tonegawa 1982). The CDR3 length is defined as the number of amino acids between the last amino acid encoded by the V_H gene (two residues after the invariant cysteine) and the invariant tryptophan residue encoded by all J_H genes.
[a] The V_H sequence of 25-3 does not allow us to assign it specifically to any particular SP-2 gene, as all members of this D family share homology in this region.

A

Block 1 (positions 1–110)

FR1 .... CDR1 .... FR2
1   10   20   30   40   50   60   70   80   90   100   110

CONSENSUS
Glu Val Gln Leu Gln Gln Ser Gly Pro Glu Leu Val Lys Pro Gly Ala Ser Val Lys Met Ser Cys Lys Ala Ser Gly Tyr Thr Phe Thr Asp Tyr Met Asn Trp Val Lys Gln
GAG GTC CAG CTG CAA CAG TCT GGA CCT GAG CTG GTG AAG CCT GGG GCT TCA GTG AAG ATG TCC TGT AAG GCT TCT GGA TAC ACA TTC ACT GAC TAC ATG AAC TGG GTG AAG CAG

Clone	Substitutions
VH10-3	—
VH15-1	—
VH3-1	---T (Met Asn); —
VH44-3	Ile (Thr); ---T
VH5-1	-TC; --A
VH23-9	Ile; --A
	-T-; --A
VH43-2	Asn A--; Ile -T-; --A
VH25-3	Asn -A-; --A

Block 2 (positions 120–230)

CDR2 .... FR3 .... FR2
120   130   140   150   160   170   180   190   200   210   220   230

CONSENSUS
Ser His Gly Lys Ser Leu Glu Trp Ile Gly Arg Val Asn Pro Ser Asn Gly Thr Gly Thr Tyr Asn Gln Lys Phe Gly Lys Ala Thr Leu Thr Val Asp Lys Ser Leu Ser Thr Ala
AGT CAT GGA AAG AGC CTT GAG TGG ATT GGA CGT GTT AAT CCT AGC AAT GGT GGT ACT TAC AAC CAG AAG TTC AAG GCC ACA TTG ACA GTA GAC AAA TCC AGC ACA GCC

Clone	Substitutions
VH10-3	—
VH15-1	—
VH3-1	—
VH44-3	Asp G--; Asp G--; —
VH5-1	-C Tyr TA-; Arg -GG Arg; Arg C-- --T; -G Asn
VH23-9	-C Arg C--; Arg -GG; -A- Asn; -A-
VH43-2	—
VH25-3	--T

Block 3 (positions 240–320)

CDR3 .... FR4
240   250   260   270   280   290   300   310   320

CONSENSUS
Tyr Met Gln Leu Asn Ser Leu Thr Ser Glu Asp Ser Ala Val Tyr Tyr Cys Ala Arg Gly Tyr Tyr Phe Asp Tyr Ala Met Trp Gly Gln Gly
TAC ATG CAG CTC AAC AGC ACA GAC TCT GAG GAC TCT GCG GTC TAT TAC TGT GCA AGG GGC TAC TAT TTT GAC TAC GCG ATG TGG GGC CAA GGC

Clone	Substitutions
VH10-3	—
VH15-1	—
VH3-1	Ser; —
VH44-3	Ile Ser -C-; —
VH5-1	-A -C-; --T
VH23-9	Ile Ser -C-; --T
VH43-2	Arg Asp A-G --A; Ala Met GC- ATG; --A; Asp Tyr --T
VH25-3	Arg Asp A-G --A; Ala Met GC- ATG; --A; --T

B

(Immunoglobulin VH gene nucleotide and amino acid sequence alignment)

First block (positions 1–115):

```
                      FR1
                      1                   10                  20                  30                  40                  50                  60                  70                  80                  90                  CDR1 100                 FR2 110
VH 33-2   Glu Val Lys Leu Val Glu Ser Gly Gly Gly Leu Val Lys Pro Gly Gly Ser Leu Lys Leu Ser Cys Ala Ala Ser Gly Phe Thr Phe Ser Tyr Thr Met Ser Trp Val Arg Gln
          GAA GTG AAG CTG GTG GAG TCT GGG GGA GGC TTA GTG AAG CCT GGA GGG TCC CTG AAA CTC TCC TGT GCA GCC TCT GGA TTC ACT TTC AGT AGC TAT ACC ATG TCT TGG GTT CGC CAG
3E12      --- --- --- --- --- --- --- --- --- --- --- --- --- --- --- --- --- --- --- --- --- --- --- --- --- --- --- --- --- --- --- --- --- --- --- --- --- ---
VH 82-3   Glu Ile Gln Leu Gln Gln Ser Gly Ala Glu Leu Val Lys Pro Gly Ala Ser Val Lys Ile Ser Cys Lys Ala Ser Gly Tyr Ser Phe Thr Gly Tyr Lys Met Asn Trp Val Lys Gln
          GAG ATC CAG CTG CAG CAG TCT GGA GCT GAG CTG GTG AAG CCT GGG GCT TCA GTG AAG ATA TCC TGC AAG GCT TCT GGT TAC TCA TTC ACT GGC TAC AAG ATG AAC TGG GTG AAG CAG
A52       --- --- --- --- --- --- --- --- --- --- --- --- --- --- --- --- --- --- --- --- --- --- --- --- --- --- --- --- --- --- --- Asn --- --- --C --- --- --- ---
VH 8-1    Val Gln Leu Gln Gln Ser Gly Pro Glu Leu Val Lys Pro Gly Ala Ser Val Lys Met Ser Cys Lys Ala Ser Gly Tyr Thr Phe Thr Ser Tyr Val Met His Trp Val Lys Gln
          GTC CAG CTG CTG CAG TCT GGA CCT GAG CTG GTA AAG CCT GGG GCT TCA GTG AAG ATG TCC TGC AAG GCT TCT GGA TAC ACA TTC ACT AGC TAT GTA ATG CAC TGG GTG AAG CAG
                                                                                                                          Ile
D30       Glu                                                                                                              --T --A                         --- --- --- ---
          GAG --- --- --- --- --- --- --- --- --- --- --- --- --- --- --- --- --- --- --- --- --- --- --- --- --- --- --- --- --- --- --- --- --- --- --- --- --- ---
```

Second block (positions 120–230):

```
          CDR2                                                            FR3
          120                 130                 140                 150                 160                 170                 180                 190                 200                 210                 220                 230
VH 33-2   Thr Pro Ala Lys Arg Leu Glu Trp Val Ala Thr Ile Ser Ser Gly Gly Gly Thr Tyr Tyr Pro Asp Ser Val Lys Gly Arg Phe Thr Ile Ser Arg Asp Ala Arg Asn Thr Leu
          ACT CCG GCG AAG AGG CTG GAG TGG GTC GCA ACC ATT AGT AGT GGT GGT ACC TAC TAT CCA GAC AGT GTG AAG GGC CGA TTC ACC ATC TCC AGA GAC AAT ACC CTG
                                                Asn                 Arg Arg
                                                                    --A C--
3E12      --- --- --- --- --- --- --- --- --- ---  -A-                 --A C-- --- --- --- --- --- --- --- --- --- --- --- --- --- --- --- --- --- --- --- --- ---
VH 82-3   Ser His Gly Lys Ser Leu Glu Trp Ile Gly Asn Ile Asn Pro Tyr Tyr Gly Ser Thr Ser Tyr Asn Gln Lys Phe Lys Gly Lys Ala Thr Leu Thr Val Asp Lys Ser Ser Thr Ala
          AGC CAT GGA AAG AGC CTT GAG TGG ATT GGA AAT ATT AAT CCA TAC TAC TAT AGT AGT ACT AGC AAT CAG AAG TTC AAG GGC AAG GCC ACA TTG ACT GTA GAC AAA TCT AGC ACA GCC
                                                Lys                                                                   Gln
                                                --G                                                                   C--
A52       --- --- --- --- --- --- --- --- --- --- --- --- --- --- --- --- --- --- --- --- --- --- --A --- --- --- --- --- --- --- --- --- --- --- --- --- --- ---
VH 8-1    Lys Pro Gly Gln Gly Leu Glu Trp Ile Gly Tyr Ile Asn Pro Tyr Asn Asp Gly Thr Lys Tyr Asn Glu Lys Phe Lys Gly Lys Ala Thr Leu Thr Ser Asp Lys Ser Ser Thr Ala
          AAG CCT GGG CAG GGC CTT GAG TGG ATT GGA TAT ATT AAT CCT TAC AAT GAT GGT ACT AAG TAC AAT GAG AAG TTC AAA GGC AAG GCC ACA CTG ACT TCA GAC AAA TCC AGC ACA GCC
D30       --- --- --- --- --- --- --- --- --- --- --- --- --- --- --- --- --- --- --- --- --- --- --- --- --- --- --- --- --- --- --- --- --- --- --- --- --- ---
```

Third block (positions 240–335):

```
          240                 250                 260                 270                 280                 290      CDR3     300                 310                 320                 330
VH 33-2   Tyr Leu Gln Met Ser Ser Leu Arg Ser Glu Asp Thr Ala Met Tyr Tyr Cys Ala Arg Arg Arg Gly Ala Tyr Asp Gly Tyr Leu Asp Tyr Trp Gly
          TAC CTG CAA ATG AGC AGT CTG AGG TCT GAG GAC ACG GCC ATG TAT TAC TGT GCA AGA AGA CGA CGG GGA GCC TAT GAT GGT TAC CTT GAC TAC TGG GGC
                                                              Val                                       Asp Val Trp Gly
                                                              G-A                                       A-T CA- --GG TTC TTC
3E12      --- --- --- --- --- --- --- --- --- --- --- --- --- --- --- --- --- --- --- Val                 Asp Val Trp Gly
                                                                                       G-A                 A-T CA- --GG TTC TTC
                                                                                                           Asp Phe Phe
                                                                                                           --T G-- --- --
VH 82-3   Tyr Met Gln Leu Asn Ser Leu Thr Ser Glu Asp Ser Ala Val Tyr Tyr Cys Ala Arg Asp Gly Asp Gly Asp Leu Tyr Tyr Ala Met Asp Tyr Trp Gly Gln
          TAC ATG CAG CTC AAC AGC CTG ACA TCT GAG GAC TCT GCA GTC TAT TAC TGT GCA AGA AGG GAT GGT GAC CTT TAC TAT GCT ATG GAC TAC TGG GGT CAA
                                                                                  Gly Arg Arg Gly Tyr Phe
                                                                                  G-- AGG TTA CGA -GA GGA GGC TAC T-T --- --C ---
A52       --- --- --- --- --- --- --- --- --- --- --- --- --- --- --- --- --- --- --G
                                                                                  G--
VH 8-1    Tyr Met Glu Leu Ser Ser Leu Thr Ser Glu Asp Ser Ala Val Tyr Tyr Cys Ala Arg Gly Tyr Tyr Asp Tyr Tyr Ala Met Asp Tyr Trp
          TAC ATG GAG CTC AGC ACC CTG AGC TCT GAG GAC TCT GCG GCC TGT GCA GGT TGT AGG TAC GAC CGG GGC TAT TAC GCT ATG TGG
                                                              Asp                                   Arg Cys Arg Phe Ala     Tyr Trp
                                                              --A                                   C-G A-C CGG TTT GCT     --- --
D30
```

Figure 2. *(See following pages for parts C and D and legend.)*

C

```
        FR1                                                                                          CDR1
        1           10           20           30            40           50           60             70           80           90            100          110
        |            |            |            |             |            |            |              |            |            |             |            |
        Asp Val Leu Met Thr Gln Thr Pro Leu Ser Leu Pro Val Ser Leu Gly Asp Gln Ala Ser Ile Ser Cys  Arg Ser Ser Gln Ser Ile Val His Ser Asn Gly Asn Thr Tyr Leu Glu
VK10-3  GAT GTT TTG ATG ACC CAA ACT CCA CTC TCC CTG CCT GTC AGT CTT GGA GAT CAA GCC TCC ATC TCT TGC  AGA TCT AGT CAG AGC ATT GTA CAT AGT AAT GGA AAC ACC TAT TTA GAA

VK15-1  --- --- --- --- --- --- --- --- --- --- --- --- --- --- --- --- --- --- --- --- --- --- ---  --- --- --- --- --- --- --- --- --- --- --- --- --- --- --- ---

VK3-1   --- --- --- --- --- --- --- --- --- --- --- --- --- --- --- --- --- --- --- --- --- --- ---  --- --- --- --- --- --- --- --- --- --- --- --- --- --- --- ---

VK44-3  --- --- --- --- --- --- --- --- --- --- --- --- --- --- --- --- --- --- --- --- --- --- ---  --- --- --- --- --- --- --- --- --- --- --- --- --- --- --- ---

VK5-1   --- --- --- --- --- --- --- --- --- --- --- --- --- --- --- --- --- --- --- --- --- --- ---  --- --- --- --- --- --- --- --- --- --- --- --- --- --- --- ---

VK23-9  --- --- --- --- --- --- --- --- --- --- --- --- --- --- --- --- --- --- --- --- --- --- ---  --- --- --- --- --- --- --- --- --- --- --- --- --- --- --- ---

            Ile Val Leu         Ser     Thr Thr     Ser     Thr Pro         Arg Val     Leu              Ala                                                     His
VK43-2  --- A-- G-- C-A --T --G T-- --- AC- A-- --- T-- --G -C- -CA --- --- AG- -T- AGT C-T --C ---  --G G-C --C --A --T ---         --C --C             --C C-- C-C
            Ile Val Leu         Ser     Thr Thr     Ser     Thr Pro         Arg Val     Leu              Ala                                                     His
VK25-3  --- A-- G-- C-A --T --G T-- --- AC- A-- --- T-- --G -C- -CA --- --- AG- -T- AGT C-T --C ---  --G G-C --C --A --T ---         --C --C             --C C-- C-C


        FR2                                                          CDR2                         FR3
         120           130          140          150            160          170          180          190          200         210           220
          |             |            |            |              |            |            |            |            |           |             |
        Trp Tyr Leu Gln Lys Pro Gly Gln Ser Pro Lys Val Leu Ile Tyr  Lys Val Ser Asn Arg Phe Ser  Gly Val Pro Asp Arg Phe Ser Gly Ser Gly Ser Gly Thr Asp
VK10-3  TGG TAC CTG CAG AAA CCA GGC CAG TCT CCA AAG GTC CTG ATC TAC  AAA GTT TCC AAC CGA TTT TCT  GGG GTC CCA GAC AGG TTC AGT GGC AGT GGA TCA GGG ACA GAT

VK15-1  --- --- --- --- --- --- --- --- --- --- --- --- --- --- ---  --- --- --- --- --- --- ---  --- --- --- --- --- --- --- --- --- --- --- --- --- ---

VK3-1   --- --- --- --- --- --- --- --- --- --- --- --- --- --- ---  --- --- --- --- --- --- ---  --- --- --- --- --- --- --- --- --- --- --- --- --- ---
                                                    Leu
VK44-3  --- --- --- --- --- --- --- --- --- --- --- C-- --- --- ---  --- --- --- --- --- --- ---  --- --- --- --- --- --- --- --- --- --- --- --- --- ---
                    His                             Leu
VK5-1   --- --- --- --C --- --- --- --- --- --- --A C-- --- --- ---  --- --- --- --- --- --- ---  --- --- --- --T --- --- --- --- --- --- --- --- --- ---
                    His                             Leu
VK23-9  --- --- --- --C --- --- --- --- --- --- --A C-- --- --- ---  --- --- --- --- --- --- ---  --- --- --- --T --- --- --- --- --- --- --- --- --- ---

                Gln         Ser His Glu         Arg Leu         Lys  Tyr Ala     Gln Ser Ile          Ile     Ser         Gly     Arg
VK43-2  --- --T -AA --A --- T-- CAT G-- --- --- -G- C-T --C --- A-G  T-T -C- --- C-G TCC A-C ---  --- A-- --C TC- --- --- G-- --- C-- --- --- --- --- ---
                Gln         Ser His Glu         Arg Leu         Lys  Tyr Ala     Gln Ser Ile          Ile     Ser         Gly     Arg
VK25-3  --- --T -AA --A --- T-- CAT G-- --- --- -G- C-T --C --- A-G  T-T -C- --- C-G TCC A-C --- ---  A-- --C TC- --- --- G-- --- C-- --- --- --- --- ---


                                                                        CDR3
        230          240              250          260          270             280          290
         |            |                |            |            |               |            |
        Phe Thr Leu Lys Ile Ser Arg Val Glu Ala Glu Asp Leu Gly Val Tyr Tyr Cys  Phe Gln Gly Ser His Val
VK10-3  TTC ACA CTC AAG ATC AGC AGA GTG GAG GCT GAG GAT CTG GGA GTT TAT TAC TGC  TTT CAA GGT TCA CAT GTT

VK15-1  --- --- --- --- --- --- --- --- --- --- --- --- --- --- --- --- --- ---  --- --- --- --- --- ---

VK3-1   --- --- --- --- --- --- --- --- --- --- --- --- --- --- --- --- --- ---  --- --- --- --- --- --A

VK44-3  --- --- --- --- --- --- --- --- --- --- --- --- --- --- --- --- --- ---  --- --- --- --- --- ---

VK5-1   --- --- --- --- --- --- --- --- --- --- --- --- --- --- --- --- --- --T  --- --- --- --- --- ---

VK23-9  --- --- --- --- --- --- --- --- --- --- --- --- --- --- --- --- --- --T  --- --- --- --- --- ---

                    Ser     Asn Ser     Asp Thr         Phe     Met     Phe      Leu     Ser Asn Ser Trp
VK43-2  --- --T --- -GT --- -A- --T --- --T A-- --A --- T-T --- A-G --- -T- --T  C-A --G A-- AAC AGC TGG
                    Ser     Asn         Asp Thr         Phe     Met     Phe      Leu     Ser Asn Ser Trp
VK25-3  --- --T --- -GT --- -A- --T --- --T A-- --A --- T-T --- A-G --- -T- --T  C-A --G A-- AAC AGC TGG
```

D

Block 1 (FR1 / CDR1), positions 1–100

```
                                                                                              CDR1
FR1
1        10            20            30            40            50            60            70           80            90           100
Asp Ile Lys Met Thr Gln Ser Pro Tyr Ser Met Tyr Ala Ser Leu Gly Glu Arg Val Thr Ile Thr Cys   Lys Ala Ser Gln Asp Ile Ser Asn Tyr Leu Ser
GAC ATC AAG ATG ACC CAG TCT CCA TAT TCC ATG TAT GCA TCT CTA GGA GAG AGA GTC ACT ATC ACT TGC   AAG GCG AGT CAG GAC ATT AAT AGC TAT TTA AGC
VK33-2
                                                                                               Arg                              Ser      Asn
VK8-1                                                        --C           --G                  -G- --A  ---  --T  ---  -GC  -AT  ---  ---  -A-
VK82-3
```

Block 2 (FR2 / CDR2), positions 110–160

```
FR2                                                                            CDR2
110           120            130            140            150           160
Trp Phe Gln Lys Pro Gly Lys Ser Pro Lys Thr Leu Ile Tyr   Arg Ala Asn Arg Leu Val Asp
TGG TTC CAG AAA CCA GGG AAA TCT CCT AAG ACG CTG ATC TAT   CGT GCA AAC AGA TTG GTA GAT
VK33-2
                        Asp Gly Thr Val      Leu                   Tyr Thr Ser            His Ser
                        --AT GG- A-- GT-      --A CT-              TAC A-- TCA  ---  --A CAC TCA
VK8-1       --AT                                                   Tyr Thr Ser            Ala Ser
                        Ser Asp Ala           Leu Trp              TAC A-- TC-  -AC  C--  -CT TC-
VK82-3      T-- --AT GCC  --C  --A CTA TG-  --T ---
```

Block 3 (FR3), positions 170–220

```
FR3                                                                                        CDR1
170           180            190            200            210           220
Gly Val Pro Ser Arg Phe Ser Gly Ser Gly Ser Gly Gln Asp Tyr Ser Leu Thr Ile Ser
GGG GTC CCA TCA AGG TTC AGT GGC AGT GGA TCT GGG CAA GAT TAT TCT CTC ACC ATC AGC
VK33-2  Gly                                                     Thr
        Gly                               --G                   AC-         ---  ---
VK8-1   --A   ---       Ala                                     Thr Ser
              --A  ---  G-T T-C C--  --C  ---  ---  --G  ---  ---  ACC TC-  ---  --A  ---
VK82-3
```

Block 4 (CDR3), positions 230–290

```
                          CDR3
230           240           250            260            270            280            290
Ser Leu Glu Tyr Glu Asp Met Gly Ile Tyr Tyr Cys   Leu Gln Tyr Asp Glu Phe Pro Pro Thr
AGC CTG GAG TAT GAA GAT ATG GGA ATT TAT TGT   CTA CAG TAT GAT GAG TTT CCT CCC ACG
VK33-2  Asn               Pro      Ile Ala Thr      Gln          Ser Lys Leu    Trp
        A-- --- --A CC-  ---  --- -T  --C  C--  ---  -AG  ---  AG- A--  C--  ---  -G  TGG  ---
VK8-1   Val               Ala Ala Ser          Gln          Phe Thr Ser  Ser
        G-- --- --A GCT  --C  --- --- GCT C--  ---  -AG  ---  C--  AG-  ---  -CC  --A  T---
VK82-3  G-- --- --- GC-  --- --- --C  --C  -C-  ---  -AG  ---  -T-  AC-  AGT  -CC  --A  T---
```

Figure 2. Nucleotide sequences of heavy and light chains of anti-DNA antibodies. Identities of DNA sequences are indicated by horizontal bars. Amino acid translations are presented above the consensus. Identical amino acids at each position are omitted. The start of the FR region and CDRs (defined by Kabat et al. 1987) are offset from preceding sequences by a space and designated by abbreviations above the first codon in each region. V_H nucleotide sequences of clone H and I members are grouped and compared to their consensus sequence (A), and sequences of single isolates are compared to V_H sequences for which a homology search indicated highest homology (B). V_κ sequences of clone H and I members (C) or single isolates (D) are illustrated as above. Spaces are introduced to maximize alignment.

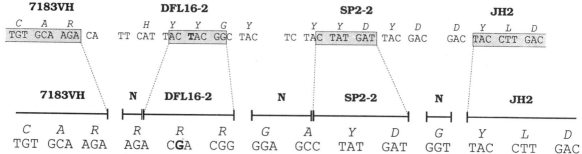

Figure 3. CDR3 region of antibody 33-2. (*Top*) The nucleotide sequence and amino acid translation (one-letter code) of portions of the V_H, D_H, and J_H gene segments used in the assembly of antibody 33-2 are shown. Shaded boxes designate regions of the gene segments used in the functionally rearranged gene (*bottom*). The CA nucleotides immediately adjacent to the canonical arginine codon at the end of V_H are the first two nucleotides of the heptamer recombinatorial signal sequence. The DFL16-2 and SP2-2 nucleotide sequences (*top*) are normally translated in the reading frame that favors tyrosine codons. In 33-2, the reading frame of DFL16-2 is shifted during assembly by one nucleotide from this preferred reading frame. Nucleotides resulting from N addition are designated. The T-to-G transversion in the DFL16-2-coding sequence is indicated by letters in boldface type.

anti-DNA antibodies in our survey are representative of the disease-associated specificity for dsDNA. This is demonstrated by a novel method (see above) that allows formation of antibody-DNA complexes in solution and measures the amount of antigen bound during this incubation (M.Z. Radic and M. Weigert, in prep.). With several antibodies that have been shown to recognize either ssDNA only or dsDNA and ssDNA (Pisetsky and Peters 1982; Stollar et al. 1986), our method produced parallel results.

Results of DNA binding by serial dilutions of supernatants from clone H hybridomas measured by the solution phase assay are shown in Figure 4. The six members of clone H are the same in affinity to ssDNA (Fig. 4A). On the other hand, clone H members fall into at least two categories with respect to dsDNA affinity (Fig. 4B). Clone members 3-1, 10-3, 15-1, and

44-3 bind dsDNA with low affinity, although they bind consistently above background levels seen for control antibodies, whereas clone members 5-1 and 23-9 have high affinity for dsDNA. The two members of clone I, 25-3 and 43-2, show a high preference for dsDNA, whereas the single isolates exhibit high (8-1 and 33-2) or exclusive (82-3) preference for ssDNA (data not shown).

Somatic Mutation

Sequence comparisons of members of clone H (Fig. 2A,C) show considerable diversity. This must be due to somatic mutation, as all clone members express the same V_H and V_κ genes. Assuming that clones H and I express the same V_H gene, somatic mutation must also account for V_H differences between these clones. In

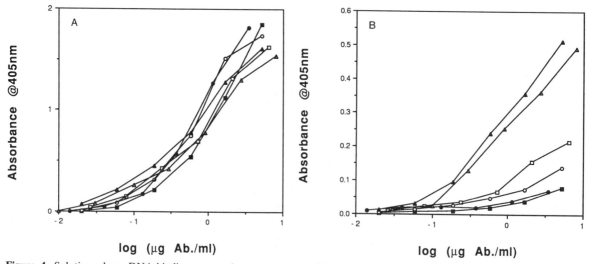

Figure 4. Solution phase DNA-binding assay of monoclonal anti-DNA antibodies. Denatured (*A*) and native (*B*) DNA specificity was assayed according to the procedures outlined in Methods. Duplicate determinations were performed for each concentration of antibody. The confidence interval for a value of the independent variable (antibody concentration), on the basis of a single dependent variable, was determined by simple linear regression using the IMSL subroutine RINPF, as discussed by Graybill (1976), and found in each case to be less than 10% of the measured absorbance. Members of clone H are designated as follows: 44-3 (□); 10-3(■); 3-1(○); 15-1(●); 23-9(△); 5-1(▲).

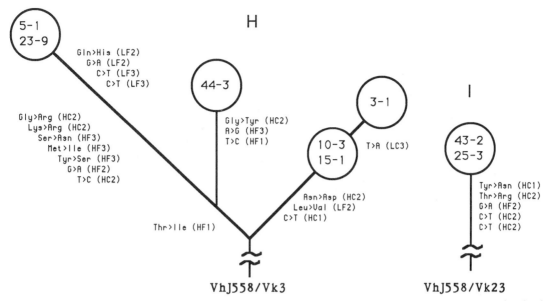

Figure 5. Genealogy relations between members of clones H and I. This genealogy was constructed from all shared and unique mutations observed in V_H sequences of clones H and I, and V_κ sequences from clone H hybrids. The pattern of mutations reflects the assumption that the same germ-line V_H gene is used by both clones. It reflects the assumption that mutations are single events and not parallel mutations. The lengths of the branches are roughly proportional to the number of mutations. Mutations along each branch are given in the direction of germ line to mutant; replacement mutations are shown as amino acid changes, and silent mutations as nucleotide changes. The chain ([H] heavy; [L] light) and domain (either F [framework] or C [complementarity-determining], along with the appropriate number) are indicated in parentheses.

Figure 5, we have indicated mutations in clone I that are based on differences from a consensus sequence derived from the V_H sequences of clones H and I. Because this consensus is derived from just two V_H sequences, the assignment of the mutations to clone I is arbitrary. These mutations may instead belong to clone H, in the reverted direction as that shown in Figure 5 for clone I. We prefer the direction of mutations shown in Figure 5, because this alternative yields residues that are unusual with respect to the extended consensus derived from all members of the V_H J558 family (Table 2; Kabat et al. 1987). It is also important to stress that mutations shared by these clones would escape our attention, as we do not know the germ-line sequence of the V_H gene expressed in clones H and I. This is also the case for the V_κ genes expressed in either clone H or I; hence, mutations shared by all members of a clone would be missed.

DISCUSSION

Oligoclonality of B cells participating in an autoimmune response has been found for rheumatoid factors (Shlomchik et al. 1987a) and anti-DNA antibodies (Shlomchik et al. 1987b, 1989; Marion et al. 1989). In a previous study of five MRL/*lpr* mice, we have found evidence for one to three anti-DNA cell clones per mouse, which account for the majority of anti-DNA antibodies. Here, we present sequences from 11 anti-DNA hybridomas from a single MRL/*lpr* mouse, the majority of which (8 of 11) are derived from two single B cells. This again demonstrates the dramatic prolifer-

ation of autoreactive B-cell clones. Given fusion efficiencies of 1 of 10^4 to 1 of 10^5 splenic B cells (Andersson and Melcher 1978; Claflin and Williams 1978), the clones contain between 10^5 and 10^6 anti-DNA B cells. Thereby fusion can easily capture clonal relatives in the form of hybridoma lines. In the cases where these clonal relatives show affinity or specificity differences, we have an opportunity to assess the influence of somatic mutation on specificity.

The distribution of replacement (R) mutations in clones H and I indicate selection: The percentage of replacement mutations in FR is low, suggesting that deleterious mutations were lost from the clone; the percentage of R mutations in CDR (R_{CDR}) is high, suggesting positive selection for the effect of these mutations on specificity. Indeed, the likelihood of obtaining at random the skewed distributions of mutations seen here is 0.07 for clone H and 0.05 for clone I, according to the method of Shlomchik et al. (1987b). Furthermore, the nature of replacement mutations observed argues for antigen selection. From theoretical considerations, Seeman et al. (1976) suggest a prominent role for arginine and asparagine in the interaction of proteins with DNA. Arginine is thought to be particularly suited for dsDNA binding because it has the potential to form two hydrogen bonds with bases in the major or minor groove, or with the sugar-phosphate backbone of DNA. Recently, direct evidence for such contacts has been obtained from X-ray crystallography of complexes between DNA and the *Eco*RI endonuclease (McClarin et al. 1986) or the phage 434 repressor (Aggarwal et al. 1988). Arginine and asparagine

Table 2. Comparison of Anti-DNA V_H J558 CDRs

Hybridoma	31	32	33	34	35	50	51	52	52a	53	54	55	56	57	58	59	60	61	62	63	64	65	76*	CDR 3
D20(a)	S	S	W	M	N	R	I	Y	P	G	D	G	D	T	N	Y	N	G	K	F	K	G	S	SGLRQLGLPFAY
DP7(a)	Ⓡ	–	–	–	–	–	–	–	–	–	–	–	–	–	–	–	–	–	–	–	–	–	Ⓡ	GGNRW–––
DP11(a)	Ⓝ	–	–	–	–	–	–	–	–	–	–	–	–	–	–	–	Y	–	–	–	–	–	Ⓡ	GGNRW–––
4H8(b)	–	–	–	–	–	–	–	–	–	–	–	–	–	–	–	–	–	–	–	–	–	D	–	ARSKYSYVLD–
1A11(b)	–	–	–	–	–	–	–	–	–	–	–	–	–	–	–	–	–	–	–	–	–	D	–	ARSKYSYVLD–
3H9(b)	–	–	–	–	–	–	–	–	–	Ⓡ	–	–	–	I	–	–	–	–	–	–	–	D	–	ARSKYSYVLD–
6N(a)	–	–	–	–	–	W	–	–	–	–	–	–	–	–	–	–	–	–	–	–	Ⓡ	–	–	YRRLFP–D–
3-1	D	Y	Y	–	–	–	V	N	–	S	N	–	G	–	T	–	D	Q	–	–	–	–	–	–YY–D–
44-3	D	Y	Y	–	–	–	V	N	–	S	N	–	Y	–	T	–	–	Q	–	–	–	–	–	–YY–D–
23-9	D	Y	Y	–	–	–	V	N	–	S	N	–	Ⓡ	–	T	–	–	Q	–	–	Ⓡ	–	Ⓝ	–YY–D–
25-3	D	Y	Ⓝ	–	–	–	V	N	–	S	N	–	G	–	Ⓡ	–	D	Q	–	–	–	–	–	RDYAMD–
H130(c)	G	Y	F	–	–	–	–	N	–	Y	N	–	–	–	F	–	–	Q	–	–	–	–	–	SRIYSNYYAD–
82-3	G	Y	K	–	–	N	–	N	–	Y	Y	–	S	–	S	–	–	Q	–	–	–	–	–	RDGLYYAMD–
A52(d)	G	Y	N	–	–	K	–	N	–	Y	Y	–	S	–	S	–	–	Q	–	–	–	–	–	GRLRR–GY–D–
8-1	S	Y	V	–	H	Y	–	N	–	Y	N	D	G	–	K	–	–	E	–	–	–	A	–	CRYDRGYYYAMD–
D30	S	Y	V	I	H	Y	–	N	–	Y	N	D	G	–	K	–	–	E	–	–	–	–	–	––A–

Amino acid residues are given in the single-letter code. Their positions are numbered according to the system adopted by Kabat et al. (1987). Replacements identified by comparison to clonal relatives or assumed on the basis of comparison to other clones that use the same germ-line gene, resulting in arginine or asparagine residues, are circled. D20 is thought to be identical (in the positions shown) to a germ-line sequence used by the top six hybridomas (Shlomchik et al., 1989) Sequences from clone members are arranged closer together than sequences from unrelated hybridomas. CDR3 sequences are aligned at their amino-terminal positions. Asterisk indicates that position 76 is not part of a conventional CDR; however, it may be involved in antigen binding (see text). Sources of sequence information are as follows: (a) Shlomchik et al. (1989); (b) Shlomchik et al. (1987b); (c) Trepicchio et al. (1987); (d) Eilat et al. (1988).

are the most frequent residues introduced into anti-DNA antibodies by somatic mutation. This is illustrated by members of one branch of clone H (represented by 5-1 and 23-9), which have higher specific binding to dsDNA than their siblings (Fig. 3B) and have R_{CDR} mutations to arginine (Fig. 5). Antibodies 5-1 and 23-9 also share an R mutation to asparagine at position 76 of FR3. This is the third instance in which a mutation at this codon has led to an arginine or asparagine substitution. DP7 and DP11 (Table 2) have mutated independently to arginine at this site. Because this FR site is highly variable (Kabat et al. 1987), mutations to arginine or asparagine are not the only substitutions allowed. Instead, the trend of these mutations suggests that residue 76 may play a role in antigen binding. This idea is plausible as residue 76 is located near the conventional CDR in antibody crystal structure (see Fig. 6). The trend toward residues relevant for DNA specificity is also found among the presumed R mutations of clone I, all of which are to arginine or asparagine. This remarkable enrichment in CDRs (or other potential binding sites) of residues capable of DNA binding gives strong support to the hypothesis that dsDNA is selecting for these mutants.

Here, as in the earlier survey, the majority of anti-DNA antibodies use members of the large J558 family, but other V_H families such as V_H 7183, as in the case of 33-2, are also used. Although different members of the J558 family are found, we have previously observed three independent examples that use a particular V_H J558 gene. Because of the high number of V_H genes (≥ 100 genes), recurrent use of a V_H cannot be a coincidence. Here, we find that a different member of the J558 family has been used in clones H and I. These repeats have prompted us to consider whether anti-DNA selects from just a subset of the J558 family. On the basis of the frequency of repeats in our entire sample, the number of J558 genes that contribute to anti-DNA is estimated to be 15 (15 is the maximum likelihood estimate; the range at 95% confidence is 9–42 [see Weigert and Riblet 1976]). Because the number of functional J558 genes is thought to be higher (Dildrop 1984), anti-DNA antibodies may use just a subset or prefer certain V_H genes of this family. The CDRs of V_H J558 genes used in anti-dsDNA antibodies are shown in Table 2. Although most CDR sites have residues found often in other V_H J558 genes, the arginine residue at site 50 is found in only a few germ-line V_H J558 genes (Dildrop 1984). Because of the role this residue can play in DNA binding, it may account for the preferential selection of these V_H regions.

In contrast to V_H, there is no evidence for preferential use of a V_κ gene. Fourteen V_κ groups are represented in our sample of 20 anti-DNA antibodies of independent clonal origin. The V_κ diversity is particularly interesting among anti-DNA antibodies that use the same V_H. Clones H and I share virtually the same V_H sequence, but their V_κ genes are from different groups (Fig. 2A,B). In our previous survey, three clones used the same V_H gene but used V_κ genes from

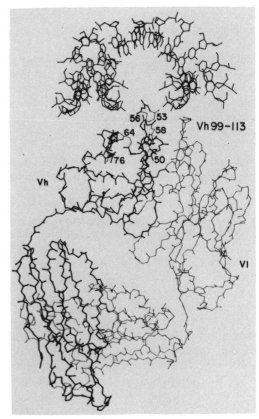

Figure 6. Hypothetical interaction between antibody and dsDNA. The Fab R19.9 fragment structure, as determined by X-ray crystallography (Lascombe et al. 1989), is simplified to represent the peptide backbones of the heavy chain (Vh, bold lines) and light chain (Vl, lighter lines). V_H residues discussed in the text are identified according to the numbering system of Kabat et al. (1987) and displayed by lighter lines. The 16-bp model structure of poly(dG)-(dC) (McCall et al. 1985) is displayed above the Fab fragment. The axis of the DNA is tilted out of the plane of view to emphasize the large major groove seen in this model.

different groups. Because these anti-DNA antibodies have similar specificities, it seems likely that most of the relevant contact residues are contributed by V_H. The patterns of mutation support this idea. The mutations that we presume to be important for dsDNA binding occur in the heavy, not the light, chain.

Table 2 displays CDR sequences of 16 anti-DNA antibodies with V_H J558. The replacements resulting from somatic mutation are highlighted. Substitutions giving rise to arginine occur at positions 53, 56, 58, and 64 of CDR2. Each CDR2 sequence may dictate a site at which arginine can contact DNA. Alternatively, each site at which arginine is found may have the potential to form a contact, regardless of CDR2 sequence. Support for the latter comes from antibodies 6N and 23-9 (Table 2), in which a mutation to arginine occurs at the same site. Assuming that this arginine was selected for by the DNA antigen, this site may be functional in spite of the eight CDR2 differences between these antibodies. CDR2 can also have more than one arginine or asparagine mutation (Table 2). Because these mutations may have been selected for sequentially by antigen, it also appears that the CDR2 is not limited to just one contact residue.

Mutations to arginine or asparagine also occur in different CDRs. Sites 31 and 33 of CDR1 and position 76 of FR3 are candidates for additional contact residues. Furthermore, junctional diversification is a mechanism capable of generating arginine residues in CDR3. With the exception of clone H (3-1, 44-3, and 23-9, Table 2), all CDR3s have at least one arginine residue. This is in sharp contrast with CDR3 compositions reported for antibodies with other specificities (0.3 arginines/CDR3; Shlomchik et al. 1989). As was found for CDR2, the precise location of arginines within CDR3 is not fixed, and even the size of this region can be extremely variable. Moreover, we often observe two or more arginines per CDR3, all of which may contribute incrementally to binding. An extreme example is shown here; antibody 33-2 has three contiguous arginine residues.

The location of arginine residues suggests that contacts with DNA can involve different sites in a CDR, as well as sites in different CDRs. This idea is plausible when one considers the structure of DNA. DNA is a polymer with recurrent epitopes (e.g., phosphodiester bonds). Therefore, arginines at different locations in the combining site may have the chance to bind the same epitope. In addition, arginine and asparagine can bind different epitopes in DNA. This is illustrated by the 3H9 antibody (Shlomchik et al. 1987b), in which a mutation to arginine increases affinity for ssDNA and creates specificity for dsDNA. This can be explained by a dual role for arginine: binding to phosphates (an epitope shared between ssDNA and dsDNA) and to base pairs (a feature that distinguishes dsDNA from ssDNA). Arginines at different anti-dsDNA combining sites may be limited to a particular dsDNA epitope. This is seen in 5-1 and 23-9 of clone H. In that case, the mutations to arginine increase affinity only for dsDNA. Thus, the orientation of these arginines may preclude binding to structures common to both dsDNA and ssDNA.

To gain a more accurate spatial view of antibody-dsDNA interactions, we have used computer modeling. As a first approximation to the structure of anti-DNA antibodies, we have chosen the X-ray crystal coordinates of Fab R19.9, a recently described fragment from an anti-arsonate antibody that is composed of a J558 heavy chain and a $V_\kappa 10$ light chain (Lascombe et al. 1989). Figure 6 shows the trajectory of the peptide backbones of those two subunits and identifies the positions corresponding to arginine 50 at the start of CDR2 and somatic replacements found in CDR2 and FR3 of anti-DNA antibodies. In addition, the relative position of CDR3 is indicated. It should be remembered that the reliability of our comparison is most compromised in this region, as CDR3 lengths and composition are extremely variable among different antibodies and thus lead to considerable structural differ-

ences. Nevertheless, the structure of Fab R19.9 (Lascombe et al. 1989) is useful in that it reveals that most of the CDR2 replacements observed in anti-DNA antibodies are clustered along the outside of the combining site and are thus suitably oriented for binding. This model also allows us to determine the distance between sites on the antibody that are thought to play a role in DNA binding and to ask whether they are compatible with the dimensions of the DNA molecule. These studies will be useful guides for the directed mutagenesis of sites presumed to be important for binding and X-ray analyses of antibody-DNA cocrystals.

CONCLUSION

Specificity for DNA is controlled by several genetic mechanisms. Certain V genes are preferentially selected. Thus, the germ-line repertoire can contribute, albeit to a modest extent, to the formation of anti-DNA. The amino acid sequence of CDR3 also plays a role, as seen by the correlation between arginine content and DNA specificity. Many anti-DNA antibodies have at least one arginine in CDR3, whereas the frequency of arginine is low in other antibodies. Superimposed upon anti-DNA V regions are somatic mutations, and one or more of the R_{CDR} mutations are to arginine or asparagine in all clones examined. The substitutions lead to increased affinity for DNA and can lead to dsDNA specificity.

These mechanisms contribute to DNA specificity at different phases of B-cell differentiation: Anti-DNA V regions resulting from V gene choice and junctional diversification mechanisms arise prior to clonal expansion; anti-DNA specificities resulting from somatic mutation arise in the phase of hypermutation as it occurs during clonal expansion. Because the contribution of these mechanisms can be disassociated in certain anti-DNA antibodies (Table 2), regulation of anti-DNA antibodies must occur both before and after antigen selection.

ACKNOWLEDGMENTS

Great thanks go to Dr. Condie E. Carmack for computer and illustration help, to Dr. Samuel Litwin for statistical analysis, to Ms. Anita Cywinski for sequencing assistance, to Ms. Violet Hay for tissue culture, and to Ms. Joni Brill-Dashoff for binding assays. This research was supported by grants from the National Institutes of Health (NIH, GM-20964 and CA-06927) and from an appropriation from the Commonwealth of Pennsylvania. M.Z.R. was supported by an NIH postdoctoral training grant (CA-09035), M.A.M. received research funds from the Cancer Research Institute through the Herman Vander Berg Fellowship, and J.E. was the Genetic Systems fellow of the Life Sciences Research Foundation.

REFERENCES

Aggarwal, A.K., D.W. Rodgers, M. Drottar, M. Ptashne, and S.C. Harrison. 1988. Recognition of a DNA operator by the repressor of phage 434: A view at high resolution. *Science* 242: 899.

Andersson, J. and F. Melchers. 1978. The antibody repertoire of hybrid cell lines obtained by fusion of X63-AG8 myeloma cells with mitogen-activated B-cell blasts. *Curr. Top. Microbiol. Immunol.* 81: 130.

Arana, R. and M. Seligmann. 1967. Antibodies to native and denatured deoxyribonucleic acid in systemic lupus erythematosis. *J. Clin. Invest.* 46: 1867.

Badley, J.E., G.A. Bishop, T. St. John, and J.A. Frelinger. 1988. A simple, rapid method for the purification of poly A + RNA. *Biotechniques* 6: 114.

Brodeur, P. and R. Riblet. 1984. The immunoglobulin heavy chain variable region in the mouse I. 100 IgH-V genes comprise 7 families of homologous genes. *Eur. J. Immunol.* 14: 922.

Claflin, J.L. and K. Williams. 1978. Mouse myeloma–spleen cell hybrids: Enhanced hybridization frequencies and rapid screening procedures. *Curr. Top. Microbiol. Immunol.* 81: 107.

Clarke, S., K. Huppi, D. Ruezinsky, L. Staudt, W. Gerhard, and M.G. Weigert. 1985. Inter- and intraclonal diversity in the antibody response to influenza hemagglutinin. *J. Exp. Med.* 161: 687.

Coleclough, C., D. Cooper, and R.P. Perry. 1980. Rearrangement of immunoglobulin heavy chain genes during B-lymphocyte development as revealed by studies of mouse plasmacytoma cells. *Proc. Natl. Acad. Sci.* 77: 1422.

Datta, S.K., Y. Naparstek, and R.S. Schwartz. 1986. In vitro production of an anti-DNA idiotype by lymphocytes of normal subjects and patients with systemic lupus erythematosus. *Clin. Immunol. Immunopathol.* 38: 302.

Dildrop, R. 1984. A new classification of mouse V_H sequences. *Immunol. Today* 5: 85.

Dixon, F.J., M.B.A. Oldstone, and G. Tonietti. 1971. Pathogenesis of immune complex glomerulonephritis of New Zealand mice. *J. Exp. Med.* 134: 65.

Eilat, D., D.M. Webster, and A.R. Rees. 1988. V region sequences of anti-DNA and anti-RNA autoantibodies from N2B/NZW F_1 mice. *J. Immunol.* 141: 1745.

Geliebter, J., R.A. Zeff, R.W. Melvold, and S.G. Nathanson. 1986. Mitotic recombination in germ cells generated two major histocompatibility complex mutant genes shown to be identical by RNA sequence analysis: K^{bm9} and K^{bm6}. *Proc. Natl. Acad. Sci.* 83: 3371.

Graybill, F.A. 1976. *Theory and application of the linear model*. Dixburg Press, North Scituate, Massachusetts.

Harbeck, R.J., E.J. Bardana, P.F. Kohler, and R.I. Carr. 1973. DNA:anti-DNA complexes: Their detection in systemic lupus erythematosus sera. *J. Clin. Invest.* 52: 789.

Kaartinen, M. and O. Makela. 1985. Reading of D genes in variable frames as a source of antibody diversity. *Immunol. Today* 6: 324.

Kabat, E.A., T.T. Wu, M. Reid-Miller, H.M. Perry, and K.S. Gottesman. 1987. *Sequences of proteins of immunological interest.* U.S. Government Printing Office, Bethesda, Maryland.

Kurosawa, Y. and S. Tonegawa. 1982. Organization, structure, and assembly of immunoglobulin heavy chain diversity DNA segments. *J. Exp. Med.* 155: 201.

Lascombe, M.-B., P.M. Alzari, G. Boulot, P. Tougard, C. Berek, S. Haba, E.M. Rosen, A. Nisonoff, and R.J. Poljak. 1989. Three-dimensional structure of Fab R19.9, a monoclonal murine antibody specific for the p-axobenzenearsonate group. *Proc. Natl. Acad. Sci.* 86: 607.

Marcu, K.B., N.A. Banerji, R. Penncavage, and N. Arnheim. 1980. 5' Flanking region of immunoglobulin heavy chain constant region genes displays length heterogeneity in germlines of inbred mouse strains. *Cell* 22: 187.

Marion, T.N., A.L.M. Bothwell, D.E. Briles, and C.A. Janeway, Jr. 1989. IgG anti-DNA autoantibodies within an individual autoimmune mouse are the products of clonal selection. *J. Immunol.* 142: 4269.

McCall, M., T. Brown, and O. Kennard. 1985. The crystal structure of d(G-G-G-G-C-C-C-C); a model for poly(dG), poly(dC). *J. Mol. Biol.* 182: 385.

McClarin, J.A., C.A. Frederick, B.-C. Wang, P. Greene, H.W. Boyer, J. Grable, and J.M. Rosenberg. 1986. Structure of the DNA-*Eco*RI endonuclease recognition complex at 3Å resolution. *Science* 234: 1526.

McKean, D., K. Huppi, M. Bell, L. Staudt, W. Gerhard, and M. Weigert. 1984. Generation of antibody diversity in the immune response of Balb/c mice to influenza virus hemagglutinin. *Proc. Natl. Acad. Sci.* 81: 3180.

Morimoto, C., H. Sano, T. Abe, M. Homma, and A. Steinberg. 1982. Correlation between clinical activity of systemic lupus erythematosus and the amounts of DNA in DNA/anti-DNA antibody immune complexes. *J. Immunol.* 139: 1960.

Newell, N., J.E. Richards, P.W. Tucker, and F.R. Blattner. 1980. J genes for heavy-chain immunoglobulins of mouse. *Science* 209: 1128.

Notman, D.D., N. Kurata, and E.N. Tan. 1974. Profiles of antinuclear antibodies in systemic rheumatic diseases. *Ann. Intern. Med.* 83: 464.

Pankewycz, O.G., P. Migliorini, and M. Madaio. 1987. Polyreactive autoantibodies are nephritogenic in murine lupus nephritis. *J. Immunol.* 139: 3287.

Pisetsky, D.S. and D.V. Peters. 1982. A simple enzyme-linked immunosorbent assay for antibodies to native DNA. *J. Immunol. Methods* 41: 187.

Pisetsky, D.S., S.A. Caster, J.B. Roths, and E.D. Murphy. 1982. *lpr* gene control of the anti-DNA response. *J. Immunol.* 128: 2322.

Potter, M., J.B. Newell, S. Rudikoff, and E. Haber. 1982. Classification of mouse V_κ groups based on the partial amino acid sequence to the first invariant tryptophan: Impact of 14 new sequences from IgG myeloma proteins. *Mol. Immunol.* 19: 1619.

Raz, E., M. Brezis, E. Rosenmann, and D. Eilat. 1989. Anti-DNA antibodies bind directly to renal antigens and induce kidney dysfunction in the isolated perfused rat kidney. *J. Immunol.* 142: 3076.

Reed, K.C. and D.A. Mann. 1985. Rapid transfer of DNA from agarose gels to nylon membranes. *Nucleic Acids Res.* 13: 7207.

Seeman, N.C., J.M. Rosenberg, and A. Rich. 1976. Sequence-specific recognition of double helical nucleic acids by proteins. *Proc. Natl. Acad. Sci.* 73: 804.

Shlomchik, M.J., A.H. Aucoin, D.S. Pisetsky, and M.G. Weigert. 1987a. Structure and function of anti-DNA autoantibodies derived from a single autoimmune mouse. *Proc. Natl. Acad. Sci.* 84: 9150.

Shlomchik, M.J., A. Marshak-Rothstein, C.B. Wolfowicz, T.L. Rothstein, and M.G. Weigert. 1987b. The role of clonal selection and somatic mutation in autoimmunity. *Nature* 328: 805.

Shlomchik, M.J., D. Nemazee, V. Sato, J. Van Snick, D. Carson, and M.G. Weigert. 1986. Variable region sequences of murine IgM anti-IgG monoclonal autoantibodies (Rheumatoid Factors): A structural explanation for the high frequency of IgM anti-IgG B cells. *J. Exp. Med.* 164: 407.

Shlomchik, M., M. Mascelli, H. Shan, M.Z. Radic, D. Pisetsky, A. Marshak-Rothstein, and M. Weigert. 1989. Anti-DNA antibodies from autoimmune mice arise by clonal expansion and somatic mutation. *J. Exp. Med.* (in press).

Souroujon, M., M.E. White-Scharf, J. Andre-Schwartz, M.L. Gefter, and R.S. Schwartz. 1988. Preferential autoantibody reactivity of the preimmune B cell repertoire in normal mice. *J. Immunol.* **140:** 4173.

Stollar, B.D., G. Zon, and R.W. Pastor. 1986. A recognition site on synthetic helical oligonucleotides for monoclonal anti-native DNA autoantibody. *Proc. Natl. Acad. Sci.* **83:** 4469.

Tan, E.M. 1982. Autoantibodies to nuclear antigens (ANA)—Their immunobiology and medicine. *Adv. Immunol.* **33:** 167.

Tan, E.M., P.H. Schur, R.I. Carr, and H.G. Kunkel. 1966. Deoxyribonucleic acid (DNA) and antibodies to DNA in the serum of patients with systemic lupus erythematosis. *J. Clin. Invest.* **45:** 1732.

Trepicchio, W., A. Maruya, and K.J. Barrett. 1987. The heavy chain genes of a lupus anti-DNA autoantibody are encoded in the germ line of a nonautoimmune strain of mouse and conserved in strains of mice polymorphic for this gene locus. *J. Immunol.* **139:** 3139.

Weigert, M. and R. Riblet. 1976. Genetic control of antibody variable regions. *Cold Spring Harbor Symp. Quant. Biol.* **32:** 161.

Winfield, J.B., I. Faiferman, and D. Koffler. 1977. Avidity of anti-DNA antibodies in serum and IgG glomerular eluates from patients with systemic lupus erythematosus: Association of high avidity anti-native DNA antibody with glomerulonephritis. *J. Clin. Invest.* **59:** 90.

Wysocki, L., T. Manser, and M. Gefter. 1986. Somatic evolution of variable region structures during an immune response. *Proc. Natl. Acad. Sci.* **83:** 1847.

Summary: The New Pragmatics of Immunology

J.C. HOWARD

Agricultural and Food Research Council, Institute of Animal Physiology and Genetics,
Cambridge Research Station, Babraham, Cambridge CB2 4AT, United Kingdom

Even allowing for various readings of his famous title, it must be admitted that Jerne had a point (Jerne 1968). Does the antibody problem not still look, with all the mitigations of hindsight, to have been the most important issue in immunology? There was something both teasing and high-minded in the paradox of a finite and, for all we knew, hard-pressed genome, bound to colinearity and structural determinism by the Central Dogma, bursting its bounds to provide an antibody repertoire of virtually infinite dimensions. The antibody problem went to the heart of the matter; it was a profound problem, and it would have a profound solution. Once known, however, the rest of the subject would, it seemed, quickly unravel as a succession of lesser and dependent problems were solved in its light. In 1967 at Cold Spring Harbor, then, with clonal selection already ten years old and, if not fully demonstrated, then certainly not refuted, and with the outline structure of the antibody molecule delineated, we might well accept that a visionary like Jerne was already Waiting for the End.

By saying what he said, then, there, and in that way, Jerne created a kind of agenda for any summarizer at a Cold Spring Harbor symposium on immunology. We are, it seems, destined to ask at this stage in the proceedings where we stand in relation to the end, and by the same token, to come to terms with the idea that immunology has an end, a stage when outstanding problems are trivial or no longer distinctive to the field. My job today is not to ask whether Jerne was right to be waiting for the end—I take it for granted that he was—but rather to focus the vast range of material from this magnificent meeting under a few headings and then to see how the great problems of immunology stand in the light of it.

TELEOLOGY

Can there be any doubt that the selective force that drives the evolution of the immune system is resistance to exogenous disease organisms? Parasites create exceptional problems for their hosts. Parasite genomes are wildly unpredictable: Viruses, bacteria, protozoa, and fungi are not threats that can be predicted in any molecular detail. They evolve at a formidable rate relative to their hosts, so host strategies of resistance are always at risk of being breached. Because the penalty for failure is so severe, selective forces in host-parasite interactions are as intense as any confronted by most animal and especially mammalian species. The evolution of massive polymorphism in host resistance systems is direct evidence for the genetic load imposed on vertebrate populations by pathogens. One of the many delights of the Bjorkman–Wiley[1] class I MHC molecule structure is the revelation in detail of one molecular target for pathogen-dependent selection. Histocompatibility antigens, we now know, make direct molecular contact with the pathogenic environment via peptide binding. The selective demands made by this confrontation result in intense dynamism in the underlying genes, exacerbated, as Parham pointed out (Parham et al.), by the intimate relationship between thymic histocompatibility antigen expression and the T-cell repertoire. It seems likely that here is to be found at least a part of the explanation for the continuing existence and dynamics of nonclassic class I genes.

The sheer prodigality of invention that has gone into the construction of the adaptive immune system is astonishing. As Hood pointed out in his opening remarks (Hunkapiller et al.), although the endpoint of a diverse repertoire is achieved in all three cases, and although the principles and machinery of rearrangement and allelic exclusion are held in common, the genomic and epigenetic bases for antibody diversity in shark, bird, and mammal are amazingly different. The (at least) mammalian ability to hunt the antigen while an immune response is going on, by somatic hypermutation of the rearranged heavy- and light-chain V regions, is a further refinement. I used to think of this mechanism simply as a device for the progressive improvement of affinity of response against a stable antigen. I was therefore enlightened by Rajewsky's suggestion (Rajewsky et al.) that the adaptive significance of the mutator system may rather derive from its ability to track microbial evolution occurring in vivo under selective pressure from the immune system. We already know that the immune system exerts a strong reciprocal pressure on pathogens in vivo, and that trypanosomes and other organisms, threatened by the power of the rearranging genes of the vertebrate immune system, have gone to the length of evolving their own rearranging gene system in return.

This was not a meeting marked by controversy, so the heat was especially noticeable when Maizels pro-

---

[1] Except in this one case, which needs no other description, undated references are to work presented by speakers at the symposium. Dated references help to make specific points, but are far from exhaustive.

posed (David and Maizels) that V-gene somatic hypermutation is due to mitotic gene conversion rather than to simple base replacement. Despite forceful arguments against this position, however, it is admittedly in harmony with the avian mechanism of V-gene repertoire generation and is well-documented also in the class I MHC multigene family. If targeted, tissue-specific, and developmentally regulated somatic hyperconversion is a mechanism in one part of the immune system, it would be wise to explore the possibility that it may operate in other relevant contexts.

I want to come back to the question of polymorphism in the immune system and to remind myself that the MHC, certainly the *locus classicus*, is not the only case we have. Indeed, whereas MHC polymorphism is reasonably well explained, at least in general terms, there is perhaps only a single well-documented case where a change in MHC allelic frequency can be directly attributed to differential resistance to a specific pathogen (Briles et al. 1977). In this context, the properties of staphylococcal enterotoxins are of exceptional interest (Kappler et al.), first because they identify a specific group of pathogens that may be a cause of polymorphism in the wild, and second because they illustrate the bizarre opportunism that intense selection pressures generate. On the one hand, we have bacteria dropping their enterotoxic hand grenades down the very barrel of the T-cell receptor gun, whereas on the other, we have the mammalian hosts apparently inventing the *Mls* loci to wipe out whole batteries of T-cell receptors by self-tolerance before the enterotoxins can get at them. The whole story is extremely odd, and no doubt much of it is not properly understood. Why, for example, is it in the staphylococcal interest to have the immune system blow up in its face? Are the additional non-MHC-linked loci that seem to fine-tune V_β ratios both by negative and positive selection (Palmer et al.) also part of a pathogen-related polymorphism?

I want to deal briefly, as the symposium did, with a different legacy from Jerne, namely the network. Surely, few would dispute that this idea is one of the most intelligent that anyone has ever had about the immune system. However, even if network considerations are generally applicable and causative, one can often get along surprisingly well without them. Attitudes to the network fall into the empiricist and structuralist schools. The empiricist immune response is imposed on an immune system in a state of rest by the introduction of a foreign antigen to which the organism is not tolerant. The response is self-limited by negative feedback via competition for limiting antigen. Affinity maturation is an adaptive consequence of the self-limitation process. Apart from the induction of stable memory, the immune system reverts to a state of rest. The structuralist immune response is an adjustment to a dynamic equilibrium whose moving parts are the specific receptors of the immune system. All receptors are both paratope and epitope, antigen is just another epitope, and self-limitation, that is, restoration of the approximate state before antigen, can hardly be

achieved because all specific components of the lymphon are in principle involved. The signs at this symposium seemed favorable for the best possible resolution between these two opposed visions, namely that both are partly right. It is the clear delineation of the Ly-1 (CD5)-positive B-cell subset (Herzenberg and Stall; Rajewsky et al.) that seems set fair to break the impasse. This B-cell subset develops early from a distinct precursor, is self-sustaining in the periphery, and favors IgM antibodies expressing germ-line V genes normally associated with natural autoantibodies. Early natural autoantibodies are connected by a set of anti-idiotypic relationships not seen in typical induced antibodies of the empiricist immune response (Coutinho et al.). It is a natural, but not yet formal, conclusion that the low-affinity natural antibody network is a distinctive product of the CD5 B-cell subset. The network is thus a part of the immune system, but not the whole. Although at least some idiotypic components of the adult immune response can be influenced by neonatal exposure to antigen (Kearney et al.), in the absence of evidence for full idiotypic connectivity between the two immune systems it seems unlikely that the network is absolutely required for the development of the adult system. A specific B-cell subset with distinctive properties suggests a distinctive function. The existence of the adult immune system shows that connectivity is not a prerequisite for immune function. My guess is that the special function of the juvenile network is to be preadaptive for bacterial infection. Surely it is important and relevant to this question that so many of the connected idiotypes of the juvenile network are components of antibodies with known specificity for bacterial polysaccharide coat structures. Even though responses against at least some bacterial polysaccharides are notoriously inefficient in newborns, the idea of a preadaptive network for constitutive protection against juvenile bacterial infection is attractive. The preadaptation, according to this idea, consists in the anti-idiotypic autoactivation of this cell population, producing a natural serum pool of antibacterial antibodies in the absence of infection. Presumably, the germ-line sequences of antibodies involved in the juvenile network must be selected both on the basis of their potential activity against carbohydrate moieties and as participants in an idiotypic network: a formidable package of structural conditions, but as already emphasized, pathogen-dependent selection is a hard taskmaster.

The network antedated the discovery of the CD5 B-cell subset. For γ/δ T cells, the delineation of the subset (Tonegawa et al.; Houlden et al.; Bluestone; Cooper et al.; Hünig et al.; Winoto and Baltimore; P. Bleicher, pers. comm.) has antedated the function. γ/δ cells appear before α/β cells in thymic ontogeny, drawing their receptors from a distinctive pool of V genes with little or no junctional diversity. γ chain usage, at least, seems to be remarkably ordered both in time and space, a challenging problem in regulated differentiation. T cells with γ/δ receptors occupy distinctive niches in the tissues, especially associated with epithelia. γ/δ cells provide no help for antibody formation and are unable to participate in the induction of adjuvant arthritis or skin graft rejection. So what do they recognize? It has been pointed out (Janeway et al. 1988) that since γ/δ cells are, if anything, $CD8^+$, they may have a predisposition to recognize class I molecules. Since nonclassical class I molecules represent a ligand without an obvious cell to recognize it, and since γ/δ cells have no obvious ligand to recognize, it is tempting to relate the one to the other. Certainly, it seems surprising how many of the relatively small number of γ/δ recognition specificities identified have turned out to be nonclassical class I molecules. Is this result informative about function? We shall need to know much more about the ontogeny of γ/δ cells before answering. Cooper et al. showed that chicken γ/δ cells express high levels of receptor very early in ontogeny, apparently not passing through a recognizable phase of low expression. Furthermore, they seem to rush through the thymic cortex at a tremendous rate. They are certainly never seen as $CD4^+/CD8^+$ double positives. Do these properties mean that they are not subject to thymic selection? We need to know the specificities generated by random combinations of T-cell receptor chains. Marrack and colleagues (Blackman et al. 1986) made a start in this direction a few years ago, but this experiment could be done better now, using randomly selected germ-line V regions in random combinations. Are they alloreactive? If so, how accurately? That is, do they specialize in class II or class I in the absence of CD4 or CD8 co-receptors? We do not know the answers to these important questions for α/β cells, let alone for γ/δ cells. The spectrum of reactivity of γ/δ cells may reflect a general adaptive propensity for germ-line T-cell receptors, whether α/β or γ/δ, to recognize molecules built on Bjorkman–Wiley principles. There are, after all, more different nonclassical class I molecules expressed in a mouse than all the classical class I and class II put together, so on a random hit basis one would expect more nonclassical class I receptors than anything else. At the moment, there is no reason to believe that the γ/δ T-cell-receptor repertoire is intrinsically different from the α/β repertoire. What *is* different, however, is the apparent homogeneity of the γ/δ constant and variable segment usage in certain tissue sites, notably the dendritic epithelial cells of skin and the intraepithelial cells of the genital tract. Do these cells represent the product rather than the precursors of a γ/δ immune response? Otherwise, by the absence of diversity we know that we are not dealing with a Burnetian immune system at all. If they are generated as the products of an immune response, where is that response induced, and by what antigen? We have far more questions than answers. At least we can be sure from the epithelial distribution of γ/δ cells that the γ/δ system will not break the generalization of an outward-looking immune system.

Immunology always has the capacity to surprise, but the categorical identification of what amounts virtually to two new immune systems, the CD5 B-cell network and the γ/δ T-cell system, within the last three years must count as remarkable even by immunology's standards.

ANTIGEN PRESENTATION

Watson proposed in his opening remarks that if 1967 was the antibody symposium and 1976 was T cells, then 1989 was the symposium on antigen presentation. Certainly, it would be difficult to overstate the impact on the antigen presentation problem of the solution of the crystal structure of HLA-A2. It is fair to say that this impact had been pretty much assimilated by 1989, but, nevertheless, this symposium was, to a great extent, a celebration of it.

The HLA-A2 molecular structure provides a focus for three grand explanations that have come to maturity in the post-Bjorkman–Wiley era. One must remember that the published structure of HLA-A2 contained the unexplained density in the groove. Now Wiley and colleagues have presented the structure of HLA-Aw68 as well, and the mysterious stranger is there again. The explanatory power of the structure would have been similar without the extra density, but perhaps it would have left a larger residue of skepticism.

First, the HLA-A2 structure with the extra density seems to embody the essential basis of the relationship between the nominal antigen and the MHC molecule, a question so long a matter of more or less clumsy hand-waving and tedious blackboard symbols. There is, as we know, only one variable T-cell receptor, and Davis and Bjorkman (1988) have pointed out that it must interact both with the nominal peptide and with the helices of the MHC molecule, although in the absence of any precise information, there is still enough room to speculate about exactly how (Kourilsky et al.). Evidently the focus of polymorphic substituents on the groove suggests the physical basis for the cellular phenomenon of MHC restriction.

Second, the molecular structure explains the evolutionary strategy of the MHC glycoproteins. The distribution of variation in MHC molecules has been largely if not totally accounted for. In particular, the localization of intensely polymorphic residues in groove-oriented positions, as I indicated above, seems to be perfectly explained by their key property of making direct contact with peptide sequence of pathogenic origin.

Third, the existence of the extra density has caused an almost universally accepted redefinition of the concepts of self-tolerance and allo-aggression. If MHC molecules present autologous peptides derived from a whole range of self-proteins, then the unresponsiveness of self-tolerance is only completely defined if both components of these complexes are specified. Kourilsky and colleagues have designated this vision "the peptidic self." It follows from this model that if tolerance is complex and MHC restricted, then so is alloreactivity. A major alloantigen is redefined as the modified set of endogenous complexes presented by a different restriction element. I do not want to reawaken old quarrels at a time when we are basking in a mood of consensus and reconciliation, but it still seems worth pointing out that this model has been available in all its essential details and implications for a decade (Matzinger and Bevan 1977; Matzinger 1981). How powerful the visual image of the HLA-A2 structure has been in focusing attention on this subtle and illuminating interpretation of tolerance and alloreactivity!

Altered-self models of MHC restriction had terrible difficulty with the formation of multiple antigen/MHC complexes from antigens with determinate structures. Randomly cleaved peptides, however, do not necessarily have fully determinate structures and can use the binding groove of the MHC molecule as a template during folding. One would guess from the promiscuity of so many analyzed restriction elements that MHC restriction must in part reflect the conformational plasticity of peptide sequences. In view of the close similarity between the α carbon traces of the peptide-binding domains of HLA-A2 and HLA-Aw68, and the high relative density of mass adjacent to the groove, it is unlikely that there is much reciprocal plasticity. MHC molecules may be stabilized by the presence of a binding peptide, but there is little ambiguity about the stable structure once achieved. It is the peptide that has to conform, not the MHC molecule.

There is an historical irony about this conclusion. One of immunology's greatest theoretical victories was its escape from template models of antibody function. The clonal selection theory was the result, born of a rigid post-Central Dogma structural determinism, in which antibody and antigen obeyed the same rules, and selection from a large repertoire was used to make the one conform to the other. The consequence of that was to change the focus of the antibody problem from the antibodies themselves to the cellular and genetic mechanisms underlying their formation. The selectionist paradigm has completely dominated immunology since then; yet the proposed relationship between the MHC molecule and the peptide is attractively close to the model originally proposed by Pauling (1940) for the antigen-antibody relationship, where a structurally indeterminate antibody was stabilized by interaction with a random determinate antigen.

There are, of course, very good reasons to try to establish rules by which binding and thus potentially antigenic peptides might be defined a priori. However, after an enormous amount of peptide making, the only rule seems to be that there is not going to be a structural rule. Maryanski et al. definitively disposed of an already troubled α-helix theory by showing that a pentaproline-substituted peptide could replace the native peptide in her restricted presentation system, a result consistent with Wiley's vision of the importance of subsites in determining peptide-binding specificity. The distinct optimized motifs for I-A and I-E binding peptides described by Grey et al. suggest that structural

features of the MHC molecule may influence which peptides bind, but do not reveal the principle. Clearly, this important subject needs new theory and new experimentation (Dornmair et al.), and unique peptide MHC complexes will have to be crystallized, a goal that seems closer for class II molecules than for class I.

ANTIGEN PROCESSING

The principle that antigens presented to T cells are normally more or less structurally disordered peptides stabilized in Bjorkman grooves applies equally to class I and class II MHC molecules. We now know that this similarity at the endpoint hides a profound difference between the biological roles and cell biology of these two classes of molecules. The original distinction was between protein of endogenous biosynthetic origin processed for access to class I, and protein of exogenous origin processed for access to class II (Morrison et al. 1986). New experiments by Braciale et al. on the processing of influenza virus hemagglutinin biosynthesized in human cells show that this form of words was simplistic. The necessary condition for access to a processing compartment destined for class II presentation is that the protein must be competent to reach the cell membrane. Thus, it is likely that peptides of endogenous proteins presented by class II will normally be derived from proteins that are destined for membrane expression. Immunoglobulin is a well-documented example (e.g., Weiss and Bogen 1989), and perhaps minor histocompatibility antigens restricted by class II such as H-Y are also proteins destined for the membrane. There appears to be no such limitation on access to the class-I-dependent processing pathway. Any protein or even peptide (Fischer Lindahl et al.; Braciale et al.; Boon et al.) synthesized in the cell seems to have access to class I presentation. One would like to be able to generalize that even transient presence in the cytoplasm, and not endogenous biosynthesis as such, is both necessary and sufficient for access to the class I pathway. As Bevan has shown (Carbone et al.), typical exogenous proteins such as bovine serum albumin can be presented as peptides through class I molecules, as long as they are introduced, exogenously, directly into the cytoplasm. For membrane and secreted proteins a proportion of biosynthesis is certainly from free ribosomes, and this anomalous material presumably provides the source of peptides presented by class I. Fischer Lindahl's *Mtf* raises an acute version of this problem, since the nonclassical class I restricted peptide is extremely hydrophobic and is presumably inserted into the inner membrane of the mitochondrion, where the protein is synthesized. In this case, is the mitochondrially synthesized material released into the cytoplasm during mitochondrial turnover?

How much subsidiary molecular and cellular apparatus is devoted to enabling protein derivatives to gain access to MHC molecules? Certainly catabolic systems are involved in processing through both pathways, and one would anticipate that these will turn out to be old and familiar. So far, this expectation seems to be fulfilled for the class II pathway, where cathepsins B and D have both been implicated in endocytic processing and colocalized with recently internalized antigen (Blum et al.; Brodsky et al.; Berzofsky et al.). The degradative mechanism that contributes peptides to the class I pathway is unknown. Initial enthusiasm for the ubiquitin-dependent protein degradation pathway must be tempered by Bevan's demonstration that bovine serum albumin delivered to the cytoplasm with all its ϵ-NH$_2$ groups fully methylated, and presumably inaccessible to lysine-dependent ubiquitination, is processed and presented through class I quite normally (Carbone et al.).

The peptide-loading process is a mystery in both pathways. N. Koch and colleagues (pers. comm.) implicate invariant chain (Ii) as an essential participant in the access of peptides derived from an exogenous antigen to class II molecules, but this cannot be shown in all systems. Cresswell et al. showed that Ii is associated with multimeric complexes of recently synthesized class II α and β chains in a post-Golgi "delay" compartment, release from which is associated with detachment of Ii mediated by a specific proteolytic step. Although this event is probably an immediate precondition for peptide loading, it still fails to clarify what precisely the invariant chain is doing. Despite the normally cytosolic origin of the peptides, loading in the class I pathway presumably happens in the endoplasmic reticulum (ER). The biosynthesis of class I MHC molecules seems to be perfectly conventional; the protein shows a typical leader sequence, and translation is from membrane-bound polysomes. Thus, the nascent protein is presumably translocated directly into the ER and has no opportunity to interact with peptides in the cytosol. The presentation of cytosolic peptides on class I molecules seems, therefore, to demand the existence of a transporter capable of translocating peptides of unpredictable sequence from the cytosol into the ER lumen. There is presently no direct information as to the identity of such a transport system, but it seems unlikely to be signal recognition particle (SRP), both because of the absence of a clear requirement for hydrophobic structure in peptides presented by class I molecules, and also because from Bevan's results (Carbone et al.) we know that it is not necessary that the protein be in the process of biosynthesis, making the ribosome-binding specificity of SRP inappropriate. Townsend et al. proposed that the behavior of the MHC class I expression mutant, RMA-S, was consistent with the defect being in the peptide transporter system, and in vitro complementation of this defect suggests strategies for identification of the protein via molecular cloning. It is possible that heat shock and related molecular chaperones (Pelham 1986) may be involved at some level in the management of the translocation and loading processes (Braciale et al.). Intriguingly, two heat shock protein loci have recently been mapped into the MHC chromosomal region (Romano et al. 1989; Wurst et al. 1989). The properties of RMA-S also suggest that in the absence of peptide, recently synthesized class I heavy chains fail to associate with β_2-microglobulin and remain in the ER. That free peptide added exogenously can induce chain association and class I expression on the membrane in an antigenically active form seems to imply that peptides contribute directly to the normal assembly of the class I molecule. This extraordinary result is also the best direct evidence that peptide/class I association normally occurs in the ER. It also implies that exogenous soluble peptides in sufficient concentration can reach the lumen of the ER, a retrograde traffic that is, to say the least, a surprise.

The properties of the RMA-S cell seem likely to contribute to the resolution of another key immunological problem. For if the class I molecule that is expressed on RMA-S in the presence of excess peptide is indeed a single-peptide/MHC complex, then it is a matter of great interest whether this material behaves like a major alloantigen or not. If Matzinger and Bevan (1977) are right, then a single-peptide complex should be no more than a minor antigen, and will not contain the antigenic complexity that even the simplest allogeneic reactions are known to contain (Sherman 1980). As a further bonus, such single-peptide complexes may provide material suitable for structural studies.

Our understanding of key immunological events has been profoundly influenced by our new grasp of antigen processing and presentation. In 1976, models of MHC-restricted T-B interaction were a complete mess. Now we know that the Ig receptor is a constitutively recycling receptor, internalized with or without ligand via the endocytic pathway; antigen fragments generated in the usual way are then re-presented in association with class II molecules on the B-cell surface. Thus, T-helper cells activated by an MHC-restricted complex on a macrophage or dendritic cell ought to find the same complex on the surface of a specific B cell. In practice, this may not always be so (Berzofsky 1983; Manca et al. 1985), and the experiments of Watts et al. suggest why not, since the specificity of the Ig receptor actively influences the identity of the stable fragments that result from endocytic processing. This result reminds one that antigen uptake by professional antigen-presenting cells (APCs) must sometimes be via opsonizing antibody, thus ensuring a degree of conformity between MHC-restricted structures on APC and on B cells (Thomas et al.). The cases described by Lanzavecchia (Panina-Bordignon et al.) where apparently normal human APC from certain individuals fail to generate a particular peptide/MHC complex from tetanus toxin may reflect fine structure in the pool of natural opsonins available for this antigen, causing differences in the direction of processing. More generally, as Sercarz argued (Ametani et al.), antigen processing effects may contribute in a number of different ways to the crypticity and dominance of particular protein epitopes.

THE RECOGNITION OF ANTIGEN

Antibody combining sites interacting with protein antigens to generate an affinity in the range of 10^{-7} M to 10^{-8} M are complex, closely complementary surfaces with an area of around 700–800 Å^2 (Davies et al.; Bentley et al.; Tulip et al.). Contact residues may be contributed from all three hypervariable loops from both chains, and occasionally from the framework as well. The Bjorkman–Davis T-cell receptor model gives a similar contact area with the top surface of a peptide/ MHC complex. Hypervariable junctional regions are primarily in contact with peptide, whereas genetically determinate variable region residues primarily contact MHC helices. This is, then, a cryptic "two-receptor" structure, in which the recognition of peptide and of MHC are quasi-independent. It is an attractive model, and the component of independent recognition of MHC is convenient for thymic positive selection. As further support for such a model, there is now direct evidence for specific affinity between T-cell receptors and helical regions of MHC molecules (both HLA-A2 and H-K^b) in the absence of a nominal peptide (Clayberger et al. 1987; Munitz et al.), although in both cases the receptors are alloreactive rather than self-restricted.

Janeway is surely right to emphasize in his introductory paper that the specific T-cell receptor is only one of a family of more or less specific adhesion molecules on the T-cell surface, and it is an attractive proposition that the evolution of T-cell function as we now see it may have been preceded by a precursor phase in which nonspecific receptors did all the work on perhaps a few differentiated types of cytotoxic or cytopathic cells. Nevertheless, the number of potential nonspecific ligands involved in T-cell function has made the specificity of most T-cell function progressively harder to account for. As long as the CD3/Ti complex was the only receptor directly involved in signal transduction, other ligands could be supposed to function simply to increase the avidity of the cell-cell interaction, and thus provide an opportunity for the specific receptor to encounter antigen. The situation is now more complex than that, and we need to understand how the distinctive signaling functions of several T-cell surface molecules are organized. Furthermore, any receptor/ligand complex that affects the likelihood of signaling by a given specific antigen concentration must be said operationally to affect the affinity so long as its function is measured with cellular response as the readout.

It is obviously essential to distinguish between machinery that has no direct contact with the T-cell receptor/ligand complex and machinery that does contribute directly. For the time being, the LFA-1/ICAM complex, at least, falls into the first category (however, see below), and the α/β T-cell receptor, the CD4 and CD8 co-receptors, and class I and class II MHC molecules fall into the second category. The CD2/LFA-3 complex is ambiguous. It is certainly capable of acting as a signal-transducing receptor, and new data (Brown et al.) suggest that it may be physically associated, albeit weakly, with the CD3/T-cell receptor complex, an association that provides an opportunity of contributing directly to T-cell-receptor-mediated signaling. That CD3 is critically involved in the signaling activity of CD2 is suggested by the observation that CD3-deficient cells cannot be triggered through CD2. The endogenous superantigens (*Mls* products) are now being implicated as a further co-ligand in the T-cell receptor/ligand complex (Janeway et al.). In the absence of any molecular information about their identity and properties, however, I remain skeptical. The fact that *Mls* products have not so far been recognized serologically, despite their explicit polymorphism, strongly suggests that they will prove, like the equally serologically invisible minor histocompatibility antigens, to be poorly conformed peptides that exist as determinate structures only in association with MHC molecules. By analogy with the enterotoxins (Dellabona et al.), and to account for their preferential interaction with the T-cell receptor β chain, we might suppose that their association with MHC molecules is atypical in some way and may not only involve the peptide-binding groove. There is at present no reason to suppose that they normally contribute to the overall affinity of receptor/MHC interactions, and their apparent absence from dendritic cells or from interactions involving CD8 cells seems to argue against a normal role in T-cell triggering in vivo.

CD4 and CD8 co-receptor molecules work only if they bind to MHC molecules that are also engaged with an α/β T-cell receptor (Parnes et al.). Exactly what that work consists of is still not clear. On the one hand, by direct interaction with the T-cell-receptor complex they behave like an additional binding chain and thus enhance the effective affinity of the T-cell receptor for MHC molecules. On the other hand, they play a more dynamic role in activation by associating with the T-cell-specific tyrosine kinase, p56^{lck}. Nevertheless, there are situations in which T-cell triggering is independent of co-receptor engagement (primed cells, for example); in these cases does T-cell triggering not depend on ζ chain phosphorylation? I am also baffled by the in vivo mechanism of CD3/Ti cross-linking, which looks like an essential precondition for activation. The formation of monovalent receptor/co-receptor/ligand complexes uniting T cells and APCs must initiate the process, but why should the density of these complexes become very high locally on the cell surface except by diffusion, which is surely too slow? Perhaps T cells exploit cytoskeletal activity to reduce the surface area of contact actively, leaving local "adhesion plaques" in which engaged ligand complexes are highly focused. Since LFA-1 is concentrated with cytoskeletal components in localized adhesion complexes, there could be a context here for Springer's demonstration that T-cell receptor cross-linking initiates an energy-dependent increase in the avidity of LFA-1 interaction with ICAM (Dustin et al.).

Although cooperative, the many ligand-receptor interactions that occur at the T-cell surface undoubtedly play specialized parts in the recognition, adhesion, and activation process. The Springer phenomenon suggests that the key to understanding the relationship between so many participants may be that distinct interactions are assembled and function sequentially. Understanding T-cell recognition means not just identifying the molecular components of the recognition process, but disentangling their relationships with one another in both space and time. A precisely similar argument has been developed to relate the Ig-mediated and class II MHC-mediated induction signals during B-cell activation (Cambier et al. 1987), an argument that seems to deserve more attention generally in these complex signaling events.

RESPONSIVENESS, UNRESPONSIVENESS, AND ONTOGENY

It is difficult to disentangle questions of lymphocyte function from questions of ontogeny. If this meeting had a hidden agenda, it was to point to the relationship between the differentiation of cell signaling machinery and the delineation of functional staging in lymphocyte ontogeny. In T cells, it is already reasonable to list five clearly distinct receptor-mediated processes that need complete functional analysis (Table 1). For B cells, the situation is less well resolved, but still distinctive consequences of antigen contact can be defined. The distinction between Ly-1 and "regular" B cells also needs to be integrated into this crude scheme, since prima facie the consequences of receptor engagement seem to be distinct. For T cells, the position of γ/δ cells in this scenario is absolutely obscure, and functional distinctions between CD4 and CD8 α/β cells need to be much

more carefully drawn, especially in relationship to lymphokine requirements.

For all its superficial character, Table 1 strongly urges the idea that the antigen-specific receptor in both T and B cells is the trigger for several different functional processes defined by the differentiation state of the cell, and usually, environmental conditions as well. Thus the receptor-mediated clonal anergy described by Schwartz et al. in CD4 T cells is conditional on the absence of costimulator activity (whatever that is). Again, unresponsiveness in $CD8^+$ T cells in the in vivo system described by Matzinger (Guerder and Matzinger) is dependent on ligand engagement by the CD8 cell in the absence of help.

These two examples also remind one how many of the distinct responses of lymphocytes are, in fact, unresponses, and this in turn shows that mechanisms for the avoidance of autoimmunity are hard-wired into lymphocyte ontogeny. The ontogenetic cases that seem adaptively straightforward are thymic negative selection and, presumably, B-cell clonal abortion (Nossal and Pike 1978). In both these cases, the tolerance mechanism operates on a functionally immature cell, certainly in a relatively sequestered environment for T cells, and to the extent that clonal abortion also occurs in the primary lymphoid organs, also for B cells. In both cases, the effect is to purge the repertoire before the cells carrying it are functionally mature. The cellular biochemistry of programed cell death in lymphocytes is only beginning to be approached. In T lymphocytes, the effector mechanism seems to involve nucleolytic chromosome fragmentation. There is a tantalizing hint that the receptor-mediated signal to induce nucleolysis may require the participation of the η chain

Table 1. Antigen-specific Receptors Signal Many Different Things

Signaling event	Location	Outcome
T cells:		
Negative selection	thymus	death?
Positive selection	thymus	permission to proceed, co-receptor selection
Primary antigen contact	lymph nodes, spleen	G_0–G_1 transition; functional differentiation; "memory"
Effector antigen contact	anywhere?	lymphokine release; perforin release
Incomplete antigen contact (absence of lymphokine, professional APC, "co-stimulator activity," help)	anywhere, except lymph node or spleen?	functional anergy
B cells:		
Primary antigen contact at high dose	immature B cells; yolk sac, fetal liver, marrow, spleen?	clonal anergy or death
Antigen contact	mature B cells	G_0–G_1 transition; "memory" susceptibility to isotype switching
Excessive antigen, mature cell	unknown	membrane μ modulation

of the CD3 complex (R. Klausner, pers. comm.), but this information is not yet available for CD4/CD8 double-positive thymocytes, which presumably are the target population for negative selection in vivo. This exciting finding suggests the testable generalization that at least a part of the differential responses of lymphocytes to antigen at different ontogenetic stages will be correlated with ontogenetic regulation in the biosynthesis of receptor components with signaling properties. CD45 (leukocyte-common antigen), already well known to exist in a number of differential splice isoforms associated with distinct lymphocyte differentiation states and now identified as an active tyrosine phosphatase, looks like another example to hang this generalization on.

How do mature cell anergies, such as those described by Guerder and Matzinger, Schwartz et al., and Waldmann et al. for T cells, and by Nossal et al. and Goodnow et al. for B cells, serve the interests of self-tolerance? In all these cases, except arguably Schwartz's, there is a prima facie failure of T-cell help, for one reason or another, and several speakers noted the similarity in principle to the Bretscher and Cohn (1970) two-signal model of immune induction, where first-signal-alone was tolerogenic. What needs clarification is why peripheral autoantigens that have failed to induce tolerance during the negative selection or clonal abortion stage should necessarily provide only a first signal. The problem is especially acute for helper cells themselves, since it is difficult to see why Schwartz's costimulator activity should not normally be present in vivo. In many experimental examples of peripheral unresponsiveness, there is no obvious explanation in terms, for example, of structural simplicity of the antigen, which would account for the tolerance on a first-signal-only basis. Le Douarin, for example, described a degree of tolerance to major alloantigens in chicks grafted with allogeneic nonthymic tissue (wingbud) in ovo (Le Douarin et al.). Why should such grafts entail a first-signal-only stimulus in this context any more than they do when grafted to an adult? Again, the minutely localized expression in pancreatic β cells of antigens driven by the insulin promoter (Burkly et al.; Hanahan et al.; Miller et al.) seems capable of inducing peripheral unresponsiveness at some level, but it is not clear, or at least not specified, why these small sequestered stimuli should entail first signals only.

In the absence of an alternative, it is tempting to return to the position of many years ago (Lafferty et al. 1980) and argue that a key distinction, although not necessarily the only distinction, between immunogenic and tolerogenic antigen in vivo is whether or not it is expressed on a professional APC, presumably a dendritic cell. There are problems about restricting the immunogenic pathway wholly to a single rare cell type, especially when considering the stimulation of class-I-restricted CD8 cells by endogenous virus antigens. However, although Mitchison's intercellular exchange of loaded class I molecules may be awkward, it has the great advantage of exposing this issue to experimental

investigation (Fisher et al.). If the APC indeed makes the difference, then the ready induction of anergy to *Mls* incompatible cells in vivo (Rammensee et al. 1989; Waldmann et al.) would confirm that *Mls* products are not normally expressed on dendritic cells. As pointed out above, this in turn further weakens the view that *Mls* products form an integral component of the inductive T-cell receptor/class II ligand complex.

A NOTE ON SUPPRESSION

This meeting was, by and large, a triumphal procession and not calculated to reveal examples of unexplained phenomena suggesting the existence of specific suppression. So solid is the mood against suppression at the moment that when obvious opportunities to consider the proposition arose, they were usually missed. With one eye on the future, therefore, it seems appropriate to remember, for example, Le Douarin's experiment showing that tolerance of allogeneic and xenogeneic tissue grafts could be obtained in birds if more than one third of the resident thymus mass was replaced by donor-specific thymus primordium. How the presence of donor thymus affects the immunological activity of cells differentiating in the resident host thymus is not explained; a paradoxical situation already well-established in the mouse (Zamoyska et al. 1989). There may be relatively uninteresting explanations for such phenomena, for example, transfer of antigen between the two thymuses; but let the problem be squarely confronted.

REPERTOIRE SELECTION

The most difficult problem still on the table in immunology is to identify the principles and mechanisms involved in repertoire selection in vivo. In B cells, the issues are less convoluted, but the issues are as explicit, as Rajewsky et al. emphasized. How do certain receptors become associated with the self-sustaining CD5 (Ly-1) B-cell lineage? Is it self-selected by its own connectivity? Or does the surface phenotype identify a population set on one side a priori, with a distinctive mechanism of V-gene rearrangement? Or does exogenous antigen initiate the network? Again, what forces select the resident pool of long-lived recirculating B cells from the enormous numbers of newly formed B cells emerging from the primary lymphoid organs, a pool of cells long-claimed (Howard 1972; Sprent and Basten 1973), frequently denied (Freitas et al. 1982), and now reinstated beyond doubt (Rajewsky et al.)?

Positive selection in the thymus is an extraordinary process, but the evidence in favor of it is surely now overwhelming. In case the T-cell-receptor transgenic experiments could be suspect (although I do not see how, relevantly), the dominant MHC-linked distortions in V_β usage in F_1 hybrids are subject to no such reservations. In three cases out of three, transgenic T-cell receptors specific for MHC class I "allo" (Loh et al.), an endogenous minor antigen H-Y restricted by class I (von Boehmer et al.), and an exogenous soluble protein antigen restricted by class II (Davis et al.), the expression of a specific MHC allele during thymic development is necessary for progress of cells bearing the transgenic receptor into the mature (single co-receptor-positive) phenotype. In no case is the expression of the nominal antigen required; indeed, in the two cases where the experiment is feasible, the expression of the nominal antigen causes the elimination of the transgenic clone by negative selection. If the nominal antigen is not required for positive selection, then the triggering event must be effectively heterologous (Marrack et al.). Three heterologous stimuli can be considered: (1) "empty" MHC molecules, presenting helical structure but no peptide, (2) MHC molecules loaded with essentially the same complex variety of peptides that we should consider in relation to self-tolerance, and (3) MHC molecules loaded with "special" structures of one kind or another. Apart from the inherent structural implausibility of empty molecules, at least for class I, there is for the time being no compelling reason to choose between these possibilities.

Let us be clear, positive selection imposes a statistical bias on the preferred restriction element for subsequent antigen presentation, not an absolute specificity. If there were any debate on this key issue, recall that one of the three examples of positive selection with a transgenic T-cell receptor is with a receptor positively selected on H-2K^b and alloreactive on H-2L^d (Loh et al.). Whichever heterologous ligand is responsible for the phenomenon, the pragmatic view of its structural basis expressed by Bjorkman and Davis has a lot to recommend it.

Thymic epithelium, expressing class I and class II MHC molecules, is the tissue responsible for positive selection (Sprent et al.). Early thymocyte maturation occurs in this environment, physically and temporally separated from the medulla, where dendritic cells known to be prepotent in their ability to cause tolerance (Matzinger and Guerder 1989) reside. It is difficult not to agree with Loh and Weissman that positive selection must normally occur, if anything, before negative selection, and the data implicate the double-positive blast cell with low T-cell-receptor expression as the target for this key event. The target of negative selection is less clear, but since thymic epithelium is fairly tolerogenic (Sprent et al.; Le Douarin et al.), and since there is ambiguity in the experimental data on timing from transgenic and other systems, we might propose that double-positive cells may be tolerized by certain ligands expressed on the epithelium, whereas up-regulation of receptor expression in young cells that are becoming single-positive coincides with a second window of negative selection mediated through dendritic cells.

Possibly the most unpalatable feature of thymic selection is the constraint it imposes on the effective repertoire. How serious is this? Quantitatively, negative selection via endogenous superligands seems to be a major effect, causing the virtual disappearance of at least some V$_\beta$ chains from the mature repertoire, presumably without regard to V$_\alpha$ usage (Kappler et al.). Nevertheless, as Sprent et al. point out, positive selection is likely to be a more stringent limitation on repertoire usage than negative selection. There is room for negotiation on the numbers, but one might suggest that the degeneracy in the repertoire of receptors for any MHC haplotype is of the order of 10%, that is, about 10% of such a repertoire will be functionally cross-reactive (for positive as for negative selection) with any other haplotype on average. It follows that only about 10% of the repertoire is positively selected by any haplotype, and of this, perhaps a further 10% may be eliminated by negative selection. As Hood et al. point out, because of junctional diversity the potential T-cell repertoire is almost infinite, and the most important variable in determining the actual repertoire is the absolute number of cells available to put it in. We want to know the number of cells in which V$_\alpha$ rearrangement occurs, since this fixes the primary repertoire size. Obviously, neither negative nor positive selection can occur until V$_\alpha$ is rearranged and a receptor is expressed on the membrane. Equally, no further diversification of the repertoire occurs after V$_\alpha$ rearrangement. The first expression of $\alpha\beta$ receptor is probably in early CD8$^+$ blasts, representing at most 10^6 cells in the young adult mouse thymus. If this compartment is replaced every 12 hours, then a maximum of 2×10^6 new receptors is generated every day. Furthermore, if V$_\beta$ rearrangement occurs at an earlier cell division than V$_\alpha$ in the same exponentially growing lineage of blasts, the total number of V$_\beta$ rearrangements must be substantially less than V$_\alpha$. This population of 10^6 new receptors per 12 hours is the substrate for positive selection, which we have set at a permissiveness of 10%, that is, one double-positive blast out of ten passes the test of positive selection. Thus, of a total repertoire production of 2×10^6 cells bearing new receptors per day, only 2×10^5 are likely to mature to the periphery; among these there could be as few as 2×10^4 new V$_\beta$ rearrangements if V$_\beta$ rearrangement occurs three cell divisions before V$_\alpha$. An input of about 2×10^5 new receptors per day is surprisingly small. Although the peripheral lymphocyte pool of an adult mouse at 100 days of age may contain 2×10^8 T cells, the repertoire is unlikely to contain more than 2×10^7 different T-cell receptors and only about 2×10^6 different V$_\beta$ sequences. The numbers become even smaller if either positive or negative selection is more stringent than 10%. Incidentally, because V$_\gamma$ rearrangement occurs even earlier in thymic ontogeny than V$_\beta$, and therefore in a smaller population of cells again, the actual pool of V$_\gamma$ sequences must be correspondingly smaller than the population of V$_\beta$ sequences, perhaps by another order of magnitude. How is co-receptor loss orchestrated? If positive selection occurs at the double-positive stage, is the loss of one co-receptor actively induced by successful participation of the other in a ligand-binding complex with the T-cell receptor? Or do co-receptors get lost at random, so that only half of all peripheralized cells have the co-receptor that was responsible for their positive selection? Although specific induced co-receptor loss seems more reasonable on teleological grounds, it implies some pretty fancy gene regulation; T-cell receptor/CD4 ligand binding has to transduce a signal that permits CD4 transcription and/or suppresses CD8, whereas T-cell receptor/CD8 ligand binding has to transduce the complementary effect. However, the stochastic alternative looks inefficient, since about half of all receptors will be predisposed to interact with an MHC molecule for which their co-receptor is inappropriate. Such cells, if positive selection means anything, must be less likely to participate in an immune response than cells whose receptors and co-receptors were selected on the same MHC molecule. Thus, if co-receptor selection is stochastic, it implies, in effect, a further 50% reduction in the useful repertoire.

CONCLUSION

The immune system is not as complicated as the nervous system, and it is a comparatively recent invention in evolutionary terms, being more or less contemporary with the vertebrates. This means that the idea of getting a complete solution to the principles of immune mechanism seems realistic. I cannot agree with the optimists (pessimists?) who believe that immunology will run and run, and that an unending succession of challenging and distinctively immunological problems are still ahead. I predict that most of the proteins that were evolved to serve the needs of the immune system have now been discovered. There are already a lot of them, and the mammalian genome codes for only about 10,000 different proteins altogether. I see the immune system as a specialized adaptation superimposed on a much older machine. As immunological investigations become more probing, the ancient roots of immune mechanisms appear. As was inevitable, transcriptional regulation of immunologically important proteins is proving to involve factors active in many other systems as well. The enzymes so far shown to be involved in antigen processing in the endocytic compartment are as old as phagocytosis, and it is a fair prediction that catabolic machinery generating cytosolic peptides will be ancient, too. The transduction systems that handle lymphocyte activation, differentiation, and division, the central acts of clonal selection, are all universal eukaryotic mechanisms. In terms of molecular machinery, immunology certainly has an end, and it is getting near.

In his summary of the 1976 symposium, Edelman (1977) ventured three specific predictions for work sure to be completed before the next symposium. The T-cell receptor has indeed been characterized, and the function of the major histocompatibility complex understood. However, Edelman was surprisingly wrong when he predicted that we should see "the origin of diversity reasonably well-ensconced within a detailed analysis of particular enzymes and their mechanisms." Although the VDJ recombinase system will unravel

soon, there is still no enzyme to work on. Of the diversification mechanisms, only terminal deoxynucleotidyl transferase has been worked out, and that was already on the table for the 1976 meeting (Baltimore et al. 1977); somatic hypermutators, in which I include gene conversion, have no worked out enzymology at all. Perhaps some of this machinery will turn out to be distinctive to the immune system, but as in other parts of the field, the deep solution to the immunological problem will be found to include ancient, profound, and general mechanisms as well, in this case presumably concerned with DNA recombination and repair.

Questions of specificity have dominated immunology since the discovery of antibodies. The antibody problem, the repertoire, clonal selection, MHC restriction, alloreactivity, tolerance, and the network are typical of the distinctively immunological problems whose end Jerne was waiting for in 1967. Now, if not ended, they have reached a level of maturity at which they attract only specialists. If the millennial Cold Spring Harbor Symposium in 2000 is on immunology, what will it be about? Certainly, by then, the enzymology of the generation of diversity and its ontogenetic control. Certainly, the orchestration of post-rearrangement lymphocyte ontogeny by receptor-mediated signals. The cell biology of antigen processing and presentation will be completed, and the true nature of *Mls* and minor histocompatibility antigens will be known. There will be crystal structure for T-cell receptor/ligand complexes, so the structural basis for positive selection and MHC restriction will be clear. The dynamics of the interaction of peptide with MHC will be understood in terms of a more general solution to the protein folding problem. Whole animal immunology will be back in business, partly because so many profound organismic problems have been left out from recent gains and partly because transgenic biology will have been extended into regulated expression and targeted gene disruption. The nature of immunological memory in T- and B-cell systems, a striking gap in present understanding, will be known. The deployment of lymphocyte populations in space and time in vivo will be an area of growth; I take it that classic lymphocyte recirculation will have been worked out, and the functional and mechanistic basis for subset localization in inflammatory sites, skin, gut, etc. will be known. I hope that the undifferentiated area of research loosely called "immunoregulation" will be resolved into a specific set of issues concerned with quantitative and qualitative aspects of antigen presentation, lymphokines, and lymphocyte differentiation states, and I expect that many if not all the outstanding problems of functional choice (that is, tolerance versus immunity, IgA versus IgG1, etc.) will sort themselves out in the light of this.

The great hope in all this fundamental work is that profoundly important, difficult, and painful problems in human immunopathology will at last have succumbed to innovative approaches. Clinically significant autoantigens will have been identified, and the T-cell repertoires for particular autoimmune diseases will have been described. For the several reasons outlined by Heber-Katz, Hood et al., and Cohen, this kind of information ought to offer a basis for direct immunological intervention in the autoimmune process.

Last, we shall expect to see dramatic advances in the construction of artificial ligands for the manipulation of biological processes. Lerner (Iverson et al.) and Paul, in the present symposium, were the heralds of the new technology of abzymes, whereas Winter (Güssow et al.) showed that the hypervariation principle can be applied to a single immunoglobulin domain to generate binding proteins, we must suspect, of any specificity under the sun.

I think we are at the end of immunology as Jerne meant it in 1967. What I look forward to for the 2000 symposium is fascinating, important, and difficult work, but it lacks the shapeliness of the original problem. Somehow I suspect that the pleasures in the next decade will come not from the elegance of the problems but from the ingenuity of their solutions.

It remains only to congratulate John Inglis and Jim Watson for organizing this outstanding meeting. If Jernian criteria alone decide, then this will have been the last in its line, although certainly the finest. If, on the other hand, immunology is accepted in its new colors as a privileged branch of evolutionary, developmental, and cell biology, endowed by the special character of its material with exceptional opportunities for the relief of human suffering, then we shall have another symposium in this beautiful laboratory before too long.

ACKNOWLEDGMENT

I thank Geoffrey Butcher for his valuable comments on this paper.

REFERENCES

Baltimore, D., A.E. Silverstone, P.C. Kung, T.A. Harrison, and R.P. McCaffrey. 1977. Specialized DNA polymerases in lymphoid cells. *Cold Spring Harbor Symp. Quant. Biol.* **41:** 63.

Berzofsky, J.A. 1983. T-B reciprocity. An Ia-restricted epitope-specific circuit regulating T cell-B cell interaction and antibody specificity. *Surv. Immunol. Res.* **2:** 223.

Blackman, M., J. Yague, R. Kubo, D. Gay, C. Coleclough, E. Palmer, J. Kappler, and P. Marrack. 1986. The T cell repertoire may be biased in favor of MHC recognition. *Cell* **47:** 349.

Bretscher, P. and M. Cohn. 1970. A theory of self-non-self discrimination. Paralysis and induction involve the recognition of one and two determinants on an antigen, respectively. *Science* **169:** 1042.

Briles, W.E., H.A. Stone, and R.K. Cole. 1977. Marek's disease: Effects of B histocompatibility alleles in resistant and susceptible chicken lines. *Science* **195:** 193.

Cambier, J.C., L.B. Justement, M.K. Newell, Z.Z. Chen, L.K. Harris, V.M. Sandoval, M.J. Klemsz, and J.T. Ransom. 1987. Transmembrane signals and intracellular "second messengers" in the regulation of quiescent B-lymphocyte activation. *Immunol. Rev.* **95:** 37.

Clayberger, C., P. Parham, J. Rothbard, D.S. Ludwig, G.K. Schoolnik, and A.M. Krensky. 1987. HLA-A2 peptides can regulate cytolysis by human allogeneic T lymphocytes. *Nature* **330:** 763.

Davis, M.M. and P.J. Bjorkman. 1988. T-cell antigen receptor genes and T cell recognition. *Nature* **331:** 627.

Edelman, G.M. 1977. Understanding selective molecular recognition. *Cold Spring Harbor Symp. Quant. Biol.* **41:** 891.

Freitas, A.A., B. Rocha, L. Forni, and A. Coutinho. 1982. Population dynamics of B lymphocytes and their precursors: Demonstration of high turnover in the central and peripheral lymphoid organs. *J. Immunol.* **128:** 54.

Howard, J.C. 1972. The life span and recirculation of marrow-derived small lymphocytes from the rat thoracic duct. *J. Exp. Med.* **135:** 185.

Janeway, C.A., Jr., B. Jones, and A. Hayday. 1988. Specificity and function of T cells bearing γ/δ receptors. *Immunol. Today* **9:** 73.

Jerne, N.K. 1968. Waiting for the end. *Cold Spring Harbor Symp. Quant. Biol.* **32:** 591.

Lafferty, K.J., L. Andrus, and S.J. Prowse. 1980. Role of lymphokine and antigen in the control of specific T cell responses. *Immunol. Rev.* **51:** 279.

Manca, F., A. Kunkl, D. Fenoglio, A. Fowler, E. Sercarz, and F. Celada. 1985. Constraints in T-B co-operation related to epitope topology on *E. coli* β-galactosidase. I. The fine specificity of T cells dictates the fine specificity of antibodies directed to conformation-dependent determinants. *Eur. J. Immunol.* **15:** 345.

Matzinger, P. 1981. A one-receptor view of T cell behaviour. *Nature* **292:** 497.

Matzinger, P. and M.J. Bevan. 1977. Why do so many lymphocytes respond to major histocompatibility antigens? *Cell. Immunol.* **29:** 1.

Matzinger, P. and S. Guerder. 1989. Does T cell tolerance require a dedicated antigen presenting cell? *Nature* **338:** 74.

Morrison, L.A., A.E. Lukacher, V.L. Braciale, D.P. Fan, and T.J. Braciale. 1986. Differences in antigen presentation to MHC class I- and class II-restricted influenza virus-specific cytolytic T lymphocyte clones. *J. Exp. Med.* **163:** 903.

Nossal, G.J.V. and B.L. Pike. 1978. Mechanisms of clonal abortion tolerogenesis. I. Response of immature hapten-specific B lymphocytes. *J. Exp. Med.* **148:** 1161.

Pauling, L. 1940. A theory of the structure and process of formation of antibodies. *J. Am. Chem. Soc.* **62:** 2643.

Pelham, H.R.B. 1986. Speculations on the function of the major heat shock and glucose-regulated proteins. *Cell* **46:** 95.

Rammensee, H.-G., R. Kroschewski, and B. Frangoulis. 1989. Clonal anergy induced in mature T lymphocytes on immunizing Mls-1^b mice with Mls-1^a expressing cells. *Nature* **339:** 541.

Romano, J.W., M.F. Seldin, and E. Appella. 1989. Linkage of the mouse Hsp84 heat shock protein structural gene to the H-2 complex. *Immunogenetics* **29:** 142.

Sherman, L. 1980. Dissection of the B10.D2 anti-H-2K^b cytolytic T lymphocyte receptor repertoire. *J. Exp. Med.* **151:** 1386.

Sprent, J. and A. Basten. 1973. Circulating T and B lymphocytes of the mouse. II. Lifespan. *Cell. Immunol.* **7:** 10.

Weiss, S. and B. Bogen. 1989. B lymphoma cells process and present their endogenous immunoglobulin to MHC-restricted T cells. *Proc. Natl. Acad. Sci.* **86:** 282.

Wurst, W., C. Benesch, B. Drabent, E. Rothermel, B.-D. Benesch, and E. Guenther. 1989. Localization of heat shock protein 70 genes inside the rat major histocompatibility complex close to class III genes. *Immunogenetics* **30:** 46.

Zamoyska, R., H. Waldmann, and P. Matzinger. 1989. Peripheral tolerance mechanisms prevent the development of autoreactive T cells in chimaeras grafted with two minor incompatible thymuses. *Eur. J. Immunol.* **19:** 111.

Appendix

The Impact on Ideas of Immunology

F. M. Burnet

School of Microbiology, University of Melbourne, Victoria, Australia

I expect that I resemble most scientists in being vastly more interested in other people's experimental results than in their theories to account for them. So that I have a delicate task in front of me if I am to provide anything that will interest you about the origin and fate of ideas on the nature of the immune process during the last ten years or so. We are all egotists at heart and I shall be largely concerned with the genesis and subsequent development of selection or genetic theories, particularly in the form that I called Clonal Selection.

I have found it absorbing over the decade to concentrate my interest in immunology on watching its development in terms of the theory of immunity which I outlined in 1957 and elaborated in the Flexner Lectures at Vanderbilt in 1958. In part this was a fairly unsophisticated desire to see how what seemed a good and fruitful idea would stand up to the development of the science, with, of course, a naive hope that it was the answer. But there was a lot more to it than that. To have what seemed to be a proprietary interest in one particular point of view made the general developing pattern of experimental and clinical immunology a far more living and meaningful experience than it would otherwise have been. I think it is true to say that every paper I have read in a journal or listened to in a lecture room has been looked at critically first from the point of its relevance to selective as against instructive theory and, more recently, in regard to the alternative ways in which a selective or genetic theory can be applied in the various fields of current experimental interest.

Like every theoretical statement, the 1957 theory of clonal selection was made in terms of contemporary knowledge. As such it is outmoded. It can be shown to be incomplete in a dozen places, and here and there to be expressed in terms that have now become meaningless. Nevertheless, it has proved easy and natural to keep the theoretical structure updated and in line with new experimental results. I have almost completed a full length book on theoretical immunology and the picture it presents is very different from that of 1957. I believe hopefully that 90% of it would be acceptable to most immunologists and that dissent would mainly concern matters currently accepted as still subject to future experimental decision.

Irrespective of how the change has taken place over the ten years, there has in fact been a sharp and fundamental break with the instructive theories generally accepted around 1955.

It has been a common opinion that the production and propagation of selective theories of immunity has provided a significant stimulus to experimental work. Although, for reasons I shall discuss, I doubt whether the work so stimulated has been particularly helpful to the development of immunology, this is probably true. The form in which the clonal selection hypothesis was stated made it easy to envisage experimental ways in which it could be tested, and supplied a connection between cellular and serological approaches. In these respects it had definite advantages over both Jerne's initial formulation and the various hypotheses of subcellular selective processes which tried to make the best of both worlds.

May I remind you that scientific truth can be defined as that corpus of facts and provisional generalizations which, in the consensus of competent scholars, has not yet been shown to be wrong. It is always provisional and the consensus of opinion changes with the outlook of the times. Today's climate of interest in biology with its concentration on the interplay of genetics and biochemistry has brought a much more sympathetic attitude to a genetic approach to antibody production. In fact, I think I can say that there is very nearly unanimity amongst immunologists on three fundamental points: (a) that the specific pattern of antibody is determined by genetic and somatic genetic factors, (b) that there is an absolute or near absolute phenotypic restriction in the type of immunoglobulin and antibody that a given clone of immunocytes can produce, and (c) that the population of lymphocytes and plasma cells is an extremely labile one from which individual cells can be selected for proliferation and others for destruction. There is immense scope for detailed elaboration of each of those points. How does the genetic variability arise? What is the mechanism of phenotypic restriction? Can immunological information be transferred from one cell to another by subcellular entities? What are the receptors and the signals which allow antigen to affect an immunocyte? There is possibility for infinite elaboration

1

within every biological field and the question could go on forever.

Yet, however much has still to be learned, something real has been achieved. The clonal selection approach is incompatible with the picture that the great biochemists from Landsteiner onwards in the 1930's and '40's developed to account for the specificity of antibody. That combination of genetics with the physical sciences which has been so specially characteristic of Cold Spring Harbor activities and symposia has now swept away the simple mechanism of the chemists. I suspect that in another ten years' time new and more subtle ideas of the interplay of genetic and biochemical factors on the process of differentiation may lead to another cycle of change in theoretical ideas about immunity and make clonal selection look as old-fashioned as the direct template theories do now.

If my name of Clonal Selection Theory can be accepted as a reasonable one for the broad present day approach to immunity, then you may find it of interest for me to attempt a sketch of developments in the ten years since I coined the phrase.

Perhaps I should begin by confessing a little sadly that I belong to a past generation, the generation of the physician-naturalist—the amateur biologists who picked up the new techniques as they emerged but never quite mastered them. I am not too apologetic about that. From Darwin onward (who you will remember was a drop-out from medical school) to Archibald Garrod (who founded biochemical genetics) and many others, there have been notable contributions from that fraternity of amateur biologists who were mostly physicians by training. There may still be a use for people who believe there is more in life and in biology than the applied biochemistry of the nucleic acids, always provided that they pay due regard to the man who has been trained to wield modern methods with precision and apply modern logical and mathematical facilities to the interpretation of his results.

With this preliminary, I should like to trace the origin and development of the clonal selection approach. As I hope I have always been careful to say, its "onlie begetter" was Niels Jerne. His "Natural Selection Theory of Antibody Formation" (1955) had a verve and a sweep that made the self-marker ideas I was struggling with at the time look clumsy and artificial. But there was one aspect that I could not possibly accept. Jerne postulated that gamma globulin molecules are continuously being synthesized in an enormous variety of different configurations. The origin of the diversity is left unexplained. When an antigen intrudes into the body, sooner or later globulin molecules of the appropriate natural pattern will become attached

to the antigenic molecules or particles. The complex is then taken up by a phagocytic cell where, by hypothesis, the globulin can be released from the antigen. Such globulin molecules either in the macrophage or after transfer to another cell were said to serve as a "signal for the synthesis or reproduction of molecules identical to those introduced, i.e., of specific antibodies." Even in 1955 this seemed wholly inadmissible. Most other aspects of the new theory were highly acceptable but the basic flaw seemed to be a fatal one.

Just at that period, two lines of experimental work in the Hall Institute were impressing the cellular aspect of immunity on me. The first was the Simonsen phenomenon in which adult chicken leucocytes, inoculated intravenously into a chick embryo, provoke *proliferative* cellular lesions in the spleen and thymus. The second was the finding by Mackay and Gajdusek (1958) that a case of Waldenstron's macroglobulinemia had an extremely high titer in Gajdusek's AICF test. It is immaterial what the real interpretation of these phenomena may be but both suggested that cells with immunological capacity could actively proliferate.

It gradually dawned on me that Jerne's selection theory would make real sense if cells produced a characteristic pattern of globulin for genetic reasons and were stimulated to proliferate by contact with the corresponding antigenic determinant. This would demand a receptor on the cell with the same pattern as antibody and a signal resulting from contact of antigenic determinant and receptor that would initiate mitosis or other cellular reaction. Once that central concept was clear, the other implications followed more or less automatically and were published in September, 1957. Just before that was written, Talmage's (1957) review was seen, in which a brief suggestion of the same type was made. His subsequent development of the idea moved a long way away from mine.

The next step was taken when Lederberg was a guest in my laboratory in November–December, 1957. He had come to work on influenza virus genetics but he found more interest in the newly born Clonal Selection Theory—the name, by the way, dates from the first preliminary paper. It was in fact the first significant attempt to bring genetic ideas into immunology and we were both excited about the possibilities. It is a happy dispensation of providence that when a new approach to investigation emerges there always seems to be someone of first rate quality around to get on with the job. This time it was Gus Nossal. Lederberg had had plenty of experience in the isolation of single bacteria for genetic work and his first suggestion was that the hypothesis could be tested quite simply by doubly immunizing an animal and seeing whether isolated cells produced one or both antibodies. Who was there in my laboratory who could get on with it? The answer, of course, was Nossal. So, instead of Lederberg and Burnet working on a problem in influenza virus recombination, it became a matter of Nossal and Lederberg (1958) modifying bacteriological methods to allow the detection of antibody production by isolated single cells from lymph nodes or spleen. It was from their work together in those few weeks that clonal selection really got off the ground.

In 1958 I had two months at Vanderbilt which I enjoyed enormously and, incidentally, where I elaborated the Flexner lectures into a book which was published the following year. On the whole, I think that book has stood up reasonably well to the passage of time. As many of you know, I have been in America and Europe most years since then, always talking clonal selection in one form or another. It was a fairly tough job and at times I felt a bit like Galileo confronting the Church.

There is one aspect of the ten years I am talking about that has interested me enormously. Most of the crucial experiments designed to disprove clonal selection once and for all, came off. Attardi et al. (1959) showed that the same cell could often produce two different antibodies if the rabbit providing it had been immunized with two unrelated bacteriophages. Nossal much more rarely found a double producer in his rats. Trentin and Fahlberg (1963) showed that, by using the Till-McCulloch method, a mouse effectively repopulated from the progeny of a single clone of lymphoid cells could produce three different antibodies. Szenberg et al. (1962) found too many foci on the choriollantois to allow a reasonable number of clones amongst chicken leucocytes and so on.

But, on the other hand, every new heuristic advance in immunology in that decade—and it has been a veritable golden age of immunology—fitted as it appeared easily and conformably into the pattern of clonal selection. With each advance some minor ad hoc adjustment might be necessary, but no withdrawals or massive re-interpretations. Sometimes the new discovery was actually predicted. The statement (Burnet, 1959, p. 119) that the lymphocyte "is the only possible candidate for the responsive cell of clonal selection theory" was validated by Gowans' work in vivo and by Nowell (1960) and many subsequent workers, especially Pearmain et al. (1963), in vitro. The thymus as a producer of lymphocytes must have immunological importance and Miller's work in 1961 was the *effective* initiation of the immunological approach to the thymus (Miller, 1962). The origin of thymic cells from the bone marrow was the logical extension of this.

In quite different directions, Jerne and Nordin's (1963) development of the antibody plaque technique provided a precise demonstration of two very important presumptions of the theory that in a mouse a few cells capable of producing anti-rabbit or anti-sheep hemolysin are present before immunization and that on stimulation with sheep cells a wholly different population of plaque-forming cells develops from what appears if rabbit cells are used as antigen.

The findings by several authors in 1964–65 that pure line strains of guinea-pigs responded to some synthetic antigens but not others; the analysis of the classic Felton paralysis by pneumococcal polysaccharide which showed that in the paralyzed mice there was a specific *absence* of reactive cells—these facts just don't fit any instructive theory.

Finally, there is the immensely productive field that opened when the work of Putnam and his collaborators led to a progressive realization of the monoclonal character of myelomatosis and the uniformity of the immunoglobulin produced. I have said somewhere else that, given the established facts of human myelomatosis, you have almost a categorical demonstration of (a) clonal proliferation, (b) phenotypic restriction and precise somatic inheritance, (c) the random quality of somatic mutation, and (d) the complete independence of specific pattern on the one hand and mutation to a metabolic abnormality such as failure of maturation of the plasmablast, on the other. Almost all the essential features of clonal selection are explicitly displayed.

The current phase, the delineation of variable and stable segments in light and heavy chains of myeloma globulins, is from one point of view merely giving us clues as to the machinery involved; the biological processes of antibody production are already clear. I said *merely* in that last sentence but I assure you that I am as excited as anyone else at the extraordinary potentialities of understanding that lie in the details of sequence and structure of the immunoglobulins. People are already wondering to what extent stochastic as well as deterministic processes play a part in differentiation.

This is far too sophisticated an audience for me to draw schoolboy morals from this contrast between the relative infertility of the experiment designed to disprove an hypothesis and the productiveness of experimental work arising from serendipity or the simple exploratory urge. But it is worth thinking about.

I have had and still have much enjoyment from playing with ideas. It is a pity in some ways that I have just had to point out that the development of immunology over the past decade has been strikingly little influenced by preconceived ideas.

To me, it has been superficially gratifying to watch the way that immunological thought moved as if it were following the path I had laid down, but I never quite believed it. I suspect that if we were honest we would have to admit that if any one of us had never been, our science would not have been quite the same but it would be awfully hard to see the difference.

Being no longer an active worker at the bench, I have no new experimental work to present and instead I should like to use the license of a senior citizen to talk a little about the future of immunology. That will of course grow out of our current understanding at the three levels of molecular biology, cytology, and functional and evolutionary significance. As one whose main interest is in the third of these, I am perhaps over-ambitious in guessing at the future developments in the molecular biology of immunity. Nevertheless I would hold strongly that all three levels must be integrated if a clear picture of the human significance of immunology is to emerge.

There is no reasonable doubt that in the next year or two we shall have a substantial series of myeloma proteins whose amino acid sequences are known either fully or over what will be established as the vital segments. I will predict that with appropriate study, many myeloma proteins will be shown to be antibodies of low avidity for definable antigenic determinants. More, like the three Zettervall et al. (1966) have described, will be easily recognized antibodies against a conventional antigen. Once sequences and avidity against defined antigenic determinants are on record, the physical chemists and their computers should soon give us the answer as to the nature of the combining site

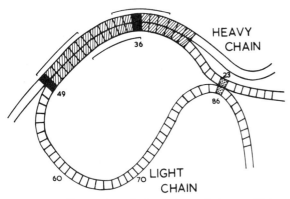

FIGURE 1. Suggestion of the nature of the combining region in which a portion of the "variable" region of light chain is associated with a portion of the heavy chain of generally similar quality. It is assumed that tyrosine residues on the light chain (black) are associated with corresponding tyrosine residues on the heavy chain. Three different combining sites involving 6 or 7 units are suggested. Cysteine (dotted) and tyrosine residues on the light chain as shown for Bence-Jones protein Ag by Putnam et al. (1966).

and the forces concerned in binding the antigenic determinant.

The process of filling out the Porter diagram is going on very actively. My own attempts to keep up to date have probably been always six months behind the growing edge of knowledge but I would like to think that the particular approach I want to talk about is not too critically dependent on guessing structural details correctly. At the risk of being proven wrong within the week, I want to outline a few very general concepts which may be helpful in fitting together the experimental findings as they emerge.

The diagram I am showing (Figure 1) assumes (a) that the combining site of antibody or of any type of specific cell receptor is produced by the interaction of portions of the variable segments both of the light chain and of the Fd portion of the heavy chain. The regions involved are assumed to be of generally similar character, perhaps specially in relation to tyrosine residues. I have accepted the evidence that the two regions will be found *not* to be identical, thereby ruining a prediction I made last year.

(b) It also assumes that the actual combining site is probably considerably smaller than the combining region where juxtaposition of the light and heavy chains provides the physical conditions necessary for specific adsorption. This introduces the possibility, as I have indicated in the diagram, that there may be several unrelated combining sites on the one antibody.

(c) The third and perhaps the only important aspect of the concept is that no combining site is in any evolutionary sense adapted to a particular antigenic determinant. The pattern of the combining site is there and *if it happens to fit*, in the sense that the affinity of adsorption to a given antigenic determinant is above a certain value, immunologically significant reaction will be initiated.

In ten years' time there will be another diagram equivalent to that—based not on imagination but on definite physical measurements. It will certainly be very different but I shall be surprised if it does not still contain these essential features: (a) that each combining site involves both light and heavy chains, (b) that the "variable" sector of both chains are concerned, (c) that there is some special and unique relationship of the 2 chains in the combining site—my duplex idea being the simplest of such possible relationships, and (d) that the combining site is small and therefore we may expect to find more than one combining site at each combining region.

I do not want to discuss the origin of the diversity of specific pattern at any length, largely because it

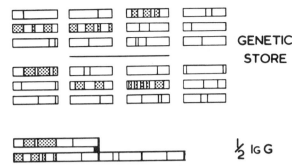

GENETIC
STORE

½ IgG

FIGURE 2. A suggestion as to the nature of the genetic store of duplicated cistrons from which the components to be used in a given clone of immunocytes are drawn by a combination of deterministic and stochastic processes. Cistrons are depicted in terms of the nature of the polypeptide subchains [of 100–115 residues] they code for. "Variable" subchains are shown with broad stippled bars, "constant" with a few narrow bars only.

is becoming operationally irrelevant. Undoubtedly there is genetic polymorphism and there has been accumulation of a certain number of duplicated cistrons over the period of vertebrate evolution. With equal certainty the genes concerned are subject, like any other genes, to somatic mutation and there is unique opportunity for a somatic mutation involving immune pattern to prosper when circumstances are right.

I have tried as an exercise in logic to devise an experimental program by which the parts played by processes evolved at the level of the organism as a whole, on the one hand, and by somatic mutation in the individual's life-time, on the other, could be quantitatively assessed. I have failed completely even if I made the two assumptions (a) that single antibody-producing cells could be cloned and allowed to produce antibody in culture, and (b) that sequence analyses of the immunoglobulins produced by such clones could be made in unlimited numbers.

Already in referring to the stability of the pathogenic clones of myelomatosis I have indicated the major difficulty—the strict phenotypic restriction that seems to operate for every immunoglobulin-producing cell. The phenomena of tolerance only make sense if the emergence of diversity of pattern during the differentiation of the immunocytes is by a random process of phenotypic restriction. Undoubtedly there are genetic potentialities in each human cell for at least 16 antigenic subtypes of Ig G but in fact only one is produced. The process may well be similar to that giving rise to the Lyon phenomenon. Those 16 types are not known to be concerned with immune pattern: there are certainly other types of genetic potentiality which are, and it would be ridiculous to exclude a major influence of somatic mutation on the variable segments particularly. We are dealing, then, with

randomized differentiation by the stochastic selection of one functional set out of a number with the further certainty that within the genes so selected, somatic mutation has been occurring since the zygote began to divide (Fig. 2). On general grounds, and relying on biological intuition rather than available facts, I should think of the genetic factors as providing a coarse adjustment, somatic mutation a fine adjustment, and again on general grounds I should expect the first to be more important in small short-lived animals like mice and the second more important, in large long-lived animals like men.

Returning to my points about the combining site I should like to speak about two other diagrams which are complementary to it. Figure 3 is an attempt to show for a given antigenic determinant the distribution of immunoglobulin molecules in a "standard" mammalian plasma according to their degree of affinity. Most of the molecules will show a minimal adsorptive affinity, not necessarily always due to the combining region, while only an occasional combining site pattern will show a high affinity. The rarity of the high affinity immunoglobulins is for precisely similar reasons that four aces are rarely dealt in a poker hand.

Figure 4 attempts to indicate the conditions under which receptors carrying immune pattern—cell bound antibody if you wish—will react, in relationship to the avidity of reaction with antigenic determinant and the effective concentration

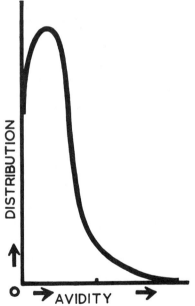

FIGURE 3. To represent the distribution, in a standard population of immunocytes or of immunoglobulin molecules, of individual cells or molecules according to their affinity for a given antigenic determinant. Specificity is only characteristic of the right hand side of the distribution but there can be no definite line of demarcation.

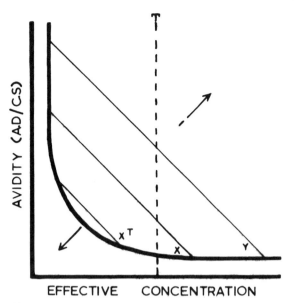

FIGURE 4. To illustrate the concept that the result of specific contact of antigenic determinant (AD) and immunocyte may be either destructive or stimulating to specific activity, depending (a) on the affinity of receptor AD union, (b) on the "effective concentration" of the antigenic determinant, and (c) on the physiological state of the immunocyte.

Destruction is more likely above and to the right of the diagonal line; proliferation and antibody production, below and to the left.

of antigen present. For reasons I need not elaborate, effective concentration will probably be a complex function of concentration, time of exposure and the mode of presentation of the antigen. Broadly speaking there are two extremes of response by an immunocyte to contact with antigen. Destruction and damage: proliferation to plasma cells and antibody production. In the diagram there is a diagonal line to mark the hypothetical conditions where the two responses are equally likely. Above and to the right, destruction will predominate; below and to the left, proliferation and antibody production. The position of the diagonal on the diagram will depend on the physiological state of the immunocyte which can be modified by its degree of maturity, the local internal environment and the presence of drugs or somatic mutations (Fig. 5).

Rightly or wrongly, I believe that those four diagrams contain the essentials of a modern selec-

tion theory of antibody production and that they are in a sufficiently generalized form to have a good chance of remaining valid indefinitely.

Now may I move from the controversial present to the wholly speculative future. If what is developing today is at all near the truth, we are on the verge of one of the most humanly important discoveries in history—the rules by which a double sequence of perhaps twice 5–7 amino acids in peptide linkage can provide a complementary steric pattern to virtually any significant biological molecule. At about the same time we shall also have clarified the structures of the active centers of the common enzymes and the toxic moiety of the potent protein toxins such as botulinus, the snake venoms and that of our Australian sea wasp (Chironex) which may be the most lethal of them all.

This brings me to a general point of great importance. In one sense there are only two major aspects of living structure. There is the maintenance and replication of genetic information and its translation into functioning substance, and at another level there is the *control* of these functioning substances to maintain a viable organism. The first function is based on nucleic acids, the second on specific pattern in protein. At the fundamental level they are best studied experimentally in bacterial viruses and in antibody structure, respectively.

With the best intentions in the world, I have spent my professional life in the study of viruses and antibodies; and I have watched both emerge from hypothetical entities needed to explain otherwise inexplicable gross phenomena to objects with structure and meaning. And at the end I find myself a Cassandra seeing dangers where I should be exulting in success. We are on the verge of knowing the nucleotide sequences which determine virulence and antigenicity of polio virus. The other small viruses such as yellow fever and foot and mouth disease are nearly equally accessible. There are doomsday weapons in the making here as well as spine-chilling possibilities of accident. Detailed analysis of some phage DNA and RNA is well under way and polio might, if anything, be simpler. But, beyond the small viruses we shall probably always have to be content with general ideas based

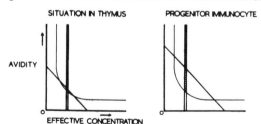

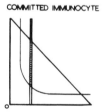

FIGURE 5. To show the use of Fig. 4 under the three circumstances: 1. On differentiation in the thymus; 2. Progenitor (uncommitted) immunocyte; 3. Committed immunocyte. The result with a standard level of effective concentration is shown as white—no effect, dots—proliferation and/or antibody production, black—destruction of the stimulated cell.

on the smaller models. To synthesize a mammalian genome is a task for 1,000 million years of evolution, not for a biochemistry laboratory.

The second great achievement of molecular biology in the making, the specification of functional action between proteins to which immunology is leading us, will in more subtle ways have equally great potentialities for evil and maybe many for good. We are in sight of understanding how to interfere effectively with any aspect of biological control in the developed organism. All control is a matter of the interplay of patterns on polypeptide chains and each control will be susceptible to specific damage by material we can synthesize. Those materials will be used therapeutically; they will also be studied as potentially lethal weapons; and in between they will be administered in good faith to produce some desirable effect. But they may have alarmingly unexpected consequences.

At the cellular level I think we are all agreed that the next major advance in theoretical and experimental biology is to be the analysis of differentiation. At times I feel pessimistic—people have been knocking hard at that door for many years and though we have many precise accounts of what happens during differentiation there are no keys yet to open up a real advance in understanding. As an immunologist I am interested in one rather tiny area of the maintenance of organic form but one which could be of great human importance. It concerns the need for and the probable existence of a mechanism to recognize and destroy aberrant cells arising by somatic mutation within the body. There are two competing conceptions, that of immunological surveillance which has been current in one form or another for a long time, and the more recent concept of allogeneic inhibition.

There is a variety of evidence both experimental and clinical that malignant disease can be prevented, aborted or even cured by immunological means. And, as Thomas (1959) was the first to point out, there are good evolutionary reasons why this should be so. It is an interesting thought that but for the heterogeneity of our histocompatibility antigens and the ability of our lymphocytes to recognize such differences, cancer would be a highly contagious disease. This would hold whether the "seek and destroy" function of the lymphocytes is based on immune reactivity or on allogeneic inhibition. Since the latter is also based apparently on differences in histocompatibility *antigens*, I am strongly inclined to think that immune processes are concerned in this surveillance.

Is there any application of all this to the question of ageing? There are insistent indications that some people live longer, age more slowly and seem to be intrinsically more healthy than others. Then there is the result which, being honest, I always have to mention when I am propagandizing against cigarettes—that 80% of heavy cigarette smokers do *not* die of lung cancer. Neither phenomenon may have a determinable cause, each being dependent on the interaction of many genetic and environmental factors. But it is stimulating to ponder on the hypothesis that what makes the healthy long-lived man is a greater effectiveness of his immune surveillance by which aberrant cells can be recognized and eliminated silently and completely. Those aberrant cells would include, as the most important component, cells on the way toward malignancy, but I see no reason why other somatic mutants doing no more than clogging the works should not also be routinely removed much as effete red cells are. This could well help to maintain health.

There are some interseting possibilities here for an eventual experimental approach. The thymus may well play a key role. It fades away after middle life to a shred of fibro-fatty tissue and perhaps this is Nature's way of seeing to that evolutionary necessity that men and mammals generally should age and die. Metcalf (1965) and others have shown that without a thymus old mice are poor at producing new types of antibody, and Miller et al. (1963) have given more direct evidence about the increased susceptibility of the neonatally thymectomized mouse to cancer induction by virus or carcinogen.

Longevity is very clearly an inheritable characteristic and if the beneficial effect of those "good" genes affects the body as a whole, it seems likely that the effect is mediated by some unitary mechanism, i.e., by something not representing an inherited quality in every cell. One thinks immediately of a heightened functional activity of that process of immunological surveillance which I have been discussing. Here and there in the literature there are hints that the activity of immune process has broader implications. Our postulated mechanism may or may not be concerned with thymic hormones but if the genetic influence is mediated through some diffusible agent it should in principle be capable of isolation, synthesis and therapeutic use. This is admittedly almost but not quite irresponsible speculation. It is developed merely to suggest another area where experimental and theoretical immunology may impinge in double-edged fashion on human affairs. Our present rate of population growth is bad enough but if, in addition, we were all to become centenarians it would throw our whole social and economic life into disorder.

I am not basically as pessimistic as I sound but I do believe that we must look absolutely squarely at what we are doing in biological science. If we are working in the genetics of animal viruses, that should be known to and discussed by both World Health Organization and national health authorities. If a means of producing a semi-synthetic antibody is devised, the results may call for an even more careful scrutiny of projected clinical applications than those applying to today's less sophisticated drugs. However much one feels that the world would be a safer place if scientists could define and interdict action toward "knowing what should not be known," this is utterly impossible. All we can hope is to keep the threat, if there is one, in the open. After all, the nerve gases, anthrax aerosols and the hydrogen bomb have all been available in quantity for a long time now and none have yet been used in the struggle for power. Nor is there yet on record a major accident involving nuclear technology.

It is always easier to destroy than to create and the more we understand about what evolution has created, the more readily we can destroy it. We must, as biologists, accept the responsibility of keeping our discoveries in the open, of being aware of any potential dangers they imply and of taking the precautions that may be necessary. On the whole the record says that we are capable of accepting that responsibility. The one thing we can be certain of is that there is no power of Church or State that can say that at this point, research must stop. It will go on in every field but we shall have to think harder and more effectively about its implications.

REFERENCES

ATTARDI, G., M. COHN, K. HORIBATA, and E. G. LENNOX. 1959. On the analysis of antibody synthesis at the cellular level. Bact. Rev. 23: 213.

BURNET, F. M. 1957. A modification of Jerne's theory of antibody production using the concept of clonal selection. Austr. J. Sci. 20: 67.

——. 1959. The clonal selection theory of immunity. Vanderbilt and Cambridge University Presses.

JERNE, N. K. 1955. The natural selection theory of antibody formation. Proc. Natl. Acad. Sci. 41: 849.

JERNE, N. K., and A. A. NORDIN. 1963. Plaque formation in agar by single antibody forming cells. Science 140: 405.

MACKAY, I. R., and D. C. GAJDUSEK. 1958. An "auto-immune" reaction against human tissue antigens in certain acute and chronic diseases. II. Clinical correlations. Arch. Intern. Med. 101: 30.

METCALF, D. 1965. Delayed effect of adult thymectomy on immunological competence. Nature 208: 1336.

MILLER, J. F. A. P. 1962. Effect of neonatal thymectomy on the immunological responsiveness of the mouse. Proc. Roy. Soc. B 156: 415.

MILLER, J. F. A. P., C. A. GRANT, F. J. C. ROE. 1963. Effect of thymectomy on the induction of skin tumors by 34 benzopyrene. Nature 199: 920.

NOSSAL, G. J. V. and J. LEDERBERG. 1958. Antibody production by single cells. Nature 181: 1419.

NOWELL, P. C. 1960. Phytohemagglutinin an initiator of mitosis in culture of normal human lymphocytes. Cancer Research 20: 462.

PEARMAIN, G. E., R. R. LYCETTE, and P. H. FITZGERALD. 1963. Tuberculin induced mitosis in peripheral blood leucocytes. Lancet 1: 637.

PUTNAM, F. W., K. TITANI, and E. WHITNEY, Jr. 1966. Chemical structure of light chains: amino acid sequences of type K Bence-Jones proteins. Proc. Roy. Soc. B 166: 124.

SZENBERG, A., N. L. WARNER, F. M. BURNET, and P. E. LIND. 1962. Quantitative aspects of the Simonsen phenomenon. II. Circumstances influencing the focal counts obtained on the chorioallantoic membrane. Brit. J. Exptl. Path. 43: 129.

TALMAGE, D. W. 1957. Allergy and immunology. Ann. Rev. Med. 8: 239.

THOMAS, L. 1959. Discussion, p. 530. In H. S. Lawrence [ed.] Cellular and humoral aspects of hypersensitive states. Hoeber, New York.

TRENTIN, J. J., and W. J. FAHLBERG. 1963. An experimental model for studies of immunologic competence in irradiated mice repopulated with clones of spleen cells, p. 66. In Conceptual advances in immunology and oncology. Hoeber, New York.

ZETTERVALL, O., J. SJOQUIST, J. WALDENSTROM, and S. WINBLAD. 1966. Serological activity of myeloma type globulins. Clin. Exptl. Immunol. 1: 213.

Summary: Waiting for the End

NIELS KAJ JERNE
Paul Ehrlich-Institut,
Frankfurt am Main, Germany

These early days of June remind me of Kierkegaard's anecdote (1843) about an artist who was asked to paint a mural of the passage of Moses across the Red Sea. He painted the entire wall red and explained: "the point in time that I have chosen to consider is when the Jews had already crossed and the Egyptians were already drowned." My present point in time is similar with respect to the passage of the trans- and cis-immunologists across the stage of this Cold Spring Harbor Confrontation, and I am afraid that my picture may show a similar lack of detail.

First, speaking for all participants, I thank our host, Dr. John Cairns, Director of the Cold Spring Harbor Laboratory of Quantitative Biology, for having organized this symposium and for having brought together this representative group of immunologists at the moment in history when we are experiencing the massive impact of molecular biology on immunology and the smaller recoil impact of immunology on molecular biology. The definitive solution of the antibody problem is approaching, and there is no doubt of the deep effect this will have on medicine, on the understanding of allergic and degenerative disorders and cancer, and on immunization, transplantation and other procedures.

We all regretted that the political situation prevented Dr. Feldman and Dr. Sela from being with us at Cold Spring Harbor.

CIS- AND TRANS-IMMUNOLOGISTS

The formation of antibodies by an animal after antigenic exposure is a phenomenon that proceeds by several steps. It is a story that unfolds over days and weeks, months and years. At the beginning, antigen is introduced or appears in the tissues of the animal. At the end, cells of this animal secrete globulin molecules that have the remarkable property of being able to recognize, and to stick to, the antigen that provoked their formation.

The antibody problem thus has a beginning and an end, and the people approaching this problem can, accordingly, be divided into two groups: (1) the trans-immunologists that start at the end, with the structure of antibody molecules, hoping to work their way backwards, and (2) the cis-immunologists that start at the beginning, with the effects of antigenic exposure, hoping to work their way forwards.

This dichotomy can be related to a saying attributed to Francis Crick: "if you cannot study function, study structure." I do not know where to place the correct emphasis, whether "if you *cannot* study function, study structure," or "if *you* cannot study function, study structure." Anyway, the trans-immunologists appeared on the scene about ten years ago, when decades of experimentation had demonstrated that immunologists, indeed, were unable to study function. The precise dividing point between cis and trans is the receptor molecule on the antigen-sensitive lymphocyte. The interest of the trans-immunologist wanes when confronted with tales about the vicissitudes of the antigen in the tissues before reaching the triggering point, whereas the cis-immunologist becomes sceptical at stories of inexorable mechanisms leading from the origin of the vertebrates to the endowment of a lymphocyte with genes for producing only a single foreordained antibody. The result is that the two hardly speak to each other. Or rather, a cis-immunologist will sometimes speak to a trans-immunologist; but the latter rarely answers.

TRANS-IMMUNOLOGY: ANTIBODIES AS GENE PRODUCTS

ANTIBODY DIVERSITY

The recognition, in 1890, of antibody specificity (Behring and Kitasato) marks the birth of the antibody problem. It was clear from the start that the range of antibody diversity, i.e. the number of different antibody molecules which one animal can synthesize, must be very large. It is still not possible to determine this number. An early guess of one million (Jerne, 1955) may be orders of magnitude too low. Evidence is accumulating that even antibody molecules having combining sites specific for the same antigen, and composed of polypeptide chains of the same classes, can display different allotypic and idiotypic markers, and can vary with respect to net electric charge and to avidity toward the antigen (Sela and Mozes, 1966; Jerne, 1951; Finkelstein and Uhr, 1966; Eisen, 1965; Steiner and Eisen, 1966). Among these

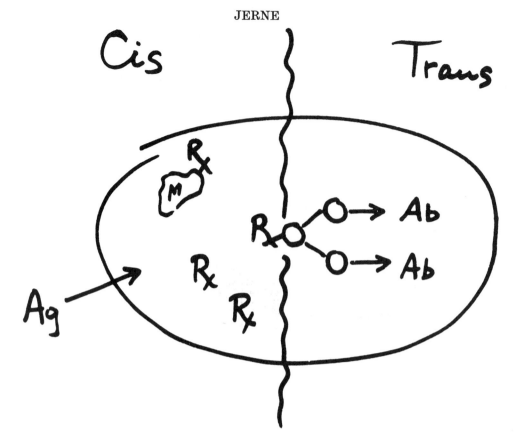

FIGURE 1. *Cis:* Antigen is introduced into an animal and meets with macrophages (M), fixed and free receptor molecules (R) before the antigenic stimulus triggers the final receptor on the antigen-sensitive cell. *Trans:* After proper triggering the antigen-sensitive lymphocyte becomes the ancestor of a clone of cells that synthesize and secrete antibody.

different sorts of diversity, those related to classes and subclasses of polypeptide chains and to their allotypic markers have been studied extensively during recent years. Some allotypic differences have been traced back to differences in amino acid sequence (Milstein, 1966; Appella and Ein, 1967), and genetic studies represented at this symposium by the reports of Potter and Lieberman[1], Kunkel and Natvig[1], Herzenberg, Minna, and Herzenberg[1], and Hamers[1], are clarifying the genetic linkage of polypeptide chain classes, and the genetics of allotypic expression.

By 1959, when antibodies had been known for seventy years, the wrinkled features of immunology were definitely in need of a face-lifting. This delicate operation was performed by Porter (1959) and Edelman (1959) whose revelation of the basic structure of immunoglobulins was followed by a burst of structural analysis in many laboratories:

1962: Bence-Jones proteins are light chains of immunoglobulins (Edelman and Gally, 1962).
1963: Different Bence-Jones proteins have common as well as distinctive peptides (Putnam, Easley, and Helling, 1963; Potter, Dreyer, Kuff, and McIntire, 1963).

[1] This volume

1964: Antibody specificity is determined by amino acid sequence (Haber, 1964; Whitney and Tanford, 1965; Freedman and Sela, 1966).
1965: Light chains have a variable N-terminal half and a constant C-terminal half (Hilschmann and Craig, 1965; Titani, Whitley, Avogardo, and Putnam, 1965; Putnam, Shinoda, Titani, and Wikler, 1967).

In the first place, these findings resolved a question that had always haunted immunology: Does the specificity of an antibody molecule reside in its primary structure, or can different combining sites arise by different folding of identical polypeptide chains? The answer, in the words of Freedman and Sela (1966a, b), is: all of the information required for the correct reformation leading to the initial conformation of the combining sites as well as the various antigenic determinants of an antibody molecule is contained in the amino acid sequence of its polypeptide chains. In the second place, the discriminating features were pinpointed to variable amino acid residues in the N-terminal halves of the chains. In about one-half of the 107 N-terminal positions different light chains show different amino acid residues. Not only did the basis of antibody diversity become immediately clear, but it also became apparent that proposals for a random generation of diversity had to contain restrictions in order to prevent the range of diversity from vastly outnumbering the 10^{12} lymphocytes of man.

That restrictions are indeed imposed on the variability of the variable parts of light and heavy polypeptide chains is becoming clear from the increasing knowledge of amino acid sequences, to which Putnam, Titani, Wikler, and Shinoda[1]; Milstein, Frangione, and Pink[1]; Appella and Perham[1]; Press and Piggot[1]; Waxdal, Konigsberg, and Edelman[1]; Cebra[1]; Koshland[1]; Hood, Gray, Sanders, and Dreyer[1] made further contributions at this symposium. Moreover, it appears that the variable positions in the chains of amino acid residues are interspersed with stretches that are conserved, and that are even identical across chain classes and across animal species. The sets of different residues occurring at each of the variable positions suggest mutations. It therefore seems most straightforward to imagine that the elements involved are phylogenic duplication and mutation of genes subject to selection, followed by an ontogenic diversity-generating process which must have two characteristics: it must partly rearrange and partly conserve the amino acid sequence of the gene product. There is one known process which accomplishes just that: crossing-over.

Two theories invoking crossing-over to explain antibody diversity were discussed. One, proposed by Edelman and Gally (1967), requires a few dozen genes each encoding the variable part of a polypeptide chain, whereas the other, proposed by Smithies[1] (1967), makes do with one and a half genes, the half gene being a "scrambler" gene specially invented to bring about a reassortment in the nucleotide sequence of the "master gene" by a crossover process during the differentiation of a cell. The discussion revealed that Edelman and Gally, in accord with Milstein (1966), have found that two genes do not suffice to generate, by somatic recombination, all variations so far observed, and that a larger set of genes is therefore needed; whereas Smithies similarly finds that two germ-line genes with many alleles do not explain all data, but prefers, with Crick's support, to attribute the remaining oddities to superimposed frills of nature. One of these frills may be the presence in the germ line of genes for more than one class of kappa chains and of lambda chains (Niall and Edman, 1967). Another crossover model for the somatic generation of antibody diversity has been proposed by Whitehouse (1967).

Mach[1] presented a variant of an earlier proposal by Potter, Appella, and Geisser (1965), placing the generation of antibody diversity at the translational level by exploiting the degeneracy of the genetic code. This idea of making different plasma cells speak different dialects did not find much favor in the discussion, because it would either reserve a large set of "unusual" codons for the special benefit of immunology, or introduce instability; antibody-forming cells proliferate and therefore must maintain a stable translation system. The case for a translational mechanism has recently been stated by Campbell (1967).

The point to which structural analysis has led us then seems to be, at the present moment, that somatic recombination by the scrambling of two germ-line genes, or rather two sets of genes, could be the crucial step marking the differentiation of a stem cell into a committed antigen-sensitive cell. According to the studies of Till, McCulloch, Phillips, and Siminovitch[1], and the work of Trentin et al. (1967) and others, the decisive crossover step would have to occur at the transition of a nonrestricted bone marrow cell into a lymphocyte, whereas Metcalf's work[1] would suggest that the event is triggered by a thymic hormone.

The genetic mechanisms proposed to account for antibody diversity thus leave us with an equally diverse population of antigen-sensitive lymphocytes. Each of these cells, even before encountering an antigenic stimulus, is committed to the production of antibody molecules of one particular specification, and each cell will transmit this single commitment to its progeny of antibody-secreting cells and memory cells. This is Burnet's Dogma (1959) in its uncompromising form.

ANTIBODY-PRODUCING CELLS

I shall now turn to the studies of cells that are already producing immunoglobulins. The possibility that these cells have separate genes for the variable and the constant portions of the polypeptide chains was considered by Hood, Gray, Sanders, and Dreyer[1], and the question whether these two portions are synthesized contiguously or whether they are joined after having been made separately has been examined by Baglioni, Cioli, Gorini, Ruffilli, and Alescio-Zonta[1]; Fleischman[1]; and Lennox, Knopf, Munro, and Parkhouse[1]. The evidence presented leads to the conclusion that both heavy and light chains are made in one piece instructed by RNA messengers each encoding an entire chain.

Several investigators have followed up the classical work of Helmreich, Kern, and Eisen (1961, 1962) on the mechanism and time scale of antibody production by isolated lymphoid cells. The reports by Askonas and Williamson[1]; Sharff, Shapiro, and Ginsberg[1]; and Ralph, Becker, and Rich[1], confirmed that synthesis of H and L chains proceeds on separate polyribosomes. Newly synthesized light chains are released into a pool. The association of free light chains, drawn from this pool, with nascent heavy chains leads to the release of half-globulin molecules which rapidly assemble pairwise. Kern and Swenson[1] reported that these assembled globulin molecules remain confined to a microsomal compartment, whereas only molecules to which carbohydrate has been attached are found in the cell sap. Further studies by Greenberg and Uhr[1] and an analysis by Melchers and Knopf[1] indicate that carbohydrate attachment proceeds by several steps requiring more than eight minutes, and is probably requisite to secretion. Fahey and Finegold[1] have studied the rate of immunoglobulin production in cultures of human lymphoid cell lines. From the amount of lambda chain produced by a million cells during one day, assuming that only those 10% of cells participate that are stainable with fluorescent antilambda antibody, a rate of secretion of about 1000 molecules per cell per second can be calculated. By order of magnitude, this confirms earlier estimates of the rate of antibody formation by a single cell.

The classical question whether all antibody molecules produced by one cell are identical must be answered in the affirmative. Earlier studies by Cebra et al. (1966), Pernis et al. (1965), and others using specific fluorescence have brought out the rule that a single cell produces one class of heavy chain and one class of light chain only, and that, in animals that are heterozygous for globulin allotypes, individual cells make only the product of either one or the other of the parental alleles. The studies by Gell and Sell (1965) on the provocation of blast transformation of peripheral lymphocytes by anti-allotype sera are compatible with the idea that this phenotypic restriction precedes the antigenic stimulation of a cell.

The one cell—one antibody rule appears to hold also for the specificity of the antibody combining site. Mäkelä[1] has immunized rabbits and rats with two types of bacteriophage. He reported his failure to find any double producer among 205 single cells that released neutralizing antibodies. The rule is confirmed by the recent work of Green, Vassalli, Nussenzweig, and Benacerraf (1967a, b) who studied cells producing antibodies against one or the other of two antigenic determinants situated on the same antigenic molecule. None of the 1569 cells observed produced antibodies against both. Papermaster[1] and many other workers are examining Nossal's troublesome question (Nossal et al., 1964) whether cells of one clone switch from IgM to IgG production. It seems as yet not definitely settled. Evidence for the production of both γ-heavy chains and μ-heavy chains by one cell line

was reported by Fahey and Finegold[1]. Apparently there do exist circumstances in which a clone can depart from the rule of restricting its synthesis to one product. The observations of Sell (1967) are relevant to this point. Pernis[1] has prepared a fluorescent antilambda chain antibody which, after absorption with normal light chains, reacts only with a particular human Bence-Jones protein. Among one million plasma cells from normal persons he found 12 stainable cells. Presumably, these cells produced lambda sharing an idiotypic determinant with the Bence-Jones chains. This is evidence for the enormous heterogeneity among a normal population of lymphoid cells with respect to the particular immunoglobulin they produce. The probability that two randomly chosen cells produce identical lambda chains may thus be less than 10^{-5}. This cellular heterogeneity is reflected by the heterogeneity of antibody molecules in the serum of animals immunized with one antigen. The reports by Reisfeld[1] and by Fazekas de St. Groth[1] brought out the difficulties of an orderly approach to this heterogeneity problem. It has been known since the work of Landsteiner (1947) that, obviously, there is not a one-to-one correspondence between antibody combining sites and antigenic determinants. On the contrary, one antigenic determinant can elicit the production of a large set of antibody-combining sites, each of which would embody a spectrum of affinities to a large set of antigenic determinants. The question raised by Eisen, Little, Osterland, and Simms[1] as to the lowest association constant that would still make us call a globulin an antibody once more focussed attention on this degeneracy problem in antigen-antibody relationships.

It might, therefore, seem very unlikely that antibody of only one molecular species can ever be isolated in an amount sufficient for studying the detailed structure of a combining site to a known antigenic determinant. Several reports, however, were more optimistic in this respect. Haber, Richards, Spragg, Austen, Vallotton, and Page[1], by using well-defined large antigenic structures, have succeeded in evoking the production of antibodies of greater homogeneity and of high binding affinity that does not, as usually observed, increase with time. Nisonoff, Zappacosta, and Jureziz[1] have been able to crystallize a homogeneous antibody from a hyperimmune rabbit. Another approach to this problem is to screen myeloma proteins and other pathological, homogeneous immunoglobulins for their antibody properties toward selected antigens. This approach was discussed by Eisen, et al.[1]; Stone and Metzger[1]; Metzger 1967; Cohn[1], and Potter and Lieberman[1], and it is remarkable that pathological immunoglobulins with antibody activity are suddenly being found in several laboratories, though Cohn had not succeeded in enticing mice to develop myelomas with phage neutralizing activity by offering them a set of bacteriophages during the myeloma-induction period. The human IgG-myeloma protein found by Eisen's group after screening 59 myeloma sera appears to be a homogeneous anti-DNP antibody with an intrinsic association constant of 2×10^4 M^{-1} for ε-DNP-lysine.

The affinity labeling experiments reported by Singer, Slobin, Thorpe, and Fenton[1] and by Wofsy and Parker[1] point to a possible classification of combining sites of different types, and to common structural features. The experiments also indicate that both heavy and light chains participate in combining site structure. This is in accordance with recent findings of Yoo, Roholt, and Pressman (1967) and of Raynaud (pers. commun.) that not only heavy chains but also isolated light chains of antibodies retain some specific binding activity toward the antigen.

ANTIBODY-FORMING CLONES

Proliferation

The proliferation of antibody-forming cells after an antigenic stimulus has recently been studied in many laboratories, including my own. Though there is no doubt that these cells can proliferate rapidly, I agree with Ellis, Gowans, and Howard[1]; Dutton and Mishell[1]; Papermaster[1]; and Claflin and Smithies (1967) that the observed doubling time, which can be less than seven hours, may be shorter than the actual generation time. If this is true, the observed rate of multiplication must be the sum of the rate of proliferation of antibody-secreting cells and the rate of recruitment of such cells from another proliferating but nonsecreting population.

The technique worked out by Dutton and Mishell[1] for stimulating lymphoid cells in culture appears to have many potentialities. In their system the appearance of antibody-forming cells after a primary stimulus is closely similar to the kinetics in animals, though the proliferation of the cells in culture appears to escape the regulatory factors which limit this process in the animal. Dutton and Mishell (1967) and Mishell and Dutton (1967) have demonstrated that two non-cross-reacting antigens address themselves to two different populations of target lymphocytes. This is in accordance with our findings.

Precursors

Various reports dealt with the precursor cells of antibody-forming clones. Till, McCulloch, Phillips, and Siminovitch[1] traced back the ancestry of these cells to a stem cell in the bone marrow and examined the question whether this stem cell is the joint progenitor of the hemopoietic and the granulopoietic as well as the lymphopoietic systems. The stem cell appears not to be antigen sensitive, but to acquire that property after having migrated to the lymphoid organs, where it may multiply with a doubling time of about 36 hours.

The antigen-sensitive cell which is the target of a primary antigenic stimulus was identified by Ellis, Gowans, and Howard[1] as a circulating, long-lived small lymphocyte which may be of a different type from the small lymphocyte that Gowans and Uhr (1967) have found to be a memory cell. The responsiveness of an irradiated rat to sheep red cell antigen can be restored by an injection of small lymphocytes from a normal but not from an immunologically tolerant donor. The fluorescence studies of van Furth, Schuit, and Hijmans (1966) likewise implicate the small lymphocyte. With a chromosome marker, Nossal, Shortman, Miller, Mitchell, and Haskill[1] have demonstrated that circulating lymphocytes from a donor rat can develop into antibody-producing plasma cells in an irradiated recipient rat. They do not exclude the possibility that medium and large lymphocytes may also be virgin target cells, either for particular classes of antigen or for the production of particular classes of antibody, and their results suggest that the population of small lymphocytes is heterogeneous with respect to control by the thymus or by another central lymphoid tissue. Methods for fractionating populations of lymphocytes from the thoracic duct, peripheral blood, and lymphoid organs are being developed to clarify this cellular heterogeneity.

Several workers have approached the question of the number of target cells present in an animal at a given moment which can respond to a primary stimulus by one antigenic determinant, or by an antigen presenting a small bundle of antigenic determinants. Papermaster[1] reported that the spleen of an untreated mouse appears to contain about 2000 cells capable of responding to sheep red cell antigen by producing progeny cells which secrete hemolytic antibody. This is about one cell per 10^5 cells present in the mouse spleen, a figure not very far from the estimates of Albright and Makinodan (1966), Kennedy, Siminovitch, Till, and McCulloch (1965, 1966), Šterzl[1], ourselves, and others, but about 100-fold lower than the number of cells capable of forming specific rosettes as shown by Biozzi, Stiffel, Mouton, Liacopoulos-Briot, Decreusefond, and Bouthillier (1966), and Zaalberg, van der Meul, and van Twisk (1966).

THE EMERGING PICTURE

I shall briefly outline the tentative general picture that emerges from the work of the groups so far mentioned.

Somewhere back in evolution, when the vertebrates emerged, a primordial gene, by duplications and mutations, developed into a set of genes coding for antibody polypeptides of various classes. A somatic crossover mechanism evolved whereby a structural gene of this set achieves the definitive base sequence determining its phenotypic expression. These developments preceded the separation of mammalian species. Phylogenically, this set of germ-line genes responded to selection pressure toward a large range of synthetic potentialities of the population of lymphocytes, including antibodies against tumor antigens and invading microbes, and incidentally including antibodies to artificial antigens and even components of the animal itself. Minor advantages of novel mutations in these genes and random drift led to a stable polymorphism with many alleles. Ontogenically, at a certain stage of cell differentiation, when a bone marrow cell becomes a lymphocyte under influence of a thymic factor, the crossover step takes place by which each cell is randomly endowed with its definitive commitment. This leads to the development of a heterogeneous population of lymphocytes that can be selectively triggered at antigen-sensitive receptor sites to proliferate and to synthesize one species of light chain and one species of heavy chain. The amino acid sequences of these chains, that were determined at the crossover step, in turn determine the structure of the antibody combining site. At full synthetic rate a cell may turn out 2000 antibody molecules per second. As each molecule has about 1300 peptide bonds, and assuming that one ribosome can make 13 peptide bonds per sec (Kepes and Beguin, 1966; Maaløe, 1966), a cell needs about 200,000 ribosomes or 10,000 polysomes for each type of polypeptide chain. These must be served by 10,000 mRNA molecules for each chain, and as the producing cell may proliferate with a generation time of about 10 hr, each structural gene must be transcribed once every 5 sec. A pool of about 10^6 free light chains is maintained in which a light chain spends an average of 3 min and from which 4000 light chains are withdrawn per sec in order to combine with nascent heavy chains to form globulin molecules. The cell may hold about 10^7 completed globulin molecules, most of which are in the process of being provided with their carbohydrate components before being released into the secretory compartment. Because of the degeneracy of antigen-antibody relationship, the set of cells triggered by a given antigenic determinant turns out a heterogeneous product. Further antigenic stimuli select among the cells of the developing clones. Many of these cells become mature plasma cells and die, others regress to become small lymphocytes of the memory class. Losses to the population are restored by proliferation and by recruitment of newcomers from the bone marrow.

From the discussions I gained the impression that this general outline is backed up by an impressive number of facts, and at least fits practically all known facts, if we disregard a few disturbing findings, such as the possibility that a cell may switch from producing one type of heavy chain to producing another (Nossal et al., 1964), and the finding by Edelman, Olins, Gally, and Zinder (1963), Roholt, Radzinski, and Pressman (1965a, b, 1967), Mannik (1967), Dorrington, Larlengo, and Tanford (1967) and others, that the heavy and light chains produced by one antibody-forming cell show a better mutual fit than a random pair of heavy and light chains; and if we refuse to pay attention to a number of experimental results that appear to be totally at odds with the above picture and that I shall refer to in turning to the cis-immunologists.

CIS-IMMUNOLOGY: ANTIBODIES AS ANTIGEN RECEPTORS

Whereas the main interest of trans-immunology is to clarify the genetic mechanisms and cellular dynamics for maintaining a population of lymphocytes capable of synthesizing an enormous range of different antibody molecules, cis-immunology is mainly concerned with the regulatory factors which permit or forbid an antigen to trigger this system successfully. Many cis-immunologists are only marginally interested in the general picture just outlined, except for the assertion that each antigen-sensitive cell is precommitted to the production of a single antibody. They would not be a bit surprised if it should turn out that a given cell can be induced by an adequate stimulus to make any one of thousands of antibodies. In immunological interpretation at the present stage of the game, however, —as in chess when a pinned piece must not be moved—Burnet's dogma of cellular precommitment must remain unimpeached.

HERESY

There is a group of workers whose findings appear to contradict this dogma. Fishman and Adler[1] presented data which imply not only that macrophages mediate in transferring the antigenic stimulus to the executive lymphocytes, but also that in doing so the macrophage transfers information concerning antibody structure in the form of RNA molecules of about 300 bases in length. Thus, macrophage RNA from a donor animal of one allotype induced lymphocytes of a recipient animal of a different allotype to produce antibodies exhibiting the allotypic markers of the donor (Adler, Fishman, and Dray, 1966). Simonsen[1] presented data that seem incompatible with single cellular commitment, in that cells capable of responding against particular histo-incompatibility antigens with a graft-versus-host reaction appear to be present in a random sample of as few as 50 donor lymphocytes. Furthermore, he cast doubt (Nisbet and Simonsen, 1967) on the proposition that cellular proliferation is a necessary component of the primary immune response, as did Bussard[1] who, on the basis of experiments with peritoneal-exudate cells, reported that at least one of every thousand, and perhaps one of a hundred of such cells can be induced in vitro to produce hemolytic antibodies against sheep red cells without undergoing cell division. This again suggests multipotentiality of individual cells.

It remains to be seen whether or not these observations, and other findings of this kind, will bring about a reconsideration of the dogma of single cellular commitment. It is clear that this would give the trans-immunologists great difficulties, because in that case an antigen-sensitive cell would have to make a choice among many genes coding for different antibody polypeptides, and to postpone this acceptance of its definitive commitment until it has recognized an antigen. In spite of the suggestions of Dreyer, Gray, and Hood[1], it seems to me that the cell would face the impossible task of evolving a set of regulator genes as large as the set of its antibody structural genes in order to produce repressor molecules that would have to discriminate between many structural genes differing only slightly in base sequence.

ANTIGEN RECEPTORS

Antigen receptors are antibody molecules. This simplifying statement is based on the propositions that agents capable of recognizing antigens must have antibody combining sites, and that antigens must be recognized as antigens before the sequence of events leading to the triggering of antigen-sensitive cells can get underway (Jerne, 1960). This is strengthened by the evidence of Sela, Schechter, Schechter, and Borek[1], Haber et al.[1], and Freedman and Sela (1966), showing that the immunogenic identity of a protein molecule is determined by its tertiary conformation, i.e., by its fit into an antibody combining site. I shall first consider the antigen receptor on the antigen-sensitive lymphocyte.

The Final Receptor

The receptor on the target lymphocyte that is triggered by an antigenic stimulus assumes the shape of an antibody molecule representing those that the cell is capable of synthesizing. This is in accordance with the findings of Gell[1] and Sell (1967) who have shown that a fraction of the small lymphocytes from a heterozygous rabbit can be triggered to blast transformation in vitro by antibody against one allotypic marker, and an additional fraction by antibody against the allelic allotypic marker. This suggests not only that a target lymphocyte carries receptors that resemble antibody molecules, but also that one cell may display receptors of one parental allotype only.

The introduction into an embryonic or newborn heterozygous animal of antibody directed against one allotypic marker suppresses the phenotypic expression of this marker, probably by eliminating the entire subpopulation of precursor cells which exhibit receptors of this allotype. Dubiski[1], Mage[1], Chou, Cinader, and Dubiski[1], and Herzenberg, Minna, and Herzenberg[1] presented results of allotypic suppression experiments. Suppression is compensated by the production of immunoglobulins that do not carry the suppressed marker. It is astonishing that this situation can persist for a period of about a year, long after the anti-allotypic antibody has disappeared from the recipient animal. Mage suggested that this persistence may result from a homeostatic mechanism whereby the immune system tends to continue to produce the types of globulin it is already producing. This is an intriguing possibility for which it is hard to imagine a satisfactory mechanism. The prolonged effect of allotypic suppression may simply be the consequence of a slow recruitment of novel, unaffected precursor cells from the bone marrow into the lymphoid system. If this were so, the recovery from allotypic suppression might be comparable to the recovery from those forms of immunological tolerance that are associated with the absence of a subset of lymphocytes as shown by Ellis, Gowans, and Howard[1], and the low rate of recovery might be related to the findings reported by Metcalf[1] indicating that precursor cells are exported by the thymus at a low rate. We may also see a relation with the prolonged effect of the Original Sin, evoked by Fazekas de St. Groth[1]. The experimental results reported by Weigle and Golub[1] contribute to a determination of the time scale for the induction of tolerance and recovery. Sell and Gell (1965) have shown that allotypically suppressed rabbits, at a time when they have no immunoglobulin molecules of the paternal allotype, do have small lymphocytes that respond with blast transformative to antibody directed against the paternal allotype. This might seem to contradict the contention that allotypic suppression is caused by destruction of precursor cells carrying receptors of the suppressed allotype. The population of immunoglobulin molecules circulating in an animal at a given time, however, does not reflect the population of precursor cells present at that time, but reflects the composition of the clones of producing cells which have arisen from earlier precursors. An analysis of this situation would require further knowledge of the population dynamics of the lymphoid system.

The Intervening Macrophage

It would be simplest to imagine that an antigenic particle elicits an antigenic stimulus by addressing itself directly to the receptor on a target lymphocyte. Matters appear to be more complicated, however. The experimental evidence of Mitchison[1], Feldman and Gallily[1], Gallily and Feldman (1967), Harris and Littleton (1966), Frei, Benacerraf, and Thorbecke (1965), and many others demonstrates that a phagocytic cell intervenes in the primary as well as in a secondary immune response. Ada, Parrish, Nossal and Abbot[1], and Litt[1] reported on the fate of antigenic material in lymph nodes. Ada confirmed that cells actually producing antibody usually do not contain detectable antigenic material (Nossal, Ada, and Austin, 1965; McDevitt, Askonas, Humphrey, Schechter, and Sela, 1966). He also presented data on the degree of immunogenicity and tolerogenicity of a given amount of antigenic material as related to the size of the particles of this material presented to the animal. Larger particles are more immunogenic and less tolerogenic than smaller particles. This is in accordance with the findings of Dresser (1962), Biro and Guadelupe (1965), and Frei, Benacerraf, and Thorbecke (1965) and appears related to macrophage involvement in the immune stimulus (Thorbecke, Maurer, and Benacerraf, 1960). Macrophages are a heterogeneous population, and the macrophages involved in the immune stimulus must compete for antigenic material with other types of macrophages that are scavengers. The ingestion of antigen by macrophages is promoted by specific antibody that either opsonizes the antigen prior to a macrophage encounter or is cytophilically attached to the macrophage (Boyden and Sorkin, 1960; Berken and Benacerraf, 1966; Uhr, 1965; Ada and Lang, 1966). Macrophage intervention, therefore, involves antibody molecules that, apart from their antigen-receptor sites, have other sites that can attach to macrophage membranes, probably by the action of a structure in the Fc-region (Berken and Benacerraf, 1966; Uhr, 1965) similar to that reported by Sjöquist, Forsgren, Gustafson, and Stalenheim[1].

As a first approximation to understanding macrophage involvement in the immune stimulus it would, therefore, seem most economic to limit the role of the macrophage to the capture, concentration, and transport of antigen by attaching it to specific antibody molecules, i.e., to initial antigen receptors situated on its membranes that can be involuted and evoluted for presentation of the antigen to the final receptor on target lymphocytes. This would be compatible with the studies of Nossal, Ada, and Austin (1964) and McDevitt, Askonas, Humphrey, Schechter, and Sela (1966), and others on the follicular localization of antigens. Antigenic stimulation would then require that the antigenic particle is attached by means of one or more antibody molecules to a membrane while presenting its free antigenic determinants to the lymphocytes.

Inhibiting and Enhancing Receptors

Wigzell[1] reported observations of the effect of passively injected 7 S antibody on primary antigenic stimulation and on immune responses already in progress. In all cases he found a depression of antibody synthesis that manifested itself not later than two days after the antibody is injected, except for the synthesis of "natural" macroglobulin antibody which appeared to be unaffected. The suppression of the primary immune response by small amounts of hyperimmune antibody has been noted by several workers (Uhr and Baumann, 1961; Finkelstein and Uhr, 1964; Rowley and Fitch, 1964; Möller and Wigzell, 1965; Wigzell, 1966; Sahiar and Schwartz, 1964; Dixon, Jacot-Guillarmod, and McConahey, 1967). The antibody appears to be suppressive simply by covering antigenic determinants. Brody, Walker, and Siskind (1967) have recently shown that the suppression of one antigenic determinant by passive antibody does not necessarily entail suppression of another determinant on the same antigenic molecule. In connection with apparently conflicting reports on the effect of specific 19 S antibody, and on enhancement of the immune response by small amounts of both 7 S and 19 S antibodies (Rowley and Fitch, 1964; Möller and Wigzell, 1965; Segre and Kaeberle, 1962; Pearlman, 1967; Clarke, Donohue, McConnell, Woodrow, Finn, Krevans, Kulke, Lehane, and Sheppard, 1963), I shall briefly report a few of the observations that have been made by Henry (Henry and Jerne, 1967a,b) in my laboratory.

The control experiment is to inject 4×10^5 sheep red cells (SRC) intravenously into a mouse and to determine, six days later, the number of plaque-forming cells (PFC) present in the spleen, and secreting 19 S hemolytic antibody. In our inbred mice this number is, on the average, 4000

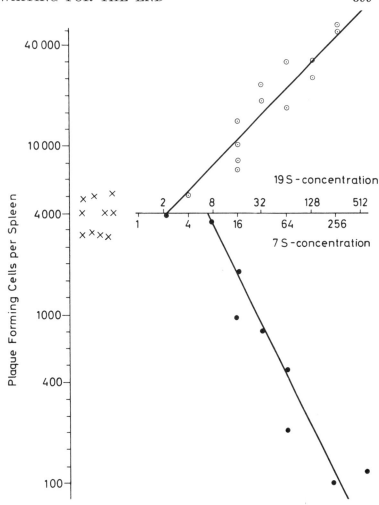

FIGURE 2. The ordinate gives the logarithm of the number of plaque forming cells per mouse spleen six days after the injection of 4×10^5 sheep red cells. The crosses represent the average normal response of groups of 20–50 mice. The abscissa, drawn at this response level, gives the relative molar concentrations of passively injected 19 S and 7 S antibody. The open circles represent the average responses of groups of mice that had received specific 19 S antibody, the closed circles give the average responses of groups of mice that had received specific 7 S antibody. Lines have been drawn through the experimental points with slopes of 0.5 and 1.0, respectively.

PFC per spleen. When specific anti-SRC antibody obtained from immunized mice is injected one hr prior to the SRC, this primary response is either enhanced or depressed. It is enhanced by 19 S antibody obtained from other mice within five days after a primary SRC stimulus and separated from 7 S antibody either by sucrose gradient centrifugation, or by euglobulin precipitation; it is depressed by 7 S antibody obtained from hyperimmune mice. Figure 2 shows the experimental results with this antigen dose and with various doses of 19 S and 7 S antibody.

The degree of enhancement as well as the degree of suppression depend, of course, on the amount of antibody injected, and when a dose of 19 S antibody, which by itself would have enhanced the response tenfold, is given together with a dose of 7 S antibody, which by itself would have depressed the response tenfold, a response in the normal range results. To a somewhat lesser degree, these effects can also be obtained by injecting mice with specific 19 S and 7 S antibody from animals of a different species. We do not know by which

mechanism the 19 S antibody acts, but it seems that a competition of 19 S and 7 S molecules for antigenic determinants is involved. Obviously, antibody already produced exercises a feed-back influence on the response to corresponding antigen.

The Receptor Puzzle

I imagine that a molecule can be immunogenic only if it presents at least two properly spaced antigenic determinants, one (the carrier) for accommodating the initial antigen receptor that places the molecule in position on a macrophage membrane, and one (the hapten) for triggering the final antigen receptor on a target lymphocyte. It follows that there are at least four deficiencies, each of which can result in unresponsiveness: (1) deficient antigenic molecules, e.g., the classical haptens, (2) lack of macrophages, (3) lack of specific initial antigen receptors, and (4) lack of target lymphocytes exhibiting the required final antigen receptors. These matters were explored in the reports by Mitchison[1], by Rajewsky and Rottländer[1], and by Benacerraf, Green, and

Paul[1]. Mitchison had used haptenic hydroxyiodo-phenyl, dinitrophenyl and diiodophenyl groups coupled to an albumin or globulin carrier. His studies of the "adoptive" secondary stimulus, by in vitro exposure of lymphoid cells from a primed animal to the hapten-carrier conjugates, have shown that stimulation can be completely in-hibited by free hapten, free carrier molecules, and by anti-immunoglobulin antibody. These ob-servations imply competition for antigen receptors. His finding that a structurally related free hapten can inhibit the appearance of the class of anti-bodies best fitting this determinant suggests that inhibition by free hapten occurs by competition for the final antigen receptors on the target lymphocytes, whereas inhibition of the response to hapten by free carrier molecules probably occurs by competition for the initial antigen receptors.

Rajewsky worked with porcine lactic dehydro-genase isozymes that have four protein subunits per molecule. Subunits of type A are immunogenic in all rabbits. In rabbits that cannot respond to type B subunits, B behaves as a hapten in the sense that antibodies to A and B appear when the rabbits are presented with molecules containing A and B together. In Rajewsky's as well as Mitchison's systems a successful secondary response to the hapten requires the same carrier that was used for the priming stimulus. These observations indicate that the animals have the target lymphocytes exhibiting the requisite hapten receptor, but depend on carrier oriented initial antigen receptors for placing the haptenic determinants *in situ*. Benacerraf dealt with dinitrophenyl-poly-L-lysine to which certain "nonresponder" guinea pigs lacking one dominant autosomal gene cannot respond, unless the substance is coupled to albumen or to another carrier. Even when responding with antibody formation to the "haptenic" part of this conjugate, these animals do not develop delayed hypersensitivity, nor can delayed hypersensitivity of that specificity be transferred to them with lymphocytes from a delayed hypersensitive "re-sponder" animal. In responder guinea pigs an anti-DNP response to DNP-poly-L-lysine is ob-tained only if there are at least eight lysine residues (Schlossman, Ben-Efraim, Yaron, and Sober, 1966). This is also the number of residues needed by Valentine and Green (1967) for linking two anti-DNP combining sites together. Cogno-scenti may wish to confront these observations with the ideas of Eisen and Karush (Karush and Eisen, 1962; Eisen and Karush, 1964) on the antigenic stimulus and on antibody molecules involved in delayed hypersensitivity, and with the mechanisms more recently proposed by Schlossman and Levine (1967) and by Leskowitz (1967). The

subject has been reviewed by Borek (1967). How can the presence of an initial antigen-receptor molecule, exhibiting a particular combining site created by random "scrambling," be controlled by one dominant autosomal gene? It is possible that this gene controls the synthesis of a self-component that, when present, eliminates the incriminated initial receptor molecules. Both Rajewsky and Benacerraf have found that there is no response to their "haptens" if the animal has acquired tolerance for the carrier. This tolerance to the haptenic determinants, therefore, does not imply the absence of competent lymphocytes but rather the dis-appearance of an initial antigen receptor for the carrier antigen. It would thus seem that certain forms of tolerance are not a consequence of the lack of specifically endowed lymphocytes as in the system of Ellis, Gowans, and Howard[1].

The experiments of Kerman, Segre, and Myers (1967) on the induction of tolerance in the off-spring of tolerant mice are relevant to this issue. Nossal[1] confirmed the discovery by Mitchison (1964) that tolerance can be provoked by ex-tremely low doses of antigen. This is possibly related to the observations of Šterzl[1] and ourselves suggesting that, in the normal antibody response, the progeny of triggered target cells need further antigenic stimuli for proliferation. A continued antigen sensitivity of the cells of triggered clones would also be needed, of course, for the selection of cells that produce the best fitting antibody (Jerne, 1951; Finkelstein and Uhr, 1966; Steiner and Eisen, 1966). It is conceivable that absence of repeated stimuli after an initial triggering can lead to an abortive response and to "low dose" tolerance. It is also possible that, under certain conditions, antigen-sensitive cells can be impaired by a direct encounter with antigen (Nossal, 1966), as when triggered by phytohemagglutinin, anti-immunoglobulin (Sell, 1967) or antilymphocytic serum (Woodruff, Reid, and James, 1967; Levey and Medawar, 1967; Brent, Courtenay, and Gowland, 1967). The reports of Gell[1], and Weigle and Golub[1] and the many observations by Sela's group have contributed further data to the solution of the receptor puzzle. Interpretation in this area of experimentation, concerned with the different immunological effects of presenting the same anti-genic determinants to an animal in different ways, requires further analysis of the set of antigen receptors and their function. I have proposed that all antigen receptors are fixed or free antibody molecules. Tentatively, five such antigen receptors have been evoked: (1) a final receptor on the target lymphocyte, (2) inhibiting 7 S antibody, (3) enhancing 19 S antibody, (4) an initial receptor for fixing antigenic molecules onto a macrophage membrane, (5) an initial receptor for explaining "carrier" functions. Some of these may be identical. It is possible that these receptors can be related to different properties of the various classes of immunoglobulins.

If, as a mathematician has said, five parameters suffice for the description of an elephant, then surely five types of antigen-receptor molecules, each with a wide range of affinities for a given antigenic determinant, and all competing for the antigen, would suffice to explain regulatory phenomena at the antigen level.

At this point I shall stop my biased summary, well aware that it is impossible to encompass in a few words all the enormous immunological advances of the last few years that were reflected at this symposium. The tortuous road that immunology followed until its molecular elements came into better focus was historically reviewed by Dr. Haurowitz[1] who himself has contributed so much to this development.

Sir Macfarlane Burnet[1] must have been pleased not only to witness at this symposium the vindication of his Clonal Selection Theory of Acquired Immunity, but also to see how his stimulating ideas have led to a great proliferation of immunologists, and to know that the fate of immunology is deposited in so many capable hands.

As this younger generation of professionals is pressing rapidly toward the definitive solution of the antibody problem, we older amateurs had perhaps better sit back, waiting for the End.

REFERENCES

ADA, G. L., and P. G. LANG. 1966. Antigen in tissues. II. State of antigen in lymph node of rats given isotopically labelled flagellin, haemocyanin or serum albumin. Immunology 5: 431.

ADLER, F. L., M. FISHMAN, and S. DRAY. 1966. Antibody formation initiated in vitro. III. Antibody formation and allotypic specificity directed by ribonucleic acid from peritoneal exudate cells. J. Immunol. 97: 554.

ALBRIGHT, J. F., and T. MAKINODAN. 1966. Growth and senescence of antibody-forming cells. J. Cell. Physiol. 67: Suppl. 1, 185.

APPELLA, E., and D. EIN. 1967. Two types of lambda polypeptide chains in human immunoglobulins based on an amino-acid substitution at position 190. Proc. Natl. Acad. Sci. 57: 1449.

BEHRING, E., and S. KITASATO. 1890. Über das Zustandekommen der Diphtherie-Immunität und der Tetanus-Immunität bei Thieren. Deutsche Med. Wochenschr. 16: 1113.

BERKEN, A., and B. BENACERRAF. 1966. Properties of antibodies cytophilic for macrophages. J. Exptl. Med. 123: 119.

BIOZZI, G., C. STIFFEL, D. MOUTON, M. LIACOPOULOS-BRIOT, C. DECREUSEFOND, and Y. BOUTHILLIER. 1966. Etude du phénomène de l'immuno-cyto-adhérence au cours de l'immunisation. Ann. Inst. Pasteur 110: 7.

BIRO, C. E., and G. GUADELUPE, 1965. The antigenicity of aggregated and aggregate-free human gamma-globulin for rabbits. Immunology 8: 411.

BOREK, F. 1967. Delayed-type hypersensitivity to synthetic antigens. Current Topics Microbiol. and Immunol., in press.

BOYDEN, S. V., and E. SORKIN. 1960. The adsorption of antigens by spleen cells previously treated with antiserum in vitro. Immunology 3: 272.

BRODY, N. I., J. G. WALKER, and G. W. SISKIND. 1967. Studies on the control of antibody synthesis. Interaction of antigenic competition and suppression of antibody formation by passive antibody on the immune response. J. Exptl. Med. 126: 81.

BRENT, L., T. COURTENAY, and G. GOWLAND. 1967. Immunological reactivity of lymphoid cells after treatment with anti-lymphocytic serum. Nature 215: 1461.

BURNET, M. 1959. The clonal selection theory of acquired immunity. University Press, Cambridge.

CAMPBELL, J. 1967. Permissive translation of nucleic acid: a mechanism for antibody synthesis. J. Theoret. Biol. 16: 321.

CEBRA, J. J., J. E. COLBERG, and S. DRAY. 1966. Rabbit lymphoid cells differentiated with respect to alpha, gamma, and mu heavy polypeptide chains and to allotypic markers Aa 1 and Aa 2. J. Exptl. Med. 123: 547.

CLAFLIN, A. J., and O. SMITHIES. 1967. Antibody-producing cells in division. Science 157: 1561.

CLARKE, C. A., W. J. A. DONOHUE, R. B. McCONNELL, J. C. WOODROW, R. FINN, J. R. KREVANS, W. W. KULKE, D. LEHANE, and P. M. SHEPPARD. 1963. Further experimental studies on the prevention of Rh haemolytic disease. Brit. Med. J. i: 979.

DIXON, F. J., H. JACOT-GUILLARMOD, and P. J. McCONAHEY. 1967. The effect of passively administered antibody on antibody synthesis. J. Exptl. Med. 125: 1119.

DORRINGTON, K. J., M. H. ZARLENGO, and C. TANFORD. 1967. Conformational change and complementarity in the combination of H and L chains of immunoglobulin-G. Proc. Natl. Acad. Sci. 58: 996.

DRESSER, D. W. 1962. Specific inhibition of antibody production. II. Paralysis induced in adult mice by small quantities of protein antigen. Immunology 5: 378.

DUTTON, R. W., and R. I. MISHELL. 1967. Cell populations and cell proliferation in the in vitro response of normal mouse spleen to heterologous erythrocytes. Analysis by the hot pulse technique. J. Exptl. Med. 126: 443.

EDELMAN, G. M. 1959. Dissociation of gamma globulin. J. Amer. Chem. Soc. 81: 3155.

EDELMAN, G. M., and J. A. GALLY. 1962. The nature of Bence-Jones proteins. Chemical similarities to polypeptide chains of myeloma globulins and normal gamma globulins. J. Exptl. Med. 116: 207.

——, ——. 1967. Somatic recombination of duplicated genes: an hypothesis on the origin of antibody diversity. Proc. Natl. Acad. Sci. 57: 353.

EDELMAN, G. M., D. E. OLINS, J. A. GALLY, and N. D. ZINDER. 1963. Reconstitution of immunologic activity by interaction of polypeptide chains of antibodies. Proc. Natl. Acad. Sci. 50: 753.

EISEN, H. N. 1965. The immune response to a simple antigenic determinant. Harvey Lectures, Ser. 60: 1.

EISEN, H. N., and F. KARUSH. 1964. Immune tolerance and an extracellular regulatory role for bivalent antibody. Nature 202: 677.

FINKELSTEIN, M. S., and J. W. UHR. 1964. Specific inhibition of antibody formation by passively administered 19 S and 7 S antibody. Science 146: 67.

——, ——. 1966. Antibody formation. V. The avidity of

gamma-M and gamma-G guinea pig antibodies to bacteriophage φX174. J. Immunol. *97:* 565.

FREEDMAN, M. H., and M. SELA, 1966a. Recovery of antigenic activity upon reoxidation of completely reduced polyalanyl rabbit immunoglobulin-G. J. Biol. Chem. *241:* 2383.

——, ——. 1966b. Recovery of specific activity upon reoxidation of completely reduced polyalanyl rabbit antibody. J. Biol. Chem. *241:* 5225.

FREI, P. C., B. BENACERRAF, and G. J. THORBECKE. 1965. Phagocytosis of the antigen, a crucial step in the induction of the primary response. Proc. Natl. Acad. Sci. *53:* 20.

FURTH, R. VAN, H. R. E. SCHUIT, and W. HIJMANS. 1966. The formation of immunoglobulins by human tissues in vitro. IV. Circulating lymphocytes in normal and pathological conditions. Immunology *11:* 29.

GALLILY, R., and M. FELDMAN. 1967. The role of macrophages in the induction of antibody in X-irradiated animals. Immunology *12:* 197.

GELL, P. G. H., and S. SELL. 1965. Studies on rabbit lymphocytes in vitro. II. Induction of blast-transformation with antisera to six IgG allotypes and summation with mixtures of antisera to different allotypes. J. Exptl. Med. *122:* 813.

GOWANS, J. L., and J. W. UHR. 1967. The carriage of immunological memory by small lymphocytes in the rat. J. Exptl. Med. *125:* in press.

GREEN, I., P. VASSALLI, and B. BENACERRAF. 1967a. Cellular localization of anti-DNP-PLL and anti-conveyor albumin in genetic non-responder guinea pigs immunized with DNP-PLL albumin complexes. J. Exptl. Med. *125:* 527.

GREEN, I., P. VASSALLI, V. NUSSENZWEIG, and B. BENACERRAF. 1967b. Specificity of the antibodies produced by single cells following immunization with antigens bearing two types of antigenic determinants. J. Exptl. Med. *125:* 511.

HABER, E. 1964. Recovery of antigenic specificity after denaturation and complete reduction of disulfides in a papain fragment of antibody. Proc. Natl. Acad. Sci. *52:* 1099.

HARRIS, G., and R. V. LITTLETON. 1966. The effects of antigens and of phytohemagglutinin on rabbit spleen cell suspensions. J. Exptl. Med. *124:* 621.

HELMREICH, E., M. KERN, and H. N. EISEN. 1961. The secretion of antibody by isolated lymph node cells. J. Biol. Chem. *236:* 464.

——, ——, ——. 1962. Observations on the mechanism of secretion of gamma-globulins by isolated lymph node cells. J. Biol. Chem. *237:* 1925.

HENRY, C., and N. K. JERNE. 1967a. The depressive effect of 7 S antibody and the enhancing effect of 19 S antibody in the regulation of the primary immune response, p. 421. *In* J. Killander [ed.] Gamma globulins. Nobel Symp. 3. Almquist and Wiksell, Stockholm.

HENRY, C., and N. K. JERNE. 1967b. Competition of 19 S and 7 S antigen-receptors in the regulation of the primary immune response. J. Exptl. Med. (submitted).

HILSCHMANN, N., and L. C. CRAIG. 1965. Amino acid sequence studies with Bence-Jones proteins. Proc. Natl. Acad. Sci. *53:* 1403.

JERNE, N. K. 1951. A study of avidity based on rabbit skin responses to diphtheria toxin-antitoxin mixtures. Acta Path. Microbiol. Scand. Suppl. *87:* 99.

——. 1955. The natural selection theory of antibody formation. Proc. Natl. Acad. Sci. *41:* 849.

——. 1960. Immunological speculations. Annual Rev. Microbiol. *14:* 341.

KARUSH, F., and H. N. EISEN. 1962. A theory of delayed hypersensitivity. Science *136:* 1032.

KENNEDY, J. C., J. E. TILL, L. SIMINOVITCH, and E. A. McCULLOCH. 1965. Radiosensitivity of the immune response to sheep red cells in the mouse, as measured by the hemolytic plaque method. J. Immunol. *94:* 715.

——, ——, ——, ——. 1966. The proliferative capacity of antigen-sensitive precursors of hemolytic plaque-forming cells. J. Immunol. *96:* 973.

KEPES, A., and S. BEGUIN. 1966. Peptide chain initiation and growth in the induced synthesis of β-galactosidase. Biochim. Biophys. Acta *123:* 546.

KERMAN, R., D. SEGRE, and W. L. MYERS. 1967. Altered response to pneumococcal polysaccharide in offspring of immunologically paralyzed mice. Science *156:* 1514.

KIERKEGAARD, S. 1843. Enten-Eller. Et Livs-fragment. Ed. Victor Eremita. C. A. Reitzel, Copenhagen, p. 14.

LANDSTEINER, K. 1947. The specificity of serological reactions. Howard Univ. Press, Washington.

LESKOWITZ, S. 1967. Mechanism of delayed reactions. Science *155:* 350.

LEVEY, R. H., and P. B. MEDAWAR. 1967. Further experiments on the action of antilymphocytic antiserum. Proc. Natl. Acad. Sci. *58:* 470.

MAALØE, O., and N. O. KJELDGAARD. 1966. Control of macromolecular synthesis, p. 91. W. A. Benjamin, New York.

MANNIK, M. 1967. Variability in the specific interactions of H and L chains of γG-globulins. Biochemistry *6:* 134.

McDEVITT, H. O., B. A. ASKONAS, J. H. HUMPHREY, I. SCHECHTER, and M. SELA. 1966. The localization of antigen in relation to specific antibody-producing cells. I. Use of a synthetic polypeptide [(T, G)-A-L] labelled with iodine-125. Immunology *11:* 337.

METZGER, H. 1967. Characterization of a human macroglobulin. V. A Waldenström macroglobulin with antibody activity. Proc. Natl. Acad. Sci. *57:* 1490.

MILSTEIN, C. 1966. Variations in amino acid sequence near the disulphide bridges of Bence-Jones proteins. Nature *209:* 370.

MISHELL, R. I., and R. W. DUTTON. 1967. Immunization of dissociated spleen cell cultures from normal mice. J. Exptl. Med. *126:* 423.

MITCHISON, N. A. 1964. Induction of immunological paralysis in two zones of dosage. Proc. Roy. Soc. B *161:* 275.

MÖLLER, G., and H. WIGZELL. 1965. Antibody synthesis at the cellular level. Antibody induced suppression of 19 S and 7 S response. J. Exptl. Med., *121:* 969.

NIALL, H. D., and P. EDMAN. 1967. Two structurally distinct classes of kappa-chains in human immunoglobulins. Nature *216:* 262.

NISBET, N. W., and M. SIMONSEN. 1967. Primary immune response in grafted cells. Dissociation between the proliferation of activity and the proliferation of cells. J. Exptl. Med. *125:* 967.

NOSSAL, G. J. V. 1966. Immunological tolerance: a new model system for low zone induction. Ann. N.Y. Acad. Sci. *129:* 822.

NOSSAL, G. J. V., G. L. ADA, and C. M. AUSTIN. 1964. Antigens in immunity. IV. Cellular localization of ^{125}I- and ^{131}I-labelled flagella in lymph nodes. Aust. J. Exptl. Biol. Med. Sci. *42:* 311.

——, ——, ——. 1965. Antigens in immunity. IX. The antigen content of single antibody-forming cells. J. Exptl. Med. *121:* 945.

NOSSAL, G. J. V., A. SZENBERG, G. L. ADA, and C. M. AUSTIN. 1964. Single cell studies on 19 S antibody production. J. Exptl. Med. *119:* 485.

PEARLMAN, D. S. 1967. The influence of antibodies on immunologic responses. I. The effect on the response to particulate antigen in the rabbit. J. Exptl. Med. *126:* 127.

PERNIS, B., G. CHIAPPINO, A. S. KELUS, and P. G. H. GELL. 1965. Cellular localization of immunoglobulins with different allotypic specificities in rabbit lymphoid tissues. J. Exptl. Med. *122:* 853.

PORTER, R. R. 1959. The hydrolysis of rabbit gamma globulin and antibodies with crystalline papain. Biochem. J. *73:* 119.

POTTER, M., E. APPELLA, and S. GEISSER. 1965. Variations in the heavy polypeptide chain structure of gamma myeloma immunoglobulins from an inbred strain of mice and a hypothesis as to their origin. J. Mol. Biol. *14:* 361.

POTTER, M., W. J. DREYER, E. L. KUFF, and K. R. McINTIRE. 1963. Hereditable variation in Bence-Jones protein structure in Balb/C mice: Relation to gamma globulin. Fed. Proc. *22:* 649.

PUTNAM, F. W., C. W. EASLEY, and J. W. HELLING. 1963. Structural study of human gamma globulin through the analysis of the tryptic peptides of Bence-Jones proteins. Biochim. Biophys. Acta *78:* 231.

PUTNAM, F. W., T. SHINODA, K. TITANI, and M. WIKLER. 1967. Immunoglobulin structure: variation in amino acid sequence and length of human lambda light chains. Science *157:* 1050.

ROHOLT, O. A., G. RADZINSKI, and D. PRESSMAN. 1965a. Polypeptide chains of antibody: effective binding sites require specificity in combination. Science *147:* 613.

——, ——, ——. 1965b. Preferential recombination of antibody chains to form effective binding sites. J. Exptl. Med. *122:* 785.

——, ——, ——. 1967. Recovery of antibody activity from inactive hybrids of H and L chains. J. Exptl. Med. *125:* 191.

ROWLEY, D. A., and F. W. FITCH. 1964. Homeostasis of antibody formation in the adult rat. J. Exptl. Med. *120:* 987.

SAHIAR, K., and R. W. SCHWARTZ. 1964. Inhibition of 19 S antibody synthesis by 7 S antibody. Science *145:* 395.

SCHLOSSMAN, S. F., S. BEN-EFRAIM, A. YARON, and H. A. SOBER. 1966. Immunochemical studies on the antigenic determinants required to elicit delayed and immediate hypersensitivity reactions. J. Exptl. Med. *123:* 1083.

SCHLOSSMAN, S. F., and H. LEVINE. 1967. Immunochemical studies of delayed and Arthus-type hypersensitivity reactions. I. The relationship between antigenic determinant size and antibody combining site size. J. Immunol. *98:* 211.

SEGRE, D., and M. L. KAEBERLE. 1962. The immunologic behaviour of baby pigs. I. Production of antibody in three week old pigs. J. Immunol. *89:* 782.

SELA, M., and E. MOZES. 1966. Dependence of the chemical nature of antibodies on the net electrical charge of antigens. Proc. Natl. Acad. Sci. *55:* 445.

SELL, S. 1967. Studies on rabbit lymphocytes in vitro. V. The induction of blast-transformation with sheep antisera to rabbit IgG subunits. J. Exptl. Med. *125:* 289.

——. 1967. Studies on rabbit lymphocytes in vitro. VI. The induction of blast transformation with sheep antisera to rabbit IgA and IgM. J. Exptl. Med. *125:* 393.

SELL, S., and P. G. H. GELL. 1965. Studies on rabbit lymphocytes in vitro. IV. Blast-transformation of the lymphocytes from newborn rabbits induced by anti-allotype serum to a paternal IgG allotype not present in the serum of the lymphocyte donors. J. Exptl. Med. *122:* 923.

SMITHIES, O. 1967. Antibody variability. Science *157:* 267.

STEINER, L. A., and H. N. EISEN. 1966. Variations in the response to a simple determinant. Bact. Rev. *30:* 383.

THORBECKE, G. J., P. H. MAURER, and B. BENACERRAF. 1960. The affinity of the R.E.S. for various modified serum proteins. Brit. J. Exptl. Path. *41:* 190.

TITANI, K., E. WHITLEY, JR., L. AVOGARDO, and F. W. PUTNAM. 1965. Immunoglobulin structure: partial amino acid sequence of a Bence-Jones protein. Science *149:* 1090.

TRENTIN, J., N. WOLF, V. CHENG, W. FAHLBERG, D. WEISS, and R. BONHAG. 1967. Antibody production by mice repopulated with limited numbers of clones of lymphoid cell precursors. J. Immunol. *98:* 1326.

UHR, J. W. 1965. Passive sensitization of lymphocytes and macrophages by antigen-antibody complexes. Proc. Natl. Acad. Sci. *54:* 1599.

UHR, J. W., and J. B. BAUMANN. 1961. Antibody formation. I. The suppression of antibody formation by passively administered antibody. J. Exptl. Med. *113:* 935.

VALENTINE, R. C., and N. M. GREEN. 1967. Electron microscopy of an antibody-hapten complex. J. Mol. Biol. *27:* 615.

WHITEHOUSE, H. L. K. 1967. Crossover model of antibody variability. Nature *215:* 371.

WHITNEY, P. L., and C. TANFORD. 1965. Recovery of specific activity after complete unfolding and reduction of an antibody fragment. Proc. Natl. Acad. Sci. *53:* 524.

WIGZELL, H. 1966. Antibody-induced suppression of 7 S antibody synthesis. J. Exptl. Med. *124:* 953.

WOODRUFF, M. F. A., B. REID, and K. JAMES. 1967. Effect of antilymphocytic antibody and antibody fragments on human lymphocytes in vitro. Nature *215:* 591.

YOO, T. J., O. A. ROHOLT, and D. PRESSMAN. 1967. Specific binding activity of isolated light chains of antibodies. Science *157:* 707.

ZAALBERG, O. B., V. A. VAN DER MEUL, and J. M. VAN TWISK. 1966. Antibody production by single spleen cells: a comparative study of the cluster and agar-plaque formation. Nature *210:* 544.

The Common Sense of Immunology

N. K. JERNE

Basel Institute for Immunology, CH-4058 Basel, Switzerland

Common sense was defined by Einstein as the set of prejudices that we have acquired by the age of eighteen. Good common sense tells us that this is an extreme definition, and that common sense is likely to contain both correct and wrong propositions.

When we study a discipline such as immunology, we not only study a set of biological objects and phenomena, but we are also disciplined in our approach by the notions that have gained general acceptance at the time—which we might call the "common sense" of the discipline. Since common sense strives to be coherent in spite of extensive areas of ignorance, it is likely to include several wrong propositions. A discipline thus distorts, to some extent, the objects it studies.

Correct propositions add to the joy of science because they make us feel that we at least know something. Moreover since correct theories are always incomplete, we have the possibility of demonstrating that there is more to them. Wrong propositions can likewise add to the joy of research if experiments can be devised that prove them wrong. Doing this successfully gives us the pleasure of throwing the coherence of common sense into a crisis with which some, but not all, of us find it hard to live. I am glad to say that this is the present state of immunology— most conspicuously so in the attempts to make sense of the relationships between the major histocompatibility complex and the recognition machine that we call the "immune system."

Cold Spring Harbor 1958

Several of us participated in the first Cold Spring Harbor symposium on immunology in 1967. Its topic was the diversity of antibodies. We have now participated in the second symposium, dealing with the diversity of lymphocytes. Biochemists have become cell biologists. It is important to note that Cold Spring Harbor continues to focus on the origin of diversity, which remains the central problem of immunology. The antibody molecule dominates the immune system and could well be said to be the most interesting of all proteins. Even so, research may have to digress from time to time. At present, regulatory problems and histocompatibility problems are in the foreground. Histocompatibility antigens, however, have functions that go beyond the immune system. Looking back at the 1967 symposium, we might well ask: Why was there not an earlier Cold Spring Harbor symposium on immunology, say nine years before, in 1958?[1]

This can be understood as one of the harmful side effects by which a wrong theory delays useful activities. The common sense of immunology in 1958 included the instructive theory of antibody formation. The convincing argument for the instructive role of antigen was that the number of different antibodies that an individual can make seemed far to exceed the number of different genes that could be imagined to be present in the genome. It is interesting to note the similarity with present arguments for a somatic origin of antibody diversity. The difference is merely that the latter theory proposes to generate diversity somatically at the level of genes (that cannot be instructed by antigen), whereas the instructive theories proposed to generate diversity somatically at the level of protein folding. If cells receive the necessary information for antibody structure from external antigen, then antibody diversity has no genetics. And since Cold Spring Harbor was dedicated to genetics, there was no place here for immunology in 1958.

The following discoveries in the 1960's changed all this:

1. Antibody-secreting plasma cells were shown to be the descendants of small lymphocytes. In other words, lymphocytes *are* the immune system. Immunology had discovered the cells responsible for the phenomena it had studied for 70 years.
2. All antibody molecules released by a single cell appeared to have identical specificity (and allotype). This insight was needed for the development of a plaque assay for single-antibody-secreting cells.
3. Antibody-secreting cells were shown to arise in vitro after the addition of antigen to a suspension of lymphocytes from an unprimed animal. The lymphocyte system is autonomous.
4. The removal by antigen of a small set of lymphocytes from a lymphocyte suspension was shown

[1] An "antibody workshop" took place at Cold Spring Harbor in 1959. Although its proceedings were not recorded, it is clear that what became the established common sense of immunology in 1967 was already present in statu nascendi much earlier among the ideas open to debate at that time. To quote an example from a 1955 paper (PNAS **41**: 851), in a paragraph concerning the diversity of antibodies I stated that ". . . it seems reasonable to assume that a great variety of configurations, due, perhaps, to various amino acid sequences at the specific site of the globulin molecules, may develop at random."

to remove the responsiveness of the remaining lymphocytes to that antigen.

5. Last, and most important, the analysis of the primary structure of antibody molecules showed that antibody specificity is determined by amino acid sequences which are the expression of nucleotide sequences in DNA. Antibody polypeptide chains are made by ribosomes as instructed by messenger RNA. Antibodies turned out to be gene products, and instruction by antigen had to be given up.

Because of the enormous size of the antibody repertoire in a single animal, the question immediately arose whether this diversity of genes in the lymphocyte population is of evolutionary or mainly of somatic origin. Consensus in this matter could not be reached then and has not quite been reached even today.

Cold Spring Harbor 1967

The controversy over the origin of such diversity of genes, however, showed that immunology had acquired an important genetic aspect. It thus qualified as the topic for the 1967 Cold Spring Harbor Symposium, which marked the farewell to antigen instruction and saw the emergence of a new common sense which included the clonal selection theory.

Clonal selection is based on two laws. The first law simply states that one lymphocyte makes only one antibody; or that all antibody molecules released by a single plasma cell have identical combining sites. The second law is an extension of the first. It states that all lymphocytes belonging to the same cell clone synthesize antibodies of identical specificity; or that all antibody-like molecules displayed on the membrane of a small lymphocyte have identical combining sites, and that this combining site is conserved in the antibody molecules synthesized by all cells that arise upon proliferation of this lymphocyte. These laws of clonal selection suggest that the immune system is made up of a large number of lymphocyte clones that differ with respect to the specificity of the antibody that the cells of a clone are committed to synthesize.

The number of different clones in the immune system of an animal equals the number of different antibody variable domains that this animal makes. Upon entering the system, antigen will select (for stimulation or suppression) cells of clones presenting antibodies that show a sufficient fit to the antigen. In other words, the total immune system is regarded as a large set of small, uncoupled immune systems independently driven by external antigen. Although regulatory problems were rarely discussed at the time, the clonal selection theory suggested that modifications in the cellular composition of a stimulated clone would be controlled by feedback mechanisms within that clone. These were

the notions that the common sense of 1967 adopted and which then seemed to accommodate most known facts so comfortably.

On closer inspection, however, it is clear that the seeds for modification of the simple picture derived from the clonal selection laws were already present in the findings reported at Cold Spring Harbor in 1967.

One disturbing finding was that the induction of antibody formation against a hapten requires recognition of the carrier as well as of the hapten, presumably by two different interacting cells. In the prevailing common sense of 1967, clonal selection took care of lymphocyte clones producing anti-hapten antibodies. The carrier-recognizing cell might therefore be a non-lymphocyte, for example a macrophage, that could present the hapten to an effector lymphocyte. The macrophage has always had a place in the common sense of immunology. The trouble with macrophages (as with mast cells, complement, etc.), however, is that they have no private specificity. In spite of this, the macrophage has played a very useful role throughout this century. Whenever experimental results did not make sense, the macrophage was readily available to straighten out the difficulties, only invariably to be dropped when no longer needed. Soon after the 1967 symposium it became obvious that lymphocytes fall into two classes, and that cooperative cell interaction in the hapten-carrier situation is between B and T lymphocytes. In other words, lymphocyte clones are not independent of each other.

The 1967 symposium also included reports on anti-idiotypic antibodies and on allotype suppression initiated by antiallotypic antibodies. These reports implied that it is also not true that the immune system is solely driven by external antigens. Allotype suppression (and idiotype suppression, which was subsequently studied) involves only molecules and cells that belong to the immune system itself. The system thus displays an Eigen behavior resulting from interactions between its own elements. It has turned out that the suppressed states are maintained by specific lymphocytes that suppress cells of other clones.

The last but not least disturbing element was the finding that animals of an inbred strain could be deficient in their response to a given antigen while responding well to other antigens. Responsiveness to that given antigen appeared to require the presence of one dominant autosomal gene. Deficiency with respect to antibody formation to this antigen could be overcome by attaching the antigen to a carrier molecule, but deficiency with respect to cellular immunity remained. Immunology thus became even more deeply involved with genetics, and extensive studies of the control of cell interaction by genes of the major histocompatibility complex have since complicated greatly the simple picture that clonal selection offered.

Cold Spring Harbor 1976

The seeds for modification have grown since 1967, and each of the disturbing findings I have mentioned has pointed to cell interaction. The common sense of immunology in 1976 retains clonal selection as one of its simpler notions, but cooperative and suppressive clonal interactions have now become the dominant themes. Regulatory feedback is no longer thought to proceed only within clones: it is now clear that different clones speak to one another. Admitting that important notions, whether antigen instruction or clonal selection, have determined the direction of immunological research, it is worthwhile to examine briefly what clonal interaction implies.

The most conspicuous examples of cell interactions in vertebrates are those studied in endocrinology and neurology. Best understood are hormonal interactions. Here the cells of one tissue secrete hormones that stimulate or inhibit the cells of another tissue. Within the immune system, the equivalent might be that T cells produce factors that stimulate or inhibit B cells, and perhaps vice versa. The existence of such T-cell factors has been demonstrated, but their effect is focused on a small set of B cells, selected by specific recognition. The endocrinological model is therefore not of much use for describing the net of cell interactions in the immune system. In the central nervous system, cells interact by synaptic contact. Here every cell interacts with a set of other cells, and as these sets overlap, we are confronted with a network. This looks a little more like the immune system, in which fixed synaptic contacts are not needed because lymphocytes travel and can seek out fitting partners. B lymphocytes that recognize the hapten of a hapten-carrier complex interact with T lymphocytes that recognize the carrier. The same set of B cells would interact with another set of T cells if the hapten were placed on a different carrier molecule. In this way, the introduction of an external antigen brings about clonal interactions not yet manifest in the immune system itself. It is the discovery of clonal interactions involving idiotype recognition that has produced a major change in perspective.

The enormous diversity of idiotypes leads us to admit that every antibody molecule must be an anti-idiotypic antibody fitting some idiotypic determinants that occur in the immune system itself. This follows from the reasonable assumption that the repertoire both of idiotypes and of combining sites is of the same order of magnitude as the repertoire of variable antibody domains and from the degeneracy of precision in antigen-antibody recognition. It also follows directly from experiments showing the production of anti-idiotypic antibodies by the same animals that produced the idiotype. This being the case, phenomena such as the induction of idiotype suppression by minute concentrations of anti-idiotypic antibody and the transfer of this suppressed state to other animals by transferring lymphocytes show that clonal interaction necessarily implies that the immune system is a functional network. The system displays an internal behavior that can be modulated by external antigen. Such is the implication that common sense forces us to face, and this is a rather stunning conclusion, indeed, since it is not clear how networks should be dealt with nor what experiments would be meaningful in a network context. The notion of cell interaction now leads us to consider the organization and stability of networks. Networks are stable only if suppressive interactions exceed stimulatory interactions. Suppressor cells themselves should not escape suppression. The necessity for suppressive interactions, many examples of which have been uncovered during the 1970's, suggests that lymphocyte diversity is restricted in its range by suppression, and this from the very onset, in the early ontogeny of the immune system. Thus immunology is forced to return to embryology in order to study the starting conditions for diversity generation and to clarify the rules and restrictions governing the expansion of the incipient network.

Since cell interaction requires recognition of membrane structures, the emphasis on cell interaction has made the cell membrane a main target for structural studies. It has become clear that, apart from antibody-like receptors at the cell surface, lymphocyte recognition also involves membrane molecules that are products of genes of the major histocompatibility complex. Allogenic histocompatibility antigens and antigen-coupled histocompatibility antigens appear to be the targets of recognition by T lymphocytes. One immediate problem is to determine the structure of the receptor molecule that enables T lymphocytes to recognize these targets. It seems unlikely that the T cell synthesizes two receptors belonging to two different recognition repertoires, as this would require a final repertoire that would be the product of the two. We should like to retain unispecificity. One receptor could recognize an antigen-modified histocompatibility molecule. I find it hard to accept a protean modification of molecules by antigen, however. It looks too much like a step back to antigen instruction of polypeptide folding. Rather, the T cell might borrow a cytophilic molecule, in addition to its indigenous receptor. Some of the discussions in this volume are devoted to these questions.

It is remarkable that basic immunology, in spite of its enormous range, seems to resist a splitting up into specialized areas. It is as if every facet of the immune system impinges on all others. None can be excluded when considering the origin of lymphocyte diversity, and thus all fall within the framework of this symposium.

Cold Spring Harbor 1985

What can we look forward to? Immunology has come a long way. It used to be an esoteric subject employing its own terminology (immunity, sensitivity, tolerance, avidity, etc.) to deal with problems that seemed scarcely related to other fields of biology. Because of vaccination, allergy, and serological diagnosis, immunology had a private line to medicine, which compensated for its isolation.

We have seen how the 1967 Cold Spring Harbor Symposium marked the confrontation of immunology with genetics, and how clonal interactions occupy a large part of this volume. In order to penetrate deeper into the meaning, origin, and mechanics of the immune system, future studies must come to grips with embryology, differentiation, membrane structures, network analysis, etc. We might conclude that immunology is losing its status as an isolated discipline and is being absorbed into classical biology. Even so, immunology comes into the fold with considerable assets and achievements:

1. It has contributed some astonishing facts to molecular genetics, such as the joining of V genes and C genes.
2. It may well contribute to the understanding of the central nervous system, with which the immune system has so many general properties in common, e.g., network structure and the ability to learn and to memorize.
3. The lymphocyte is not only one of the most interesting vertebrate cells, but it has also become the cell that can be most easily studied in vitro by a wide variety of methods.
4. And finally, if antibody diversity results from a mechanism of somatic gene modification in lymphocytes, immunology will have discovered an important extension to Darwinian evolution. We seem to have no germ-line genes specifying antibodies against particular viruses; likewise, the brain does not have germ-line genes specify-

ing mathematical propositions. Nature has been obliged to solve such problems in a different way. It is useless to develop germ-line genes for antibodies against viruses which can evolve much faster than vertebrates. As the future evolution of viral opponents cannot be predicted from past experience, it may well be that the optimal strategy in this genetic game is to make random somatic moves that the opponents cannot foresee. If true, this supra-Darwinian idea is obviously of far-reaching importance to our understanding of biology. Immunology may have discovered an early instance of the original sin, somatic mutation, by which the individual ceases to rely solely on the wisdom of its zygotic genes. Because it is frightening to give up the heaven of precise parental instructions, it is unlikely that those who wish to place all antibody genes in the germ line or those that propose that somatic permutations of antibody genes are genetically controlled will be convinced by the arguments presented in this volume for a mainly somatic, random origin of lymphocyte diversity. What we could all agree upon, I think, is that a definitive solution of this controversy of phylogeny versus ontogeny can be obtained only by analysis at the DNA level. It seems clear to me from the progress reported in this volume by DNA chemists that the proponents of a germ-line theory are fighting a losing battle.

Descending from these higher regions of biology, we could ask: Will progress in immunology have a further impact on medicine comparable to the tremendous success of prophylactic immunization? Current findings, such as the correlations of histocompatibility types with susceptibility to specific diseases, may well lead to important medical advances. In any event, basic immunology should receive adequate long-term support, to develop as it may. I believe that even if it takes a long time, basic research is the most rapid way to medical applications.

In this volume we have in hand the common sense of immunology emerging from a week of discussions. I can only hope that nine years from now Dr. Watson will be able to arrange a third Cold Spring Harbor symposium on immunology to focus on the diversity of lymphocyte networks.

Summary: Understanding Selective Molecular Recognition

G. M. EDELMAN

Laboratory of Developmental and Molecular Biology, The Rockefeller University, New York, New York 10021

Let me begin by thanking the organizers and planners of this Symposium, in particular, Dr. Watson and all of his colleagues at Cold Spring Harbor who made our coming together so convenient, pleasant, and interactive.

Over the course of a week, we were challenged to understand the most extensively studied and interesting molecular recognition machine. I was asked to put together a picture of this biological machine based on the many beautiful papers that we heard. I can only paraphrase Samuel Johnson to give you some idea of my attitude towards all of this. He said that when a man knows he is to be hanged in a fortnight, it concentrates his mind wonderfully. Although I have really tried very hard to concentrate, I obviously cannot review here all of the papers and hope that I am not to be hanged twice for those to which I do not refer.[1] My overall impression, gained from all of the presented papers, is that things are going swimmingly. By 1984 or so, presumably when the next meeting will be held here, we should have satisfactory answers to many of the major questions of immunology.

The coincidence of this second Cold Spring Harbor meeting on immunology with America's bicentennial prompts me to remind you of the horror with which Henry Adams of the great Adams family viewed the diversity of a world under the sway of science and machines. In his autobiography, *The Education of Henry Adams* (1918), he describes how the physicist Langley, who was trying to make a working airplane, took him through the exhibits of the Great Exposition of 1900 in Paris. Langley was mainly interested in motors to make his new airplane feasible. When Langley showed Adams the great 40-foot dynamos in the Hall of Machines, it was almost too much for Adams. He felt that the great unifying moral forces of the past were being replaced by mechanisms and multiplicities of forces with no human reference and therefore by ultimate human confusion.

I cannot help but wonder whether he would not have been reassured in his views of science if he knew what modern immunologists know about the machinery of specificity and recognition. Here we see how diversity is made valuable as a repertoire to meet future occasions. The subtle immunological machines that carry out this function are particular variants of informational machines. They carry out selective molecular recognition on a scale that makes dynamos and even computers seem trivially simple. But the ideas generated by studying selective recognition in the immune system are very unusual and beautiful. These ideas are likely to have far-reaching consequences for our understanding of all biological systems that can recognize new patterns and particularly for our understanding of the human brain.

PREDICTIONS AND FULFILLMENTS

At the time of the last Cold Spring Harbor meeting in 1967, two large events were taking place — the elaboration in its main outlines of the theory of clonal selection, and the development of a massive attack on antibody structure. That meeting had great significance, I believe, for it was the first important indication of the general acceptance of the theory of clonal selection. The second achievement of that meeting was to bring to the attention of immunologists at large the enormous power of structural methods in refining the ideas of clonal selection and, indeed, in clarifying the choices that had to be made in putting details into that theory. This structural work eventually provided us with the essential picture of the antibody molecule, a picture that will, I believe, remain as the central reference for all further thinking in the field.

It is worth mentioning, however, that the cellular immunologists were not inactive at this time, although the structural work dominated many people's thinking. The experiments of Jim Gowans (1970) had already provided us with the key evidence for the idea that the lymphocyte was the immunocompetent cell and that lymphocyte populations were extraordinarily heterogeneous. Jacques Miller (1962) gave us an extraordinarily important insight into the function of the thymus, a development that led to the appreciation of the bifurcation of the immune system into T and B cells. Henry Claman et al. (1966) already had made the first gestures towards indicating some kind of T-B cooperation, and Avrion Mitchison (1968) was already talking about concepts of antigen presentation and help. Of particular importance were the elegant

---

[1] Very few references are cited in this summary and those that are cited are for historical purposes, to make a fine point, or to give a hint as to a source of primary references. No specific attempt has been made to achieve scholarly balance. All names cited without a date refer to papers read or comments made at the meeting.

experiments of Gus Nossal and Oli Mäkelä (1962; Mäkelä 1968) showing that one cell makes just one antibody specificity. The subsequent development of the Jerne plaque technique (Jerne et al. 1963) opened up the possibilities of our understanding of the detailed responses of the B cell. All of this work gave a real basis for the central ideas of selection advanced by Niels Jerne (1955) and Macfarlane Burnet (1959).

Clonal selection, it now appears, has three main requirements (Fig. 1):

1. *Repertoire:* The creation, existence, and renewal of a repertoire of diverse antigen-binding cells having different V regions presented on their surfaces. We know the basis of the diversity of the repertoire – the V regions of antibody molecules. But we do not yet know the genetic origin of V-region diversity and we are just beginning to understand the "zero[th]" stage of clonal selection – the ontogeny of antigen-binding cells.

2. *Encounter:* The means for assuring encounter of proper subsets of these cells with antigens and with each other. We are now aware of a great hierarchy of complex cellular interactions among T and B cells both for help and suppression. These mechanisms are not understood at the molecular level, but we now suspect that genetic control of key surface molecules is involved.

3. *Triggering:* A mechanism for stimulating the cells to mature, divide, secrete antibodies, or directly mediate effector functions. We know how to trigger T and B cells with a variety of substances but know next to nothing of the biochemical details or of the causal chains that lead to key cellular responses.

Repertoire building involves the molecular biology of diversification and of differentiation. The analysis of encounter has resulted in a definition of a new physiology of the immune response, the physiology of regulation to which Jerne devoted many of his important opening remarks. The study of triggering brings us to confront the general questions of the molecular biology of growth and maturation.

Which of these is distinctive to immunology? I believe that the origin of diversity is the idiosyncratic or distinctive feature. It is difficult to say whether encounter mechanisms will be found to be general, but of course triggering and mitogenesis are certainly a general feature of many different cellular systems. In any case, immunology can satisfy collectors of the unique as well as inveterate generalists. Whatever their predilections, I think that most people will agree that the satisfactory answers will come from a molecular analysis of each of the requirements of clonal selection. Let us look at some of the past predictions and present predicaments that were brought to our attention in this volume.

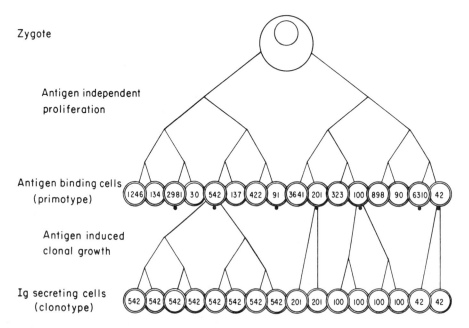

Figure 1. A model of the somatic differentiation of antibody-producing cells according to the clonal selection theory. The number of immunoglobulin genes may increase during somatic growth so that in the immunologically mature animal, different lymphoid cells are formed, each committed to the synthesis of a structurally distinct receptor antibody (indicated by an Arabic numeral). A small proportion of these cells proliferate upon antigenic stimulation to form different clones of cells, each clone producing a different antibody. This model represents bone-marrow-derived (B) cells, but with minor modifications it is also applicable to thymus-derived (T) cells.

FULFILLING THE FIRST REQUIREMENT

Antibody Molecules

The requirement for repertoire has to be looked at in two ways, as is shown in several papers in this volume. First, we have to look at the generation of diversity at the molecular level, and second, we have to look at the actual repertoire as it develops in the cells of the embryo, a process that I will call the zero[th] stage of clonal selection.

The basis of the diversity of the repertoire has now, I think, been securely established. You should remember that at the last meeting, we were still struggling for a complete molecular structure of the immunoglobulins. Sometime afterwards, when the structure was completed, it appeared likely that the molecule was arranged in domains (Edelman 1970), V domains for antigen binding and C domains for effector functions. The work of the X-ray crystallographers, Davies and Poljak (and others not present, Edmondson and Huber [see Davies et al. 1975]), now provides us with verification of this hypothesis. Immunoglobulins are indeed arranged in domains. Thanks to their work, we see a couple of other things that were previously suspected but not solidly proved. The antigen-binding site consists of contributions from both the V_H and V_L domains. We also see that this site is capable of the degree of degeneracy that the theorists said it should have, which is consoling.

Once and for all, this work makes clear the distinction between antibodies and enzymes. Even though both kinds of proteins follow the same physical-chemical principles, antibodies have obviously evolved in a manner much different from that of enzymes. The crystallographic work has also brought us new and intriguing information that deserves mention, although I cannot dwell upon it. There is, for example, a characteristic Ig fold. The similarity of this β structure with that of the enzyme superoxide dismutase is an intriguing observation. It implies either that this kind of fold is highly stable and generally useful, and therefore that this is a case of convergent evolution, or that immunoglobulins are, in fact, evolutionarily related to an early enzyme.

Some other impressive features of the crystallographic work are the detailed rules of symmetry and the way that the V's and C's resemble each other, details that could not have been predicted by any kind of hypothesis based on sequence work alone. One of the classical hopes of immunochemistry, literally to see how different hapten antigens fit the combining site, has now been completely realized. Landsteiner would have been greatly pleased to see this ultimate fulfillment of his work.

This information provides workers such as Haber and Givol with the possibility of attempting to build a site. We will not hear the end of these efforts very soon, but we should note that they employ remarkable combinations of technology that will be of extreme use in applications as well as in fundamental matters.

In these days of multiple receptors, it is not too trite at this point to remind ourselves again that antibodies are the key molecules of immunology. As a result of the structural work on antibodies, the bridge was built from immunology to molecular genetics, a transition marked by great clarifications. But the marks of heterodoxy were inflicted on immunology by just these satisfying developments. Conventional evolutionary and genetic models did not appear to account for the diversity of V regions, and it became clear that there was either a need for an enormous number of germ-line V genes or for a process of somatic variation in lymphocyte precursors. Moreover, how was one to account for the need to fuse information from a V gene to that from a C gene, as well as for the association of different C regions with the same V region? Who does not remember the great Talmudic disputes (see Gally and Edelman 1972 for references) of the late 60's on these issues? As is obvious from the papers in this volume, these questions are still not fully resolved, but thanks to the gene-counting people, we have made real headway.

Genes and Gene Counting

We all knew, of course, that the talk had to stop sometime, and that the issue of the origin of diversity had to be ceded to the DNA and RNA chemists. We even suspected that hybridization methods would be attempted after isolation and characterization of mRNA. But we hardly suspected the elegance that would be achieved by these methods in the hands of Milstein, Leder, and Tonegawa.

Using these and other approaches, we have to account for the origin of the diversity of cells with different V regions and, as reported at this meeting, we have to account for the mechanism of formation of a complete VC gene. Are these processes separate or linked? Is there a single, common mechanism that will relieve us of the necessity of assuming two independent exotic mechanisms? Whatever the answer, I shall first discuss these processes as if they were independent, although, as Leder suggests, they may share enzymes in common.

All of the work on hybridization provides satisfying but not conclusive evidence for the inference that there is a very small number of germ-line genes for V regions in a subgroup. In the case of the mouse λ chain, the evidence of Leder begins to be particularly persuasive. Moreover, the genetic indications of a small number of C-region genes are now reasonably well confirmed. These developments put us in a better position to suggest that the proponents supporting somatic variation of a few germ-line V genes are probably right. Hybridization data are not proof of the process, however, and the details of the mechanism still remain mysterious.

Here, Baltimore has made, I think, the key point about where one should look: one has to look at enzymology. What kind of enzymes might be involved? So far, I believe, three candidates have been presented, one of which may already be ruled out by the experiments of Dr. Tonegawa. Baltimore suggested the terminal transferase of Bollum as a very good candidate because that enzyme is template-independent and because it will add on any of the four bases. It therefore would be a perfect mutator in consort with the appropriate complex of enzymes, particularly the polymerases. If this is correct, however, there has to be a quite nice matching of the transferase and polymerase activities. I have raised the demurrer that the transferase might stutter a bit, and if that happened for runs greater than three bases, one might expect a curious (and anomalous) accumulation of paired mutations, an event not observed in actual sequences. Perhaps it would be fun to set up an in vitro system with transferase, polymerase, and a defined template to see if there were a need for stringent control to avoid this possibility. Whatever the outcome, of course, the final mechanism has to be shown in lymphoid tissue, not in model systems.

The second kind of enzyme was mentioned by Dr. Leder. I think his is a fascinating suggestion because an appropriate set of restriction-modification enzymes might make mutation and VC joining *both* part of a common mechanism. There is no reason to assume, however, there would have to be only one restriction-modification enzyme. Leder has already gone through the kinds of palindromes that *might* be required, and Milstein has already made clear that he has so far found no evidence for them. But perfect palindromic sequences may not be necessary.

A third enzymic system — an error-prone polymerase, and a faithful reverse transcriptase, with multiple insertion of V regions into C regions — has had some doubt cast on it by Dr. Tonegawa's experiments on VC fusion.

My main purpose in making these remarks is to direct your attention to the likelihood that we are going to see a wave of enzymology in basic immunology. The question then becomes: Where will the people who plan to ride that wave have to look? Will it be sufficient to look in the embryo, or will they have to look elsewhere? In order to answer this question, I think that, before long, we are going to see the exploitation of modern techniques such as recombinant DNA technology, a procedure that has become subject to the kind of societal difficulties that Henry Adams was worried about. It is fairly obvious that if you could take out the V genes *from* the appropriate organism and put them *into* the appropriate organisms to enhance

their replication and then see how various enzymes and restriction enzymes work on this DNA sequence as compared to C-region sequences, we might make a great leap forward. Another possibility, of course, is to use virally transformed cells at the right stage of development, in the hope that the requisite enzymes will be caught in flight by the transformation.

What about the coordination problem relating to diversification and VC fusion? Pernis, Cooper, Uhr and Vitetta, and others have certainly provided convincing evidence that two classes of heavy chains with the same V regions can coexist in the same cell. In all likelihood, this cannot be explained by the persistence of messenger RNA. Tonegawa's elegant experiments have given us the first direct suggestion of the reality of the fusion event. Of course, it is important that he extend his search to adult tissues as well as to various transformed cell lines.

The major problem is to determine the mechanism for forming a complete VC gene. At present, his experiment cannot distinguish between integration, inversion, or deletion. It is very important to determine whether a cell can make just two classes of immunoglobulins with the same V_H regions or more than two. If there are just two, then perhaps paternal and maternal chromosomes may be involved (along with some fanciness involving their proper distribution to daughter cells). But if someone shows that there are indeed three or even four classes simultaneously expressed for a time greater than the survival time of a messenger, I think we will have to look elsewhere for the mechanism of insertion or deletion that accounts for VC fusion.

Even after we understand these events, there is much that remains to be understood about the expression of antibody receptors in the earliest clones of the repertoire. For this we must turn to an analysis of the ontogeny of the repertoire at the level of cellular populations in individual animals.

Ontogeny and the Zero[th] Stage of Clonal Selection

Clonal selection has two sets of stages — a beginning stage in ontogeny which is almost certainly not antigen-driven and a continuing set of stages in which the repertoire expands and responds to antigen (Fig. 1). Much study has gone into the continuing stages, enough in fact to generate a new physiology of the immune response. But we still know relatively little of how the repertoire first arises.

The classic work of Silverstein, Sterzl, and Uhr (see Sterzl and Silverstein 1967) has given us some bearings, and we also owe much to the work of Owen together with Moore. Only recently, however, have we been able directly to address the problem of the repertoire of antigen-binding cells. Nossal and Pike (1973) and Spear (Spear et al. 1973) have given a description of the rates of appearance of T and B cells in the liver and spleen. The antigen-binding cells for a variety of antigens all appear in the mouse at about the same time, with no strict evidence of order (D'Eustachio and Edelman 1975). In contrast, Cooper has reported in this volume that clonal diversity in the bursa is generated sequentially in a programmed sequence. The same conclusion was also reached by Klinman, who described a sequence of stimulated response in the mouse along with a similar sequence of tolerance induction. These observations raise the idea of a program for repertoire expression of V regions that must be under evolutionary control, particularly because Klinman implies that it occurs in the same order in different individuals.

This is a radical idea whatever the origin of diversity since it requires some control over the expression of antigenic specificities before encounter with antigens. But it must be said that there are experimental limitations even in the elegant methods that Klinman has used. For example, his procedures involve a complex transfer experiment in which he is already selecting certain clones. Moreover, sequential expression of clones in different mice is not seen in the classic work described by Askonas. In the ideal experiment, I suppose one must compare antigen binding and antigen responsiveness for a similar avidity range. Both Melchers and others (D'Eustachio et al. 1976) found that the ratios of antigen-*binding* cells for different antigens are constant in both adult and fetus, and this discrepancy with the changes in ratios found by Klinman and Cooper must be resolved. In addition, one must be sure that the programmed sequence is really the same in different individuals. Furthermore, frequency differences may be missed because they are not detected below a certain threshold of detection.

I therefore suspect that the order observed in Cooper's and Klinman's experiments is related to the way the repertoire is being sampled and to the order in which certain cells *respond* to antigen. But it must be admitted that if both binding and response methods give an ordered appearance of cells during ontogeny, then our view of clonal selection is in for an overhaul. Independent of the expression of specificities, there is now some evidence that overall growth regulation of the repertoire is genetically controlled in different strains of mice, as mentioned by D'Eustachio. This is perhaps not surprising; the main point of mentioning it here is to emphasize that it must be distinguished from *specific* programmed expression.

After repertoire building, there is certainly evidence for maturational steps that guarantee response. This is evident in the progression from IgM-, to IgM + IgD-, to IgD-bearing cells noted by Pernis and Uhr and Vitetta. Moreover, there is evidence for a new type of T cell appearing at about 10 days after birth, a time when responsiveness

appears in the intact mouse (Spear and Edelman 1974). In line with all of these developmental changes are the marked differences in B-cell tolerance and feedback responses to anti-IgM described in this volume by both Nossal and Raff. It is clear that modulation *could* account for B-cell tolerance, and that early cells are much more susceptible than adult cells. Furthermore, Nossal made a good case for clonal abortion as a mode of tolerance to be considered in addition to T-cell factors. Tolerance still remains a physiological matter concerned with cell populations and possibly stochastic factors involving the balance of a variety of mechanisms. But at least there is now some indication that early cell response differs from adult cell response, and I believe that is important for our thinking.

All of this interest in ontogeny is occurring at a time when there is also very active work on the differentiation of both T-cell and B-cell lineages and an enormous increase in our ability to classify, name, and functionally categorize these cells. The result has been a physiology of the immune response which emerges from a consideration of a hierarchical series of interactions of genes, their products, and the cells that bear these products. This physiology has to do with fulfillment of the second requirement of clonal selection, i.e., the nature of the regulatory interactions that time the selective recognition machine and keep it from exploding.

FULFILLING THE SECOND REQUIREMENT

Cell Interactions and the New Physiology of the Immune Response

Early ideas on the control of the immune response involved feedback of specific antibody molecules of IgM and IgG to incite or repress a response. As reported by Nossal, Jerne, Pernis, and others, this kind of mechanism must still play a role, particularly for B cells. The modern era began, however, when the role of the thymus was first grasped and when T-B interactions were appreciated. This really just grazed our consciousness at the last Cold Spring Harbor meeting, but it was already there. Now the matter has been brought to a very sophisticated level of intellectual analysis by Jerne, who proposes to describe the new physiology as a network. Most of us tend to think of a static structural network, but Jerne, I believe, implies a dynamic network. It is therefore important that the time constants and response characteristics of this kind of network be defined. This, I believe, is the operational challenge posed by his idea.

All of this new physiology of encounter depends upon our ability to distinguish one lymphocyte from another. We have made real progress in this area as a result of the efforts by Boyse (see Boyse and

Bennett 1974) to classify lymphocytes by a variety of antigenic markers and by several laboratories to relate this classification to lymphocyte function. Out of all of this has come a kind of lymphocyte bestiary in which the chief beasts of the moment are T lymphocytes. We now know, as Cantor and Feldmann report, of a variety of T lymphocytes carrying out helper, suppressor, amplifier, and killer functions, each with a somewhat different set of markers and a slightly different history of differentiation. Throw in a real beast, the macrophage, as Paul and Pierce have done, and the zoo becomes even more exotic.

As Gershon, Basten, Claman, and Feldmann have revealed, we can now mark a reasonable beginning in relating the various Ly classes to lymphocyte function. Of course, it will be important to look at the chemistry of the T markers themselves; we already have reports from Williams on the Thy-1 marker and from Gottlieb on Ly-3. Classification of this kind is also useful in defining the differentiation pathway of lymphocytes, as indicated by Goldstein and Weissman, whose work, along with that of Cantor and Boyse, puts the classification on a dynamic footing.

What about the interactions of these various cells? Here there may be profit in considering the informational hierarchy that constitutes the immune system (Fig. 2). This hierarchy consists of components concerned with repertoire and components concerned with response, and it is clear that, altogether, the products of genes on at least five different chromosomes play upon the surfaces of the cells involved. At the right moment, the various receptors and factors can alter the metabolic states of the different cells to give a variety of functional responses. There are genes with a unique mechanism of diversification and integration for repertoire and genes on different chromosomes specifying regulatory factors for response. Moreover, the gene products interact at the surfaces of various cells, including macrophages.

It must not be forgotten, however, that these interactions take place in a system of pipes, tubes, and sinuses, as well as defined anatomical structures, in which the chief actors are the cells subject to bulk transport, death, and varying fluid flow. There are two immune systems, an artificial one in glass, which Mishell and Dutton have shown can operate surprisingly well without the anatomy, and the one inside the animal. The one inside the animal is a system that is far from thermodynamic equilibrium. It is still a mystery how such a system can behave to select high-affinity cells for preferential stimulation, even though we have *apparent* explanations in terms of equilibrium thermodynamics. Clonal filtering acts *as if* the system were close to equilibrium (Edelman 1974). We must try to understand this better and, as Jerne insists, to understand at least qualitatively the part processes of regulation.

We have seen that the key issues in this domain have been focused around two questions, one related to repertoire and the other to response, in the sense that response involves controls on cellular interactions from genes other than V and C genes. These questions are: What is the nature of the T-cell receptor? And what is the nature and function of the Ir gene products and major histocompatibility antigens? The two questions are connected because it appears more and more likely that one of the consequences of the fact that the T-cell receptor is cell-linked is that molecules other than antigen and the receptor must also be involved for T cells to function.

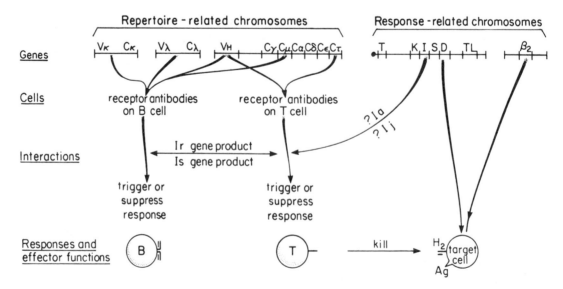

Figure 2. Informational and functional hierarchies in the immune system. The complex informational pathways call upon related and unrelated gene products from different chromosomes, some of which have genes linked in clusters. It is not known whether I-region products also constitute a repertoire.

The T-cell Receptor

For a while, this subject has been a center of debate, but as we can see from the papers by Binz and Wigzell, Eichmann, and Rajewsky, we may now be approaching some unanimity. It appears that the T-cell receptor is an immunoglobulin, at least in the sense that it has V_H regions at its active site. We are thus relieved of the repellent possibility of having to invoke two separate origins of diversity, one for B cells and one for T cells. The experiments used to identify the T-cell antibody are ingenious, and they run the gamut of immunological approaches to a difficult problem.

If we accept the data from these workers that the receptor consists of two disulfide-linked chains, each of molecular weight 72,000 and each containing a V_H region, we may risk several guesses that are useful for the problem of understanding T-cell function. I think it is likely that the receptor molecule will be arranged in domains, and, of course, it is also very likely to be a symmetrical structure consisting of identical heavy chains. How many domains is a question of some speculation, depending upon how much carbohydrate is found to be present; in any case, there will probably be four or five pairs of C domains. This assumption, of course, implies the existence of appropriate C_τ genes on the translocon for heavy chains and, in accord with the domain hypothesis, it also implies a set of different constant-region functions. Moreover, inasmuch as the molecule lacks light chains, the repertoire cannot be *identical* to that of B-cell antibodies, although the two repertoires might be very similar. Indeed, as reported by Rajewsky, there are both similarities and differences.

Because of its reactivity with anti-idiotype antibodies, and the domain hypothesis, and provided the evidence on the absence of light chains is confirmed, I would guess that the T-cell receptor exists in form A (Fig. 3), which is univalent. This is reminiscent of the artificial heavy-chain structures that can be reconstituted from B-cell heavy chains in

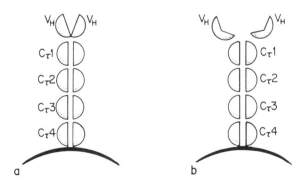

Figure 3. A model for the T-cell receptor. *(a)* The preferred univalent model. V_H, variable-region domain; $C_\tau 1$ and $C_\tau 4$, assumed constant-region domains. *(b)* Bivalent structure with "naked," noninteracting V_H domains.

vitro (Björk and Tanford 1971). Of course, the alternative form B, which is bivalent and contains two "naked" V_H domains is possible, but it seems much less likely. To make the decision, we must go back to classical immunochemistry and determine whether the T-cell receptor is univalent or divalent. One other point of chemistry is of some interest in relation to function: if all of these structural assumptions are correct, the T-cell receptor is a long, flexible, rod-shaped molecule. It is clear that we must press on with structural verification of these hypotheses and, in particular, we must concentrate on the C region.

If the T-cell receptor is a long, flexible molecule with V_H and separate C_τ domains, we have to consider the interactions of these domains with the surface molecules of other cells and with factors produced by these cells. Here we enter the response side of the hierarchy and hear the sound of truly modern immunological music. If the sound is a bit cacophonous, it is still exciting. This music comes out of the convergence of two separate biological searches, one concerned originally with transplantation antigens, and the other with the basic nature of the immune system itself. What is remarkable is how these two separate searches have become intertwined in a compelling and unexpectedly striking way. This is one of those tantalizing cases of scientific correlation, beginning in empirical explorations with varying motives but ending with a beautiful logical closure.

Histocompatability Loci and the Genetics of the Immune Response

Any hope that the new physiology of the immune response would be a simple feedback loop between elicited antibody molecules and antibody-producing cells was dispelled by the in-depth study of the interaction between T cells and B cells. The detailed exploration of the relationship of the immunogenetics of histocompatibility loci and the MHC to the immune response, which comprises so much of this volume, really makes this point with a vengeance. The roles of this system in the function of killer T cells and in immune surveillance, in the genetic control of immune responses, and in connection with differentiation antigens are all fascinating subjects that were largely unseen at the time of the first Cold Spring Harbor meeting.

As can be seen from the work presented in this volume, the story is still far from complete. It has, of course, been known since the pioneering work of Gorer and Snell (see Klein 1975) that the MHC is an extraordinary immunogenetic system. The elegant work of Shreffler and Klein, and their postulate of gene duplication to account for K and D loci with multiple allelism as the basis for this largely polymorphic system are now classic (Klein 1975). However, aside from the implication of this system in a variety of lymphocyte reactions such as the MLR, the function of this extraordinary gene complex was not known. As knowledge developed, it became clear that the human HL-A system (and other systems in various species) has many similarities to the mouse system, although the genes are arranged differently. The implications of the human system for population genetics and medicine were deeply explored by workers such as Bodmer, Bach, and van Rood.

Only recently, however, have we been able to throw some light on the function of this system as a group of linked genes. A line of work beginning with Arquilla's observations in guinea pigs (Arquilla and Finn 1963, 1965) and extensively pursued by Benacerraf (see McDevitt and Benacerraf 1969) indicated that immune responses in the guinea pig were under genetic control. Similar work by Mc-Devitt and Sela (1965) using synthetic antigens in the mouse extended the range of these observations, and it was soon clear that Mendelian genes seemed to be controlling certain aspects of the immune response in the intact organism. McDevitt made the important observation (see McDevitt and Benacerraf 1969) that, in the mouse, these genes were linked to the major histocompatibility loci. Since then, as we all know, the IX linkage group on chromosome 17 of the mouse has been intensively explored, but it is still wise to caution that there is much genetic material still left unaccounted for in the MHC. In this connection, it is worth noting that Bodmer's theory, discussed here, that there may be pseudoallelism in the H-2 system and that the genetics reflect the action of linked regulatory genes is still tenable or at least not disproved.

This intriguing background prompted a number of laboratories to attempt to determine the structure of the products of H-2 and HL-A genes. As a result of the work of Cunningham, Hood, Nathenson, Uhr, Crumpton, Bodmer, and Strominger and their coworkers, we have a nice model of these products and also enough amino acid sequences to reach some satisfactory preliminary conclusions. H-2 antigens consist of β_2-microglobulin noncovalently bonded to a heavy chain which contains the carbohydrate and the private and public antigenic specificities. There is a strong sequence homology between H-2 and HL-A gene products, but a bit of a paradox about the order of gene duplication and speciation. The sequence variation is consistent with the observed genetic polymorphism. Much should be made of the fact that the products of the D and K loci are homologous since it confirms the nice prediction by Shreffler and Klein that these loci arose by gene duplication. This opens up, almost promiscuously, the obvious temptation to propose that the whole chromosome arose by gene duplication. In any case, there is a suggestion based on Uhr and Vitetta's observations and those of Cunningham and his colleagues that the T_L antigen may be homologous to H-2.

All of this is very satisfying, but it deserves to be pointed out that 30 residues out of 400 are hardly a basis for grand generalization and that the use of the sequenator alone risks partial sequence pollution. Methods of peptide surgery will have to be combined with microchemistry to get a glance at the middle of the structure. Surprises may be in store.

There is, of course, another experimentally accessible mystery to be resolved. What is an immunoglobulin domain like β_2-microglobulin doing on the surface of a great variety of nonlymphoid cells in association with H-2 and T_L antigens? Gally and I have suggested (Gally and Edelman 1972) that perhaps the genes at the MHC were primitives for Ig genes. This would imply that the H-2 heavy chain is Ig-like. Of course, there are other alternatives. For example, β_2 might be bound to the heavy chain in the way that complement is bound to the CH_2 domain of Ig. In that case, β_2 might be serving a masking function for a site on the H-2 heavy chain. Alternatively, it might induce an active conformation for H-2 heavy-chain function or even be part of a site for binding of a complement-like molecule from the outside or from the same cell. In any case, no homology with Ig has so far been found on the heavy chain of H-2 or HL-A. It is only a question of time—either sequencing or serology will provide the answer.

This brings us to the larger problem of the function of the histocompatibility antigens. Past surmises have ranged far and wide, but the most intriguing guesses stem from the observations of Zinkernagel and Doherty that, somehow, H-2 recognition is implicated in the anti-viral activity of T cells. The work of Shearer and Bevan also focuses our attention on the fact that alteration of H-2 changes T-cell recognition. The closely similar work of Shrader and coworkers, and Germain et al. (1975) supports the idea for killer T cells. Schrader has shown that it is the H-2 antigen on the target cell that is important and, with Cunningham et al., has found evidence to support molecular interaction between H-2 and viral Ag. Koszinowski, Zinkernagel, Schrader, and others have reported on the most likely models: (1) some kind of interaction complex is formed between H-2 and the viral antigen, which is then recognized by the T-cell receptor, or (2) the H-2 and viral antigens are separately recognized by two different receptors. The main evidence tends to support the first model, but conclusive proof remains to be obtained.

All of this leads me to speculate that one function of H-2 antigens is perhaps to bring the antigen (virus) together with the H-2 heavy chain and β_2-microglobulin so that the recognition function can be tied to that of killing without invoking additional humoral factors. Unlike the Ag–Ab–complement complex, killing must be done directly by cells and cell-surface-linked molecules. Presumably such a delicate and potentially dangerous function might require establishment of a ternary complex before it can be activated. The selective advantage of polymorphism in the population would come from the need to favor interactions with viral variants and mutations. Indeed, one should not neglect the possibility that some H-2 antigens are viral receptors.

Other linked gene products of the MHC have now been implicated in suppressor and helper functions. It is good to see that increasing attention is being focused on the region and that some chemistry is beginning to emerge for its gene products. The key questions are: What is their relationship to the Ir gene products? And what is their relationship to the various helper and suppressor factors we have heard about?

I do not think we can get a clear picture of the role of these factors until we are sure whether or not they bind antigens specifically. Furthermore, it is also important to show whether these factors interact with each other or with the T-cell receptor. We must note the contributions of workers such as Tada, who have isolated I-region-related factors with intriguing properties, and such as Pierce and Paul, who are bringing in macrophage interactions via IA products. These are valiant efforts to map the T-B and T-T interactions in terms of molecules, and they must be encouraged. But it should also be said that to get satisfactory answers requires some excellent biochemistry. The factors must be more highly purified in order to make sure, for example, that their apparent antigen-binding properties are not due to a fragment of T-cell receptor stuck to the factor. We also have to get hold of assays that show larger changes so that we are not so much in the margin.

None of this is intended to diminish the pioneering work of all these people who bring these factors to our attention as there is no doubt that factors exist. Indeed, the genetics serves as an indicator that there *must* be molecules and gene products that can do these tasks. In interpreting the assays, however, we need to know whether cells themselves interact with cells, i.e., whether T cells actually interact with B cells and themselves *directly*. We need to know these things whether or not cells export specific or nonspecific factors. Except for killing by cytotoxic lymphocytes, I believe we lack the answers.

One very satisfying resolution of the complex set of interactions required of cells and factors would be via the T-cell receptor. The factors might bind to C_τ regions and act to enhance or block responses (Fig. 4a). A similar role for C_τ regions might be envisioned for killing events involving H-2. The V_H site might recognize the antigen–H-2 complex, and a third molecule on the killer cell might then interact with that complex (Fig. 4b).

In any case, it does seem clear that the histocompatibility restriction in cell interactions is not by any means absolute, and we have reports here of examples that range from tight, to lax, to nonexistent restriction. The key issue here is to determine whether restriction exists at all in a *primary* encounter. If restriction is mainly a reflection of choices from the repertoire in secondary reactions, the difficulty of explaining the relative nature of restriction disappears. In that case, selection from the T-cell repertoire could encompass all possibilities, and the H-2 barriers and restrictions would not have to be universal. Instead, they would merely reflect whether or not the original selection in immunization was for a complex involving the H-2 antigen. I believe that this will turn out to be the case.

Whatever the fate of these factors and models, the

Figure 4. Some possible interactions of cellular factors and H-2 antigens with the T-cell receptor. *(a)* Suppressor or helper factors from T cells may interact with C_τ domains, enhancing or preventing subsequent interaction with a hypothetical cell-bound triggering molecule (t). *(b)* Cytotoxic T lymphocyte is assumed to recognize H-2–viral antigen complex by V_H domains. This may be followed by interaction with the complex of a hypothetical cell-bound effector molecule (K) to carry out killing.

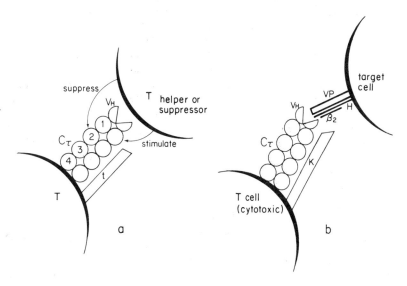

genetics is not dubious, thanks to the work of Benacerraf and his colleagues. There is one key issue that I believe must be raised about the larger evolutionary significance of the Ir genes. Why are they there at all? Obviously, one answer relates to their function in regulation. But there is another interesting possibility. If an immune response requires somatic generation of a degenerate V-gene repertoire, it is difficult to see how evolution can rapidly alter particular responses of organisms in a particular environment. By selecting Is and Ir genes, however, it could alter the emergence of the *response* specificity of the system in a quite rapid and neat way without having to alter *binding* specificities in the V-gene repertoire. It has become increasingly apparent that clonal selection acts by filtering the response out of the binding repertoire, favoring higher affinities and specificities (see Edelman 1974). Understanding the nature of the high-pass filter that carries out this task requires an understanding of the molecular mechanisms of cell triggering.

FULFILLING THE THIRD REQUIREMENT

Triggering, Maturation, and Mitogenesis

If the origin of diversity and the particular tricks of T-B interaction are sui generis and not to be found elsewhere, it would still be parochial and foolish to ignore the third requirement, which is more likely to share its molecular mechanisms with all cells. Here, Möller has done us a service by presenting so extreme a view, for even after a knowledge of the 3D structure of antibody receptors, it is difficult to see how binding an antigen at the sites conveys a signal through to the terminal C_H domain of a single receptor and thereby to the cell. In all likelihood, an additional molecule is involved. A simple cross-linkage hypothesis seems to be excluded by the finding that monovalent Con A and Fab fragments of anti-carbohydrate antibodies are mitogenic for T cells, although cross-linkage can induce inhibition of cell-surface mobility and account for the inhibitory effects of higher doses of lectins (Edelman 1976). The adequate initial signal and the molecules that mediate it remain to be defined. At present, however, there is no reason to exclude antibodies from the roster as Möller has done.

Whether the lymphocyte is stimulated by antigens or lectins, we also want to know the biochemistry of mitogenesis and maturation. Here we must consider the lymphocyte as a G_0 or resting cell and try to determine the biochemical pathway for mitogenesis. The problem is that we just do not have enough relevant assays, nor do we have the appropriate cell cycle mutants. It would certainly be helpful to have assays that connect to the key events such as initiation of DNA replication or of maturation and protein synthesis.

Table 1. Distribution of "Initiation" and DNA Polymerase Activities in Stimulated Lymphocytes and Other Cell Sources

Source of cytosol	Units/ml of	
	initiation activity	polymerase activity
Unstimulated spleen cells	0	0
Con-A-stimulated spleen cells	0.18	0.06
P388 lymphoid cell line	0.32	2.92
Fetal mouse liver	0.18	0.29
Adult liver	0	0
Adult brain	0	0
3T3 cells (confluent)	0	0.06
SV3T3 cells (confluent)	0.27	1.26
RSV-*ts*68 chick embryo fibroblasts (confluent at 41°C)	0	—
RSV-*ts*68 chick embryo fibroblasts (confluent at 37°C)	0.19	—

Assays. Initiation: measures incorporation of dTTP into chromosomal DNA in a cell-free system initially containing frog liver nuclei, deoxynucleoside triphosphates, and appropriate ions and buffers. Polymerase: measures incorporation of dTTP in presence of poly(dA[dT])$_{10}$ and salmon testis DNA. See Jazwinski et al. (1976) for details.

We have recently developed one such system (Jazwinski et al. 1976). This is a cell-free assay based on the stimulation of DNA replication in nuclear extracts after the addition of cytoplasmic extracts from mitogenically stimulated cells or from transformed cells of lymphoid or other origin. For example, cytoplasmic extracts of the proliferating lymphoid cell line P388 stimulate dTTP incorporation which is dependent on ATP and incorporates into Okazaki fragments that can be chased into high-molecular-weight DNA. Furthermore, a tenfold increase in replication eyes is detectable by electron microscopy of nucleochromatin from the stimulated assay preparation. The factor or factors appear to be proteins with molecular weights greater than 50,000, and their activity may be separate from that of DNA polymerase.

All proliferating cells so far tested (Table 1) have these factors, whereas resting cells do not. Of particular interest is the finding that stimulation of lymphocytes by Con A induces the factor. This is one example of what we might want to develop in order to untangle the complex stimulation pathways of lymphocytes. Assays such as these will be of some use to people who are studying the mechanisms of tolerance because the suppression might occur before or after the induction of such factors. Biochemical studies of this kind are certainly going to be among the main future directions of immunology.

THE GENERALIZATION OF IMMUNOLOGY

On that note, I want to make some final comments on immunology as a model system and as the provenance of chemical tools for research in many areas. At the beginning of these summary remarks, I said that the immune system is one of the most startling and beautiful molecular recognition machines. Through the application of technological achievements based on the properties of that machine, the field will pretty soon pay back its debts to molecular biology, developmental biology, and cell biology. It will do so, I believe, not only conceptually, but also through applications of antibody-based microchemistry (ABM). This inexpensive and peaceful ABM will be employed increasingly to characterize biochemically both populations of cells and single cells. The work of Phillips and Morrison (1970), Marchalonis, and Uhr and Vitetta, employed together with radiochemical approaches such as those of Niall (Jacobs et al. 1974) and Sanger, has already been remarkably successful, as we have seen in the examples of structural work on histocompatibility antigens described in this volume.

Immunology breeds new subjects and makes new series of alliances in each decade: first medicine and microbiology, then chemistry, then molecular biology. I believe that now the connection will be with developmental biology, for the message of clonal selective systems centers on ontogeny, gene expression, cell interaction, and population dynamics. Indeed, the recent work on ontogeny suggests that there are general genetic influences on the formation of the immune repertoire. This and work on allophenic systems (Mintz 1971) raises the possibility that there will be a new field of study—population embryology—a field concerned with frequencies, interactions (clonal and otherwise), and overall influences on morphogenesis with emphasis on the stochastic features of developing cell populations. This field will owe much and give much to immunology.

Finally, I want to raise the possibility that even apparently remote subjects may come to owe a large conceptual debt to immunology. I am thinking particularly of the relationship of immunology to that other lateralizer of possibilities for confrontation of future events, the brain. I am also thinking of the subject of human language. Like immunology, these subjects may also involve selective systems based on generation of a repertoire from a given innate or genetic basis.

It is not a trivial observation to note that immunology, like language, is reflexive. It can refer to itself via antibodies to antibodies. It is also, like language, full of degenerate cases and possibilities. For these reasons, the immune system, like a linguistic system, can be ambiguous. This point is important because it suggests that we cannot hope to achieve an absolutely complete description of the immune system. It is not necessary for the physiologists to describe the response in each case down to the last molecule, nor is it particularly fruitful

to enter into extensive efforts to produce an endless clustered nest of idiotypes, one against the other.

What I am getting at in emphasizing these properties of the immune system is that immunology may be the first of a whole field of disciplines concerned at the molecular and cellular level with recognition of previously unencountered phenomena that could not have been dealt with during evolution. This field, which we might call *cognology*, may come to include many aspects of higher nervous systems, certain detoxification systems, and various aspects of developmental biology.

Perhaps I should end, however, by making somewhat more detailed and less fanciful predictions. By the next meeting at Cold Spring Harbor, I think it is likely that we are going to see the T-cell receptor characterized, the major histocompatibility complex understood in terms of its functions, and the origin of diversity reasonably well ensconced within a detailed analysis of particular enzymes and their mechanisms. We shall, of course, hear of more surprising discoveries. It is a heady experience to make a discovery, but in some ways it is a more lasting privilege to watch a field grow, to let it fuel our imaginations, and, above all, to see younger people enter it as new practitioners with new ideas. These are signs of the enormous health of science. All of us share this privilege and are brought together in a reaffirmation of the belief that, whether its picture of the world is mechanical or not, science truly does progress. And we can reassure the descendents of Henry Adams that by no means is it malign. There are some machines, like the immune system, that are truly beautiful, eminently practical, and valuable to the human race.

To all who contributed to the meeting—participants, speakers, and chairmen—and especially to those whose papers are presented in this volume, we owe an expression of our thanks and appreciation for their devotion and effort.

REFERENCES

ADAMS, H. 1918. *The education of Henry Adams.* Houghton Mifflin, New York.

ARQUILLA, E. R. and J. FINN. 1963. Genetic differences in antibody production to determinant groups on insulin. *Science* **142:** 400.

———. 1965. Genetic control of combining sites of insulin antibodies produced by guinea pigs. *J. Exp. Med.* **122:** 771.

BJÖRK, I. and C. TANFORD. 1971. Gross conformation of free polypeptide chains from rabbit immunoglobulin G. I. Heavy chain. *Biochemistry* **10:** 1271.

BOYSE, E. A. and D. BENNETT. 1974. Differentiation and the cell surface. Illustrations from work with T cells and sperm. In *Cellular selection and regulation in the immune response. Society of General Physiologists Series* (ed. G. M. Edelman), vol. 29, p. 155. Raven Press, New York.

BURNET, M. 1959. *The clonal selection theory of acquired immunity.* Vanderbilt University Press, Nashville, Tennessee.

CLAMAN, H. N., E. A. CHAPERON and R. F. TRIPLETT. 1966. Thymus-marrow cell combinations. Synergism in antibody production. *Proc. Soc. Exp. Biol. Med.* **122:** 1167.

DAVIES, D. R., E. A. PADLAN and D. M. SEGAL. 1975. Three-dimensional structure of immunoglobulins. *Annu. Rev. Biochem.* **44:** 639.

D'EUSTACHIO, P. and G. M. EDELMAN. 1975. Frequency and avidity of specific antigen-binding cells in developing mice. *J. Exp. Med.* **142:** 1078.

D'EUSTACHIO, P., J. E. COHEN and G. M. EDELMAN. 1976. Variation and control of specific antigen-binding cell populations in individual fetal mice. *J. Exp. Med.* **144:** 259.

EDELMAN, G. M. 1970. The covalent structure of a human γG-immunoglobulin. XI. Evolutionary and functional implications. *Biochemistry* **9:** 3197.

———. 1974. Origins and mechanisms of specificity in clonal selection. In *Cellular selection and regulation in the immune response. Society of General Physiologists Series* (ed. G. M. Edelman), vol. 29, p. 1. Raven Press, New York.

———. 1976. Surface modulation in cell recognition and cell growth. *Science* **192:** 218.

GALLY, J. A. and G. M. EDELMAN. 1972. Genetic control of immunoglobulin synthesis. *Annu. Rev. Genet.* **6:** 1.

GERMAIN, R. N., M. E. DORF and B. BENACERRAF. 1975. Inhibition of lymphocyte mediated tumor-specific lysis by alloantisera directed against H-2 serological specificities of the tumor. *J. Exp. Med.* **142:** 1023.

GOWANS, J. 1970. Lymphocytes. In *The Harvey Lectures 1968–1969,* Series 64, p. 87. Academic Press, New York.

JACOBS, J. W., B. KEMPER, H. D. NIALL, J. F. HABENER and J. T. POTTS, JR. 1974. Structural analysis of human proparathyroid hormone by a new microsequencing approach. *Nature* **249:** 155.

JAZWINSKI, S. M., J. WANG and G. M. EDELMAN. 1976. Initiation of replication in chromosomal DNA induced by extracts from proliferating cells. *Proc. Nat. Acad. Sci.* **73:** 2231.

JERNE, N. K. 1955. The natural selection theory of antibody formation. *Proc. Nat. Acad. Sci.* **41:** 849.

JERNE, N. K., A. A. NORDIN and C. HENRY. 1963. The agar plaque technique for recognizing antibody producing cells. In *Cell bound antibodies* (ed., B. Amos and H. Koprowski), p. 109. Wistar Institute Press, Philadelphia.

KLEIN, J. 1975. *Biology of the mouse histocompatibility-2 complex.* Springer-Verlag, New York.

MÄKELÄ, O. 1968. The specificity of antibodies produced by single cells. *Cold Spring Harbor Symp. Quant. Biol.* **32:** 423.

McDEVITT, H. O. and B. BENACERRAF. 1969. Genetic control of specific immune responses. *Adv. Immunol.* **11:** 31.

McDEVITT, H. O. and M. SELA. 1965. Genetic control of the antibody response. I. Demonstration of determinant-specific differences in response to synthetic polypeptide antigens in two strains of inbred mice. *J. Exp. Med.* **122:** 517.

MILLER, J. F. A. P. 1962. Effect of neonatal thymectomy on the immunological responsiveness of the mouse. *Proc. Roy. Soc. B.* **156:** 415.

MINTZ, B. 1971. Clonal basis of mammalian differentiation. In *Control mechanisms of growth and differentiation. Society of Experimental Biology Symposium* (ed. D. D. Davies and M. Balls), vol. 25, p. 345. Cambridge University Press, Cambridge, England.

MITCHISON, N. A. 1968. Antigen recognition responsible for the induction *in vitro* of the secondary response. *Cold Spring Harbor Symp. Quant. Biol.* **32:** 431.

NOSSAL, G. J. V. and O. MÄKELÄ. 1962. Kinetic studies on the incidence of cells appearing to form two antibodies. *J. Immunol.* **88:** 604.

NOSSAL, G. J. V. and B. PIKE. 1973. Studies on the differentiation of B lymphocytes in the mouse. *Immunology* **25:** 33.

PHILLIPS, D. R. and M. MORRISON. 1970. The arrangement of proteins in the human erythrocyte membrane. *Biochem. Biophys. Res. Comm.* **40:** 284.

SPEAR, P. G. and G. M. EDELMAN. 1974. Maturation of the humoral immune response in mice. *J. Exp. Med.* **139:** 249.

SPEAR, P. G., A. L. WANG, U. RUTISHAUSER and G. M. EDELMAN. 1973. Characterization of splenic lymphoid cells in fetal and newborn mice. *J. Exp. Med.* **138:** 557.

STERZL, J. and A. M. SILVERSTEIN. 1967. Developmental aspects of immunity. In *Advances in immunology* (ed. F. J. Dixon, Jr. and J. H. Humphrey), vol. 6, p. 337. Academic Press, New York.

Author Index

Subject Index

A

Abzymes. *See* Antibodies, catalytic
Accessory molecules. *See* T-cell accessory molecules
Adenovirus
E1, oncogenicity of, 597
E1A, antigen model, 600
Adhesion molecules, 81, 83, 611, 620–623, 667
antigen presentation, role in, 295–297, 667
CD2/LFA-3 interaction, 620–623
ICAM-1, 753–766
ICAM-2, 753–766
integrin family of, 83, 755
LFA-1 (CD11a/CD18), 753–766
LFA-1/ICAM-1 interaction, regulation of adhesion, TCR-mediated, 759–763
Adjuvant, complete Freund's, 6–7
Allergens, response to, molecular aspects of, 459–470
Allergies, HLA-D phenotypic association with, 459
Allergy, 459
Alloreactivity, 93
MHC class I, murine, mutants, analysis of, 527
peptide, possible involvement of, 93, 527
Amb a V, antigen model (allergen), 459–470
Antibodies. *See also* Immunoglobulin
anti-DNA, 933–946
nucleotide sequences of, 935–939
structural model of DNA recognition, 943
anti-idiotype, 203–208, 241
antigen epitope mimicry, 239, 243–244
auto-, catalytic, 283–286. *See also* Antibodies, anti-DNA
basic structure, 17–18
catalytic, 273–281, 957
assay systems for screening, 279
cleavage of peptide bonds, 283–286
naturally occurring, 283–286
reactions catalyzed by, 274–275
monoclonal
anticlonotypic, to 2C TCR, 147
for HLA-typing, 471
to IL-5R, 748
to invariant chain (POP.I4.3), 310
to lymphocyte homing receptor, peripheral lymph node (MEL-14), 81
to murine γδ-T-cell receptors, 31
to self-peptide/MHC complex, 94–95, 657
to TCR of MBP-specific hybridoma, 875
to V$_\beta$5 + TCR, 136–137
Antibody-antigen complex structure. *See* X-ray crystallography, antibody-antigen complex structure

Antigen competition. *See* T-cell antigen epitopes, MHC peptide binding, competition for
Antigen endocytosis. *See* Endocytosis
Antigen epitope
immunoglobulin, 239
characteristics of, 236
definition of, 249
influenza virus, neuraminidase, 259
T-cell. *See* T-cell antigen epitopes
Antigen, haptens, 4
Antigenic determinants. *See* T-cell antigen epitopes; Antigen epitope, immunoglobulin
Antigenicity. *See also* Antigen processing, determinant selection; Immunoglobulin, antigen recognition
accessibility, role of, 236
mobility, role of, 236
Antigenic variation
antibody escape, mechanism of, 257
gene conversion in, 227–229
Antigen peptides. *See* T-cell antigen epitopes
Antigen presentation, 949–950. *See also* Antigen-presenting cells; Antigen processing; MHC; T-cell antigen epitopes
accessory molecules, role of, 539–542, 659–660, 652–653
adhesion molecules, role in, 295–297, 667
antigen-occupied MHC molecules, proportion of in antigen-pulsed cells, 397
classic versus superantigen, 375–382. *See also* Superantigens
competition for. *See* T-cell antigen epitopes, MHC peptide binding, competition for
differences between cell types. *See* Antigen-presenting cells, differences between
intracellular parasites, antigens synthesized by, 568
invariant chain, role in, 377, 390–391
MHC-independent membrane-peptide interaction hypothesis, 293–294
MHC mutations, effects of, 377–379, 422–425, 521–529
mitochondrially encoded proteins, of, 563–570
nonclassic MHC class I molecules, by, 563–570
phospholipases, effects on, 388
polysaccharides, inhibitory effects of, 389
self-, 453–458, 670. *See also* Peptidic self model
Antigen-presenting cells (APCs). *See also* Antigen presentation; Antigen processing
adhesion molecules, expression of, 295–297, 667
B cells, 319–332, 333–344. *See also* Antigen processing, B cells

immunoglobulin uptake, route of, 320–329
T-cell help, mechanism of recruiting antigen-specific, 348
dendritic cells, 6–7, 667
differences between, 387
differential expansion of T$_H$1 versus T$_H$2 cells, 503
relevance of, 497
mutants of
class I-dependent, reversal by peptide addition, 299–308
loss of adhesion molecules, 295–297
loss of MHC class I, 299
thymic, 670–671
treatment with phospholipases, loss of function upon, 293
Antigen processing, 287, 293–298, 950–951. *See also* Antigen presentation; Antigen-presenting cells; Endocytosis; Endosomes; Proteolysis; T-cell antigen epitopes
B cells, 319–333, 345–352
immunoglobulin, membrane, processing of, 349–350
immunoglobulin, role of. *See* Immunoglobulin, membrane, receptor-mediated endocytosis of
intercellular sites of, 335–338
characterization of processed peptides, 395–397
determinant selection, 293–298, 418–419
B cells, effect of immunoglobulin-fine-specificity on, 345, 349, 351
cryptic determinants, 505, 510
MHC, role in, 293, 510
minor determinants, 505
variation between antigen-presenting cell types, 445–453
endocytosis role of, 287–289, 319, 324–327, 345–347,
endosomal proteinases, role in, 287–292, 324–327, 419–420
insulin, of, 337
intercelluar MHC class I-dependent (endogenous) pathway, 479, 482–484
de novo protein synthesis not required, 552–553
exogenous antigens, introduction into, 551–553
requirement for peptide transport mechanism, 299–308
intercellular MHC class II-dependent (exogenous) pathway, 320–329, 382–383, 417–430, 479, 482–484
endogenous antigens, introduction into, 481–482, 488–489
protein synthesis inhibitors, effects of, 386–387
MHC/antigen interaction
intercellular site restrictions, 568
structural intermediates of, 409–416
timing of relative to proteinase cleavage, implications of, 508, 510
mini-gene, synthetic, studies with, 479